Cancer in
the Elderly

BASIC AND CLINICAL ONCOLOGY

Editor

Bruce D. Cheson, M.D.

National Cancer Institute
National Institutes of Health
Bethesda, Maryland

ADDITIONAL VOLUMES IN PREPARATION

Cancer in the Elderly

edited by

Carrie P. Hunter

National Institutes of Health
Bethesda, Maryland

Karen A. Johnson

National Cancer Institute
National Institutes of Health
Bethesda, Maryland

Hyman B. Muss

University of Vermont
Burlington, Vermont

MARCEL DEKKER, INC.   NEW YORK · BASEL

ISBN: 0-8247-0278-6

This book is printed on acid-free paper.

Headquarters
Marcel Dekker, Inc.
270 Madison Avenue, New York, NY 10016
tel: 212-696-9000; fax: 212-685-4540

Eastern Hemisphere Distribution
Marcel Dekker AG
Hutgasse 4, Postfach 812, CH-4001 Basel, Switzerland
tel: 41-61-261-8482; fax: 41-61-261-8896

World Wide Web
http://www.dekker.com

The publisher offers discounts on this book when ordered in bulk quantities. For more information, write to Special Sales/Professional Marketing at the headquarters address above.

Current printing (last digit):
10 9 8 7 6 5 4 3 2 1

PRINTED IN THE UNITED STATES OF AMERICA

Series Introduction

The current volume, *Cancer in the Elderly,* is the twenty-third in the Basic and Clinical Oncology series. Many of the advances in oncology have resulted from close interaction between the basic scientist and the clinical researcher. The current volume illustrates the success of this relationship as demonstrated by new insights into the changing paradigm of cancer management and the burden of cancer in the elderly.

As editor of the series, my goal is to recruit volume editors who not only have established reputations based on their outstanding contributions to oncology but also have an appreciation for the dynamic interface between the laboratory and the clinic. To date, the series has consisted of monographs on topics that are of a high level of current interest. *Cancer in the Elderly* certainly fits into this category and is a most important addition to the series.

Volumes in progress focus on tumor angiogenesis and microcirculation. I anticipate that these books will provide a valuable contribution to the oncology literature.

Bruce D. Cheson

Preface

Cancer is a disease of genetic alterations in DNA that may result from an inherited predisposition, altered host susceptibility, or an interaction between environmental factors and an individual's inherent profile of genetic susceptibility. Cancer risk increases with age, as complex molecular and biological changes occur. The greatest burden of cancer occurs in men and women aged 65 years and older, a population that suffers excess morbidity, reduced quality of life, and economic disparity due to chronic disease. Advancements in the diagnosis and treatment of cancer have been associated with modest reductions in morbidity and improved quality of life. Yet the challenges of cancer in an aging population remain.

For the better part of the twentieth century, cancer in the elderly received little attention. Screening and early detection were generally not offered to older patients. Despite the demonstrated benefit from detecting early disease in screening trials, older women were (and still are) less likely than younger women to receive screening mammography and Papanicolaou tests. More advanced disease, less aggressive surgery, fewer treatment options and interventions, and a prevailing attitude among health care professionals to offer—and among patients to accept—more conservative approaches to diagnosis and treatment characterized cancer care in elderly patients.

The aging process is better understood now than it was in the past. Shifting demographics and improved health among the persons past middle age have led to a gradual transition from palliative or conservative disease management to an emphasis on disease prevention and expanded treatment options. New attention and research support have been directed toward the problem of cancer in the older populations by federal agencies, academic and private institutions, and other public health organizations. Older individuals have participated in clinical trials, and a critical mass of information has been accumulated. This book brings together a compendium of knowledge of cancer in the elderly, and we believe it will be useful for health care professionals, researchers, educators, policy makers, and students of public health and preventive medicine.

Cancer in the Elderly is divided into six parts. Part I begins with an epidemiological review of cancer in the elderly population of the United States, then looks at U.S. multiracial/cultural cancer patterns and the global burden of cancer in the elderly. It provides new insights into trends in cancer incidence and mortality, and examines the nature and extent of cancer burden in older populations. Part II examines medical evidence that secondary and primary control of cancer can be achieved in the elderly. This part also addresses screening and prevention of breast, prostate, and colorectal cancers and discusses the cultural attitudes, social structures, and the variety of constraints imposed by the health care system that affect how our society approaches the challenges of controlling cancer. Part III contains chapters on biological markers and the inherited susceptibility to cancer.

Part IV provides in-depth reviews of site-specific cancer treatments and the results of research interventions, including discussions on breast, gastrointestinal, gynecological, genitourinary, and lung cancer, as well as melanomas, sarcomas, and the major hematological malignancies. Special considerations in surgery, chemotherapy, and radiation treatment are presented. Part IV also examines the comparability of cancer patient populations in international studies with respect to transferability of results. Multidisciplinary interaction between oncologists and geriatricians is important in caring for elderly cancer patients, and the domain of geriatric oncology is emerging. Part V addresses several aspects of the decision making process, including co-morbidity, quality of life, health service research, management of the terminally ill, and methodological and assessment issues unique to elderly patients. Part VI highlights selected health policy issues concerning cancer in the elderly that will be increasingly important in the new millennium.

Carrie P. Hunter
Karen A. Johnson
Hyman B. Muss

Contents

vii

Contributors

Matti S. Aapro Mulidisciplinary Institute of Oncology, Clinique de Genolier, Genolier, Switzerland

Robin L. Bennett Division of Medical Genetics, University of Washington, Seattle, Washington

Shulamit L. Bernard Research Triangle Institute, Research Triangle Park, North Carolina

Stephen A. Bernard School of Medicine, University of North Carolina at Chapel Hill, Chapel Hill, North Carolina

Samer E. Bibawi Department of Medicine, Hematology/Oncology Unit, University of Vermont, Burlington, Vermont

Otis W. Brawley National Cancer Institute, National Institutes of Health, Bethesda, Maryland

Wylie Burke Department of Medicine, University of Washington, and Fred Hutchinson Cancer Research Center, Seattle, Washington

Harold J. Burstein   Department of Adult Oncology, Dana–Farber Cancer Institute, and Department of Medicine, Brigham and Women's Hospital, Harvard Medical School, Boston, Massachusetts

Erna Busch-Devereaux   Prohealth Care Associates, Lake Success, New York

Elizabeth C. Clipp   Geriatric Research, Education and Clinical Center, Veterans Administration Medical Center, and Division of Geriatrics, Department of Medicine, Duke University Medical Center, Durham, North Carolina

Harvey Jay Cohen   Geiatric Research, Education and Clinical Center, Veterans Administration Medical Center, and Center on Aging, Duke University Medical Center, Durham, North Carolina

Susan S. Devesa   Biostatistics Branch, Division of Cancer Epidemiology and Genetics, National Cancer Institute, National Institutes of Health, Bethesda, Maryland

Barbara K. Dunn   Basic Prevention Science Research Group, Division of Cancer Prevention, National Cancer Institute, National Institutes of Health, Bethesda, Maryland

Martine Extermann   Division of Medical Oncology, H. Lee Moffitt Cancer Center, and Department of Internal Medicine, University of South Florida, Tampa, Florida

Patricia A. Ganz   Division of Cancer Prevention and Control Research, Jonsson Comprehensive Cancer Center, University of California, Los Angeles, California

Marc Gautier   Dartmouth Hitchcock Medical Center, Lebanon, New Hampshire

Steven M. Grunberg   Hematology/Oncology Unit, Department of Medicine, University of Vermont, Burlington, Vermont

Mary S. Harper   Departments of Nursing, Social Work, and Medicine, University of Alabama, Tuscaloosa, Alabama

William R. Hazzard   Department of Internal Medicine and J. Paul Sticht Center on Aging, Wake Forest University School of Medicine, Winston–Salem, North Carolina

Carrie P. Hunter   Office of Research on Women's Health, National Institutes of Health, Bethesda, Maryland

Hanlee P. Ji   Department of Medicine, University of Washington, Seattle, Washington

Karen A. Johnson Breast and Gynecologic Cancer Research Group, Division of Cancer Prevention, National Cancer Institute, National Institutes of Health, Bethesda, Maryland

Arnold D. Kaluzny Department of Health Policy and Administration, School of Public Health, and Cecil G. Sheps Center for Health Services Research, University of North Carolina at Chapel Hill, Chapel Hill, North Carolina

Margaret M. Kemeny Division of Surgical Oncology, Department of Surgery, SUNY Stony Brook, Stony Brook, New York

Gretchen Kimmick Division of Hematology/Oncology, Department of Internal Medicine, Wake Forest University School of Medicine, Winston–Salem, North Carolina

Jonathan E. Kolitz Don Monti Division of Medical Oncology/Division of Hematology, Department of Medicine, North Shore University Hospital, New York University School of Medicine, Manhasset, New York

William G. Kraybill Department of Surgical Oncology, Roswell Park Cancer Institute, Buffalo, New York

Stuart M. Lichtman Don Monti Division of Medical Oncology/Division of Hematology, Department of Medicine, North Shore University Hospital, New York University School of Medicine, Manhasset, New York

Dan L. Longo National Institute on Aging, National Institutes of Health, Bethesda, Maryland

Robert J. Mayer Department of Adult Oncology, Dana-Farber Cancer Institute, and Department of Medicine, Brigham and Women's Hospital, Harvard Medical School, Boston, Massachusetts

Worta McCaskill-Stevens National Cancer Institute, National Institutes of Health, Bethesda, Maryland

Paul E. McGann Department of Internal Medicine and J. Paul Sticht Center on Aging, Wake Forest University School of Medicine, Winston–Salem, North Carolina

David H. Moore Department of Obstetrics and Gynecology, Indiana University School of Medicine, Indianapolis, Indiana

Arno James Mundt Departments of Radiation and Cellular Oncology, University of Chicago Hospitals, Chicago, Illinois

Sheila A. Prindiville   Division of Medical Oncology, Department of Medicine, University of Colorado Health Sciences Center, Denver, Colorado

David B. Reuben   Division of Geriatrics and Multicampus Program in Geriatric Medicine and Gerontology, Department of Medicine, University of California, Los Angeles, California

Christopher W. Ryan   Department of Medicine, University of Chicago Medical Center, Chicago, Illinois

William A. Satariano   Division of Public Health Biology and Epidemiology, School of Public Health, University of California, Berkeley, California

Jeffrey Scott Stephens   Department of Surgery, Roswell Park Cancer Institute, Buffalo, New York

Linda M. Sutton   Triangle Hospice, Duke University Medical Center, Durham, North Carolina

Nicholas J. Vogelzang   Department of Medicine, University of Chicago Medical Center, Chicago, Illinois

Eric Paul Winer   Dana–Farber Cancer Institute and Harvard Medical School, Boston, Massachusetts

1

The Burden of Cancer in the Elderly

Susan S. Devesa
National Cancer Institute
National Institutes of Health
Bethesda, Maryland

Carrie P. Hunter
National Institutes of Health
Bethesda, Maryland

I. INTRODUCTION

In 1997, it was estimated that a total of 1,257,800 new cases of invasive cancer would be diagnosed that year in the United States (1). This estimate includes carcinoma in situ of the bladder but excludes more than 900,000 cases of basal and squamous cell skin cancers, 36,400 cases of carcinoma in situ of the breast, and 20,100 cases of melanoma carcinoma in situ. The majority of these cancers occur at three sites. In men, over 55% of new cases are due to cancers of the prostate (32%), lung and bronchus (15%), and colon and rectum (10%). In women, over 50% of new cases are due to cancers of the breast (30%), lung and bronchus (13%), and colon and rectum (11%).

II. TRENDS IN CANCER

Between 1973 and 1994, the cancer incidence rate in men rose 33% for all cancers combined, 3% for lung cancer, and 110% for prostate cancer (1). Among women, the incidence rate increased 13% for all cancers combined, 122% for lung cancer, and 23% for breast cancer. Of the three most common cancers, only the colorectal cancer incidence rate declined overall by 5% for both sexes during this period. The risk of developing most cancers increases with advancing age. Sixty-three percent

1

of all new cancers in 1990 occurred in the population aged 65 years and older (2). The population of the United States age 65 years and older is projected to increase from 12.5% in 1990, to 13.3% by year 2010, to 20.1% in the year 2030 (3), due in large part to the impact of the Baby Boom generation. The burden of cancer will likewise increase as more people live longer.

In the United States, cancer is the second most frequent cause of death, accounting in 1993 for more than 500,000 deaths (23%) and following only deaths due to heart disease (4). Cancer was the second most frequent cause of death among both males and females overall and at all ages except among males aged 15–34 years, when it fell to fifth, and among females aged 35–74 years, when it was the leading cause of death (Table 1). The most frequent cause of death due to cancer was lung cancer, followed by prostate cancer among males and breast cancer among females, with colorectal cancer third and pancreas cancer fourth among both sexes (Table 2). However, the most common cancers varied by age group. At young ages, leukemia, brain cancer, and non-Hodgkin's lymphoma predominated. At middle ages, breast cancer was the leading cause among women, with lung and colorectal cancers gaining in importance. At ages 55 years and older, the patterns resembled those seen overall. The numbers of deaths due to cancer annually rose from less than 2000 among those under age 15 years to more than 200,000 at ages 75 years and older.

In this chapter, we will draw upon descriptive data available from several sources. Much of the incidence and survival data derive from information regarding primary cancer diagnosed among residents of nine areas of the United States participating in the Surveillance, Epidemiology, and End Results (SEER) program, supported by contracts let by the National Cancer Institute, and population estimates based on data from the Census Bureau (1). The areas include the states of Connecticut, Iowa, Utah, New Mexico, and Hawaii and the metropolitan areas of Detroit, Atlanta, San Francisco–Oakland, and Seattle–Puget Sound, where quality population-based registries have existed for several decades. Specific data on racial/ethnic population subgroups are from SEER (5). Mortality data for the United States were based on death certificate information provided by the National Center for Health Statistics. Published sources were used to evaluate the international variation in mortality among the elderly (6).

The number of cases of cancer, excluding superficial skin cancers, diagnosed in the United States rose 56% from 1975 to 1990 to more than one million per year, and the number of deaths due to cancer rose 40% (Table 3a). These increases were due to several factors. The first is the growth in the population size, which increased 15%. Thus, the crude incidence rate per 100,000 population rose 36% and the crude mortality rate increased 21%. Rates for most cancers rise with age. As mortality due to other causes, notably cardiovascular disease, has declined, people have been living longer and shifting the age distribution toward older ages. A technique called age-adjustment accounts for these changes, permitting comparison of rates as if the population distribution were the same. Comparison of the age-adjusted rates reveals

Table 1 Reported Deaths for the Five Leading Causes of Death by Age and Sex, United States, 1993

Rank	All ages Male	All ages Female	Ages 0–14 Male	Ages 0–14 Female	Ages 15–34 Male	Ages 15–34 Female	Ages 35–54 Male	Ages 35–54 Female	Ages 55–74 Male	Ages 55–74 Female	Ages 75+ Male	Ages 75+ Female
	All causes 1,161,797	All causes 1,106,756	All causes 9799	All causes 6525	All causes 70,593	All causes 24,535	All causes 149,843	All causes 78,010	All causes 426,512	All causes 302,888	All causes 486,337	All causes 680,138
1	Heart diseases 367,479	Heart diseases 375,981	Accidents 3792	Accidents 2264	Accidents 21,475	Accidents 6513	Heart diseases 33,768	Cancer 30,345	Heart diseases 146,359	Cancer 111,937	Heart diseases 183,642	Heart diseases 278,010
2	Cancer 279,375	Cancer 250,529	Cancer 922	Cancer 689	Homicide 12,892	Cancer 3308	Cancer 28,782	Heart diseases 12,032	Cancer 142,057	Heart diseases 83,787	Cancer 104,037	Cancer 104,203
3	Accidents 60,117	Cerebrovascular diseases 91,060	Homicide 682	Congenital anomalies 637	HIV infection 10,040	Homicide 2810	HIV infection 19,670	Accidents 5182	Chronic obstructive pulmonary diseases 22,936	Cerebrovascular diseases 19,003	Cerebrovascular diseases 36,047	Cerebrovascular diseases 70,193
4	Cerebrovascular diseases 59,048	Chronic obstructive pulmonary diseases 46,706	Congenital anomalies 652	Homicide 438	Suicide 9337	HIV infection 1868	Accidents 16,102	Cerebrovascular diseases 3469	Cerebrovascular diseases 18,182	Chronic obstructive pulmonary diseases 16,754	Chronic obstructive pulmonary diseases 29,339	Pneumonia and influenza 36,895
5	Chronic obstructive pulmonary diseases 54,371	Pneumonia and influenza 44,824	Heart diseases 313	Heart diseases 286	Cancer 3509	Suicide 1819	Suicide 7976	HIV infection 2746	Diabetes mellitus 10,797	Diabetes mellitus 11,665	Pneumonia and influenza 26,135	Chronic obstructive pulmonary diseases 25,818

HIV, human immunodeficiency virus.
Source: Ref. 4: based on data from Vital Statistics of the United States, 1996.

Table 2 Reported Deaths for the Five Leading Cancers by Age and Sex, United States, 1993

Rank	All ages	Under 15	15–34	35–54	55–74	75+
Males	All cancers 279,375	All cancers 978	All cancers 3509	All cancers 28,782	All cancers 142,057	All cancers 104,037
1	Lung and bronchus 92,493	Leukemia 359	Leukemia 645	Lung and bronchus 8771	Lung and bronchus 55,421	Lung and bronchus 28,122
2	Prostate 34,865	Brain and ONS 255	Non-Hodgkin's lymphoma 477	Colon and rectum 2508	Colon and rectum 13,689	Prostate 22,465
3	Colon and rectum 28,199	Endocrine system 113	Brain and ONS 458	Non-Hodgkin's lymphoma 1699	Prostate 12,051	Colon and rectum 11,787
4	Pancreas 12,669	Non-Hodgkin's lymphoma 63	Colon and rectum 209	Brain and ONS 1542	Pancreas 6678	Pancreas 4580
5	Leukemia 10,873	Soft tissue 47	Hodgkin's disease 197	Pancreas 1375	Esophagus 4661	Leukemia 4076
Females	All cancers 250,529	All cancers 721	All cancers 3308	All cancers 30,345	All cancers 111,937	All cancers 104,203
1	Lung and bronchus 56,234	Leukemia 238	Breast 560	Breast 9279	Lung and bronchus 31,803	Lung and bronchus 18,802
2	Breast 43,555	Brain and ONS 205	Leukemia 441	Lung and bronchus 5501	Breast 18,937	Colon and rectum 16,137
3	Colon and rectum 29,206	Endocrine system 74	Brain and ONS 326	Colon and rectum 2064	Colon and rectum 10,861	Breast 14,778
4	Pancreas 13,776	Bones and joints 44	Cervix uteri 323	Ovary 1823	Ovary 6159	Pancreas 6909
5	Ovary 12,870	Soft tissue 37	Non-Hodgkin's lymphoma 214	Cervix uteri 1623	Pancreas 5933	Non-Hodgkin's lymphoma 4854

ONS, other nervous system.

Note: All cancers category excludes basal and squamous cell skin cancers and in situ carcinomas except bladder.

Source: Ref. 4; based on data from Vital Statistics of the United States, 1996.

Table 3a Trends in Total Cancers in the United States, 1975–1990, All Ages

	1975	1990	% Change
Number of cases	665,000	1,040,000	56.4
Number of deaths	365,000	510,000	39.7
Population	215,467,000	248,710,000	15.4
Crude incidence	308.6	418.2	35.5
Crude mortality	169.4	205.1	21.1
Age-adjusted incidence	332.4	394.1	18.6
Age-adjusted mortality	162.3	174.0	7.2

Rates per 100,000; age-adjusted using 1970 U.S. population standard.
Source: unpublished data from the SEER program.

that incidence and mortality rose a more modest 19% and 7%, respectively, which are better reflections of changes in risk.

In 1990, a total of 650,000 cases of cancer were diagnosed among the elderly aged 65 years and older, accounting for 62.5% of the 1,040,000 total cancer cases diagnosed. More than half of the cancers occurring at ages 65 and older were diagnosed among males (Table 3b). By ages 80 years and older, more cases were diagnosed among females, largely due to females having a greater life expectancy than males (2). The number of incident cancers among the elderly is projected to increase among males from 344,200 in 1990 to 905,600 in 2030, or by more than 500,000 (163%), and among females from 305,800 to 626,900, by more than 300,000 (105%), respectively. Among those aged 80 and older, the projected numerical increases are smaller, but the proportional increases are larger: 213% among males and 127% among females. It is projected that the number of incident cancers in elderly men in the U.S. population will increase faster than in women over the next few decades, owing to a faster increase in men's life expectancy (2,7). This projected

Table 3b Projected Numbers of Incident Cancers for U.S. Men and Women Aged 65 Years and Over and Aged 80 Years and Over

Year	Aged 65 years and older		Aged 80 years and older	
	Males	Females	Males	Females
1990	344,200	305,800	82,600	92,700
2000	407,100	341,500	112,300	119,300
2010	477,300	377,300	145,400	142,200
2020	660,800	484,200	168,800	152,200
2030	905,600	626,900	258,900	210,100

Note: Only invasive cancers are included except for in situ bladder tumors.
Source: Ref. 2.

change in the pattern of cancer distribution in elderly men and women is largely unrecognized, but it will be of increasing importance to clinicians, researchers, and health care administrators in planning future cancer care and research interventions, as well as health policy and public health campaigns for the elderly.

The incidence of all cancers combined among the elderly aged 65–84 years increased 33% from 2337 per 100,000 person-years during 1975–1979 to 3114 during 1990–1994 among males and 24% from 1307 to 1625 among females (Fig. 1). Total cancer mortality rose less rapidly, from 1283 to 1367 and from 671 to 794, or 7% and 18% among males and females, respectively. Among elderly males, incidence rates for prostate cancer rose most rapidly, more than doubling over the time period shown (Fig. 2), with the most marked increase occurring between 1985 and 1994, a period during which many subclinical cases of prostate cancer were diagnosed based on prostate-specific antigen (PSA) screening along with digital rectal examination (8–12). Rates also increased substantially for kidney cancer and the lymphomas, due in part to improved diagnoses. The rise in kidney cancer incidence is related to smoking (13–15). The rising lymphoma incidence may be related to occupational exposures to pesticides or solvents, possibly to hair dyes, and to acquired immunodeficiency syndrome (AIDS), particularly among young and middle-aged men (16, 17). Recent epidemiologic leads suggest that the lymphoma risk may be associated with diets that are high in animal protein and fat and low in fruits and vegetables; a prior history of blood transfusions may also increase the risk of lymphomas (18). Notably, the lung cancer incidence has not continued to increase among males in recent years as in earlier periods. This leveling off reflects the impact of a 54% decline in smoking prevalence since 1965, due in large part to successful smoking prevention and cessation public health campaigns. Colorectal cancer peaked during the late 1980s, and rates for stomach and oral cavity cancers have declined.

Among elderly females, the most rapid increases in both incidence and mortality were for lung cancer (Fig. 3). Initiation of smoking in women lagged some 25–30 years behind men. Between 1975 and 1994, the lung cancer rates in women rose faster than in men, whose peak changes had occurred earlier (19). In the early 1990s, lung cancer surpassed colorectal cancer as the second most frequent cancer among females. Breast cancer rates rose significantly until the 1990s with a more modest rise in rates since that time. As among males, incidence rates for lymphomas and kidney cancer also increased substantially. Rates declined notably for stomach and cervix uteri cancers. Among both males and females, cancer-specific mortality rates were lower than the corresponding incidence rates. Of note, in 1985, the lung cancer mortality rate for women aged 65–84 years surpassed the breast cancer mortality rate. In comparison, this lung to breast cancer mortality rate crossover point occurred for all women some 2 years later in 1987; and it was reached some 4 years later in 1989 for all black women (1).

The risk of dying from cancer generally increases exponentially with age (Fig. 4). Based on U.S. mortality data for 1970–1994, rates for all cancers combined increased linearly starting around age 20 years until about age 60, after which the

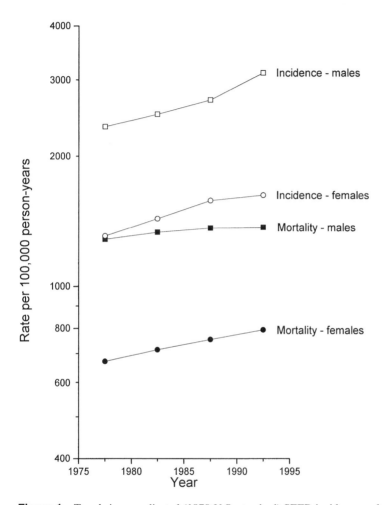

Figure 1 Trends in age-adjusted (1970 U.S. standard) SEER incidence and U.S. mortality for all cancers combined among the elderly aged 65–84 years by sex, 1975–1979 to 1990–1994.

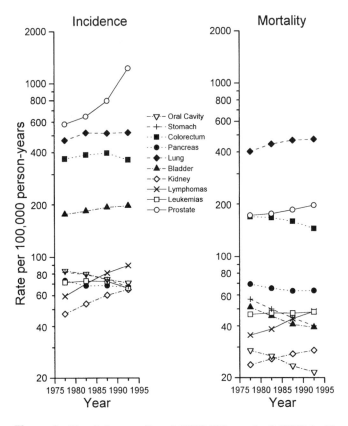

Figure 2 Trends in age-adjusted (1970 U.S. standard) SEER incidence and U.S. mortality for selected cancers among elderly males aged 65–84 years, 1975–1979 to 1990–1994.

increases were less rapid. Higher rates among males than females were most evident at ages 60 and older. This pattern was repeated for many of the specific forms of cancer, although there were exceptions. For lung cancer, the male excess was most pronounced at ages 40 years and older, with smaller differences at younger ages. Consistently higher rates among blacks than whites were evident for esophageal, stomach, cervix uteri, and prostate cancers, whereas rates among whites were notably higher for melanoma of the skin and corpus uteri cancer. Rates among young people generally were quite low, although bimodal curves were apparent for cancers of the kidney and brain and for leukemia.

At current rates, the probability at birth of ever developing cancer is 47%, or almost one out of two for males and 38%, or more than one out of three, for females (Table 4). At birth, the probability of dying of cancer is more than one out of five. By age 60, the probability of eventually developing cancer rises to 48% for males

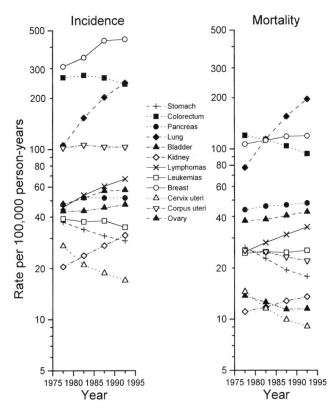

Figure 3 Trends in age-adjusted (1970 U.S. standard) SEER incidence and U.S. mortality for selected cancers among elderly females aged 65–84 years, 1975–1979 to 1990–1994.

but falls to 33% for females. A male at age 60 years has a 21% chance of being diagnosed with prostate cancer, 9% with lung cancer, and 6% with colorectal cancer during his remaining years. A 60-year-old female has almost a 10% risk of breast cancer, 6% of colorectal cancer, and 5% of lung cancer during her remaining lifetime. At current rates, 7% of males will die of lung cancer, 4% of prostate cancer, and 3% of colorectal cancer. More than 4% of females will die of lung cancer and 3% each due to breast or colorectal cancer.

There is considerable variation in cancer incidence and mortality rates according to racial/ethnic group (Fig. 5) (5).[1] The racial categories of Alaska Native,

---

[1] SEER data are used to show the general racial/ethnic patterns of cancer in U.S. population subgroups. SEER covers 14% of the total United States population. The SEER data include 78% of the Hawaiian population, 60% of the Japanese population, 49% of the Filipino population, 43% of the Chinese population, 34% of the Korean population, 31% of the Vietnamese population, 27% of the American Indian population, and 25% of the Hispanic population (5).

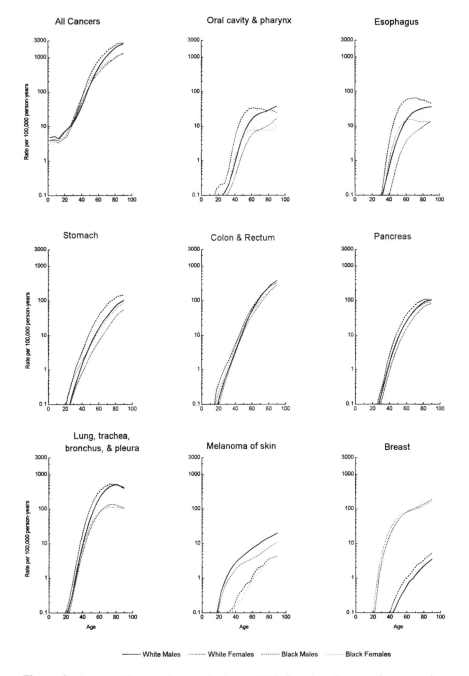

Figure 4 Age-specific mortality rates in the total U.S. for selected cancers by race and sex, 1970–1994.

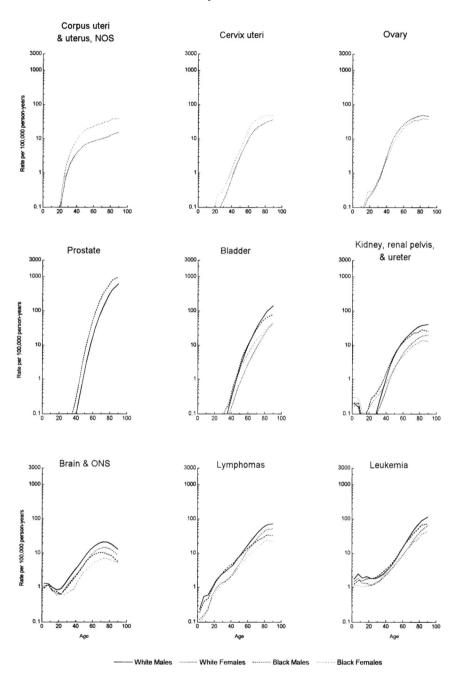

Figure 4   Continued

Table 4 Probabilities (%) of Developing (Ever or After Age 60) or Dying from Cancer by Type of Cancer and Sex: SEER areas, 1992–1994

	Males			Females		
	Developing			Developing		
Type	Ever	After age 60	Dying	Ever	After age 60	Dying
All cancers	46.64	48.46	23.85	38.00	32.75	20.63
Oral cavity and pharynx	1.52	1.22	0.43	0.74	0.60	0.25
Esophagus	0.71	0.68	0.68	0.26	0.24	0.23
Stomach	1.24	1.25	0.80	0.74	0.72	0.52
Colon and rectum	5.88	6.07	2.57	5.72	5.54	2.53
Liver[a]	0.58	0.55	0.56	0.30	0.28	0.33
Pancreas	1.18	1.19	1.11	1.25	1.23	1.21
Larynx	0.77	0.70	0.25	0.18	0.14	0.06
Lung and bronchus	8.43	8.60	7.06	5.55	5.01	4.41
Melanoma	1.46	1.07	0.30	1.07	0.59	0.19
Breast	0.11	0.10	0.03	12.52	9.43	3.46
Cervix uteri	–	–	–	0.83	0.39	0.27
Corpus uteri	–	–	–	2.66	2.17	0.51
Ovary	–	–	–	1.76	1.28	1.14
Prostate	18.85	21.19	3.64	–	–	–
Testis	0.35	0.02	0.02	–	–	–
Urinary bladder[b]	3.38	3.53	0.70	1.18	1.13	0.35
Kidney and renal pelvis	1.29	1.15	0.51	0.83	0.69	0.33
Brain and other nervous system	0.66	0.44	0.51	0.53	0.35	0.39
Thyroid	0.27	0.15	0.04	0.66	0.24	0.07
Hodgkin's disease	0.24	0.08	0.06	0.21	0.07	0.05
Lymphomas	1.96	1.55	0.93	1.68	1.43	0.87
Multiple myeloma	0.62	0.63	0.48	0.55	0.51	0.42
Leukemias	1.35	1.22	0.94	1.03	0.87	0.74

–, not applicable.
[a] Liver and intrahepatic bile duct.
[b] Urinary bladder (invasive and in situ).
Note: Invasive cancer only unless specified otherwise
Source: Ref. 1.

American Indian, black, Chinese, Filipino, Hawaiian, Japanese, Korean, Vietnamese, and white are mutually exclusive. The ethnic category Hispanic may include any race; rates are also shown for white Hispanics and white non-Hispanics. Among males, the highest total cancer incidence rates per 100,000 person-years during 1988–1992 occurred among blacks, followed by white non-Hispanics, with relatively low rates among Asian/Pacific Islander populations; these patterns were due

SEER Incidence Rates, 1988-1992

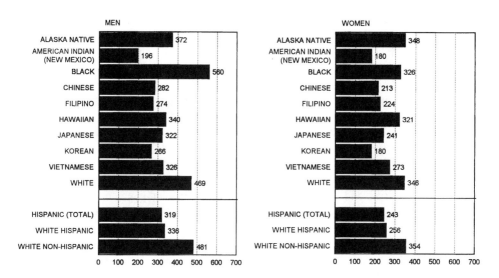

U.S. Mortality Rates, 1988-1992

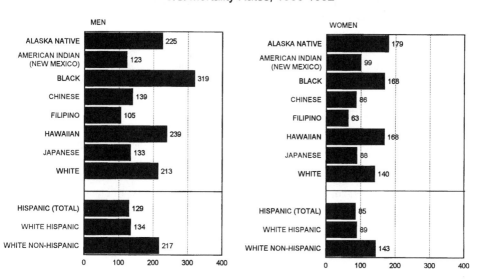

NOTE: Rates are "average annual" per 100,000 population, age-adjusted to 1970 U.S. standard; N/A = information not available.

Figure 5 Racial/ethnic variation in SEER incidence and United States mortality rates (per 100,000 person-years) for all cancers combined, 1998–1992. (From Ref. 5.)

largely to differences in the incidence of prostate, lung, and colorectal cancers. Incidence rates for prostate cancer were highest among blacks (181), white non-Hispanics (138), and white Hispanics (93), with low rates being observed among the Vietnamese (40) and Koreans (24). Lung cancer incidence rates among males ranged from highs of 117 among blacks, 89 among Hawaiians, 81 among Alaska Natives, and 79 among white non-Hispanics to lows of 44 among white Hispanics, 43 among Japanese, and 14 among American Indians (data for the latter only for New Mexico). Colorectal cancer rates were highest among Alaska Natives (80), Japanese (64), blacks (61), and white non-Hispanics (58) and lowest among American Indians (19). Black males also had relatively high rates of oral (20), esophageal (15), pancreatic (14), and laryngeal (13) cancers and multiple myeloma (11).

Among females, white non-Hispanics had the highest total cancer incidence rate, followed by Alaska Natives and blacks, with the lowest rates being among American Indians and Koreans. Differences in the incidence of breast, lung, and colorectal cancers largely account for these patterns. Female breast cancer incidence rates ranged from highs of 116 among white non-Hispanics, 106 among Hawaiians, 95 among blacks, and 74 among white Hispanics to lows of 32 among American Indians and 29 among Koreans. The highest female lung cancer incidence rates occurred among Alaska Natives (51), blacks (44), white non-Hispanics (44), and Hawaiians (43), with low rates among Filipinos (18), Koreans (16), and Japanese (15). Colorectal cancer incidence rates were highest among Alaska Natives (67), blacks (46), Japanese (40), white non-Hispanics (39), and lowest among American Indians (15). Cervix uteri cancer incidence rates were highest among the Vietnamese (43) followed by white Hispanics (17), Alaska Natives (16), Koreans (15), and blacks (13), with the lowest rate being among the Japanese (6). Among both males and females, total cancer mortality rates were high among blacks, Hawaiians, and Alaska Natives and relatively low among several of the Asian groups. Among racial/ethnic subgroups, the site-specific cancer distributions for ages 70 years and older were similar to those of their racial/ethnic category for all ages combined.

There is also substantial international variation in cancer mortality rates (6, 20). Table 5a presents age-adjusted (world standard) mortality rates during 1990–1992 for all cancers combined among the elderly, defined as ages 65–84 years. Rates among males ranged from highs in the Netherlands, Italy, England and Wales, Uruguay, and Denmark to lows in Australia, Japan, Sweden, Portugal, and Argentina. Other countries, including the United States, had rates that were intermediate. Among females, rates were highest in Denmark and in England and Wales and were lower in Germany, Canada, the United States, the Netherlands, and Uruguay, with the lowest rates being in Argentina, France, Spain, and Japan. These patterns most likely were influenced by variations in the relative frequency of the various forms of cancer.

For example, among males aged 65–84 years, lung cancer was the most common cause of cancer death in every country shown (Table 5b); rates ranged from greater than 600 in the Netherlands and 500 in England and Wales to less than 300

Table 5a International Variation in Total Cancer Mortality Rates[a] Among Elderly Males and Females, Aged 65–84 Years, Selected Countries, 1990–1992

Country	Males	Females
United States	1306.1	754.1
Canada	1356.6	754.6
Argentina	1124.9	631.4
Uruguay	1537.4	758.5
Denmark	1494.6	936.6
France	1431.2	583.6
Germany	1399.5	760.8
Italy	1525.1	673.1
Netherlands	1617.6	724.8
Poland	1433.5	688.6
Portugal	1119.1	567.8
Spain	1317.7	540.8
Sweden	1081.6	692.3
England and Wales	1513.1	860.1
Australia	1280.9	676.1
Japan	1213.8	532.8

[a] Per 100,000 person-years, age-adjusted by the direct method to the world population standard.
Source: Ref. 6.

in Japan, Argentina, Portugal, and Sweden. Intestinal cancer mortality rates were highest in Germany followed by England and Wales, with the lowest rates again being in Japan and Argentina. Prostate cancer rates exceeded 100 in all countries except in Japan, where the rate was less than 40; rates were highest in Uruguay, Sweden, Denmark, Australia, and the United States. The patterns for stomach cancer were quite different, with the rate exceeding 250 in Japan, 185 in Portugal, 175 in Poland, and 140 in Italy, in contrast to a rate less than 40 in the United States. Oral cancers were most frequent in France; pancreatic cancer in Japan, Germany, and the Scandinavian countries; and bladder cancer in Italy and Denmark.

Among elderly females, shown in Table 5c, lung cancer was the most frequent form of cancer death only in the United States, England and Wales, Denmark, and Canada; rates ranged from less than 25 in Spain to 180 in the United States. Breast cancer was the most common malignancy in the Netherlands, England and Wales, Denmark, and Uruguay, with rates all exceeding 130, in contrast to a rate of only 21 in Japan. Intestinal cancer was the first-ranked cancer in Germany, Poland, Spain, Portugal, Sweden, and Australia; rates ranged from 70 to 130. Stomach cancer was the leading cancer in Japan, with a rate of almost 100, five times that in the United States. Uterine cancer rates ranged from less than 25 in Japan and Australia to almost

Table 5b International Variation in Mortality Rates[a] for Selected Cancers Among Elderly Males, Aged 65 to 84 Years, Selected Countries, 1990–1992

Country	Mouth and pharynx	Esophagus	Stomach	Intestines	Pancreas	Lung	Prostate	Bladder
United States	22.4	33.3	39.4	144.7	60.8	460.7	173.5	34.6
Canada	26.2	34.5	57.8	170.7	62.8	466.1	169.5	39.2
Argentina	22.4	58.5	92.4	116.4	NA	250.0	132.8	53.0
Uruguay	31.4	77.0	114.3	129.6	NA	391.2	217.8	65.3
Denmark	22.0	40.7	57.2	197.2	66.8	436.3	198.2	87.5
France	56.2	63.3	68.6	178.0	56.7	322.7	163.9	58.2
Germany	24.8	26.1	122.3	186.2	65.1	378.2	162.2	65.3
Italy	32.4	27.8	143.4	164.1	59.6	453.5	122.0	84.8
Netherlands	16.0	40.3	98.5	165.3	68.1	617.5	171.3	65.3
Poland	27.6	28.9	177.1	127.2	57.3	473.1	105.5	68.9
Portugal	28.0	34.4	186.3	159.7	43.8	194.8	154.3	45.9
Spain	30.5	32.4	116.5	135.5	43.9	351.2	135.1	77.6
Sweden	16.1	22.5	71.1	130.3	70.1	194.1	212.9	36.8
England and Wales	16.7	62.1	109.6	181.9	59.0	511.2	173.5	66.9
Australia	28.2	37.5	58.1	170.5	51.4	353.3	182.0	37.3
Japan	14.9	54.0	266.1	119.8	69.3	288.2	38.4	20.7

NA, not available.
[a] Per 100,000 person-years, age-adjusted by the direct method to the world population standard.
Source: Ref. 6.

Table 5c International Variation in Mortality Rates[a] for Selected Cancers Among Elderly Females, Aged 65–84 Years, Selected Countries, 1990–1992

Country	Stomach	Intestines	Pancreas	Lung	Breast	Uterus	Ovary	Kidney
United States	17.1	91.9	44.1	179.6	118.8	30.8	41.2	13.4
Canada	25.9	110.4	45.5	152.8	126.2	30.6	37.0	13.9
Argentina	35.9	71.3	NA	36.0	116.1	49.5	NA	NA
Uruguay	51.0	109.5	NA	27.4	133.9	50.0	NA	NA
Denmark	29.3	132.4	54.8	161.5	143.0	57.3	59.2	21.1
France	26.4	94.9	31.3	34.7	100.3	34.7	36.6	13.1
Germany	59.4	131.2	45.0	56.4	113.2	41.6	45.8	21.0
Italy	64.7	100.3	37.9	54.6	101.5	35.7	24.4	11.4
Netherlands	36.4	114.2	44.0	59.2	140.2	33.0	53.1	19.1
Poland	63.8	84.3	40.1	64.1	76.3	59.6	NA	NA
Portugal	91.5	97.5	26.1	32.6	82.0	39.4	17.7	6.9
Spain	52.4	79.6	26.6	24.9	77.8	32.6	18.4	8.3
Sweden	33.4	95.4	56.5	64.0	86.4	33.5	44.5	24.6
England and Wales	42.6	113.9	43.0	166.2	144.5	37.3	49.1	12.3
Australia	22.5	107.9	37.7	99.1	100.4	24.7	36.2	17.0
Japan	98.0	70.0	41.1	67.3	20.7	24.5	14.5	6.8

NA, not available.
[a] per 100,000 person-years, age-adjusted by the direct method to the world population standard.
Source: Ref. 6.

60 in Poland and Denmark, whereas ovarian cancer rates ranged from less than 20 in Japan, Spain, and Portugal to almost 50 in England and Wales and nearly 60 in Denmark.

Among patients diagnosed with cancer (all forms combined) in the United States, the 5-year relative survival rate, which is adjusted for expected general population mortality, ranged from 41% among black males to 62% among white females (Table 6). These rates were driven by the differing relative frequency of the major forms of cancer with varying survival rates. Survival rates were relatively high among patients diagnosed with cancers of the testis, thyroid, prostate, breast, or corpus uteri or with melanoma. Patients diagnosed with liver, pancreatic, esophageal, or lung cancer fared particularly poorly. Compared with patients of all ages, those diagnosed at ages 65 years or older fared better in a few instances, such as those diagnosed with breast cancer, but more frequently they did less well. Differences were substantial for those diagnosed with cervix uteri, corpus uteri, ovarian, or especially brain cancer, Hodgkin's disease, or leukemia. Across the board, survival rates were higher among whites than blacks for most cancers. Black males diagnosed with oral cancer experienced survival rates notably lower than the other three race/sex groups; however, black males with brain or other nervous system cancers had better survival experiences than the other three race/sex groups.

The stage of disease at diagnosis varied considerably among the various solid

Table 6   Five-Year Relative Survival Rates (%) by Race, Sex, and Cancer: All Ages, Ages 65+, SEER Program, 1986–1993

Type	All ages				Ages 65+			
	WM	WF	BM	BF	WM	WF	BM	BF
All cancers	56.5	62.3	41.1	47.9	58.6	54.6	45.7	39.3
Oral cavity and pharynx	51.8	61.7	28.4	47.3	53.1	54.8	25.9	32.8
Esophagus	12.1	11.1	7.5	8.8	10.3	9.3	8.4	7.4
Stomach	16.6	24.5	16.9	25.2	17.5	22.9	15.7	22.8
Colon and rectum	62.9	61.8	51.5	53.2	63.5	61.0	49.3	49.2
Liver	4.4	9.1	3.0	6.6	2.1	4.5	2.1	0.0
Pancreas	3.6	3.9	4.5	5.7	2.0	2.7	3.0	3.3
Larynx	70.5	63.6	53.0	58.7	69.3	58.8	56.5	62.5
Lung	12.7	16.1	10.5	12.2	11.1	14.0	9.3	8.1
Melanoma of the skin	85.4	91.1	50.0	78.7	86.5	86.0	NA	71.0
Breast	–	85.5	–	70.0	–	87.7	–	73.0
Cervix uteri	–	71.4	–	57.1	–	50.6	–	50.0
Corpus uteri	–	85.9	–	55.3	–	82.1	–	44.2
Ovary	–	46.5	–	41.9	–	29.1	–	24.1
Prostate	90.2	–	75.3	–	90.9	–	74.7	–
Testis	95.3	–	86.4	–	88.3	–	NA	–
Bladder	85.1	75.1	65.0	53.6	82.1	69.7	56.8	51.2
Kidney	60.8	58.4	54.0	57.2	56.5	49.4	47.1	41.1
Brain and other nervous system	28.6	30.2	37.6	30.9	3.9	5.4	13.1	6.5
Thyroid	92.9	96.2	87.9	88.9	80.3	80.1	NA	60.4
Hodgkin's disease	79.1	85.2	71.7	75.3	44.0	47.6	NA	NA
Non-Hodgkin's lymphoma	48.7	56.6	40.0	49.0	46.3	47.8	38.1	38.7
Multiple myeloma	29.4	27.3	29.9	30.3	23.3	23.3	25.4	27.4
Leukemias	43.8	41.4	31.4	35.7	35.5	34.7	23.6	25.0

WM, white male; WF, white female; BM, black male; BF, black female; NA, not available; –, not applicable.
Source: Ref. 1.

tumors (Table 7). More than 70% of the cancers were still localized to the organ of origin for those arising in the corpus uteri or bladder and for melanomas of the skin. In contrast, about half of patients diagnosed with ovarian and nearly half of those diagnosed with lung or pancreatic cancer had distant spread of the disease. The stage of disease at diagnosis strongly influenced subsequent survival. Among females diagnosed with cervix uteri cancer, the 5-year relative survival rate exceeded 90% if the cancer was still localized, but it was less than 10% if there was distant spread; the comparable rates for females with breast cancer were 97 versus 21% and for males with prostate cancer, 100 versus 31%.

Table 7 Stage Distribution and 5-Year Relative Survival Rates (%) by Stage of Cancer (All Races, Ages, Both Sexes) for Localized, Regional, Distant Disease, SEER Program, 1986–1993

Type	Stage distribution (%)			5-Year relative survival (%)		
	Local	Regional	Distant	Local	Regional	Distant
Oral cavity and pharynx	36	43	9	80.9	41.8	17.9
Esophagus	24	24	26	22.7	10.4	1.6
Stomach	19	31	36	60.5	22.7	2.2
Colon and rectum	37	37	20	91.6	63.8	7.3
Liver	20	22	24	13.1	6.8	1.8
Pancreas	8	23	48	14.6	5.1	1.5
Larynx	49	32	13	84.6	54.7	41.6
Lung	15	25	45	48.5	18.2	1.9
Melanoma of the skin	82	8	4	95.0	60.8	15.9
Breast	60	31	6	96.8	75.9	20.6
Cervix uteri	52	33	8	91.3	49.4	9.1
Corpus uteri	73	13	9	95.5	66.1	26.8
Ovary	24	13	57	92.6	54.7	25.3
Prostate	58	18	11	100.0	94.1	30.9
Testis	66	19	12	98.5	97.1	72.3
Bladder	74	18	3	93.5	49.0	5.9
Kidney	46	23	24	87.9	59.7	9.1
Thyroid	60	31	5	99.7	93.7	44.8

Source: Ref. 1.

III. HEALTH BEHAVIORS AND RISK RACTORS

Changes in screening practices and lifestyle behaviors impact cancer incidence and mortality. For example, the use of screening procedures to detect early lesions is very important. The large declines in incidence and mortality rates for cancer of the cervix uteri were due largely to the widespread use of the Papanicolaou (Pap) smear and pelvic examination, leading to the increased detection of premalignant treatable lesions (21). Despite its widespread use, older women often go unscreened (22). In recent years, mammography screening has become more prevalent (Table 8) (23). The proportion of non-Hispanic white women aged 50–64 years who had a mammogram within the past 2 years increased from 34% in 1987 to 68% by 1994, a doubling in mammographic participation. Rates among non-Hispanic black and Hispanic women were somewhat lower but also rose substantially, showing increases of 146–161% during this period. Utilization rates among women aged 65 years and older were also somewhat lower than for women aged 50–64 years, but the use of mam-

Table 8 Trends in Mammography Utilization by Age Group, Racial/Ethnic Group, and Socioeconomic Group: Percentage of Women 50 Years of Age and Older Having a Mammogram in the Last 2 Years

	1987	1990	1994
Ages 50–64 years			
Racial/ethnic group			
White, non-Hispanic	33.6	58.1	67.5
Black, non-Hispanic	26.4	48.4	63.6
Hispanic	23.0	47.5	60.1
Ages 65 years and older			
Racial/ethnic group			
White, non-Hispanic	24.0	43.8	54.9
Black, non-Hispanic	14.1	39.7	61.0
Hispanic	13.7[a]	41.1	48.0
Poverty status			
Below	13.4	28.0	40.3
At or above	25.0	46.6	58.4
Education			
Less than 12 years	16.5	33.0	45.6
12 years	25.9	47.5	59.1
13 years or more	32.3	56.7	64.3

[a] Relative standard error greater than 30%.
Source: Ref. 23.

mography increased 129% in white non-Hispanic women, 336% in black non-Hispanic women, and 243% in Hispanic women. Both poverty status and educational level influenced the mammography utilization rate.

Cigarette smoking is the dominant cause of lung cancer (24). It also increases the risk for cancers of the larynx, oral cavity, esophagus, bladder, pancreas, and cervix uteri. The prevalence of cigarette smoking in 1965 exceeded 50% among adult males and 30% of females (Table 9) (23). Since then, the prevalence of current smoking has declined to one-third or less among males and one-quarter or less among females. At each point in time, the prevalence was higher among black than white males, with small racial differences among females. Among persons aged 65 years and older, the smoking prevalence was lower than among the corresponding age range 18 years and older. The prevalence declined consistently over time among males, whereas rates rose among females before peaking during the mid-1980s. During 1994, the prevalence of cigarette smoking among black males was more than twice that among the other three race/sex groups aged 65 years and older.

Although specific dietary factors are less well established as influencing cancer risk, high fruit and vegetable consumption appears to be protective for many cancers,

Table 9 Trends in Cigarette Smoking Prevalence in the United States by Sex and Race: Ages 18 Years and Older, and 65 Years and Older

	1965	1974	1985	1994
Ages 18 years and older				
White males	50.8	41.7	31.3	27.5
Black males	59.2	54.0	39.9	33.5
White females	34.3	32.3	28.3	24.3
Black females	32.1	35.9	30.7	21.1
Ages 65 years and older				
White males	27.7	24.3	18.9	11.9
Black males	36.4	29.7	27.7	25.6
White females	9.8	12.3	13.3	11.1
Black females	7.1	8.9	14.5	13.6

Source: Ref. 23.

whereas high fat consumption may increase the risk of breast, colon, and prostate cancer (25–27). Obesity has been associated with several cancers, including those of the corpus uteri and breast in postmenopausal women. Since the early 1960s, the proportion of the population that was overweight has increased, with the most dramatic increases occurring in the 1988–1994 period (Table 10) (23). At each point in time, the proportion overweight was higher among black females than the three other race/sex groups, and in recent years it exceeded 50%. The percentage overweight tended to increase with age before peaking around age 65 years. In addition, heredity, past reproductive experiences in women, and the cumulative effects of environmental exposures to carcinogenic agents and chemicals in genetically susceptible individuals contribute to the risk of developing cancer.

IV. FUTURE CHANGES IN TRENDS

The burden of cancer in the elderly will progressively increase in the early part of the 21st century owing to the large number of cancers that will be diagnosed as the Baby Boom generation becomes the elderly population in America. One in five persons in the United States will be age 65 years or older by the year 2030, which is a nearly two–fold increase from the 1990 level. A large segment will be from racial and ethnic subgroups. With increased longevity, a greater proportion of these cancers will occur in men.

Reducing the burden of cancer is a challenge. Cumulative effects over time of risk factors, genetic susceptibility, environmental exposures to carcinogens, and less healthy behaviors or practices increase the risk of cancer. However, several

Table 10 Trends in % of Population Ages 20 Years and Older Overweight According
to Sex, Race, and Age, United States

	1960–1962	1971–1974	1976–1980	1988–1994
Race/sex group				
White males	23.1	23.8	24.2	34.3
Black males	22.2	24.3	25.7	34.0
White females	23.5	24.0	24.4	33.9
Black females	41.7	42.9	44.3	53.0
Sex/age group				
Males (years)				
20–34	19.6	19.2	17.3	25.4
35–44	22.8	29.4	28.9	34.9
45–54	28.1	27.6	31.0	37.7
55–64	26.9	24.8	28.1	43.7
65–74	21.8	23.0	25.2	42.9
75 and older	NA	NA	NA	27.7
Females (years)[a]				
20–34	13.2	14.8	16.8	25.6
35–44	24.1	27.3	27.0	36.8
45–54	30.7	32.3	32.5	45.4
55–64	43.2	38.5	37.0	48.2
65–74	42.9	38.0	38.4	42.3
75 and older	NA	NA	NA	35.1

NA, not available.
[a] Excludes pregnant women.
Source: Ref. 23.

factors are likely to have a major effect on reducing the rates of cancer—including
the reduction of smoking and increased consumption of fruits and vegetables. Behavioral change interventions to modify lifestyle habits—e.g., smoking, diet—and improved preventive health practices can impact cancer rates. Cancer is a disease of
genetic alterations. Technological advancements in genetics research will make possible the identification of individuals at risk for cancer and will influence future
trends in cancer incidence and mortality. Advancements in chemoprevention, such
as in the tamoxifen prevention study that demonstrated a reduction in the incidence
of breast cancer in high-risk women by 45% (28), herald a new era in the primary
prevention of cancer.

The paradigm of cancer in the elderly population is changing and will continue
to shift over the next few decades. Recent data show that overall cancer incidence
and mortality rates are decreasing—a most encouraging sign (29). Compared to an
increasing cancer incidence trend during 1973–1990, the rates show an overall decrease on average of 0.7% per year during 1990–1995, most notably for cancers of

the lung, prostate, colon and rectum, and urinary bladder and for leukemia, with a leveling off for breast cancer. Declines in the incidence rates in the elderly were most striking for persons over 75 years of age. Cancer death rates overall, which had increased 0.4% per year during 1973–1990, show a decline on average of 0.5% per year during 1990–1995. Continued monitoring of trends in cancer incidence and mortality will be needed in order to determine changes in the burden of cancer due to differences in cohorts, risk factors, environmental exposures, and lifestyle habits, as well as the effects of genetic screening and early detection in the aging population.

ACKNOWLEDGMENTS

We thank Joan Hertel of IMS, Inc., Rockville, MD, for computer support and figure development; Annette Cunningham, Holly Brown, and Jennifer Donaldson for table preparation; and Dr. B.J. Stone for editorial assistance.

REFERENCES

1. Ries LAG, Kosary CL, Hankey BF, Miller BA, Harras A, Edwards BK, eds. SEER Cancer Statistics Review, 1973–1994, National Cancer Institute. NIH Pub. No. 97–2789, Bethesda, MD, 1997.
2. Polednak AP. Projected numbers of cancers diagnosed in the US elderly population, 1990 through 2030. Am J Public Health 1994; 84:1313–1316.
3. U.S. Bureau of the Census. Current Population Reports, Special Studies, P23–190, 65+ in the United States. US Government Printing Office, Washington, DC, 1996.
4. Parker SL, Tong T, Bolden S, Wingo PA. Cancer statistics, 1997. CA Cancer J Clin 1997; 47:5–27.
5. Miller BA, Kolonel LN, Bernstein L, Young Jr. JL, Swanson GM, West D, Key CR, Liff JM, Glover CS, Alexander GA, eds. Racial/ethnic patterns of cancer in the United States 1988–92, National Cancer Institute. NIH Pub. No. 96-4104, Bethesda, MD, 1996.
6. Levi F, La Vecchia C, Lucchini F, Negri E. Worldwide trends in cancer mortality in the elderly, 1955–1992. Eur J Cancer 1996; 32A:652–672.
7. Population projections of the United States by age, sex, race and Hispanic origin: 1992 to 2050. Current Population Reports, Series P-25, No. 1092. US Bureau of the Census, Washington, DC. 1992.
8. Chu TM. Prostate–specific antigen and early detection of prostate cancer. Tumour Biol 1997; 18:123–134.
9. Arcangeli CG, Ornstein DK, Keetch DW, Andriole GL. Prostate-specific antigen as a screening test for prostate cancer. The United States experience. Urol Clin North Am 1997; 24:299–306.
10. Gann PH. Interpreting recent trends in prostate cancer incidence and mortality (editorial). Epidemiology 1997; 8:117–120.
11. Merrill RM, Potosky AL, Feuer EJ. Changing trends in U. S. prostate cancer incidence rates. J Natl Cancer Inst 1996; 88:1683–1685.

12. Stephenson RA, Stanford JL. Population-based prostate cancer trends in the United States: patterns of change in the era of prostate-specific antigen. World J Urol 1997; 15:331–335.

13. US Department of Health and Human Services. Reducing the Health Consequences of Smoking: 25 Years of Progress. A Report of the Surgeon General, US Department of Health and Human Services, Public Health Service, Centers for Disease Control, Center for Chronic Disease Prevention and Health Promotion, Office on Smoking and Health, US Government Printing Office DHHS Publication No. (CDC) 89–8411, Washington, DC. 1989.

14. McCredie M. Bladder and kidney cancers. Cancer Surv 1994; 19–20:343–368.

15. Boyle P. Cancer, cigarette smoking and premature death in Europe: a review including the Recommendations of European Cancer Experts Consensus Meeting, Helsinki, October, 1996. Lung Cancer 1997; 17:1–60.

16. Devesa SS, Fears T. Non-Hodgkin's lymphoma time trends: United States and international data. Cancer Res 1992; 52:5432S–5440S.

17. Hartge P, Devesa SS, Fraumeni JF Jr. Hodgkin's and non-Hodgkin's lymphomas. Cancer Surv 1994; 19–20:423–453.

18. Cerhan JR. New epidemiologic leads in the etiology of non-Hodgkin's lymphoma in the elderly: the role of blood transfusion and diet. Biomed Pharmacother 1997; 51:200–207.

19. Travis WD, Lubin J, Ries L, Devesa S. United States lung carcinoma incidence trends: declining for most histologic types among males, increasing among females. Cancer 1996; 77:2464–2470.

20. Doll R, Fraumeni JF Jr, Muir CS, eds. Trends in cancer incidence and mortality. Cancer Surv 1994; 19–20:1–583.

21. National Institutes of Health Consensus Development Conference statement on cervical cancer. Gynecol Oncol 1997; 66:351–361.

22. Martin LM, Calle EG, Wingo PA, Heath CW Jr. Comparison of mammography and Pap test use from the 1987 and 1992 National Health Interview Surveys: are we closing the gaps? Am J Prev Med 1996; 12:82–90.

23. USDHHS. Health, United States 1996–97 and Injury Chartbook. DHHS Pub. No. (PHS) 97–1232. National Center for Health Statistics, Hyattsville, MD. 1997.

24. Shopland DR. Tobacco use and its contribution to early cancer mortality with a special emphasis on cigarette smoking. Environ Health Perspect 1995; 103(Suppl 8):131–142.

25. Steinmetz KA, Potter JD. Vegetables, fruit, and cancer prevention: a review. J Am Diet Assoc 1996; 96:1027–1039.

26. Willett WC. Diet, nutrition, and avoidable cancer. Environ Health Perspect 1995; 103(Suppl. 8):165–170.

27. Wynder EL, Cohen LA, Muscat JE, Winters B, Dwyer JT, Blackburn G. Breast cancer: weighing the evidence for a promoting role of dietary fat. J Natl Cancer Inst 1997; 89:766–775.

28. Klausner RD. Breast Cancer Prevention Trial. Statement before the Senate Appropriations Subcommittee on Labor, Health, Human Services and Related Agencies, April 21, 1998.

29. Wingo PA, Ries LA, Rosenberg HM, Miller DS, Edwards BK. Cancer incidence and mortality, 1973–1995, a report card for the U.S. Cancer 1998; 82:1197–1207.

2
Breast Cancer Screening

Worta McCaskill-Stevens
National Cancer Institute
National Institutes of Health
Bethesda, Maryland

I. SIGNIFICANCE OF THE PROBLEM

In 1999, about 176,000 new cases of breast cancer are expected to be diagnosed, and nearly 44,000 women are expected to die from the disease (1). Approximately one half of all cases of breast cancer occur in women older than 65 years of age. Cancer of all kinds is the leading cause of death for women older than 75 years old (1), and breast cancer mortality is second only to colorectal cancer as a cause of death for this age group (1). From SEER (Surveillance, Evaluation, and End-Results [Program]) data, the overall breast cancer incidence rate for women aged 65 years and older is 443 per 100,000 (460 per 100,000 for whites and 365 per 100,000 for African-Americans) (2). Comparable incidence rates for women under 65 years of age are 110 per 100,000 overall: 113.5 per 100,000 for whites and 99.5 per 100,000 for blacks. The large number of women over the age of 65 years who face the problem of breast cancer make breast cancer screening an important public health issue.

The incentive to pursue early detection of breast cancer through screening is based on a demonstrated 14–32% decrease in mortality from breast cancer secondary to screening in randomized clinical trials that included women who ranged from 40 to 74 years old at the time of entry. Screening guidelines for the age groups at the ends of the age range (women <50 years old and women 65 years old and older) are a source of controversy for women and clinicians, because women in age groups at the extremes of the age range were fewer in number than those in the age groups at the center of the age distribution. Screening recommendations are formulated for a target population, but there is a concern that age may introduce sufficient heterogeneity in screening outcomes that an adjustment in screening practices for age-related differences may be needed. Nevertheless, the early randomized screening trials were designed to obtain a result for entire study populations not for subgroups within each study population. A meta-analysis of screening studies can be performed, but the results are most robust for predicting outcomes in women between the ages of 50 and 64 years.

The 1990 National Institute of Aging's Forum for Screening in Older Women provided the following recommendations for breast cancer screening (3):

> Monthly breast self-examinations for all women age 65 years and older
> Annual clinical breast examination (CBE) for women 65–74 years old and mammography every 2 years
> Clinical breast examinations for women 75 years old and older with good health and life expectancy and mammography every 2 years

The approach summarized above is more comprehensive than the recommendations from several other organizations, which have been summarized by the U.S. Preventive Services Task Force (USPSTF) (4). The USPSTF recommends mammography every 1 or 2 years either alone or with clinical breast examination for women aged 50–69 years. Many organizations recommend that breast screening begin at the age of 40 years, with annual CBE and mammography every 1 or 2 years and continue at 50 years old with annual CBE and mammography (American Cancer Society, American College of Radiology, American Medical Association, and American College of Obstetrics and Gynecology). The American College of Physicians recommends cessation of mammography at age 75 years. Given these variations in guidelines, some physicians may take the approach of stopping at the earliest juncture consistent with any guideline. Other reasons that have been cited for avoiding a recommendation to an elderly patient for screening include the existence of comorbidity or other individual circumstances that are overriding. A major point of variability in the guidelines is the age at which to cease mammography, if ever. Some clinicians would cease recommending mammography for a reduced life expectancy, reasoning that if the life expectancy is short, the benefits of screening might not be realized. The average life expectancy of a healthy 65-year-old women is 15–20 years, of a 75-year-old is 11 years, and 5–7 years for a woman of 85 years (5).

Health care provider recommendations in favor of breast cancer screening and patient acceptance fo the recommendations are releated to the knowledge, attitudes, and beliefs of both the providers and the patients. Technical elements which have an effect on acceptance include (a) demonstration of the effectiveness of the modality by well-designed studies, (b) the perception of net clinical benefit after evaluation of the risks and benefits to the public health, and (c) evaluation of the economic impact of the intervention (6). Potential benefits to the individual woman who is screened include a wider selection of treatment options, better quality of life, and improved survival.

II. BREAST CANCER SCREENING PROCEDURES

A. Mammography and Clinical Breast Examination

Since 1963, nine major randomized trials have provided data about breast cancer screening for about 500,000 women. Although mammography was performed in all nine studies, it was not combined with CBE in all of the trials. The main results are summarized by the "Fletcher Report" (7). Although mortality due to breast cancer after screening was reduced up to 32% in these trials, the report concluded that there were too few women older than 70 years of age included in the studies to assess the effectiveness of screening in this age group. Only two randomized controlled trials included women who were 65 years old or older. The Malmö Trial included women up to the age of 69 years and the Two Counties Trial included women aged up to age 74 years (8, 9).

Tabar, et al. have discussed various factors that contribute to the effectiveness of breast cancer screening with mammography. Results from the Swedish Two-County Trial suggest that the effectiveness of mammography can be increased by adjusting the screening interval to some optimal value that is shorter than the sojourn time, which is defined as the estimated maximum duration of the detectable preclinical phase (10). The Two-County estimate of the sojourn time for women aged 40–49 years was 1.7 years: 3.3 years for women aged 50–59 years, 3.8 years for women aged 60–69 years, and 2.6 years for women aged 70–74 years. These results conform to the view that the sojourn time is longer for older women. If older women exceed current recommendations for mammographic screening every 1–2 years, the possibility of interval cancer is increased.

Although the elderly are poorly represented in randomized screening clinical trials, retrospective studies have been used to estimate the positive predictive value of mammographic screening and other characteristics. Biopsy yields and cancer detection rates following mammography have been reported to be higher in older women (11, 12). The positive predictive value (PPV) of first mammography, defined as the number of breast cancers detected per abnormal screening examination, was found to be 0.17 for women aged 60–69 years and 0.19 for women aged 70 years and older (11). These values compare with 0.03 for women aged 30–39 years and 0.04 for women aged 50–59 years. For women 70–79 years old, the false-positive rate of mammography has been reported as 4.4 and 2.2% for clinical breast examination (12). Comparable rates for women 60–69 years of age were 5.3 and 2.5%, with 7.4 and 3.5 for the 50- to 59-year-old age group.

Additional information is available that helps to define the risk versus benefit from screening mammography in the elderly. A study was conducted with a cohort of 23,171 women aged 65 years and older, who were screened with mammography from January 1995 through April 1995 (13). The women were tracked over an 8-month period for the subsequent performance of additional breast imaging and biopsy procedures. During the study period, the percentage of women receiving initial mammography ranged from 29.9% of women aged 65–69 years to lower percentages of the older age groups: 26.5% of women aged 70–74 years, 21.2% for women aged 75–79 years, 14.2% for women aged 80–84 years, and 7.9% for women aged 85–89 years. For each 1000 women aged 65–69 years, 85 had follow-up testing, 76 had additional tests for breast imaging, and 23 had biopsies performed. Some women had repeat testing, including 11% who received biopsies more than once. In this study, the positive predictive value of an abnormal screening mammogram for women aged 65–69 years was 0.08 and 0.14 for women over the age of 70 years, which is somewhat lower than the values reported above.

B. Breast Self-Examination

Monthly breast self-examination (BSE) has been widely recommended (3, 14–16), but the effectiveness of BSE has not been demonstrated. Theoretically, BSE could detect interval cancers between screening mammography and provide women with an alternate, low-cost way of detecting breast pathology. Studies have been limited and the results are inconclusive. One of these studies was a World Health Organization (WHO)–sponsored, controlled trial in the former Soviet Union that was designed to assess the effectiveness of BSE to detect breast cancer, but it demonstrated no benefit at 8 years of follow-up (17). This study included women aged 40–84 years with a sample size of 20,000 women, but compliance at 4 years was only 18%. Results have been reported from a second study, which was a randomized controlled trial in Shanghai with 267,040 women who performed BSE in the absence of mammography (18). The women were provided personalized instruction for BSE with reinforcement. Attendance at reinforcement sessions fell from 96% at baseline to 89% 4 years later. Attendance at individual sessions to demonstrate proficiency in BSE fell from 90% in 1990 to 41% in 1995. Although the women in this study reported increased levels of suspicion about breast masses, no benefit from detecting small tumors or early-stage disease or a reduction in morality was demonstrated. Cumulative breast cancer mortality rates through 5 years were 30.9 in the control compared to 32.7 in the intervention group. A large randomized clinical trial of BSE has not been conducted in the United States; however, results from controlled trials in other countries have provided insight about the potential limitations of this procedure.

Although not well studied, mitigating factors such as loss of vision, tactile sensitivity, and cognitive deficits may decrease BSE proficiency. Studies have reported that the percentage of women aged 65 years or older who had received instruction by health professionals to perform BSE is as low as 32%, and only 54% had ever performed the test (19, 20). The impact of interventions such as video self-instructions with models to improve knowledge and skill of BSE are being assessed (21), but the impact on behavior is unclear.

III. UTILIZATION OF SCREENING PROCEDURES

In the 1987 National Health Interview Survey (22), 87% of women aged 40–64 years reported ever having had clinical breast examination (CBE) by a health professional. Older age groups were less likely to report ever having had CBE: 77% of women 65–74 years old and 68% of women 75 years old and older. Utilization of mammography was reported to be less by older age groups as well. For women aged 40–54 years, 42% reported ever having a mammogram. Comparative figures for successive age groups were 41% of women aged 55–64 years, 35% aged 65–74 years, and 25% aged 75 years and older. Other studies confirm less use of mammography by successive age cohorts (23).

Older women have given a variety of reasons for avoiding mammography. Reasons for not obtaining mammograms have included (a) believing the tests are not necessary (reported as high as 37%), (b) not receiving a physician recommendation (23%), (c) not experiencing any breast problems (18%), (d) never having thought about it (12%), and (e) not wanting it (7%) (24). A retrospective analysis of supplementary data to the National Heath Interview Surveys of 1987 and 1992 evaluated correlates of breast and other cancer screening in older women (25). The study examined several sociodemographic factors to assess their relationship to the likelihood of obtaining breast cancer screening. Women with more education were more likely to report a higher use of mammograms as were women living above the poverty line or living in urban areas.

The institution of Medicare coverage of screening mammography in 1991 introduced the possibility of determining the influence of this factor on mammography utilization. In 1991 and 1993, the National Cancer Institute (NCI) Breast Cancer Screening Consortium (26, 27), conducted a survey to examine the relationship between age, level of functioning, medical history, and mammography use. At the survey sites, only 26% of women had mammograms. Hypertension, diabetes, and myocardial infarction had no significant association with mammography use; however, a history of stroke, hip fracture, or Alzheimer's disease was negatively associated with mammography use.

Consortium data provided additional insight into the use of mammography in the Medicare population by examining the influence of breast cancer risk factors on the breast cancer screening behavior of older women insured by Medicare (28). Women with a history of benign breast disease and a family history of breast cancer were surveyed. They were asked about mammography and CBE history in the previous years and whether they received a physician's recommendation for mammography. Across the various sites, the percentage of women with a family history of breast cancer who had never had a mammogram ranged from 7 to 21%. Of the women with a history of benign breast disease, only 4–12% had never had a mammogram. Among individuals without a family history of breast cancer or benign breast disease, 21–33% had never had a mammogram. Sixty-six percent of women in all risk groups reported they had received a physician's recommendation for a mammogram. Those women with a history of a benign breast biopsy were most likely to have received a physician's recommendation. For clinical breast examinations, 40–58% of women had both a family history and a benign disease history; 45–54% of women with benign breast disease and 26–37% of lower-risk women had clinical examinations performed. The coincident use of the CBE and mammography procedures was higher among higher-risk women. These results suggested that older women with additional risk factors, other than age, are more likely to participate in screening mammography; however, some elderly women remain inadequately screened despite a family history of breast cancer.

As part of their activities, the NCI Breast Cancer Screening Consortium conducted an educational intervention (education for patients, physicians; and radiologist; patient and physician prompting; and community-based public education programs) to see if the use of Medicare for mammography could be promoted (29). There was little change in mammography usage in the two time periods compared: 1991–1992 versus 1989–1990 for the Medicare age group. Nevertheless, the percentage of those women who used public sources to pay for mammography increased. In 1992, two thirds of the elderly female population were unaware that mammography was a Medicare benefit. This situation precipitated large-scale outreach efforts by Health Care Financing Administration (HCFA) to increase awareness (30).

IV. CONCLUSIONS

The burden of breast cancer in the elderly population is high, which has generated an interest in using mammography to reduce that burden where possible. Health care providers are hampered in making definitive recommendations to elderly women concerning breast cancer screening, because there is a distinct lack of information from randomized clinical trials about breast cancer screening in women over the age of 65 years. Variability in screening recommendations as well as concern about the amount of benefit that will be obtained if there are coexisting health problems contribute to the inadequate use of mammography in older women. Elderly women who obtain breast screening are likely to have follow-up tests performed, but the predictive value of these tests may be low. Tools are needed to help identify elderly women who are at an increased risk of receiving no benefit and a decreased quality of life during the process of screening for breast cancer. The diversity of the elderly population with regard to health status, motivation, and financial status presents a special challenge on the part of health care providers to provide the best available information to guide elderly women in their use of available breast cancer screening resources.

REFERENCES

1. Landis SH, Murray T, Bolden S, Wingo PA. Cancer statistics, 1999. CA Cancer J Clin 1999; 49:8–31.
2. SEER Cancer Statistics Review 1973–1994.
3. Costanza, ME. Breast cancer screening in older women: synopsis of a forum. Cancer 1992; 69:1925–1931.
4. Screening for Breast Cancer. In: Report of the United States Preventive Services Task Force: Screening in Breast Cancer. Guide to Clinical Preventive Services, 2nd ed. Baltimore: Williams & Wilkins, 1996.
5. Katz S, Branch LG, Branson MH. Active life expectancy. N Engl J Med 1983; 309: 1218–1224.
6. Smith R. Screening fundamentals. J Natl Cancer Inst Monogr 1997; 22:15–19.
7. Fletcher SW, Black W, Harris R, et al. Report of the International Workshop on Screening for Breast Cancer. J Natl Cancer Inst 1993; 85:1644–1656.
8. Tabar L, Fagerberg CJG, Baldetrop L, Holmberg LH, Grontoft O. Reduction in mortality from breast cancer after mass screening with mammography. Lancet 1985; 1:829–832.
9. Nystrom L, Rutqvist LE, Walls, Lindgre A, Lindqvist. Breast cancer screening with mammography: an overview of the Swedish randomized trials. Lancet 1993; 341:973–978.
10. Tabar L, Fagerberg G, Chen H, Duffy S. Efficacy of breast cancer screening by age: new results from the Swedish Two-County Trial. Cancer 1995; 75:2507–2517.
11. Kerlikowske K, Grady D, Barclay J, Sickles EA, Eaton A, Ernster V. Positive predictive value of screening mammography by age and family history of breast cancer. JAMA 1993; 270:2444–2450.
12. Elmore JG, Barton MB, Moceri VM, Polk S, Arena PJ, Fletcher SW. Ten-year risk of false positive screening mammograms and clinical examinations. N Engl J Med 1998; 338:1089–1096.
13. Welch H, Fisher E. Diagnostic testing following screening mammography in the elderly. JNCI 1998; 90:1389–1392.
14. American Cancer Society. 1989 survey of physicians' attitudes and practices in early cancer detection CA-A 1990; 40:77.
15. Council on Scientific Affairs. Mammographic screening in asymptomatic women aged 40 years and older. JAMA 1989; 261–2535.
16. American College of Obstetricans and Gynecologists. The obstetrician-gynecologist and primary preventive health care. Washington, DC, 1993.
17. Semiglazov VF, Moiseyenko VM. Breast self examination for the early detection of breast cancer: a USSR/WHO controlled trial in Leningrad. Bull WHO 1987; 65:391–396.
18. Thomas D, Gao D, Self S, Allison C, Porter P. Randomized trial of breast self-examination in Shanghai:methology and preliminary results. J Natl Cancer Inst 1997; 89:355–365.
19. Ruchlin H. Prevalence and correlates of breast and cervical cancer screening among older women. Obstetr Gynecol 1997; 90:16–21.

20. Field L, Wilson T. Mammographic screening in women more than 64 years old: a comparison of 1- and 2-year intervals. AJR Am J Roentgen 1998; 170:961–965.

21. Wood, R. Breast self-examination proficiency in older women: measuring the efficacy of video self instruction kits. Cancer Nurs 1996; 19;429–435.

22. Dawson DA, Thompson GB. Breasts cancer risk factors and screening: United States. 1987. Vital and Health Statistics. Department of Health and Human Services (DHHS) publication no (PHS) 90–1500. Hyattsville, MD: US DHHS, 1990:1–33.

23. Romans MC, Marchant DJ, Pearse WH, Sutton SM. Utilization of screening mammography—1990. Women's Health Iss 1991; 1:68–73.

24. Rimer BK, Resch N, Ross E, Boyce A. Multistrategy health education program to increase mammography use among women ages 65 and older. Public Health Rep 1992; 4:369–380.

25. Anderson LM, May DS. Has the use of cervical, breast, and colorectal cancer screening increased in the United States? Am J Public Health 1995; 85:840–842.

26. Breen, N, Fuer E. The effect of medicare reimbursement for screening mammography on utilization and payment, Public Health Rep 1997; 112:423–432.

27. Blustein J, Weiss L. The use of mammography by women aged 75 and older: factors related to health, functioning, and age. J Am Geriatr Soc 1998; 46:941–946.

28. Roetzheim R, Fox S, Leake B, Houn F. The influence of risk factors on breast carcinoma screening of Medicare-insured older women. Cancer 1996; 78:2526–2534.

29. Breen N, Fuer E. The effect of medicare reimbursement for screening mammography on utilization and payment,. Public Health Rep 1997; 112:423–432.

30. MMWR. 1995:44:777–781. Centers for Disease Control. Use of Mammography services by women aged >65 years enrolled in medicare—United States, 1991–1993. JAMA 1995; 274:1420–1421.

3
Prostatic Cancer Screening

Otis W. Brawley
National Cancer Institute
National Institutes of Health
Bethesda, Maryland

I. INCIDENCE

Prostatic cancer is a significant cause of human suffering and death. Overall prostatic cancer is the fourth most commonly diagnosed malignancy in men worldwide (1). Prostatic cancer incidence is quite variable among populations throughout the world. It is much higher in Western countries when compared to developing countries of the Middle East or Asia. In the United States where prostatic cancer is the most common malignancy diagnosed in men, the incidence rate is much higher among men of African heritage than among white men. Asian-American and Hispanic-American men have prostatic cancer incidence rates lower than those of whites. It is estimated that there will be 184,000 prostatic cancers diagnosed in the United States in 1999 and approximately 40,000 deaths (2). Prostatic cancer is predominantly a disease of the elderly. The median age at diagnosis in the United States is approximately 71 years for whites and 69 years for blacks. Half of all American men diagnosed with prostatic cancer are 71 years of age or older and over 80% are 65 years or older.

Modern medicine has brought about decreases in a number of competing causes of death, such as heart disease and infection, causing the life expectancy of men to increase. This success, along with the Baby Boom after World War II means that early in the 21st century there will be the largest number of men over the age of 65 years alive in history. It has been estimated that there will be a doubling of the male population over 65 years of age from 1990 to 2020, and the absolute number of diagnosed prostatic cancers is destined to rise.

In the United States, the age-adjusted incidence of prostatic cancer has been dramatically affected by prostatic cancer screening, especially by screening with serum prostate-specific antigen (PSA) since the late 1980s. A steady rise in prostatic cancer incidence in the 1970s and early 1980s can be attributed to an increase in the number of transurethral resections (TURPs) for benign prostatic hyperplasia (3). The subsequent acceleration of incidence can be attributed to the increasing use of PSA. Eventually, an equilibration is expected, because cases identified early will not be available for detection in subsequent years. Also, it should be noted that the use of TURP actually decreased during the late 1980s. Despite dramatic shifts in incidence, the prostatic cancer mortality rates for black and white Americans has been relatively stable over the past 25 years. Five-year survival rates have increased over this time. This change is consistent with lead time bias due to screening (4). There has been much discussion of a relatively small decline in mortality in the 1990s as reflected by the overall age-adjusted mortality rate for white men of 24.7 per 100,000 in 1991 compared with 22.9 per 100,000 in 1995. By comparison, incidence over the same time period was much less stable owing to longitudinal fluctuations in case detection related to factors mentioned above. In 1991, the age-adjusted incidence for white Americans was 169.1; but in 1995, it was 129.8 per 100,000.

II. HEREDITY

The role of heredity as a factor contributing to the development of prostatic cancer in the elderly remains a subject of research. In the face of limited data, a hereditary contribution to prostatic cancer incidence may be suspected when there is familial clustering with cases occurring at younger ages. Although a prostatic cancer gene has not been found, it is believed that approximately 10% of prostatic cancer patients have a genetic predisposition to develop it. Familial patterns of prostatic cancer have been identified by case-control analysis (5). A man with one first-degree relative with prostatic cancer is estimated to have a 2.1 to 2.8-fold greater risk of being diagnosed with prostatic cancer compared with a man of average risk (6). Having a first-degree and a second-degree relative with prostatic cancer may increase the prostatic cancer risk sixfold over the background level of risk established by the general population. Through study of a group of high-risk families (multiple males with prostatic cancer), a major prostatic cancer susceptibility locus has been found on chromosome 1 (1q24–25) (7). Identified as *HPC1,* this gene is felt to be involved in only 33% of hereditary prostatic cancer cases, or perhaps as few as 3% of all prostatic cancer cases. This gene may be linked to higher grade and more aggressive prostatic cancers in younger men (8). The gene was found to be common in families with an extensive history of prostatic cancer (five or more males affected) and early ages at the time of diagnosis (9).

Specific mutations of *BRCA1* or *BRCA2* genes known to be associated with breast cancer risk, may be related to an increased risk of prostate cancer (10, 11). In one study of Ashkenazi Jewish carriers of certain *BRCA1* and of certain *BRCA2* germline mutations, there was an increased risk of prostatic cancer manifesting after age 50 years (12, 13). In another study of two families, specific mutations in the *BRCA2* gene, located on chromosome 13, have been linked with an approximately threefold excess relative risk of prostatic cancer (14, 15).

III. SCREENING

Because the burden of prostatic cancer is large, interest has been directed at screening as a way of reducing that burden. Although recommendations for prostatic cancer screening are readily made, the area remains controversial (16). Many American physicians advocate annual prostatic cancer screening with a digital rectal examination (DRE) and PSA starting at age 40 or 50 years for men and continuing while life expectancy is at least 10 years, but this approach is not as popular outside the United States (17–20). Most medical organizations recommend against prostatic cancer screening or otherwise recommend obtaining consent from the patient after carefully informing him of the potential risks and potential benefits. Several studies have been completed to show that the use of DRE and PSA is effective at finding prostatic cancer in asymptomatic men, but no randomized screening study has been completed to assess the effectiveness of prostatic cancer screening for saving lives. Studies to determine if prostatic cancer screening saves lives are underway (21–23). In the PLCO (Prostate, Lung, Colorectal and Ovarian) Screening Trial, it is planned that 74,000 men aged 55 to 74 years will be randomized to receive baseline testing with DRE and PSA to be repeated annually for 3 years. At the end of September, 1998, 58,283 men had been enrolled and approximately 40% were 65 years of age or older (24). At the end of the study, subgroup analysis of results by age should allow some appreciation of whether the value of screening varies according to age.

Inherent to the screening question is a determination of the proportion of men who do not benefit from a diagnosis of prostatic cancer secondary to screening either because they have an incurable tumor or a tumor that does not need treatment. Evidence demonstrates that both groups comprise a significant proportion of men diagnosed with prostatic cancer after screening. However, even though it is not yet proven, most experts believe that there is a group of men who will benefit from prostatic cancer screening in the sense that the subsequent course of disease in this group will lead to decreased mortality from prostatic cancer and longer survival in comparison with a similar group who do not receive the screening.

If prostatic cancer screening is done, it should occur only after the patient receives an explanation of the potential risks and potential benefits (25, 26). Screening should involve a DRE and a serum PSA. Some experts advocate at least a sextant biopsy of the prostate for all men with a PSA of 4.0 ng/mL or higher. Some experts advocate the use of age-specific or age-adjusted PSA to trigger prostatic biopsy.

Older men often have elevations of PSA due to benign prostatic hyperplasia. Age-specific or age-adjusted PSAs are reported to decrease the number of negative biopsies in older men (27).

Extreme advocacy of prostatic cancer screening should be subject to caution based on conclusions derived from the application of screening principles to the epidemiology of prostatic cancer (28). Length bias is a well-described phenomenon associated with many tests used to screen asymptomatic individuals. Asymptomatic disease processes, cancer included, are on average less biologically aggressive than diseases diagnosed on the basis of symptoms. In general, a screening test is more likely to pick up prevalent, indolent cases instead of life-threatening cases.

An extreme form of length bias, known as overdiagnosis, occurs when lesions are detected that never would have come to medical attention at all were it not for screening. There are two forms of overdiagnosis: (a) detection of lesions with virtually no potential for progression and (b) detection of indolent lesions with a potential to progress but not within the remaining "natural" life span of the individual. The latter form of overdiagnosis can be substantial in a disease such as prostatic cancer, in which the average age of diagnosis is in the eighth decade of life. Competing causes of death often mean that a diagnosed prostatic cancer may not need treatment. The most significant question in a man diagnosed with prostatic cancer is: Is this specific cancer of clinical significance to this particular patient?

A number of prostatic cancers fulfill histological criteria for clinically significant disease when they are found at autopsy in men who died of noncancerous causes without a diagnosis of cancer (29). These cancers were obviously not clinically significant for these men. On the other hand, in one case series, pathologists estimated that 15% of men with a PSA-based diagnosis of prostatic cancer had tumors that did not fulfill histological criteria for clinically significant prostatic cancer. This is to say that pathologists looking at a group of men diagnosed with prostatic cancer through screening and treated with radical prostatectomy believe that at least one in seven receive unnecessary treatment based on histological criteria for malignancy and aggressiveness (30).

Population studies confirm that a number of diagnosed tumors do not need definitive therapy by showing that geographical areas with higher levels of screening have significantly higher prostatic cancer incidence rates compared to areas that screen very little. Despite the difference in incidence, both areas have very similar prostatic cancer mortalities (31, 32).

There are a number of potential adverse consequences to prostatic cancer treatment. Men who receive needless treatment (cured indolent disease or unresponding, aggressive disease) are at risk for the side effects of therapy. Indeed, these men experience all the morbidities, sooner and for a longer time, without any of the benefits. In a study of Medicare beneficiaries, less than 60% of 3,173 men aged 65 years and over who underwent radical prostatectomy from 1985 to 1991 were eventually determined to have confined disease (33). Five years after surgery, more than 35% of men received additional therapy for cancer recurrence or persistence. Even among men diagnosed with pathologically confined cancer after radical prostatectomy, the cumulative incidence of additional prostatic cancer treatment at 5 years was 25% (34).

Although all forms of localized prostatic cancer therapy have side effects, they are most clearly described for radical prostatectomy and external beam radiation. Both treatments cause sexual impotence, rectal injury, urinary incontinence, and urethral stricture. Impotence rates are 25–40% or higher, rectal injury rates are 1–3%, urinary incontinence rates are 3–6%, and urethral stricture rates are 8–18%, with radiation therapy at the lower end of the range compared to surgery. In a survey of Medicare patients undergoing radical prostatectomy from 1988 to 1992, 30% reported the chronic need for pads and urinary clamps. More than 60% reported a problem with wetness, 60% reported having no erections since surgery, and 90% reported no erections sufficient for intercourse in the month prior to answering the survey (35). Prostatectomy incurs a higher risk of treatment-related death than radiation therapy. Although individual surgeons have reported death rates of less than 0.5% depending on patient selection and the surgeon's skill, the surgical mortality rate was 2% in a national sample of Medicare beneficiaries. In that same series, 8% of men suffered major cardiopulmonary complications after radical prostatectomy.

IV. CONCLUSIONS

As a intervention, prostatic cancer screening is yet to be proven effective for any age group. With prostatic cancer screening, some men are diagnosed who do not benefit either because their life cannot be saved or because their life is not endangered by the prostatic cancer. Even if randomized trials demonstrate that prostatic cancer screening can be used to detect some cases that will benefit from treatment, it is still possible that the harm associated with screening will be found to outweigh the benefits overall.

REFERENCES

1. Parkin DM, Pisani P, Ferlay J. Estimates of the worldwide incidence of eighteen major cancers in 1985. Int J Cancer 1993; 54:594–606.
2. Landis SH, Murray T, Bolden S, Wingo PA. Cancer Statistics, 1999. CA Cancer J Clin 1999; 49:8–11.
3. Potosky AL, Miller BA, Albertsen PC, Kramer BS. The role of increasing detection in the rising incidence of prostate cancer. JAMA 1995; 273:548–552.
4. Gerber GS, Thompson IM, Thisted R, Chodak GW. Disease-specific survival following routine prostate cancer screening by digital rectal examination. JAMA 1993; 269:61–64.

5. Carter BS, Bova GS, Beaty TH, et al. Hereditary prostate cancer: epidemiologic and clinical features. J Urol 1993; 150:797–802.

6. Steinberg GS, Carter BS, Beaty TH, et al. Family history and the risk of prostate cancer. Prostate 1990; 17:337–40.

7. Smith JR, Freije D, Carpten JD, et al. Major susceptibility locus for prostate cancer on chromosome 1 suggested by a genome-wide search. Science. 1996; 274(5291):1371–1374.

8. Platz EA, Giovannucci E, Dahl DM, et al. The androgen receptor gene GGN microsatellite and prostate cancer risk. Ca Epidemiol Biomark and Prev 1998; 7:379–384.

9. Gronberg H, Xu J, Smith JR, et al. Early age at diagnosis in families providing evidence of linkage to the hereditary prostate cancer locus (HPC1) on chromosome 1. Cancer Res 1997; 57:4707–4709.

10. Arason A, Barkard RB, Egilsson V. Linkage analysis of chromosome 17q markers and breast-ovarian cancer in Icelandic families, and possible relationship to prostatic cancer. Am J Hum Genet 1993; 52(4):711–717.

11. Tulinius H, Egilsson V, Olafsd GH, Sigvaldason H.: Risk of prostate, ovarian, and endometrial cancer among relatives of women with breast cancer. BMJ. 1992; 305: 855–857.

12. Struewing JP, Hartge P, Wacholder S, et al. The risk of cancer associated with specific mutations of BRCA1 and BRCA2 among Ashkenazi Jews. N Engl J Med. 1997; 336: 1401–1408.

13. Williams BJ, Jones E, Zhu XL, et al. Evidence for a tumor suppressor gene distal to BRCA1 in prostate cancer. J Urol 1996; 155:720–725.

14. Easton DF, Steele L, Fields P, et al. Cancer risks in two large breast cancer families linked to BRCA2 on chromosome 13q12–13. Am J Hum Genet 1997; 61:120–128.

15. Sigurdsson S, Thorlacius S, Tomasson J, et al. BRCA2 mutation in Icelandic prostate cancer patients. J Mol Med 1997; 75:758–761.

16. Mandelson MT, Wagner EH, Thompson RS. PSA screening: a public health dilemma. Annu Rev Public Health 1995; 16:283–306:283–306.

17. Rose VL. ACP issues guidelines on the early detection of prostate cancer and screening for prostate cancer. Am Fam Physician 1997; 56:1674–1675.

18. Woolf SH. Should we screen for prostate cancer? BMJ 1997; 314:989–990.

19. Denis LJ, Murphy GP, Schroder FH. Report of the consensus workshop on screening and global strategy for prostate cancer. Cancer 1995; 75:1187–1207.

20. Ramsey EW. Early detection of prostate cancer. Recommendations from the Canadian Urological Association. Can J Oncol 1994; 4(Suppl 1):82–5:82–85.

21. Shroder FH, Damhuis RA, Kirkels WJ, et al. European randomized study of screening for prostate cancer—the Rotterdam pilot studies. Int J Cancer 1996; 65:145–151.

22. Schroder FH, Bangma CH. The European randomized study of screening for prostate cancer (ERSPC). Br J Urol 1997; 79(Suppl 1):68–71.

23. Gohagan JK, Prorok PC, Kramer BS, Cornett JE. Prostate cancer screening in the Prostate, Lung, Colorectal and Ovarian Cancer Screening Atrial of the national Cancer Institute. J Urol 1994; 152:1905–1909.

24. Trial Update. PLCO News. http://dcp.nci.nih.gov/PLCO/news/V1-N2/enrollment.html.

25. Brown V. Informed consent for PSA testing. J Fam Pract 1996; 43:234–235.
26. Glode LM. Prostate cancer screening: a place for informed consent? Hosp Pract (Off Ed) 1994; 29(9): 8, 11–2.
27. Oesterling JE, Jacobsen SJ, Chute CG. Serum prostate-specific antigen in a community-based population of healthy men: establishment of age-specific reference ranges. JAMA 1993; 270:860–864.
28. Kramer BS, Brown ML, Prorok PC, et al. Prostate cancer screening: what we know and what we need to know. Ann Intern Med 1993; 119:914–923.
29. Sakr WA, Haas GP, Cassin BF, et al. The frequency of carcinoma and intraepithelial neoplasia of the prostate in young male patients. J Urol 1993; 150:379–385.
30. Albertsen PC. Defining clinically significant prostate cancer: pathologic criteria versus outcomes data. J Natl Cancer Inst 1996; 88:1177–1178.
31. Brawley OW. Prostate carcinoma incidence and patient mortality: the effects of screening and early detection. Cancer 1997; 80:1857–1863.
32. Shibata A, Ma J, Whittemore AS. Prostate cancer incidence and mortality in the United States and the United Kingdom. J Natl Cancer Inst 1998; 90:1230–1231.
33. Lu-Yao GL, McLerran D, Wasson J, Wennberg JE. An assessment of radical prostatectomy. Time trends, geographic variation, and outcomes. The Prostate Patient Outcomes Research Team. JAMA 1993; 269:2633–2636.
34. Lu-Yao GL, Potosky AL, Albertsen PC, et al. Follow-up prostate cancer treatments after radical prostatectomy: a population-based study. J Natl Cancer Inst 1996; 88:166–173.
35. Fowler FJJ, Barry MJ, Lu-Yao G, et al. Patient-reported complications and follow-up treatment after radical prostatectomy. The National Medicare Experience: 1988–1990. Urology 1993; 42:622–629.

4

Screening for Colorectal Cancer in the Elderly

Sheila A. Prindiville
University of Colorado Health Sciences Center
Denver, Colorado

I. SIGNIFICANCE OF THE PROBLEM

In 1999, approximately 129,400 American men and women were expected to develop colorectal cancer and 56,600 to die of the disease, making colorectal cancer the second leading cause of cancer-related mortality in the United States (1). An average-risk individual in the United States has about a 6% lifetime risk of developing colorectal cancer (2). Colorectal cancer is predominantly a disease of the elderly, with the incidence rising sharply after age 50 years and approximately doubling every decade until around age 80 years, so that nearly 70% of cases of colorectal cancer occur in persons aged 65 years or more.

II. NATURAL HISTORY

It is well established that the majority of sporadic colorectal cancers arise from adenomatous polyps over an average duration of 5–10 years (3). A progressive accumulation of genetic alterations is thought to account for the transformation of normal colonic epithelium to small adenomas, large adenomas, and ultimately to cancer over time. Survival from colorectal cancer is strongly correlated with the stage at diagnosis, with the 5-year survival for early, localized cancers being greater than 90%, dropping to 64% after regional spread, and falling to less than 8% for distant metastatic disease (2). There is no apparent difference in the 5-year survival rate (62%) for those age 65 years and older at diagnosis compared to those under age 65 years. Consequently, colorectal cancer is an ideal screening target because of the significant burden of disease, the presence of an identifiable precancerous lesion, and the availability of effective therapy for disease detected in the early stages.

III. RISK FACTORS

About 75% of colorectal cancer occurs in people with no known predisposing risk factors. The remaining 25% occurs in individuals at higher risk for the disease, including those with a family history of colorectal cancer, a personal history of adenomatous polyps or colorectal cancer, or a predisposing medical condition such as inflammatory bowel disease (4). There are two well described hereditary autosomal dominant colorectal cancer syndromes; familial adenomatous polyposis (FAP) and hereditary nonpolyposis colorectal cancer (HNPCC). Affected individuals with FAP, who harbor hundreds to thousands of precancerous adenomatous polyps, account for less than 1% of colorectal cancer cases (5). Hereditary nonpolyposis colorectal cancer accounts for about 5% of all colorectal cancer and is characterized clinically by the early onset of colorectal cancer (median age 45 years), an increased proportion of proximal (right-sided) colon cancers, and an increased risk for cancer at other sites (6). Another 15–20% of colorectal cancer occurs in individuals who do not fit into one of the well-defined hereditary syndromes but may nevertheless have some familial evidence of elevated risk such as a first-degree relative (parent, sibling, or child) with colorectal cancer or adenomatous polyps.

The importance of family history as a risk factor for colorectal cancer may diminish with age. A prospective study of 32,085 men and 87,031 women who participated in the Health Professionals Follow-up Study or the Nurses' Health Study found a family history of colorectal cancer was associated with a significantly increased risk of the disease among younger persons but not for those over age 65 years at the time of diagnosis. (7) Additionally, the rare hereditary syndromes are not a large cause of colorectal cancer in the elderly, because over 90% of individuals with FAP and 68–75% with HNPCC develop colorectal cancer by age 65 years (5, 6). This chapter focuses on screening the asymptomatic, average-risk elderly individual. For high-risk individuals, who require intensive screening strategies, detailed recommendations can be found elsewhere (4, 6).

IV. TYPES OF SCREENING TESTS FOR COLORECTAL CANCER

Several tests are available for colorectal cancer screening, including the digital rectal examination, fecal occult blood testing, sigmoidoscopy, colonoscopy, and barium enema. The strength of the scientific literature regarding the effectiveness of these tests is highly variable, with only fecal occult blood testing having been evaluated in randomized, controlled clinical trials. Mortality from colorectal cancer is the best endpoint by which to evaluate studies, because other endpoints such as survival and shift in the stage of diagnosed cancers are subject to lead-time and length bias.

A. Digital Rectal Examination

The digital rectal examination (DRE) can detect rectal cancers within the reach of the finger. The DRE has not been studied in a randomized, controlled trial, and as a screening modality, its value is limited, because less than 10% of all colorectal cancers are within the reach of the finger (8). One case-control study from the Kaiser Permanente Medical Care Program studied 172 cases of cancer in the distal 7 cm of the rectum in patients 45 years of age or older (55% were age 65 years and older) and found no evidence that DRE reduces mortality from cancer in the distal rectum (9).

B. Fecal Occult Blood Testing

Screening for colorectal cancer with fecal occult blood testing (FOBT) is based on the supposition that cancers may bleed occultly, and of those that do, some may be detected at an earlier stage than would otherwise have occurred if FOBT had not been done. There are five controlled clinical trials that have reported that mortality from colorectal cancer can be reduced by 12–43% following the use of FOBT (10–14). These studies are described in more detail below and summarized in Table 1. Additionally, several retrospective, case-control studies also support the association between the use of FOBT and colorectal cancer mortality reduction (15–19).

One of the most commonly used fecal occult blood tests is Hemoccult II (SmithKline Diagnostics, San Jose, CA), a guaiac-based test which detects the peroxidase-like activity of hemoglobin (20). Two slides are prepared from each of three consecutive bowel movements. Screenees should avoid aspirin and nonsteroidal anti-inflammatory drugs, red meat, poultry, fish, and vitamin C, which can interfer with test performance. Individuals with a positive result in any one of the six slide windows are considered to have a positive screening test and should have a complete colorectal evaluation (colonoscopy or flexible sigmoidoscopy plus double-contrast barium enema). Several issues such as the type of fecal occult blood test and the optimal frequency of screening (annual vs biennial) are still unresolved and recommendations may change in the coming years.

1. Controlled Clinical Trials of FOBT

a. *Memorial Sloan-Kettering Cancer Center–Strang Clinic Trial*

Begun in 1975, a prospective trial conducted by the Memorial Sloan-Kettering Cancer Center in collaboration with the Preventive Medicine Institute–Strang Clinic

Table 1 Controlled Colorectal Cancer Screening Trials Using Fecal Occult Blood Testing

	Overall population size and age (in years)	Elderly population (%) (and age in years)	Overall mortality reduction (%)	Elderly mortality reduction (%) (and age in years)
Controlled Trials (Ref.)				
New York (10)	21,756	25 (60–69)	43	50 (60–69)[a]
	≥40	8 (≥70)		38 (≥70)
Minnesota (11)	46,551	42 (60–69)	33	Not reported
	50–80	17 (≥70)		
Nottingham, UK (12)	152,850	39 (60–69)	15	10 (≥65)
	45–74	15 (≥70)		
Funen, Denmark (13)	61,933	33 (60–69)	18	16 (≥60)
	45–75	16 (≥70)		
Goteborg, Sweden (14,26)	27,700	100 (60–64)	12[b]	12 (≥60)
	60–64			

[a] Values are approximate and derived from the graphic presentation of the data in the study publication for Trial group II (10).
[b] Reported by meeting abstract only (26).

involved 21,756 participants aged 40 years and older with approximately 33% of the population aged 60 years and older (10). Study subjects were recruited from two populations seen at the clinic: health-conscious volunteers who regularly underwent annual health checkups (Trial group I) and patients who were being seen for the first time at the clinic (Trial group II). All subjects had a baseline physical examination, medical history questionnaire, and 25-cm rigid sigmoidoscopy. Subsequently, subjects were assigned either to a study or control group. The study group was offered annual FOBT using predominantly nonrehydrated slides and 25-cm rigid sigmoidoscopy, whereas the control group was only offered rigid sigmoidoscopy. The overall compliance rate for FOBT was 75% on the initial screen. Test sensitivity was estimated to be 70% and specificity to be 98% (21). Positive test results (overall rate 1.7%) were evaluated with a double-contrast barium enema and colonoscopy. A significant stage shift in earlier stage colorectal cancers (Dukes' A and B cancers) was seen in the study group compared to controls (65 vs 33%). For subjects in Trial group II, colorectal cancer mortality was 43% lower in the study group compared to the control group after 10 years, although the statistical significance was marginal ($P = .053$). The mortality reduction was seen in all age groups, including those aged 70 years and older. There was no significant difference in mortality between study and control group participants in Trial group I; possibly due to the higher prevalence of examinations, including sigmoidoscopy, prior to study enrollment.

b. Minnesota Colon Cancer Control Study

The Minnesota Colon Cancer Control Study is a randomized, controlled trial in which 46,551 subjects between 50 and 80 years of age were randomized from 1975 to 1977 to FOBT once a year, FOBT every 2 years, or no screening (11). Eighteen percent of women and 16% of men were aged 70 years or older. Participants submitted two smears from each of three consecutive stools on six guaiac paper slides. Slides were rehydrated before interpretation in the majority (83%) of subjects. Those with one or more positive slides were considered to have a positive test and were further evaluated with colonoscopy. The rate of test positivity was 2.4% for nonrehydrated slides, but 9.8% when rehydrated. The rate of positivity was associated with age such that individuals aged 80 years and older at study entry had a test positivity rate double that of those aged 50–59 years at entry (16 vs 8%). The age effect was less pronounced in nonrehydrated slides. The overall compliance rate for FOBT was about 90% for the initial screen. Test sensitivity for rehydrated slides was estimated to be 92% and specificity to be 90%. A shift toward detection of colorectal cancers at an earlier stage and improved survival was seen. After 13 years of follow-up, mortality from colorectal cancer was reduced by 33% in the annually screened group. No mortality reduction was seen in the biennially screened group. A recent update after 18 years of follow-up continues to show a reduction in mortality (36%) in the annually screened group (21).

c. Nottingham, United Kingdom Trial

Another large randomized, controlled trial was conducted in the Nottingham area of the United Kingdom between 1981 and 1991 with an enrollment of 152,850 persons aged 45–74 years (12). Approximately 33% of the population in this study was age 65 years or older. Participants were randomized to nonrehydrated FOBT every 2 years for three to six rounds or usual care. The rate of test positivity was 2.1%. Subjects with positive tests were offered a colonoscopy. The overall compliance rate for FOBT was about 60% for the initial screen. Test sensitivity was estimated to be 54% and specificity to be 98% (21, 22). After a median follow-up time of 7.8 years, there was a stage shift toward earlier cancers being diagnosed in the screened group compared to the control group and a 15% reduction in colorectal cancer mortality in the screened group. There was a slight effect of age on the mortality benefit, with individuals younger than age 65 years seeing a greater mortality reduction than those aged 65 years or greater at study entry (19 vs 10%).

d. Fünen, Denmark Trial

In a study conducted in Fünen, Denmark, 61,933 people were randomized to biennial nonrehydrated FOBT or usual care beginning in 1985 (13). Approximately 31% of the study population was age 65 years or older at study entry. The proportion of positive tests ranged from 0.6 to 1.7% with the proportions being higher in men and the elderly. Participants with a positive test were offered colonoscopy. The overall compliance rate for FOBT was about 67% for the initial screen. Test sensitivity was estimated to be 48% and specificity to be 99% (23). After a median follow-up time of 10 years, there was a stage shift toward earlier cancers being diagnosed in the screened group compared to the control group. An 18% reduction in colorectal cancer mortality in the screened group was seen, with a slightly greater effect in persons younger than age 60 years as compared to those aged 60 years or greater at study entry (23 vs 16%).

e. Göteborg, Sweden Trial

In a trial begun in 1982, 27,700 residents of Göteborg, Sweden, between the ages of 60–64 years were randomly assigned to a FOBT screening or a control group (14). Two additional cohorts of subjects between the ages of 60–64 years were recruited in 1987 and 1990 for a total study population of 68,308 subjects (24). Participants in the screening arm were subdivided into a rehydrated group and a nonrehydrated group with the test positivity rate being 1.9% in the nonrehydrated group and 5.8% in the rehydrated group. Individuals with a positive test were offered proctoscopy, 60-cm rectosigmoidoscopy, and double-contrast barium enema. All participants in the screening arm were offered rescreening between 16 and 24 months (mean 20 months) after the initial screen. The overall compliance rate for completing at least one FOBT screen was 69%. Test sensitivity for nonrehydrated slides was estimated to be 52% and specificity to be 99% (21, 25). A stage shift was observed, with earlier stage cancers being diagnosed in the screened group. Preliminary results reported in a meeting abstract are consistent with other studies showing a nonsignificant 12% reduction in colorectal cancer mortality in the screened group compared to controls after 8.75 years of follow-up (26). More mature results will be needed to make firm conclusions regarding the trend toward reduced mortality in this trial.

C. Sigmoidoscopy

Endoscopic examination of the large bowel by sigmoidoscopy provides direct visualization of the bowel and is only limited by the length of the sigmoidoscope. The most commonly used instrument is the 60-cm flexible sigmoidoscope which can usually reach the descending colon or as high as the splenic flexure. Approximately 65–75% of polyps and 40–65% of colorectal cancers are located distal to the splenic flexure and can be visualized if the flexible sigmoidoscope is fully inserted (27). Polyp biopsies can be obtained during the procedure, but a follow-up colonoscopy with a full bowel preparation is necessary to remove adenomas found during flexible sigmoidoscopy and to examine the proximal colon (4). Patients in general do not receive any sedation for flexible sigmoidoscopy, and about 10–15% experience discomfort with the procedure. Serious complications are rare; the rate of intestinal perforation with sigmoidoscopy is approximately 1 to 2 per 10,000 examinations and is slightly higher when biopsies are performed.

There have been no completed randomized, controlled studies of the effectiveness of screening sigmoidoscopy in reducing colorectal cancer mortality. The PLCO (prostate, lung, colon, and ovary) screening trial, an ongoing randomized, controlled trial sponsored by the National Cancer Institute, is assessing the worth of 60-cm flexible sigmoidoscopy on colorectal cancer mortality in 148,000 subjects aged 55–74 years (28). This trial, with accrual starting in 1993, is not expected to provide definitive mortality results for several years.

The best evidence supporting the effectiveness of screening sigmoidoscopy in reducing colorectal cancer mortality comes from a case-control study in the Kaiser Permanente Medical Care Program (29). The use of screening rigid sigmoidoscopy by 261 plan members 45 years of age and older who had a fatal adenocarcinoma of the colon or rectum during 1971–1988 was compared to 868 matched controls. The mean age at diagnosis of cases was 66 years old (range 45–91 years old). A significantly lower proportion of cases than controls (8.8 vs 24.2%) had undergone rigid sigmoidoscopy screening during the 10-year period prior to diagnosis. There was a 59% reduction in mortality from colorectal cancer in individuals who had undergone one or more screening sigmoidoscopies during the 10-year period compared with those who had not. This mortality reduction was seen in all age groups. This study was well designed, and because no protective effect of rigid sigmoidoscopy was seen for fatal cancers that were beyond the reach of the scope, concerns that the results may be biased are minimized.

Other case-control studies provide additional evidence for the benefit of sigmoidoscopy (30–31). One study compared 66 members of a prepaid health plan in Wisconsin who died of fatal large-bowel cancer from 1979 to 1988 with 196 matched controls for a history of screening sigmoidoscopy (30). Fifty percent of the study population was aged 70 years or older at the time of the case diagnosis. Both rigid and flexible sigmoidoscopy were used during the time period evaluated, but the majority of subjects (66% of cases and 59% of controls) were screened with flexible sigmoidoscopy. Thirty percent of control subjects and only 10.6% of cases had undergone at least one sigmoidoscopy. Risk for death from colorectal cancer was reduced by 79% among individuals who had undergone at least one screening sigmoidoscopy compared to those who had never had one. Another case-control study in veterans provides additional evidence for a protective role of sigmoidoscopy, although it was limited by the inability to account for whether endoscopic procedures were performed for screening or diagnostic purposes (31).

Intuitively it makes sense to consider the combination of sigmoidoscopy and FOBT as a screening option as the tests may complement each other (4). The FOBT covers the entire colon, but it is limited by its sensitivity, whereas sigmoidoscopy has high sensitivity, but it only covers the distal 60 cm of the colon. Although the combination may theoretically be better than either test alone, there are limited data supporting this approach as a screening program to reduce colorectal cancer mortality. One prospective, controlled screening trial that has addressed the combination of FOBT and sigmoidoscopy is the Memorial Sloan-Kettering Cancer Center trial discussed previously in the section on FOBT (10). In this trial, 12,479 subjects 40 years of age and older were allocated to annual screening with rigid sigmoidoscopy plus FOBT or rigid sigmoidoscopy alone. Those in the combined screening group had a 43% lower mortality from colorectal cancer after 10 years of follow-up compared to those in the rigid sigmoidoscopy-only arm ($P = .053$).

D. Colonoscopy

Colonoscopy is an endoscopic procedure that provides direct visualization of the entire large bowel from the rectum to the cecum which is usually performed using conscious sedation after cleansing the bowel. It is the only screening modality that allows both total colonic visualization and removal of polyps in one examination. Studies which directly measure the sensitivity of colonoscopy are not feasible, since the pathological specimen, the only true "gold standard," would be necessary. The sensitivity for detecting colorectal cancer has been estimated to be 95% by retrospectively determining the number of colorectal cancers that develop in patients who had undergone a colonoscopy within 3 years prior to the cancer diagnosis (32). This approach assumes that the cancer was missed during the prior colonoscopy and that a significant interval cancer should not have developed during the 3-year follow-up period. In a study of tandem colonoscopies performed by two endoscopists on the same day, the reported miss rate is 27% for small adenomas ≤5 mm, 13% for adenomas 6–9 mm, and 6% for adenomas ≥1 cm. (33). Serious complications are rare, but the rate of intestinal perforation with colonoscopy is approximately 1 per 1000 examinations and is higher when polypectomy is performed (4). The elderly do not seem to be at increased risk for complications as suggested by a study of the complications in a series of 436 colonoscopies performed at one institution in patients aged 80 years or older. In this group, there were only four (0.9%) nonfatal complications in octogenarians, which was similar to the overall complication rate at that institution (34).

There is no direct evidence that colonoscopy reduces mortality from colorectal cancer, but indirect evidence is supportive. The National Polyp Study prospectively followed 1418 patients who had a complete colonoscopy during which one or more adenomas were removed (35). The incidence rates of colorectal cancer in this cohort after 5.9 years of follow-up were less than the expected population rates; suggesting a preventive effect of polypectomy. A case-control study in 32,702 veterans found a 53% reduction in colon cancer mortality in those who had undergone a colonoscopy within 6 years (31). Although this study provides additional evidence for a protective role of colonoscopy, it was limited by the inability to account for whether endoscopic procedures were performed for screening or diagnostic purposes.

E. Barium Enema

Barium enema is a radiographic contrast study in which barium is instilled into the rectum to look for mucosal filling defects from neoplastic lesions. In a single-contrast study, only barium is instilled, whereas in a double-contrast study, air in addition to barium is instilled to define better the contours of the bowel mucosa. Both barium enema techniques are felt to be equally effective in detecting large neoplastic lesions (>1 cm) in properly performed examinations; however, the double-contrast barium enema (DCBE) is better at detecting smaller lesions (36). The consensus among radiologists is that the DCBE should be the preferred approach except when it is not feasible; for example, very elderly, ill, or disabled patients who cannot fully cooperate (36, 37). The estimates of the sensitivity of DCBE come from studies conducted mostly in symptomatic populations; thus, since the likelihood of finding disease in such patients is higher, the sensitivity estimates may be biased upward. The sensitivity of DCBE is about 50–80% for polyps less than 1 cm, 70–90% for polyps greater than 1 cm, and 55–85% for Dukes' stage A and B cancers (4). The complication rate is low, with about 1:10,000 examinations being complicated by bowel perforation (38).

There is no direct evidence that barium enema reduces mortality from colorectal cancer, but the early detection and removal of adenomatous polyps found at barium enema would be expected to reduce the cancer incidence (35). A recent retrospective study suggests colonoscopy performs better than barium enema in the detection of early cancer (32). Medical records from 2193 consecutive cases of colorectal cancer (mean age 69.8 years) identified from 20 central Indiana hospitals were reviewed to see if a prior diagnostic colonic examination had been performed within 3 years of diagnosis. If a study had been performed and was negative, it was presumed to have missed the diagnosis of cancer. The sensitivity of colonoscopy was 95% compared with 82.9% for barium enema, with nearly all of the advantage in sensitivity occurring from the detection of early (Dukes' A) lesions.

Data from the Göteborg, Sweden FOBT screening study suggest DCBE alone may miss a substantial proportion of cancers and polyps in the rectosigmoid (40). Positive fecal occult blood tests in this study were further evaluated with both DCBE and sigmoidoscopy. Double-contrast barium enema alone missed about 25% of cancers and polyps >1 cm in the rectosigmoid. The sensitivity of DCBE plus flexible sigmoidoscopy was about 98% for cancer in this study. These results support the conclusion that if the rectosigmoid is not well visualized at DCBE for colorectal cancer screening, then flexible sigmoidoscopy should be performed.

The combination of DCBE plus flexible sigmoidoscopy has been compared to colonoscopy in a randomized, controlled trial in subjects with suspected lower gastrointestinal bleeding (39). Three hundred and eighty-two patients aged 40 years and older (mean age 62 years) were randomized to undergo flexible sigmoidoscopy plus DCBE or colonoscopy. Colonoscopy detected more cases of small polyps (<9 mm), but there was no difference between strategies in the detection of patients with cancers or polyps ≥9 mm.

V. CONCLUSIONS AND RECOMMENDATIONS

Based on recent evidence from randomized, controlled trials of FOBT screening and well-designed case-control studies showing a reduction in colorectal cancer mortality, the United States Preventive Services Task Force (USPSTF) for the first time in 1996 recommended screening asymptomatic persons aged 50 years and older with FOBT, or sigmoidoscopy, or both (27). Although there is agreement that screening should be recommended, considerable controversy exists as to which screening modality is most appropriate. Several other organizations, including the American Cancer Society (ACS) and the United States Agency for Health Care Policy and Research (AHCPR), have recently published guidelines which are summarized in Table 2 (4, 41). The major difference between the USPSTF and the ACS guidelines is that the latter organization recommends screening with *both* FOBT and flexible sigmoidoscopy. Additionally, the ACS and the AHCPR have included total colonic examination with DCBE or colonoscopy as alternative modalities for

Table 2 Recommendations for Colorectal Cancer Screening for Asymptomatic Persons Aged 50 or Older

Organization (Ref).	Recommendations	Periodicity
US Preventive Services Task Force (27)	FOBT and/or Sigmoidoscopy	Annual Not specified
American Cancer Society (41)	FOBT plus flexible sigmoidoscopy or DCBE[b] or Colonoscopy[c]	Annual/every 5 years[a] Every 5–10 years Every 10 years
Agency for Health Care Policy and Research (4)	FOBT testing or Flexible sigmoidoscopy or FOBT plus flexible sigmoidoscopy or DCBE[b] or Colonoscopy[c]	Annual Every 5 years Annual/every 5 years[a] Every 5–10 years Every 10 years

FOBT, fecal occult blood testing; DCBE, double-contrast barium enema.
[a] Annual FOBT and flexible sigmoidoscopy every 5 years.
[b] Flexible sigmoidoscopy should be performed additionally if the rectosigmoid colon is not well visualized.
[c] DCBE should be performed additionally if the entire colon has not be adequately visualized.

screening, whereas the USPSTF concluded there was not sufficient evidence to recommend for or against routine screening with these modalities. In concordance with the recommendations of these health care organizations, Medicare coverage was recently expanded to include colorectal cancer screening for persons aged 50 years and older (42).

The choice of a screening procedure can be made on an individual basis depending on patient and physician preference as well as the availability of trained clinicians to provide quality examinations. The FOBT is easily performed, inexpensive, and has been proven to be effective in large-scale randomized, controlled trials which included elderly populations. It is limited mainly by its low sensitivity. Individuals with a positive result in any one of the six slide windows are considered to have a positive screening test and should have a complete colorectal evaluation with colonoscopy or flexible sigmoidoscopy plus DCBE.

Flexible sigmoidoscopy is readily available, safe, highly sensitive for the area of the colorectum visualized, and has been shown in well-designed case-control studies to decrease mortality from colorectal cancer. A complete colonoscopy is recommended for patients with adenomas found during flexible sigmoidoscopy, because 30–50% of patients who present with an adenoma in the distal bowel have a synchronous adenoma or cancer in the proximal bowel (43, 44). The major limitation of flexible sigmoidoscopy is its inability to visualize the proximal colon. In studies in which asymptomatic patients had a screening colonoscopy, a substantial proportion (36–56%) of adenomas were found in the proximal bowel when there was no index lesion in the distal bowel (45–47). This may be particularly important in elderly patients, who have a higher proportion of cancers and adenomas located proximally (48–50).

Both DCBE and colonoscopy provide examination of the entire bowel and are acceptable alternatives to FOBT and/or flexible sigmoidoscopy for screening. Although both DCBE and colonoscopy provide full bowel visualization, they are more complex and costly than FOBT and/or sigmoidoscopy and require the patient to cooperate with bowel preparation and examination maneuvers. The choice of DCBE or colonoscopy is based on individual physician and patient preference. Factors to be considered include cost, local expertise, complication rate, the overall medical condition of the patient, and the likelihood of obtaining an adequate examination. Abnormalities detected by DCBE need to be further evaluated with colonoscopy; thus necessitating a second procedure. In studies of patient preference, it is not clear whether patients consider barium enema or colonoscopy more acceptable (51, 52).

Elderly patients have higher mortality rates from colorectal cancer surgery, much of which is related to comorbid conditions and emergent surgery rather than to age alone (53). In one study of elderly patients aged 70 years and older, the mortality rate was 25% for patients undergoing emergency surgery for colon cancer compared to 1.4% for elective resections (54). Screening may be an effective way to reduce mortality from colorectal cancer in the elderly by identifying lesions earlier and avoiding the need for emergent surgery for advanced, obstructing lesions. Cost-effectiveness analyses for periodic screening of persons 60–85 years old have found a program of annual FOBT or sigmoidoscopy every 5 years to be cost effective in the elderly population (55).

When is one too old to benefit from screening? The literature is not clear on this point. The progression of a polyp to a cancer usually takes 5–10 years; thus, it may not be in the patient's best interest to screen if one's life expectancy is less than this period of time or if comorbid conditions exist. The average, otherwise healthy 65-, 75-, and 85-year-old has an average life expectancy of 17, 11, and 6 years, respectively, and may often be functioning and living independently (56). The recommendation to screen should be based on the physician's assessment of the potential benefit to the patient taking into account the patient's overall health, life expectancy, and willingness and ability to complete screening and potential diagnostic testing. Other unanswered questions include when to stop screening after multiple negative tests. Some practitioners have suggested that persons with two negative sigmoidoscopies have a very low risk of developing cancer and are likely not to benefit from further screening (57).

Although data continue to accumulate about the best way to use traditional screening methods, the future will bring new approaches. Attempts to improve FOBT performance include combining Hemoccult II Sensa, a more sensitive guaiac-based test, with HemeSelect, an immunological test for human hemoglobin that is more sensitive and nearly as specific as the current Hemoccult II test (58). Active areas of investigation include the development of markers of genetic change in the stool that could possibly provide the basis for molecular screening (59). Virtual colonoscopy is a promising, novel radiographic approach that provides computer-rendered, intraluminal views of the colorectum using volumetric analysis of helical computed tomographic (CT) scan data to develop interactive, three-dimensional intraluminal views of the colorectum (60). Because virtual colonoscopy is a less invasive procedure than traditional colonoscopy and does not require sedation, it may potentially be an attractive screening modality for the elderly.

REFERENCES

1. Landis SH, Murray T, Bolden S, Wingo PA. Cancer Statistics, 1999. CA Cancer J Clin 1998; 49:8–31.
2. Ries LAG, Kosary CL, Hankey BF, Miller BA, Harras A, Edwards BK, eds. SEER Cancer Statistics Review, 1973–1994, National Cancer Institute. NIH Pub. No. 97-2789, Bethesda, MD, 1997.
3. Fearon ER, Vogelstein B. A genetic model for colorectal tumorigenesis. Cell 1990; 61: 759–767.
4. Winawer SJ, Fletcher RH, Miller L, Godlee F, Stolar MH, Mulrow CD, Woolf SH, Glick SN, Ganiats TG, Bond JH, Rosen L, Zapka JG, Olsen SJ, Giardiello FM, Sisk

JE, Antwerp RV, Brown-Davis C, Marciniak DA, Mayer RJ. Colorectal cancer screening: clinical guidelines and rationale. Gastroenterology 1997; 112:594–642.

5. Burt RW. Hereditary aspects of the polyposis syndromes. Hematol Oncol Ann 1994; 2:163–170.

6. Burke W, Petersen G, Lynch P, Botkin J, Daly M, Garber J, Kahn MJE, McTiernan A, Offit K, Thomson E, Varricchio C; for the Cancer Genetics Studies Consortium. Recommendations for follow-up care of individuals with an inherited predisposition to cancer: I. Hereditary nonpolyposis colon cancer. JAMA 1997; 277:915–919.

7. Fuchs CS, Giovannucci EL, Colditz GA, Hunter DJ, Speizer FE, Willett WC. A prospective study of family history and the risk of colorectal cancer. N Engl J Med 1994; 331:1669–1674.

8. Winawer SJ, Schottenfeld D, Flehinger BJ. Colorectal cancer screening. J Natl Cancer Inst 1991; 83:243–253.

9. Herrinton LJ, Selby JV, Friedman GD, Quesenberry CP, Weiss NS. Case-control study of digital-rectal screening in relation to mortality from cancer of the distal rectum. Am J Epidemiol 1995; 142:961–964.

10. Winawer SJ, Flehinger BJ, Schottenfeld D, Miller DG. Screening for colorectal cancer with fecal occult blood testing and sigmoidoscopy. J Natl Cancer Inst 1993; 85:1311–1318.

11. Mandel JS, Bond JH, Church TR, Snover DC, Bradley GM, Schuman LM, Ederer F. Reducing mortality from colorectal cancer by screening for fecal occult blood. N Engl J Med 1993; 328:1365–1371.

12. Hardcastle JD, Chamberlain JO, Robinson MHE, Moss SM, Amar SS, Balfour TW, James PD, Mangham CM. Randomised controlled trial of faecal-occult-blood screening for colorectal cancer. Lancet 1996; 348:1472–1477.

13. Kronborg O, Fenger C, Olsen J, Jorgensen OD, Sondergaard O. Randomised study of screening for colorectal cancer with faecal-occult-blood test. Lancet 1996; 348:1467–1471.

14. Kewenter J, Björk S, Haglind E, Smith L, Svanvik J, Åhrén C. Screening and rescreening for colorectal cancer: a controlled trial of fecal occult blood testing in 27,700 subjects. Cancer 1988; 62:645–651.

15. Selby JV, Friedman GD, Quesenberry CP, Weiss NS. Effect of fecal occult blood testing on mortality from colorectal cancer: a case-control study. Ann Intern Med 1993; 118: 1–6.

16. Wahrendorf J, Robra BP, Wiebelt H, Oberhausen R, Weiland M, Dhom G. Effectiveness of colorectal cancer screening: results from a population-based case-control evaluation in Saarland, Germany. Eur J Cancer Prev 1993; 2:221–227.

17. Lazovich D, Weiss NS, Stevens NG, White E, McKnight B, Wagner EH. A case-control study to evaluate efficacy of screening for faecal occult blood. J Med Screen 1995; 2: 84–89.

18. Saito H, Soma Y, Koeda J, Wada T, Kawaguchi H, Sobue T, Aisawa T, Yoshida Y. Reduction in risk of mortality from colorectal cancer by fecal occult blood screening with immunochemical hemagglutination test: a case-control study. Int J Cancer 1995; 61:465–69.

19. Zappa M, Castiglione G, Grazzini G, Falini P, Giorgi D, Paci E, Ciatto S. Effect of faecal occult blood testing on colorectal mortality: results of a population-based case-control study in the district of Florence, Italy. Int J Cancer 1997; 73:208–210.

20. American College of Physicians. Suggested technique for fecal occult blood testing and interpretation in colorectal cancer screening. Ann Intern Med 1997; 126:808–810.
21. Markowitz AJ, Winawer SJ. Screening and Surveillance for colorectal carcinoma. Hematol Oncol Clin North Am 1997; 11:579–608.
22. Robinson MHE, Moss SM, Hardcastle JD, Whynes DK, Chamberlain JO, Mangham CM. Effect of retesting with dietary restriction in Haemoccult screening for colorectal cancer. J Med Screen 1995; 2:41–44.
23. Møller Jensen B, Kronborg O, Fenger C. Interval cancers in screening with fecal occult blood test for colorectal cancer. Scand J Gastroenterol 1992; 27:779–782.
24. Kewenter J, Brevinge H, Engarås B, Haglind E, Åhrén C. Results of screening, rescreening, and follow-up in a prospective randomized study for detection of colorectal cancer by fecal occult blood testing: results for 68,308 subjects. Scand J Gastroenterol 1994; 29:468–473.
25. Kewenter J, Engarås B, Haglind E, Jensen J. Value of retesting subjects with a positive Hemoccult® in screening for colorectal cancer. Br J Surg 1990; 77:1349–1351.
26. Kewenter J, Brevinge H, Haglind E. The Göteborg hemoccult screening study for CRC. In Abstracts of the European Group for Colorectal Cancer Screening Meeting, Visby, Sweden, 1996.
27. US Preventive Services Task Force. Guide to Clinical Preventive Services. 2nd ed. Baltimore: Williams & Wilkins, 1996.
28. Gohagan JK, Prorok PC, Kramer BS, Hayes RB, Cornett JE. The prostate, lung, colorectal, and ovarian cancer screening trial of the National Cancer Institute. Cancer 1995; 75:1869–1873.
29. Selby JV, Friedman GD, Quesenberry CP, Weiss NS. A case-control study of screening sigmoidoscopy and mortality from colorectal cancer. N Engl J Med 1992; 326:653–657.
30. Newcomb PA, Norfleet RG, Storer BE, Surawicz TS, Marcus PM. Screening sigmoidoscopy and colorectal cancer mortality. J Natl Cancer Inst 1992; 84:1572–1575.
31. Müller AD, Sonnenberg A. Prevention of colorectal cancer by flexible endoscopy and polypectomy: a case-control study of 32,702 veterans. Ann Intern Med 1995; 123:904–910.
32. Rex DK, Rahmani EY, Haseman JH, Lemmel GT, Kaster S, Buckley JS. Relative sensitivity of colonoscopy and barium enema for detection of colorectal cancer in clinical practice. Gastroenterology 1997; 112:17–23.
33. Rex DK, Cutler CS, Lemmel GT, Rahmani EY, Clark DW, Helper DJ, Lehman GA, Mark DG. Colonoscopic miss rates of adenomas determined by back-to-back colonoscopies. Gastroenterology 1997; 112:24–28.
34. Bat L, Pines A, Shemesh E, Levo Y, Zeeli D, Scapa E, Rosenblum Y. Colonoscopy in patients aged 80 or older and its contribution to the evaluation of rectal bleeding. Postgrad Med J 1992; 68:355–358.
35. Winawer SJ, Zauber AG, Ho MN, O'Brien MJ, Gottlieb LS, Sternberg SS, Waye JD, Schapiro M, Bond JH, Panish JF, Ackroyd F, Shike M, Kurtz RC, Hornsby-Lewis L, Gerdes H, Stewart ET, and the National Polyp Study Workgroup. Prevention of colorectal cancer by colonoscopic polypectomy. N Engl J Med 1993; 329:1977–1981.
36. Smith C. Colorectal cancer: radiologic diagnosis. Radiol Clin North Am 1997; 35:439–456.

37. Gelfand DW, Chen YM, Ott DJ. Detection of colonic polyps on single-contrast barium enema study: emphasis on the elderly. Radiology 1987; 164:333–337.

38. Gelfand DW. Colorectal cancer: screening strategies. Radiol Clin North Am 1997; 35: 431–438.

39. Rex DK, Weddle RA, Lehman GA, Pound DC, O'Connor KW, Hawes RH, Dittus RS, Lappas JC, Lumeng L. Flexible sigmoidoscopy plus air contrast barium enema versus colonoscopy for suspected lower gastrointestinal bleeding. Gastroenterology 1990; 98: 855–861.

40. Kewenter J, Brevinge H, Engaros B, et al. The yield of flexible sigmoisoscopy and double-contrast barium enema in the diagnosis of neoplasms in the large bowel in patients with a positive hemoccult test. Endoscopy 1995; 27:159–163.

41. Byers T, Levin B, Rothenberger D, Dodd GD, Smith RA for the American Cancer Society Detection and Treatment Advisory Group on Colorectal Cancer. American Cancer Society guidelines for screening and surveillance for early detection of colorectal polyps and cancer: update 1997. CA Cancer J Clin 1997; 47:154–160.

42. Your Medicare Benefits. U.S. Department of Health and Human Services Health Care Financing Administration Publication No. HCFA-10116, October 1998.

43. Bond JH for the Practice Parameters Committee of the American College of Gastroenterology. Polyp guideline: diagnosis, treatment, and surveillance for patients with nonfamilial colorectal polyps. Ann Intern Med 1993; 119:836–843.

44. Read TE, Read JD, Butterly LF. Importance of adenomas 5 mm or less in diameter that are detected by sigmoidoscopy. N Engl J Med. 1997; 336:8–12.

45. Rex DK, Lehman GA, Hawes RH, Ulbright TM, Smith JJ. Screening colonoscopy in asymptomatic average-risk persons with negative fecal occult blood tests. Gastroenterology 1991; 100:64–67.

46. Foutch PG, Mai H, Pardy K, Disario JA, Manne RK, Kerr D. Flexible sigmoidoscopy may be ineffective for secondary prevention of colorectal cancer in asymptomatic average-risk men. Dig Dis Sci 1991; 36:924–928.

47. Lieberman DA, Smith FW. Screening for colon malignancy with colonoscopy. Am J Gastroenterol 1991; 86:946–951.

48. Devesa SS, Chow WH. Variation in colorectal cancer incidence in the United States by subsite of origin. Cancer 1993; 71:3819–3826.

49. Nelson RL, Dollear T, Freels S, Persky V. The relation of age, race, and gender to the subsite location of colorectal cancer. Cancer 1997; 80:193–197.

50. DiSario JA, Foutch PG, Mai HD, Pardy K, Manne RK. Prevalence and malignant potential of colorectal polyps in asymptomatic, average-risk men. Gastroenterology 1991;86: 941–945.

51. Van Ness MM, Chobanian SJ, Winters C, Diehl AM, Esposito RL, Cattau EL. A study of patient acceptance of double-contrast barium enema and colonoscopy: which procedure is preferred by patients? Arch Intern Med 1987; 147:2175–2176.

52. Steine S. Which hurts the most? A comparison of pain rating during double-contrast barium enema examination and colonoscopy. Radiology 1994; 191:99–101.

53. Berger DH, Roslyn JJ. Cancer surgery in the elderly. Clin Geriatr Med 1997; 13:119–141.

54. Keller SM, Markovitz LJ, Wilder JR, Aufses AH. Emergency and elective surgery in patients over age 70. Am Surg 1987; 53:636–640.

55. Wagner JL, Herdman RC, Wadhwa S. Cost effectiveness of colorectal cancer screening in the elderly. Ann Intern Med 1991; 115:807–817.

56. National Center for Health Statistics. Vital statistics of the United States, 1990, Vol II, Sec 6 life tables. Public Health Service, Washington, DC, 1994.

57. Atkin WS, Cuzick J, Northover JMA, Whynes DK. Prevention of colorectal cancer by once-only sigmoidoscopy. Lancet 1993; 341:736–740.

58. Allison JE, Tekawa IS, Ransom LJ, Adrain AL. A comparison of fecal occult-blood tests for colorectal-cancer screening. N Engl J Med 1996; 334:155–159.

59. Sidransky D, Tokino T, Hamilton SR, Kinzler KW, Levin B, Frost P, Vogelstein B. Identification of *ras* oncogene mutations in the stool of patients with curable colorectal tumors. Science 1992; 256:102–105.

60. Fenlon HM, Ferrucci JT. Virtual colonoscopy: What will the issues be? Am J Roentgenal 1997; 169:453–458.

5

Cancer Prevention in the Elderly

Karen A. Johnson
National Cancer Institute
National Institutes of Health
Bethesda, Maryland

I. INTRODUCTION

For 1999, the expected burden of cancer in the United States was estimated to include the diagnosis of 1,221,800 new cases of all types of cancer (1). One of every two men was expected to develop a serious malignancy during his lifetime, and for women, one of every three. Incidence trends from SEER (Surveillance, Epidemiology, and End Results) data up to 1995, and for the 5-year period from 1991 to 1995, indicated that about 60% of expected cancer cases occur in individuals who are 65 years of age or older (2). This group of elderly cancer patients represents a target population for whom interventions might be used to prevent the occurrence of invasive cancer. In opting for the preventive approach, many individuals who might never develop cancer would nevertheless go through the prevention process. The costs of prevention in terms of time, procedures, medications, and side effects, particularly in the segment of the population that would not develop cancer, must be weighed against the burden of the disease in patients who could delay or avoid its occurrence with preventive interventions. Once an older individual is diagnosed with invasive cancer, there is no doubt about the need to consider the therapeutic options; however, at that point, the more aggressive natural history of invasive cancer and the likelihood of comorbid conditions may limit the opportunity for avoiding mortality and morbidity.

Optimization of the timing of intervention in the carcinogenesis process has been guided by results from clinical treatment trials. For example, it has been demonstrated in breast cancer treatment trials that treatment is less effective for recurrent and usually disseminated tumor compared with treatment for occult residual tumor in the adjuvant setting (3). As a strategy, it is superior to administer adjuvant treatment for a reduction in mortality rather than to wait for disease recurrence and administer treatment when the tumor burden is greater and the tumor cells are more heterogeneous and fatal. Following this paradigm, intervention directed at preinvasive neoplasia should generate a similar advantage. This approach is medically comparable to treating hypertension to avoid stroke rather than waiting to treat the patient after a stroke has occurred. Especially because of the older individual's high risk of developing cancer, a prevention paradigm is the natural purview of the elderly.

The goal of controlling cancer in older age groups is a particular challenge, but the underlying principles of cancer control are similar for all age groups. Traditionally, the ways of achieving cancer control have been defined as occurring at three levels (4). The first level, or primary control of cancer, is obtained when an intervention can be used to prevent cancer; that is, to keep the disease from developing. Although a standard set of diagnostic criteria are used to establish the occurrence of a case, the diagnostic criteria are usually fulfilled after a continuum of biological and physiological changes have taken place. Although progression through this continuum may be arrested, it is possible that a so-called preventive intervention will only delay the carcinogenic process. Nevertheless, even if the carcinogenic process is not totally arrested, there is also a value from shifting the occurrence of invasive cancer to ever later age groups so that individuals will live longer before developing cancer and that, ultimately, some individuals with premalignant disease will die from other causes without ever developing invasive cancer. Either outcome, the arrest or delay of carcinogenesis, would lead to and could be measured by a reduction in the age-specific cancer incidence with an expected corresponding reduction in the age-specific mortality from the cancer in question. For some people, the value attributed to this result might be seen as related to the amount of life gained and the quality of life in those final years.

Many of the chapters in this book deal with secondary and tertiary control of cancer, that is, treatment of life-threatening invasive cancer. Secondary control of cancer can be obtained if the elderly patient at the time of diagnosis can be rendered free of cancer and maintained without recurrence until the patient dies from another disease. Under these circumstances, even though incidence has not been reduced, cancer-related mortality can be delayed and possibly avoided altogether leading to a decline in age-specific cancer mortality. Once a patient has chronic findings and symptoms of cancer, then palliative care and symptom management can be used for tertiary control. The goal of this chapter is to examine some of the existing medical evidence that primary control of cancer can be achieved in an elderly population and also to consider the merit of pursuing preventive interventions in preference to waiting for the occurrence of invasive cancer as a trigger that begins control measures at the secondary or tertiary level.

II. RATIONALE FOR CANCER PREVENTION IN THE ELDERLY

For individuals who are diagnosed with invasive cancer at an age of 65 years or older, prognosis, as usual, is recognized to be related to performance status. Even in the setting of a good-performance status, the functional and physiological reserves of older individuals may interfere with the delivery of usually effective therapies, especially when the chemotherapy of choice was developed in an investigational setting using a population that included younger individuals. For the elderly, to weigh the pros and cons of prevention in anticipation of disease versus treatment in reaction to disease, documentation for toxicities and drawbacks must be specifically obtained from an elderly population. If an individual reaches the age of 65 years without developing an invasive cancer, a risk-reducing, preventive intervention is more likely to be accepted when the preventive intervention is essentially nontoxic; that is, an attractive way to avoid the relatively higher toxicity of some of the treatments that might be assayed if invasive disease developed.

As with all age groups, the benefit from therapy with curative intent is expected to be related to the stage of disease at diagnosis. The major benefit sought by cancer screening is the identification of disease at an earlier stage consistent with an opportunity to achieve better results from treatment. Although less use of cancer screening in more senior age groups may reflect an adjustment for comorbid conditions, other factors seem to play a role. Whether physicians do not recommend screening as vigorously to the elderly or whether elderly patients avoid the use of screening services (even when cost considerations are ameliorated by Medicare), it can be anticipated that the perception of screening as a tool for initiating and tracking the results of a preventive intervention may help to reduce the barriers to screening for cancer in the elderly.

In identifying interventions with net clinical benefit including cancer prevention, the most reliable evidence is derived from randomized clinical trials, preferably placebo-controlled trials. As a condition for conducting this kind of trial, it is useful to have a screening methodology that identifies participants who are starting the trial without findings suspicious for invasive cancer; that is, triaging out people who more appropriately might be candidates for treatment following a diagnostic work-up obtained in a timely fashion. There is little evidence that chemopreventive agents are appropriate as first-line therapy for invasive cancer. After baseline studies clear participants for entry into prevention trials, repeat screening is central to the process of case ascertainment and crucial to the accounting process that determines when and if a subsequent case of invasive cancer occurs in relationship to the use of the test intervention. Therefore, it is not surprising that the development of cancer chemopreventive interventions are most developed for organ sites like the breast, colon/rectum, and prostate for which screening methods are relatively well developed or widely applied as described in the preceding chapters.

III. INTERVENTIONS FOR CANCER PREVENTION IN THE ELDERLY

In the case of breast cancer, screening technology based on mammography was demonstrated to have a role in reducing mortality from breast cancer many years ago. In the United States, the HIP (Health Insurance Plan of New York) study provided results as early as 1967 indicating that annual mammography was associated with an approxiamte 30% reduction in subsequent deaths from breast cancer (5). Although the study population at entry was between the ages of 40 and 64 years, there is no evidence that the performance characteristics of mammography in women over the age of 65 years are inferior to those for women of younger ages. A by-product of mammographic screening is the increased identification of breast carcinoma in situ, the removal of which may result in cancer prevention.

One approach to cancer prevention is to develop screening technology so that premalignant lesions are identified and removed before there is systemic spread. This approach would be especially attractive if the procedure for lesion removal was well tolerated, with limited morbidity, such as a breast lumpectomy or a colorectal polypectomy. In the breast cancer setting, there has been an increasing use of screening mammography, and the rate of diagnosis of ductal carcinoma in situ (DCIS) has more than doubled between 1983 and the present. At the end of the 1990s, around 15% of all breast cancer cases were diagnosed as DCIS (stage 0), and this figure would be expected to increase with the increasing use of mammography (6) or if technology were developed to identify breast DCIS lesions sensitively and accurately. Since not all cases identified as DCIS may be destined to progress to invasive lesions, the potential for breast cancer prevention from the mammographic identification of in situ lesions at current levels with subsequent removal is relatively small but could increase.

Theoretically, the potential for preventing colorectal cancer by removing adenomatous polyps may be substantial. This strategy depends on the percentage of invasive colorectal lesions that arise from polyps. It has been suggested by a case-control study that the use of screening sigmoidoscopy was associated with a 60% reduction in the risk of dying from colorectal cancer, with benefit presumably being derived from either polyp removal or treatment of early-stage disease (7, 8). In this study, fatality from colon cancer beyond the reach of the scope was predictably not related to sigmoidoscopic screening. It appeared that the benefit of a screening procedure might persist for up to 10 years after the last sigmoidoscopy. This result is consistent with observations from the National Polyp Study (NPS), which suggested that the transformation of small polyps into cancer took about 10 years (9).

One important hypothesis generated by the NPS is that 75–90% of colorectal cancers in adenomatous polyp formers may arise in antecedent adenomatous polyps, suggesting that many cancers could be prevented if periodic colorectal screening were used to remove colorectal adenomas (10). In the NPS, the intervention of colonoscopic screening with polypectomy was directed at participants who (a) uniformly had a history of prior adenomatous polyps and (b) can be presumed to have been healthy volunteers. Rates of colorectal cancer in the NPS were then compared with colorectal cancer rates for three reference groups who were screened less frequently. Consequently, there is an expectation that the comparison rates may have been artificially low and the estimated 75–90% reduction in cancer somewhat inflated. For colorectal cancer arising outside a circumscribed antecedent polyp, the prevention potential from colonoscopy may be limited. Nevertheless, periodic colonoscopic surveillance for the purpose of removing adenomatous colorectal lesions with high malignant potential (e.g., 1 cm or more in diameter) (11), could prove to be an attractively beneficial and tolerable intervention in the elderly. Compared with breast or colorectal cancer, existing screening technology does not lend itself to the removal of a premalignant lesion for prostatic cancer prevention, particularly since many malignant prostatic lesions in the elderly follow an essentially benign course. Cancer prevention from removal of premalignant lesions is pursued for a variety of lesions; for example, high-grade intraepithelial lesions of the uterine cervix, actinic keratoses, and oral leukoplakia. When a large field of tissue is at risk, a systemic therapy may gain in value over repeated localized therapy.

When primary control of cancer is unlikely to be achieved by removal of premalignant lesions, other approaches to cancer prevention are needed. Categories of cancer prevention include (a) avoidance of cancer-causing exposures that increase cancer risk, (b) dealing with an unavoidable exposure by blocking its effect with a protective agent that prevents carcinogenic change from occurring, or (c) reversing a defect in the cellular machinery by compensating for a missing function (12). Avoidance interventions are illustrated by avoiding tobacco use and the hypothesis that a low-fat diet may reduce cancer risk. The use of antioxidant vitamins to prevent oxidative damage illustrates the second approach. Calcium in the gut may provide a protective effect against colorectal cancer. Compensatory activity can be observed when premalignant lesions redifferentiate under the influence of pharmacological agents like retinoids. As an antiestrogen, tamoxifen may compensate for an increased rate of proliferation by an abnormal clone of cells in the breast epithelium.

In pursuing interventions for cancer prevention in the elderly, some potential leads are provided by the food and nutrition health claims recognized by the U.S. Food and Drug Administration (FDA). Included in the Nutrition Labeling and Education Act of 1990 were 10 substance–disease relationships, of which 3 involved cancer. The three claims address (a) dietary fat and cancer (13), (b) fiber-containing grain products, fruits, and vegetables and cancer (14), and (c) fruits and vegetables and cancer (15). Health claims about cancer and foods or food substances are presented in the context that many other factors may contribute to the development of cancer. Also recognized are the uncertainties surrounding the specific components of the diet or the epiphenomena linked with diet, which are responsible for the various associations between diet and cancer. Nevertheless, along with an acknowledgment of the multifactorial etiology of cancer, food manufacturers have the option to note that a diet that is either low in fat; low in fat and fiber-rich from grain, fruits and vegetables; or low in fat and rich in fruits and vegetables with fiber, vitamin A, or vitamin C may reduce the risk of some cancers or some types of cancer. Until more definitive data are obtained, the message that a diet low in fat, high in fiber, and rich in fruits and vegetables can serve as the basis for a personal cancer prevention program in the elderly as well as in other age groups.

The standard for FDA-recognized health claims that foods may reduce the risk of cancer is one of "significant scientific agreement," but the supporting evidence for these claims is largely based on retrospective data for case-control analysis, which is subject to bias and confounding and less robust than results from randomized clinical trials. As the number of studies increases, the evidence is often found to be inconsistent. For example, a combined analysis of 12 case-control studies examining the relationship between dietary factors and breast cancer concluded that the risk of postmenopausal breast cancer was associated with an increased dietary fat intake (16). A pattern has emerged that cohort studies with prospectively collected data frequently contradict the findings of the case-control studies. When prospectively collected data were pooled from seven cohort studies, there was no evidence that breast cancer risk was associated with high levels of dietary fat intake as determined by a comparison of the highest quintile with lower quintiles (17). In the most recent update of the largest of the seven cohort studies, results from the Nurses' Health Study after 14 years of follow-up support the null hypothesis that a low-fat diet is not protective against breast cancer (18). Since cohort studies may correct for flaws that occur in case-control studies, it will be helpful to have results from a large randomized clinical trial in progress that examines the hypothesis that a reduction in dietary fat can be used to decrease breast cancer risk (19). Until results from this kind of trial become available, it is reasonable to pursue a low-fat diet, recognizing that other health benefits may be obtained while additional data are being collected to clarify the effect of diet on cancer. If a low-fat diet is achieved by increasing the intake of fruits and vegetables, cancer risk reduction may occur on that basis. Furthermore, it is felt that the risk of cardiovascular disease is strongly related to the type of dietary fat, and that reduction of saturated fat in the diet may be helpful in reducing cardiovascular mortality (20, 21).

Examination of the fiber claim, again reveals controversy. In a combined analysis of 13 case-control studies examining the relationship between dietary fiber intake and colorectal cancer, it was concluded that the risk of colorectal cancer was decreased about 40% in association with the increased intake of fiber in the highest quintile compared with the lowest (22). A reanalysis of the data based on a subset of studies which met more stringent inclusion criteria (e.g., validated dietary questionnaires) dramatically diminished the previously observed fiber-associated risk reduction (23). Subsequent reports from cohort studies have failed to find an association between dietary fiber and the reduction of colorectal cancer risk (24–26); however, fruit fiber was associated with a nonsignificant 14% reduction in colorectal cancer risk in one study (16). In another study, a risk reduction was observed in association with citrus fruit, vegetable, and high-fiber grain consumption without a specific analysis of fiber content (17). Of additional concern to the hypothesis that dietary fiber reduces cancer risk are the results from randomized clinical trials where fiber interventions failed to reduce colorectal adenoma incidence (27, 28).

Beyond low-fat and high-fiber fruit and vegetable consumption, other dietary interventions may prove to be useful for preventing colorectal adenomas. In a randomized trial that compared calcium carbonate (1200 mg of elemental calcium) with placebo, the calcium intervention significantly reduced the subsequent occurrence of adenomas in patients with a history of previously removed adenomas (29). Although the effect of calcium on the colon is not fully understood, it is thought that one mechanism protective of the bowel mucosa is the binding of bile acids by calcium (30).

Given the inconsistencies of and questions raised by comparing the results from dietary case-control and cohort studies, the need for conducting randomized clinical trials (RCT) to measure the worth of preventive interventions is obvious. Inherent to the cancer prevention RCT process is a protocol that imposes a consistent definition of the diagnostic criteria for counting cancer cases and a consistent application of methods for detecting the disease. The value of an intervention is ultimately defined by using the RCT to compare the incidence outcome under controlled conditions in the group of individuals who have used the preventive intervention with a similar group of individuals who have not. Balance in patient characteristics is usually achieved with the randomization process, eliminating sources of bias and confounding that are problematic with retrospective studies. If an incidence reduction is possible and can be demonstrated, the RCT becomes the setting for measuring secondary outcomes for both good and ill, so that the net clinical benefit of an intervention can be established within the population where it is tested. In order to advise elderly patients on the merit of preventive interventions, it is imperative that prevention trials include enough elderly patients that there is confidence the result is consistent across age groups. The extent of fine tuning the intervention for elderly patients will depend on the availability of data on risks and benefits specific to the elderly population.

As mentioned above, the question of the role of a low-fat diet in preventing cancer is being addressed in part by a large RCT: the Women's Health Initiative (WHI) Clinical Trial initiated in 1992 (12). Within the clinical trial population of the WHI are 48,837 participants randomized to an intervention based on the reduction of total dietary fat to 20% of calories with saturated fat less than 7%. Along with fat reduction, the participants are trained to increase servings of fruits and vegetables to at least five a day and servings of grain products to at least six a day. Women randomized to the control arm are advised to maintain their usual eating habits and are provided with standard nutrition guidelines, but they do not participate in the intensive behavioral program that is used to establish and maintain the changed diet in the intervention group. The two main endpoints in the dietary-modification trial are prevention of breast and colon cancers. The secondary endpoint is a reduction in coronary heart disease. The dietary-modification trial population is a subset of a larger population planned to total about 64,500 women, who are allocated according to a partial factorial design. It is anticipated that the trial will last for 15 years and cost 628 million dollars. The age composition of participants was targeted to include 45% of participants in the 60–69 years age bracket with another 25% aged 70–79 years. Accrual to the overall clinical trial group was completed in September, 1998.

A second interventional study in the WHI is looking at the colorectal cancer endpoint. A subset of 32,234 women has been randomized to receive a combined supplement with 1000 mg of elemental calcium and 400 IU of vitamin D in two tablets each day versus placebo. Instructions are to take the supplement with meals in divided doses. Reduction in colorectal cancer is a secondary endpoint, with the primary endpoint being an anticipated reduction in the risk of hip and other fractures (31). Hypercalcemia with the intervention is expected only rarely, but at the initiation of such an intervention in clinical practice, it would be prudent to determine calcium levels with a subsequent check after start-up considering issues related to hyperparathyroidism or diuretic use if hypercalcemia is found.

The WHI makes an impressive start at using randomized clinical trials to determine the effect of dietary interventions on the risk of major cancers in women. These interventions have great appeal because of their apparent safety. Behavioral modifications that reduce exposure to ultraviolet radiation for skin cancer risk reduction or that increase regular exercise to reduce breast and colon cancer risk are also attractive, but they may be difficult to maintain. Cancer prevention interventions with pharmacological agents are often more controversial. Various definitions of cancer chemoprevention have been provided, and one of these is, "the prevention of cancer by the use of pharmacological agents to inhibit or reverse the process of carcinogenesis" (32). A recent review of cancer chemoprevention studies reported in the English-language literature identified more than 60 RCTs, but only 9 trials were considered to be definitive on the basis of study design. In these nine trials, 15 well-defined interventions with endpoints were tested (33). From the results of these trials, two definitive interventions were identified that reduced cancer risk. One of these, the Skin Cancer Prevention Trial, demonstrated that 25,000 IU of retinol daily could be used to reduce the risk of developing squamous cell cancer of the skin. The observed reduction was 26% with modest significance ($P = .04$ with 95% CI from 1 to 44%). The clinical implications of this trial are ambiguous, since squamous cell cancer of the skin is often classified as less than a serious malignancy and effective local treatments are available. The second definitive intervention was identified by the Breast Cancer Prevention Trial (BCPT), in which 20 mg of daily tamoxifen was found to reduce the overall risk of breast cancer by 49% in the study population.

The BCPT with tamoxifen is a randomized, placebo-controlled trial conducted by the National Surgical Adjuvant Breast and Bowel Project and opened to accrual in 1992. In 1998, results were reported that showed a highly significant reduction in invasive breast cancer among women treated with tamoxifen (34). There were 13,388 women enrolled in this trial, of whom about 30% were over 60 years of age or older. Six percent of the women participating in the BCPT were aged 70 years or older. Starting with baseline mammograms that revealed no findings suspicious for malignancy, evidence was obtained that women aged 60 years or older, who were randomized to 20 mg of daily oral tamoxifen for a planned 5 years, experienced a 55% reduction in the risk of developing breast cancer. In other subsets based on age, the reduction in invasive breast cancer was 44% in women aged 49 years or younger and 51% in women aged 50–59 years. In addition to breast cancer risk reduction, the BCPT found that fractures of the hip and spine (mostly occurring in women over age 50 years) were reduced. There were 53 fractures in the placebo group compared with 35 fractures in the women randomized to tamoxifen, a result that fell short of statistical significance.

In the BCPT, the adverse effects of tamoxifen were characterized as non–life threatening or life threatening. In the former category, increases were observed in hot flushes, with 45.7% of the women on tamoxifen reporting ''quite a bit'' or extremely bothersome hot flushes compared with 28.7% of the placebo-treated women. Vaginal discharge was quite a bit or extremely bothersome for 12.4% of the women on tamoxifen versus 4.5% of the women on placebo. More serious risks occurred infrequently and included endometrial cancer and noncardiac vascular events. For women over the age of 50 years, there was an elevated risk of developing endometrial cancer, but many American women over 50 years old have undergone hysterectomy, thereby avoiding this risk. The annual increase in endometrial cancer risk amounted to about 1.3 cases per thousand women, and all the cases that occurred in women using tamoxifen were stage I lesions. Women over the age of 50 years who used tamoxifen were also found to have increased rates of stroke (tamoxifen: 35 events; placebo: 20), pulmonary embolism (tamoxifen: 18 events; placebo 6), and deep-vein thrombosis (tamoxifen: 24 events; placebo: 14) compared with women of similar age taking placebo, but the differences did not reach statistical significance.

Approval from the FDA to market tamoxifen for the reduction of breast cancer incidence in women at high risk for the disease was obtained in 1998 soon after the results of the trial were reported. In deciding when to use tamoxifen for breast cancer prevention, a woman with her physician should consider the benefit from breast cancer reduction in its overall context, recognizing adverse consequences as well as the benefits of using tamoxifen. One place to start is by obtaining an estimate of the breast cancer risk that the woman can expect in the next 5 years and for her projected lifetime. This information will help the woman to appreciate how the use of tamoxifen changes her personal risk of developing breast cancer. A risk assessment tool for physicians is available from the National Cancer Institute. A bulletin entitled ''Estimating Breast Cancer Risk'' describes the tool on-line at http://cancer-net.nci.nih.gov.

When considering tamoxifen for breast cancer prevention, insight into the decision-making process will grow as more experience is obtained. In an analysis by Canadian investigators, a statistical model was applied to the results of the BCPT (35). For Canadian women aged 60 years or more, it was determined that the average reduction for the remaining lifetime breast cancer risk was 13 cases per 1000 women compared with an increased risk of 5 cases of pulmonary embolism and 11 cases of endometrial cancer per 1000. For individual women, the reduction in expected breast cancers would be increased for women aged 60 years who had higher than average breast cancer risk, and of course the endometrial cancer risk would drop out if a hysterectomy had been performed. Adjustment for individual factors such as these is needed to provide an assessment of the potential overall benefit that is as accurate as possible.

Results from the BCPT have provided an option for women aged 65 years or more to consider when they are looking for a way to reduce their risk of developing breast cancer. The availability of this chemopreventive intervention demonstrates the potential for developing other chemopreventive interventions. For men, the results of the Prostate Cancer Prevention Trial (PCPT) which opened for accrual in 1993 are eagerly awaited. The PCPT is being conducted by the Southwest Oncology Group, comparing an intervention with 5 mg of finasteride (a 5α-reductase inhibitor) versus placebo daily for 7 years. Although digital rectal examination and prostate-specific antigen (PSA) are performed annually, all participants are scheduled to undergo prostatic biopsy at the end of the intervention so that the opportunity for case ascertainment is balanced in the two arms of the study. Otherwise, suppression of PSA by finasteride might reduce the number of biopsies and opportunity for identification of cases in the intervention arm.

IV. FUTURE PROSPECTS

Plans are underway to follow the PCPT with a major prostatic cancer prevention trial using selenium and vitamin E as the intervention. A trial of tamoxifen versus raloxifene will follow the BCPT to see how raloxifene compares with tamoxifen as a breast cancer preventive agent. On the horizon is the prospect that cyclooxygenase-2 (COX-2) inhibitors, a lower toxicity version of nonsteroidal anti-inflammatory drugs, will show promise in reducing colon cancer risk in the elderly.

Even though the opportunities for cancer prevention in the elderly are limited by the availability of evidence to support intervention, the rationale for cancer prevention is strong and trials are in progress to augment the number of interventional options. Great care should be taken to assure that the inclusion of elderly patients in cancer prevention trials is sufficient to provide the appropriate data so that informed access to cancer prevention opportunities is available to this large high-risk segment of the population, which is growing larger.

REFERENCES

1. Landis SH, Murray T, Bolden S, Wingo PA. Cancer statistics, 1999. CA Cancer J Clin 1999; 49:8–31.

2. Ries LAG, Kosary CL, Hankey BF, Miller BA, Edwards BK, eds. SEER Cancer Statistics Review, 1973–1995, Bethesda, MD; National Cancer Institute, 1998.

3. Breast Cancer Trials Committee: Adjuvant tamoxifen in the management of operable breast cancer: the Scottish trial. Lancet 1988; 2:171–175.

4. Taylor WR, Marks JS, Livengood JR, Koplan JP. Current issues and challenges in chronic disease control. In: Chronic Disease Epidemiology and Control. Brownson RC, Remington PL, Davis JR, eds. Baltimore: American Public Health Association, 1993.

5. Shapiro S, Venet W, Strax P, et al. Ten- to fourteen-year effect of screening on breast cancer mortality. J Natl Cancer Inst 1982; 69:349–355.

6. Ernster BL, Barclay J, Kerlikowske K, Grady D, Henderson IC. Incidence of and treatment for ductal carcinoma in situ of the breast. JAMA 1996; 275:913–918.

7. Selby JV, Friedman GD, Quesenberry CP, Weiss NS. A case-control study of screening sigmoidoscopy and mortality from colorectal cancer. N Engl J Med 1992; 326:653–657.

8. Levin B. Screening sigmoidoscopy for colorectal cancer. N Engl J Med 1992; 326:700–701.

9. Winawer DSJ. Natural history of colorectal cancer. Am J Med 1999; 106(Suppl 1A): 3S–6S.

10. Winawer SJ, Zauber AG, Ho MN, O'Brien MJ, Gottlieb LS, Sternberg SS, Waye JD, Schapiro M, Bond JH, Panish JF, Ackroyd F, Shike M, Kurtz RC, Hornsby-Lewis L, Gerdes H, Stewart ET, and the National Polyp Study Workgroup. Prevention of colorectal cancer by colonoscopic polypectomy. N Engl J Med 1993; 329:1977–1981.

11. Atkin WS, Morson BC, Cuzick J. Long-term risk of colorectal cancer after excision of rectosigmoid adenomas. N Engl J Med 1992; 326:658–662.

12. Bertram JS, Kolonel LN, Meyskens FL. Rationale and strategies for chemoprevention of cancer in humans. Cancer Res 1987; 47:3012–3031.

13. Code of Federal Regulations: Title 21, Section 101.73.

14. Code of Federal Regulations: Title 21, Section 101.76.

15. Code of Federal Regulations: Title 21, Section 101.78.

16. Howe GR, Hirohata T, Hislop G, Iscovich JM, Yuan J-M, Katsouyanni K, Lubin F, Marubini E, Modan B, Rohan T, Toniolo P, Shunzhang. Dietary factors and risk of breast cancer: combined analysis of 12 case-control studies. J Natl Cancer Inst 1990; 82:561–569.

17. Hunter DJ, Speigelman D, Adami HO, Beeson L, van den Brandt PA, Folsom AR, Fraser GE, Goldbohm A, Graham S, how GR, Kushi LH, Marshall JR, McDermott A, Miller AB, Speizer FE, Wold A, Yaun S-S Willet W. Cohort studies of fat intake and the risk of breast cancer—a pooled analysis. N Engl J Med 1996; 334:356–361.

18. Holmes MD, Hunter DJ, Colditz GA, Stampfer MJ, Hankinson SE, Speizer FE, Rosner B, Willett WC. Association of dietary intake of fat and fatty acids with risk of breast cancer. JAMA 1999; 281:914–920.

19. The Women's Health Initiative Study Group. Design of the Women's Health initiative clinical trial and observational study. Control Clin Trials 1998; 19:61–109.

20. Hu FB. Dietary fat intake and the risk of coronary heart disease in women. N Engl J Med 1997; 337:1491–1499.

21. National Research Council. Diet and health: implications for reducing chronic disease risk: report of the Committee on Diet and Health, Food and Nutrition Board. Washington, DC: National Academy Press, 1989.

22. Howe GR, Benito E, Castelleto R, Cornee J, Esteve J, Gallagher RP, Iscovich JM, Dengao J, Kaaks R, Kune GA, Kune S, L'Abbe KA, Lee HP, Lee M, Miller AB, Peters RK, Potter JD, Riboli E, Slattery ML, Trichopoulos D, Tuyns A, Tzonou A, Whittemore AS, Wu-Williams AH, Shu Z. Dietary intake of fiber and decreased risk of cancers of the colon and rectum: evidence from the combined analysis of 13 case-control studies. J Natl Cancer Inst 1992; 84:1887–1896.

23. Friedenreich CM, Brant RF, Riboli E. Influence of methodologic factors in a pooled analysis of 13 case-control studies of colorectal cancer and dietary fiber. Epidemiology 1994; 5:66–79.

24. Fuchs CS, Giovannucci EL, Colditz GA, Hunter DJ, Stampfer MJ, Rosner B, Speizer FE, Willett WC. Dietary fiber and the risk of colorectal cancer and adenoma in women. N Engl J Med 1999; 340:169–176.

25. Thun MJ, Calle EE, Namboodiri M, et al. Risk factors for fatal colon cancer in a large prospective study. J Natl Cancer Inst 1992; 84:1491–1500.

26. Giovannucci E, Rimm EB, Stampfer JM, Colditz GA, Ascherio A, Willett WC. Intake of fat, meat, and fiber in relation to risk of colon cancer in men. Cancer Res 1994; 54: 2390–2397.

27. MacLennan R, Macrae F, Bain C, et al. Randomized trial of intake of fat, fiber and beta carotene to prevent colorectal adenoma: the Australian Polyp Prevention Project. J Natl Cancer Inst 1995; 87:1760–1766.

28. McKeown-Eyssen GE, Bright-See E, Bruce WR, Jazmaji V. A randomized trial of a low fat high fibre diet in the recurrence of colorectal polyps: Toronto Polyp Prevention Group. J Clin Epidemiol 1994; 47:525–536.

29. Baron JA, Beach M, Mandel JS, van Stolk RU, Haile RW, Sandler RS, Rothstein R, Summers RW, Snover DC, Beck GJ, Bond JH, Greenberg ER, for the Calcium Polyp Prevention Study Group. Calcium supplements for the prevention of colorectal adenomas. N Engl J Med 1999; 340:101–107.

30. Newmark HL, Wargovich MJ, Bruce WR. Colon cancer and dietary fat, phosphate, and calcium: a hypothesis. J Natl Cancer inst 1984; 72:1323–1325.

31. Dawson-Hughes B, Harris SS, Krall EA, Dallal GE. Effect of calcium and vitamin D supplementation on bone density in men and women 65 years of age or older. N Engl J Med 1997; 337:670–676.

32. Sporn MB, Newton DL. Chemoprevention of cancer with retinoids. Fed Proc 1979; 38: 2528–2534.

33. Lippman SM, Lee JJ, Sabichi AL. Cancer chemoprevention: progress and promise. J Natl Cancer Inst 1998; 90:1514–1528.

34. Fisher B, Costantino JP, Wickerham DL et al.: Tamoxifen for Prevention of Breast Cancer: Report of the National Surgical Adjuvant Breast and Bowel Project P-1 Study. J Natl Cancer Inst 1998; 90:1371–1388.

35. Logan D, Will BP, Berthelot J-M, Flanagan W, Tomiak E, Fung Kee Fung M, Evans WK. Economic and health impacts of administering preventative tamoxifen to women at high-risk of breast cancer in Canada. Proc ASCO 1999; 18:415a

6

Molecular Biology and Biological Markers

Barbara K. Dunn
National Cancer Institute
National Institutes of Health
Bethesda, Maryland

Dan L. Longo
National Institute on Aging
National Institutes of Health
Bethesda, Maryland

I. INTRODUCTION

Cancer is a disease of dysregulated cell growth that involves excessive proliferation of cells as well as the capacity to invade tissues and metastasize to and colonize remote sites (Fenton and Longo, 1998). Nearly all cancers arise from a single cell whose uncontrolled proliferation leads to a clone of cells that appears as a recognizable tumor. This origin of a tumor from a single clone of cells is the critical feature that distinguishes a malignant neoplasm from hyperplasia or a benign growth. The aberrant cell growth results from an interplay between environmental and genetic factors. Environmental factors include exogenous agents such as chemicals (food additives, insecticides), radiation, and infectious organisms. Environmental agents exert their impact on the cell by promoting dysregulated growth at two basic levels: first, in an extragenetic fashion by functioning directly as growth factors or by stimulating the production of growth factors; or by causing physical mutations, or changes, in genes, which result in quantitative or qualitative modifications of their expression. Thus, environmental insults may impact directly on the genome to promote carcinogenesis.

Genetic factors include endogenous products of genes which are mutated. Primarily cancer is a genetic disease in which the abnormal products expressed from mutated genes lead to dysregulated cell growth. The culprit genetic mutations may result from environmental assaults, as just described, or they may be a consequence of random replication errors or faulty DNA repair processes. Most such mutations consist of actual sequence changes in the DNA, leading, for example, to missense, nonsense, or frameshift mutations. In addition, chromosomal translocations involving the juxtaposition of previously separated DNA sequences may lead to altered expression of the repositioned genes. Amplification or deletion of DNA sequences constitutes another type of gene alteration that contributes to neoplasia. Genetic mutations may be present in the germ cells of an individual, implying that they were inherited from the parents. Alternatively, genetic mutations may be acquired in the DNA of somatic cells. In the former case, perpetuation of the cancer-causing mutation in the germline of successive generations may lead to what is conventionally cited as an ''inherited cancer.'' In the latter case, the acquisition of genetic changes in the DNA of somatic cells of an individual may result in the development of a ''sporadic cancer.'' Importantly, a single inherited cancer-causing mutation is sufficient only to predispose but not actually to cause the cancer outcome in the affected individual. Rather additional somatic mutations are required to implement the predisposition into the actual development of a cancer. In fact, a single genetic change is rarely sufficient to induce neoplastic transformation. The process of carcinogenesis generally requires the accumulation of multiple mutations, of the order of 5–10, each contributing a slight growth advantage, the net result of which is the evolution from a normal to a frank malignant phenotype (Vogelstein, 1988; Kinzler, 1996). Finally, the contributing cancer-causing mutations may be either inherited or acquired, and a combination of mutations arising in both etiological fashions may contribute to the net outcome—neoplastic growth.

II. CELLULAR PROCESSES THAT CAN BE ALTERED IN CANCER

Not just any gene will cause cancer when it is mutated. Only genes whose normal products carry out specific types of functions in the cell are candidate targets for cancer-causing mutations. For example, genes whose products participate in processes influencing cell growth in either a growth-promoting or growth-inhibiting manner are prime candidates for oncogenic mutations. Since cell growth is the final pathway of a number of key cellular operations, the genes whose products carry out these operations are, in turn, the targets of oncogenic mutations. Other cellular processes that constrain and organize growth, such as cell–cell adhesion interactions and cellular migration, are determined by genes which, when mutated, may also contribute to carcinogenesis.

A. Cell Cycle

1. Cell Cycle Phases and Checkpoints

The process of cell division has many features that are common to eukaryotic organisms ranging from yeast to humans (Beach, 1994; Nasmyth, 1996; Fenton and Longo, 1998). Early light microscopic studies recognized that the visually detectable process of cell division, or cytokinesis, was preceded by mitosis, consisting of chromosomal condensation, alignment on the spindle apparatus, sister chromatid segregation to opposite poles of the cell, and packaging into two new nuclei. The intervening stage between successive mitoses, interphase, is composed of three intervals: G1 (gap 1), S phase, and G2 (gap 2) (Fig. 1) (Stillman, 1996; Fenton and Longo, 1998). G1, the gap between mitosis (M phase) and the onset of DNA replication, is a period of cellular growth during which the chromosomes acquire the competence to initiate and commit to DNA synthesis. S phase, the period of DNA synthesis, is a process that depends on the activity of numerous enzymes. Following the unfolding of chromatin from the DNA, DNA helicase together with single-strand binding proteins open the double helix. DNA polymerase and DNA primase attach to periodically spaced replication origins along the DNA and catalyze DNA polymerization of tandem replication units. During the replication process, topoisomerases break and reseal DNA strands to prevent tangling. Following completion of replication, the replication units reassemble and chromatin binds to the nascent DNA chain, preventing more than one replication of each region. Although the replication system is relatively accurate, the occasional mistakes that are made are remedied by a variety of repair mechanisms (Hanawalt, 1994; Modrich, 1994; Sancar, 1994). G2, the gap between S and M phases, is the period during which the fidelity of DNA replication is assessed and errors are corrected. Finally, there are certain signals that the cell may receive during G1 which induce it to withdraw from the cycle into a resting state (G0) rather than to commit to progressing through another division. Recent studies have focused on identifying the factors that promote and inhibit transitions between these phases. These factors are sometimes altered in cancer, leading to dysregulated, often unchecked, progression through the cell cycle and resulting in excessive cell proliferation. Because DNA polymerase is unable to replicate the ends of DNA strands (Watson, 1972), a special mechanism has evolved whereby tandem six-nucleotide repeats are added to the ends of chromsomes, constituting telomeres. The addition of these repeat sequences is carried out by telomerase, an RNA-dependent DNA polymerase that is not found in most normal somatic cells but is expressed in germ cells as well as in cancer cells.

The four phases thus defined are viewed as major cell cycle states. The transition from each state to the next is tightly regulated. Thus, a cell cycle transition has been referred to as "a unidirectional change of state in which a cell that was performing one set of processes shifts its activity to perform a different set of processes" (Elledge, 1996). The purpose of such strict regulation is to ensure that chro-

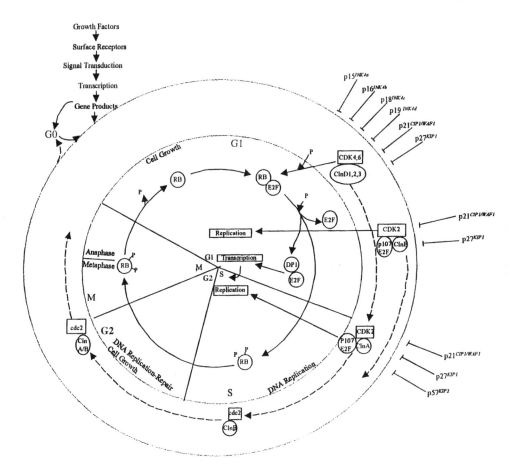

Figure 1 Cell cycle and checkpoint controls. The cell cycle consists of four phases, or major cell cycle states: G1 (gap 1); S phase (period of DNA synthesis); G2 (gap 2); and M phase (mitosis). The transition from one state to the next is induced by the activation of a class of protein kinases, the cyclin-dependent kinases (CDKs). Activation of CDKs occurs when they form complexes with the appropriate regulatory subunits, called cyclins (Cln). For example, cyclin D–CDKs trigger phosphorylation of pRB which causes it to release E2F which, in turn, heterodimerizes with the transcription factor DP-1 and activates genes required for DNA synthesis. In response to a variety of stimuli, including DNA damage, the inhibitors of the CDKs, $p15^{INK4a}$, $p16^{INK4b}$, $p18^{INK4c}$, and $p19^{INK4d}$, as well as another group of CDK inhibitors, $p21^{CIP1/WAF1}$, $p27^{KIP1}$, and $p57^{KIP2}$, block progression through the cell cycle prior to specific checkpoints. There is thus a balance between cell cycle–promoting and cell cycle–inhibiting actions, which represent the cell's response to both exogenous and endogenous signals. An example of such a signal is the growth factor eliciting activation of the generic signal transduction pathway which is shown intersecting with the cell cycle. (Adapted from Sherr, 1996 and Fenton and Longo, 1998.)

mosome duplication and segregation occur in the correct order and that a given event is initiated only when the previous event has been successfully completed (Nasmyth, 1996). This regulation is carried out at specific points in the cell cycle by surveillance mechanisms that monitor the cell for successful completion of the preceding stage and block transition to the next stage in its absence. These surveillance mechanisms that block cell cycle transitions are called checkpoints (Hartwell, 1994; Nasmyth, 1996). The biochemical pathway that constitutes a checkpoint may be either intrinsic or extrinsic. In the presence of DNA damage, for example, a functional checkpoint causes the cell to sense the DNA damage and to respond by inhibiting further progression through the cell cycle until adequate DNA repair has been completed.

2. Genes Whose Products Act During the Cell Cycle to Promote or Inhibit Transitions Between Phases

Transitions between states are induced by the activation of members of a special class of protein kinases. These are known as cyclin-dependent kinases (CDKs), because they are active only when their catalytic subunits are complexed with regulatory subunits called cyclins. Cyclins, in turn, acquired their name because they repeatedly accumulate and disappear in cycles corresponding to the cycles of cell division (Beach, 1994; Nasmyth, 1996). Each cyclin undergoes transcriptionally regulated expression followed by ubiquitin-mediated degradation at specific points in the cell cycle. There are at least seven CDK family members, each of which associates with a distinct cyclin.

Mitogenic signals induce one or more D-type cyclins (D1, D2, and D3) as cells enter phase G1 from phase G0, or quiescence (see Fig. 1) (Sherr, 1996). The D cyclins, complexed with their catalytic partners CDK4 and CDK6, then facilitate the transition from G1 to S. The normal surveillance mechanisms that operate as checkpoints at this transition merit attention, because the regulation of this transition is frequently disrupted in cancer. Potential targets of disruption include those proteins that normally function to inhibit the G1 to S transition. Thus, there are four known inhibitors of CDK4 and CDK6, the INK4 proteins (p16^{INK1a}, p15^{INK1b}, p18^{INK1c} and p19^{INK1d}), which directly block cyclin D–dependent kinase activity and cause G1 phase arrest. Furthermore, inhibition of the G1 to S transition is primarily maintained by the retinoblastoma gene product, pRB, which, in its hypophosphorylated form, binds a transcription factor called E2F (Weinberg, 1995; Kaelin, 1997). When pRB is phosphorylated, E2F is released. In this free, or unbound, form, E2F transcriptionally activates several growth-promoting genes, including c-*myc*, B-*myb*, *cdc2*, dihydrofolate reductase, thymidine kinase, proliferating cell nuclear antigen (PCNA), and the promoter of the *E2F-1* gene itself (Nevins, 1992; Levine, 1997), thus facilitating the transition from G1 to S phase (Weinberg, 1995).

Cyclin A–and cyclin B–dependent kinases maintain pRB in its hyperphosphorylated state. Cyclin A synthesis begins late in G1, and it appears to be important for the G1 to S transition, whereas cyclin B synthesis does not begin until S phase. The cyclin D–, E–, and A–dependent kinases are negatively regulated by a distinct family of CDK inhibitors that includes p21$^{CIP1/WAF1}$, p27^{KIP1} and p57^{KIP2}. Of particular interest is the fact that the *CIP1* gene is induced by the tumor suppressor p53 (El-Deiry et al., 1993). The p27^{KIP1} protein, whose expression is regulated at both the translational and posttranslational level (Pagano, 1995; Hengst, 1996; Kwon et al., 1996, 1997), appears to be the most directly involved in checkpoint control, mediating repression of cyclin E–CDK2 and cyclin A–CDK2 activity in cyclin cells. When a loss of cyclin D–dependent kinase activity is coupled with p27^{KIP1}-mediated inhibition of CDK2, arrest is observed within G1.

The transition from G2 to M, leading to initiation of mitosis, is facilitated by a complex of Cdc2, another important member of the CDK family, with cyclins A and B. Recent data suggest a model for the pathway governing surveillance at the G2 to M checkpoint in response to DNA damage (Furnari, 1997; Peng, 1997, Sanchez, 1997, Weinert, 1997). Activation of Cdc2 depends on its being dephosphorylated by the protein phosphatase Cdc25. Conversely, arrest at G2 in response to DNA damage requires inhibitory phosphorylation of Cdc2. For this to happen, Cdc25 must be inactivated, which occurs when it is phosphorylated on its serine 216 by the protein kinase, Chk1. Chk1, in turn, is activated after DNA damage by other checkpoint proteins, including Rad3 and related proteins.

Cell cycle transition–promoting proteins and the inhibitory proteins work in counterpoint to one another to ensure that cells cycle in an orderly, regulated fashion. Either overabundance of a cycle-promoting activity or deficiency of a cycle-inhibiting activity is expected to result in excessive, unrestricted passage through the cell cycle, with the consequence of unregulated cell proliferation and possible tumor growth, reflecting loss of a cell cycle checkpoint (Hartwell, 1994; Paulovich, 1997). In fact, precisely such alterations have been identified in a number of the cell cycle gene products previously described in a variety of tumor types. One of each of the four genes constituting the p16–cyclin D1–CDK4–pRB pathway, the central regulator of the G1 to S phase transition, is altered in nearly every cancer examined (Levine, 1997). For example, the gene for cyclin D1, CCND1, located on human chromosome 11q13, is overexpressed in many human cancers as a result of amplification or translocation (Hunter and Pines, 1994; Hall and Peters, 1996). In parathyroid adenomas, an inversion, inv(11)(p15;q13), results in a rearrangement that juxtaposes the parathyroid hormone gene to 11q13, the locus of the cyclin D1 gene *CCND1* (known in this work as *PRAD1* for parathyroid adenomatosis), leading to overexpression of cyclin D1 (Arnold et al., 1988; Motokura et al., 1991). Although B lymphocytes normally express only cyclins D2 and D3, in mantle cell lymphomas, the B lineage lymphoma cells express cyclin D1 as a result of the translocation t(11; 14) (q13;q32) which rearranges the cyclin D1 gene (called *BCL1* for B-cell leukemia/lymphoma-1 in this context) to the region of the immunoglobulin heavy chain enhancer on chromosome 14 (Seto et al., 1992; Williams et al., 1992; Komatsu et al., 1994). Other examples of cyclin D1 overexpression result from amplication of its chromosomal region 11q13 in head and neck squamous cell carcinomas (43% of cases), esophageal carcinomas (34%), bladder cancer (15%), primary breast carcinoma (13%), small cell lung cancers (10%), and hepatocellular carcinomas (10%). Although only 13% of breast cancers contain an amplified D1 gene, 50% of breast cancers overexpress D1. Other examples of tumors that overexpress D1 but rarely show D1 gene amplification include sarcomas, colorectal tumors, and melanomas. In addition to cyclin D1, the gene encoding CDK4, its catalytic partner, located on chromosome 12q13, is amplified in various types of sarcomas and central nervous system tumors, particularly gliomas (Hall and Peters, 1996).

Examples also exist of inactivation of inhibitory proteins in specific tumors. Thus, inactivating mutations of the *INK4a* gene (also known as *CDKN2* or *MTS1* for multiple tumor suppressor 1) are found in familial melanomas (Hussussian et al., 1994; Kamb et al., 1994) as well as biliary tract (50%) and esophageal (30%) carcinomas. Homozygous deletions of chromosome 9p21, the *INK4a* locus, are frequently found in gliomas (55%), mesotheliomas (55%), nasopharyngeal carcinomas (40%), acute lymphocytic leukemias (30%), and sarcomas, bladder, and ovarian tumors, as well as cell lines derived from tumors of lung, breast, brain, bone, skin, bladder, kidney, ovary, and lymphocytes (Kamb et al., 1994; Cairns et al., 1995). Inherited loss of *INK4a* has been associated with the familial form of melanoma (Cannon-Albright et al., 1992; Hussussian et al., 1994). Mutations in addition to deletions of *INK4a* are seen in pancreatic, head and neck, and non–small-cell lung carcinomas. An alternative mechanism of evading inactivation of CDK4, a mutation in CDK4 that abrogates its interaction with p16[INK4], is found in melanoma. Additional support for the role of p16[INK4] in tumorigenesis comes from the observation that *INK4a* nullizygous or knockout (INK4a$^{-/-}$) mice develop a variety of different tumors spontaneously by the age of 6 months (Serrano et al., 1996). INK4a$^{-/-}$ mice also show an accelerated rate of tumor formation in response to carcinogenic treatment, whereas fibroblasts from such mice do not senesce and can be transformed by the *RAS* oncogene alone, unlike corresponding wild-type fibroblasts.

One of the prime examples of cancer associated with disruption of a cell cycle inhibitory function by inactivation of the responsible gene involves the *RB* gene (Weinberg, 1995). pRB inactivation via mutation or loss is classically associated with retinoblastoma, where it occurs in both an inherited and a sporadic form (Knudson, 1993). Individuals with germline *RB* mutations also have 2000 times the normal risk of osteosarcoma and a somewhat lower risk of other tumors, including melanoma and soft-tissue sarcoma (Gallie, 1994; Kaelin, 1997). Somatic mutations of the *RB* gene are common in adult cancers, particularly small-cell carcinomas of the lung, but they are also found in non–small-cell lung carcinomas, mesotheliomas, and glioblastomas, as well as cervical, breast, prostatic, bladder, and parathyroid carcinomas (Cryns et al., 1994; Geradts et al., 1995; Weinberg, 1995; Sherr, 1996; Kaelin, 1997). Interestingly, there are data pointing to an inverse correlation between pRB and p16[INK4] expression in certain tumor types (Okamoto et al., 1994; Otterson et al., 1994; Serrano et al., 1996), which is consistent with the observation that the loss of expression of both genes in a single tumor is extremely uncommon (Geradts et al., 1995). p16^{INK4}-mediated inhibition of cellular proliferation depends on the presence of a functional pRB such that inactivation of either tumor suppressor protein is sufficient to allow cell growth and tumorigenesis (Serrano et al., 1995).

3. Genes Responsible for Sensing DNA Damage and Arresting the Cell Cycle to Allow for DNA Repair

There are specific genes whose products carry out surveillance at cell cycle checkpoints in order to detect mistakes, damage, or incompletion of earlier cell cycle events (see above). In response to the detection of a mistake, these gene products inhibit progression through the cell cycle. When the DNA damage caused by exogenous agents such as chemicals or radiation is detected by the surveillance mechanisms at the appropriate checkpoint, cell cycle arrest is induced. The ATM and p53 genes are critical to the induction of cell arrest in mammalian cells in response to DNA damage. Another example involves the surveillance mechanisms that detect the failure of sister kinetochores to be properly aligned on the mitotic spindle and in response block progression into anaphase (Elledge, 1996; Nasmyth, 1996).

a. ATM/TEL

In the disease ataxia telangiectasia (AT), mutation of the *ATM* (AT mutated) gene leads to pleiotropic effects including cerebellar degeneration, immune deficiencies, premature aging, an increased incidence of cancer, and sensitivity to ionizing radiation. The cells from AT patients have defective G1 and G2 damage checkpoints, resulting in the failure to reduce the rate of DNA synthesis and cause mitotic delay in response to DNA damage (Friedberg et al., 1995; Meyn, 1995; Elledge, 1996). This checkpoint failure leads to radiation-resistant DNA synthesis which is ultimately manifested as chromosomal instability and a decreased cellular life span. Premature cellular death, triggered by unrepaired DNA damage, is due to inappropriate p53-mediated apoptosis (see below). A typical aberration seen in AT cells is the end-to-end attachment of chromosomes. Similar chromosomal abnormalities are found in senescing human cells that have short telomeres (Counter et al., 1992), suggesting that AT cells may be defective in some aspect of telomere regulation. In support of this, mutation of the yeast (*Saccharomyces cerevisiae*) gene *tel1*, a homologue of the human *ATM* gene (Greenwell et al., 1995; Morrow et al., 1995; Savitsky et al., 1995), results in shortened telomeres. There is therefore a constellation of attributes (including defective DNA damage sensing/checkpoint, end-to-end attachment of chromosomes, shortened telomeres, cellular senescence, and cancer) which reflects the fact that a single defect in a cell cycle checkpoint, via its effect on DNA repair and telomere integrity, has etiological ramifications for both carcinogenesis and aging. It should be emphasized that there is no definitive evidence proving that the profound sensitivity to ionizing radiation that characterizes AT cells is due to a primary defect in repair of the radiation-damaged DNA (Friedberg et al.,

1995). The predominant phenotype is the failure of AT cells to delay DNA replication in the presence of DNA damage, which has been attributed to loss of G1 checkpoint control rather than defective DNA repair per se.

Malignancy develops in about 10% of AT homozygotes. Leukemia incidence is increased 70-fold and lymphomas 250-fold, with the majority occurring in children (Taylor et al., 1996). Heterozygous carriers of the *ATM* gene may be at significantly increased risk for developing cancer (Kastan, 1995). Studies of AT families have suggested that female relatives of AT patients, presumed to be carriers of the mutated gene, have a five- to eightfold increased risk for breast cancer and may account for up to 8% of all cases of breast cancer in the United States (Swift et al., 1987, 1991). This association, however, has not been consistently supported (FitzGerald et al., 1997).

b. p53

Among the checkpoint controls that are superimposed on the cell cycle is the p53-dependent G1 checkpoint (Sherr, 1996). In this capacity, p53 is a negative regulator of the cyclin D1–CDK4 complex (Levine, 1997). Levels of the p53 protein increase rapidly in response to a variety of signals reflecting cellular distress, such as the DNA damage resulting from ionizing irradiation, hypoxia, decreased ribonucleoside triphosphate pools, and possibly teratogen-induced birth defects (Levine, 1997). As an example, when p53 is upregulated in response to some forms of DNA damage, it activates transcription of one of its downstream targets, the p21 gene (*WAF1, CIP1*) (El-Deiry, 1993; Harper, 1993). p21, in turn, binds to several cyclin–CDK complexes (cyclin D1–Cdk4, cyclin E–Cdk2, cyclin A–Cdk2, cyclin A–Cdc2) and inhibits the function of the cyclin-dependent kinases, leading to G1 arrest. There may also be a role for p53 in a G2-M phase checkpoint (Cross et al., 1995). When cells are chemically blocked in G2, cells with wild-type p53 remain blocked, whereas cells lacking wild-type p53 reinitiate DNA sythesis, increasing the ploidy of the cells. Cultured fibroblasts from p53$^{-/-}$ (null) mice have abnormal numbers of centrosomes and produce spindle apparatuses with multiple poles, resulting in aneuploidy after a few cell passages. p53 Also participates at the G0–G1 checkpoint, since the *Gas1* gene, whose product maintains the cell in G0 arrest, can do so only when wild-type p53 is present in the cell (Del Sal et al., 1995).

p53 is mutated in over 50% of human cancers, more than any other single gene (Hollstein, 1991). Germline mutations of p53 are found in the Li-Fraumeni syndrome, in which affected individuals develop such cancers as breast carcinoma, soft-tissue sarcomas, brain tumors, osteosarcoma, leukemia, and adrenocortical carcinoma (Malkin et al., 1990). Somatic mutations of p53 are found in many tumor types, including cancers of the lung, both small-cell and non–small-cell, breast (58%) (Carey and Davidson, 1997), colon, esophagus, liver, bladder, ovary, and brain, as well as sarcomas, lymphomas, and leukemias (Hollstein, 1991). In contrast to the alterations observed in other tumor-suppressor genes, a very high percentage of p53 mutations (80%) are missense mutations (Harris and Hallstein, 1993). The mutant p53 products of such genes generally have much longer half-lives than the wild-type protein, resulting in immunohistochemically detectable accumulated p53 in the affected cells. The spectrum of DNA base substitutions differs for different types of cancer. Furthermore, specific environmental insults appear to be associated with particular p53 missense mutations in specific tumors. Thus, studies of p53 mutations in hepatocellular carcinoma revealed that exposure to high levels of aflatoxin B1, a fungal toxin, leads to an AGG to AGT mutation at codon 49 of p53 in 58% of hepatocellular carcinomas from Qidong, China, a region that is at high risk for this disease (Aguilar et al., 1994). Such a mutation is rarely seen in hepatocellular carcinomas from Western countries. Finally, allelic loss or accumulation of p53 protein has been correlated with prognosis in several types of cancer, including breast cancer, non–small-cell lung cancer, transitional cell bladder carcinoma, and, most recently, aggressive B-cell lymphoma (Ichikawa et al., 1997).

B. Signal Transduction

Environmental signals provide the impetus as well as the restraints to the cell for embarking on one of its potential outcomes: cell cycle progression, apoptosis, differentiation, or continued quiescence. The coupling of the cell's response to extracellular signals is carried out by a cascade of molecular interactions flowing from cellular receptors internally to the nucleus resulting in the expression of new gene products such as the molecules responsible for enabling the cell to traverse the cell cycle (Hunter and Pines, 1997; Fenton and Longo, 1998). There are multiple cascades that contribute to this process of signal transduction (Fig. 2). The signal transduction cascades converge on factors that either repress or activate transcription as a means of eliciting the appropriate cellular response (Hill and Treisman, 1995). The immediate environmental stimulus to signal transduction is a ligand, a molecule that physically interacts with receptors in or on the cell. Thus, two types of receptors, cytoplasmic and cell surface receptors, mediate interactions between environmental stimuli and the cell.

1. Cytoplasmic Receptors

The cytoplasmic receptors belong to the intracellular receptor or steroid hormone receptor superfamily. In the presence of ligand, such receptors translocate to the nucleus and bind to specific DNA sequence motifs called response elements. These response elements are located within the transcriptional promoter or enhancer regions of genes that are under the control of hormones (Mangelsdorf et al., 1995). Examples of ligands that elicit specific cellular responses by binding to cytoplasmic receptors include glucocorticoids, thyroid hormone, and retinoids (Kastner et al., 1995). Mutations or rearrangements of the genes for cytoplasmic receptors resulting in abnormal expression of the protein product have been associated with specific malignancies. Thus, the t(15;17) translocation found in acute promyelocytic leuke-

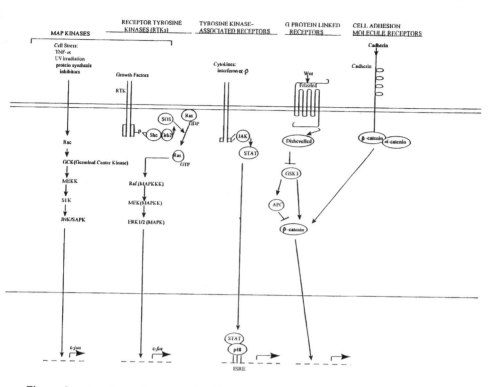

Figure 2   Signaling pathways involved in cancer. Examples of signaling pathways mediated by receptor tyrosine kinases (Ras/ERK), tyrosine kinase–associated receptors (JAK/STAT), and G protein–linked receptors (Wnt/Frizzled, β-adrenergic receptor) are diagrammed. Two signal transduction pathways which operate via a mitogen-activated protein kinase (MAPK) cascade are shown: the Ras/ERKs and the JNK/SAPKs. Also shown is a signaling pathway emanating from cadherin, a receptor belonging to the integrin family of cell adhesion molecules (CAMs). The cadherin and Wnt/Frizzled pathways intersect downstream in that both mobilize the transcriptional regulator β-catenin. (Adapted from Hunter and Pines, 1997 and Fenton and Longo, 1998.)

mia generates a chimeric protein consisting of the retinoic acid receptor-α fused to a portion of the PML (promyelocytic leukemia) protein (Warrell et al., 1993). The precise mechanism by which this translocation induces PML is not completely clear. However, in the presence of its ligand, the chimeric receptor correctly translocates to the nucleus and the malignant cells differentiate.

2. Cell Surface Receptors

The second large category of receptors includes those that span the cell membrane. Specific domains within a receptor molecule subserve specific functions. Thus, the extracellular domain operates as binding site for ligand. A lipophilic region functions as the transmembrane domain, and the intracytoplasmic region relays the signal initiated at the time of receptor–ligand interaction to the molecular component which is just downstream of the receptor in the cell, initiating a signal transduction cascade. One type of signaling system that is commonly used by cells to transduce extracellular cues into intracellular responses is the mitogen-activated protein kinase (MAPK) cascade (Cano and Mahadevan, 1995). MAPKs are activated by phosphorylation on threonine and tyrosine residues, and they in turn phosphorylate their substrates on serine or threonine residues adjacent to prolines. The result is a cascade of activating phosphorylations on successive molecules; that is, successive MAPKs, each of which relays its activated state via the mechanism of phosphorylation to the next molecule downstream (see examples below). One consequence of the activation of the MAPK cascade is the expression of AP-1 transcription factor family members, including members of the *fos* and *jun* oncogene family members (Whitmarsh and Davis, 1996; Karin et al., 1997). There are three major categories of cell surface receptors: Ion channel-linked receptors, G protein–linked receptors, and enzyme-linked receptors. Ion channel–linked receptors are involved primarily in neurotransmitter signal transduction as opposed to the other two types of receptors which are important in tumorigenesis.

a.   *G Protein–Linked Receptors*

In contrast to the enzyme-linked receptors described below, the G protein–linked receptors do not directly induce covalent modification in their substrates (Sausville and Longo, 1997). Rather, following the binding of ligand, G protein–linked receptors elaborate second-messenger molecules that in turn allosterically modify target effector molecules, such as protein kinases and phospholipases. In the prototypic example, binding of ligand to the β-adrenergic receptor leads to activation of adenylyl cyclase which converts ATP to cyclic AMP (cAMP), the second messenger (Levitzki, 1988). The cAMP in turn binds to the regulatory subunits of the target cAMP-dependent protein kinase (protein kinase A, or PKA). Following cAMP-induced activation, PKA enters the nucleus to mediate phosphorylation and thereby activation of the transcription factor cyclic AMP response element binding protein (CREB) (Ghosh, 1995). Although CREB binds specifically to a DNA consensus sequence found in the promoters of many genes, including c-*fos*, phosphorylation at specific sites on CREB is required before it can interact with the polymerase II transcription machinery to initiate transcription. The role for the ''G protein'' in this sequence of events is to act as a molecular ''switch'' which enables the ligand-bound receptor to activate the adenylate cyclase.

    The G protein, a large heterotrimeric complex of α, β, and γ subunits, interacts with the intracellular carboxyl terminal of the ligand-bound receptor, after which the Gα subunit binds to GTP and is released from the trimer. A given subtype of GTP-Gα mediates a specific function, such as stimulation of adenylyl cyclase (G_s)

and inhibition of adenylyl cyclase (G_i) in the example cited above, as well as regulation of calcium and potassium channels (G_s and G_o) and stimulation of phospholipase Cβ (G_q and G_{16}), until its GTP is hydrolyzed by a guanosine triphosphatase (GTPase) activity to yield GDP–Gα. Hydrolysis is stimulated by a GTPase-activating protein (GAP) (Millman and Andrews, 1997). The subfamily of GAPs that stimulate GTPase hydrolysis of the large heterotrimeric G proteins has been designated regulators of G protein–signaling (RGS) (Iyengar, 1997). The GDP-bound α chain then reassociates with the $\beta\gamma$ chains, and the trimer is ready for another response. Since GDP–Gα subunits have much lower affinities for effectors than do GTP–Gα complexes, hydrolysis by the GTPase terminates signaling through the Gα subunit. Other molecules besides cAMP which serve as second messengers that are induced on G protein–linked receptor stimulation include cGMP and Ca^{2+}. Thus, stimulation of Gα_q protein–linked receptors leads to activation of phospholipase Cβ (PLCβ), which hydrolyses phosphoinositide 4,5-bisphosphate (PIP2) into diacylglycerol (DAG) and inositol triphosphate (IP$_3$) (Berridge, 1995; Umemori, et al., 1997). IP$_3$, a second messenger in its own right, causes release of Ca^{2+} from intracellular stores, leading ultimately to the stimulation of DNA synthesis and cell proliferation.

The other product of PLCβ, DAG, also serves a proliferation-inducing function via activation of protein kinase C (PKC) which in turn activates the MAPK cascade and phosphorylates IκB (Nishizuka, 1992; Fenton and Longo, 1998). Just as the MAPK-signaling pathway culminates in stimulation of expression of transcription factors in the AP-1 family, phosphorylation of IκB, which normally binds to and retains transcription factors of the Rel/NF-κB family in the cytoplasm, results in its ubiquitin-mediated degradation and the nuclear translocation of Rel/NF-κB (Beg and Baldwin, 1993; Brown et al., 1995). Thus, MAPK cascade activation leads via independent pathways to upregulation of transcription, with a resulting increase in cellular proliferation. In opposition to this effect, glucocorticoids induce IκB synthesis, inhibiting NF-κB and in turn the immunoregulatory genes that are the targets of its transcriptional activation effects (Auphan et al., 1995; Scheinman et al., 1995).

The involvement of the G protein–linked receptor pathways has been documented in several tumors. A subset of growth hormone–secreting pituitary tumors (18 of 42) contain mutations of the Gα_s gene which inhibit its ability to hydrolyze bound GTP, leading to constitutive activation of the Gα_s protein (Lyons, 1990). The presence of a mutation in the Gα_{i2} gene in 3 of 11 adrenal cortex tumors and 3 of 10 endocrine tumors of the ovary suggests that the mutated Gα_{i2} protein has lost its ability to inhibit adenylyl cyclase. Evidence implicating downstream components of G protein–linked receptor pathways in carcinogenesis comes from the *bcl-3* oncogene, a member of the IκB family that was originally identified by its location adjacent to a chromosomal breakpoint associated with chronic lymphocytic leukemia (Ohno et al., 1990; Hatada et al., 1992). In another example, B chronic lymphocytic leukemia (B-CLL) and hairy cell leukemia (HCL) cells fail to generate nuclear-localized c-*jun* and c-*fos* proteins (components of AP-1) in response to mitogenic stimulation, a signal transduction defect which is believed to be due to problems in the coupling of the protein kinase C–dependent pathways (Jabbar et al., 1995).

b. Enzyme-Linked Receptors

The enzyme-linked receptors induce covalent modifications in their substrate proteins, typically the addition of phosphate groups to specific amino acid sites. At least five classes of enzyme-linked receptors have been described: receptor guanylyl cyclases, receptor tyrosine kinases, tyrosine kinase–associated receptors, receptor tyrosine phosphatases, and receptor serine/threonine kinases. The last four categories are known to play an important role in cancer.

Receptor Tyrosine Kinases. Many of the traditional growth factors bind to transmembrane receptors with tyrosine kinase activity, the protein receptor tyrosine kinases (Fenton and Longo, 1998). These receptors can be classified into families named for members showing specificity for growth factor ligands such as platelet-derived growth factor (PDGF), epidermal growth factor (EGF), fibroblast growth factors (FGFs), insulin and insulin-like growth factors (IGF) I and II, nerve growth factor, and vascular endothelial growth factor (VEGF). Binding of ligand, or growth factor, to the receptor induces dimerization of receptor subunits (Heidin, 1995). This in turn leads to activation of the receptor's tyrosine kinase activity and resulting autophosphorylation of the intracellular domains of the receptor chains. Some of the autophosphorylated sites serve as docking sites for the src-homology region 2 (SH2) domains (named for the *src* nonreceptor tyrosine kinase in which the SH2 domain was first identified) that are present in the signal transduction molecules downstream of the receptor. The association of the receptor with the SH2 domains of such downstream molecules triggers subsequent events. In the case of downstream molecules that lack a docking domain, association with the receptor is facilitated by adaptor proteins that consist solely of docking domains.

As an example, in mammalian cells, the *ras*/ERK pathway provides a common route by which signals from different growth factor receptor tyrosine kinases converge downstream to regulate the transcription of the transcription factor c-*fos* and other coregulated genes (Hill and Treisman, 1995). Ras, a 21-kDa protein, is a small G protein that belongs to the same GTPase superfamily as the $G\alpha_s$ component of the large heterotrimeric G protein discussed above. It is normally attached to the inner cell membrane via an isoprenyl lipid group that is added by the enzyme farnesyl transferase (Casey, 1995). The farnesylated Ras is bound to GDP and, as such, is inactive in unstimulated cells. Following stimulation of the receptor tyrosine kinase by its ligand, the guanine nucleotide exchange factor SOS (son of sevenless, named for its role in *Drosophila* eye development) is brought close to the membrane, and thus to Ras, by association with the adaptor protein grb2 (named "grabbed" because it grabbed phosphotyrosine-containing proteins). SOS then removes GDP from Ras and adds GTP. The GTP-bound Ras then initiates activation via phosphorylation of a sequence of proteins conforming to a MAPK-signaling system (see above), including Raf (a MAPKKK), then MEK (a MAPKK), and finally ERK 1/ ERK 2 (extracellular signal response kinases; MAPKs) (Cano and Mahadevan, 1995; Mochly-Rosen, 1995). The activated ERK molecules enter the nucleus where they target transcription factors, such as c-*fos*, that regulate expression of genes responsible for a variety of cellular outcomes (growth, differentiation, survival, growth arrest, apoptosis).

The *ras*/ERK pathways also offer examples of how mutations in components of a signal transduction cascade cause abnormal functioning, which leads ultimately to unregulated growth and tumorigenesis. Activating mutations of H-*ras*, K-*ras* and N-*ras*, all members of the *ras* family, have been found in human tumors (Hunter and Pines, 1997). In fact, the frequency of *ras* mutations is among the highest observed for any gene in human cancers, with K-*ras* being the most commonly mutated, particularly in its codon 12 (Fearon and Cho, 1996). K-*ras* mutations appear in about 50% of colorectal cancers, about 70–90% of pancreatic cancers, and about 30% of adenocarcinomas of the lung. H-*ras* mutations occur in about 10% of bladder cancers, whereas N-*ras* mutations have been detected in about 20–30% of acute nonlymphocytic leukemias but only infrequently in epithelial cancers. The oncogenic mutations at codons 12, 13, and 61 of *ras* impair the ability of the Ras protein to hydrolyze GTP to GDP as a result of a reduced affinity of Ras for Ras–GAP, its specific GTPase-activating protein (Fearon and Cho, 1996; Scheffzek et al., 1997; Sprang, 1997). As a result, the Ras protein remains in the GTP-bound, or ''active,'' state, leading to constitutive activation of the Ras-dependent signal transduction cascade and the consequent effects on cellular growth. Just as with the 50% of colorectal carcinomas mentioned above, a similar percentage of adenomas larger than 1 cm are characterized by *ras* mutations, with 80% occurring at K-*ras* codon 12 and 15% at K-*ras* codon 13. In contrast, the smaller adenomas less than 1 cm in size have *ras* mutations in only 5–10% of cases (Vogelstein et al., 1988). These findings suggest that mutation in the *ras* gene contributes to the progression from small adenomas to larger, clinically more significant adenomas. The Ras protein is involved indirectly in oncogenesis in individuals afflicted with the hereditary disease neurofibromatosis which is characterized by a variety of benign and malignant tumors (Fearon and Cho, 1996; Gutmann et al., 1997). The NF1 gene, which encodes neurofibromin, a GAP protein responsible for inactivating Ras by hydrolysis of its GTP to GDP, is mutated to an inactive form in this disease, resulting in a constitutively activated Ras protein (Basu et al., 1992; Side et al., 1997).

Members of the receptor tyrosine kinase family carry mutations in a number of epithelial cancers. Lung, bladder, breast, head and neck, gastric, and ovarian cancers have been shown to overexpress EGF receptors, IGF-I receptors, and HER-2/Neu/ErbB2 (Dickson and Lippman, 1995; Fearon and Cho, 1996). In addition, the *met* proto-oncogene, which encodes a receptor tyrosine kinase, contains missense mutations in its tyrosine kinase domain in the germline of affected individuals in families with hereditary papillary renal cell carcinoma (HPRC), as well as in a subset of patients with sporadic papillary renal carcinomas (Schmidt et al., 1997). The *met*/HGF (hepatocyte growth factor/scatter factor) proto-oncogene also offers an example of how alteration of a tyrosine kinase receptor can result in its constitutive dimerization, independent of ligand, with resultant activation of the cytoplasmic catalytic domain (Hunter and Pines, 1997). A genomic rearrangement placing *tpr* (translocated promoter region) from chromosome 1 into the *met* locus on chromosome 7 results in production of the Tpr-Met fusion protein, where the N-terminal of Tpr mediates dimerization of the attached Met/HGF receptor domain leading to constitutive activation and oncogenic transformation (Rodrigues and Park, 1993; Hunter and Pines, 1997). Similarly, fusion of *tpr* sequences to the kinase domain of the *trk*/nerve growth factor (NGF) receptor tyrosine kinase has been noted in human thyroid papillary tumors (Greco et al., 1992). Furthermore, point mutations in specific portions of other receptor tyrosine kinases, such as the transmembrane domain of HER-2/Neu/ErbB2 and the extracellular domain of the CSF-1 receptor, cause dimerization. The t(5;12) translocation which characterizes chronic myelomonocytic leukemia results in the Tel–platelet-derived growth factor-β (PDGF-β) receptor fusion protein wherein the N-terminal of Tel, a transcription factor, mediates dimerization and resulting constitutive activation of the attached cytoplasmic domain of the PDGFβ receptor tyrosine kinase. In CD30$^+$ anaplastic large cell lymphomas, fusion of NPM (nucleolar protein B/nucleophosmin) to ALK (anaplastic lymphoma kinase), a protein receptor tyrosine kinase, as a result of a t(2;5) translocation leads to oligomerization and constitutive activation of the kinase with resulting cellular transformation (Fujimoto et al., 1996; Hunter and Pines, 1997). Constitutive activation of Ret, another receptor tyrosine kinase, can also result from fusion of its cytoplasmic domain to a variety of N-terminal domains that mediate constitutive dimerization and activation (Hunter and Pines, 1997). In addition, mutations in *ret* have been noted in human tumors, including thyroid papillary carcinomas, as well as such hereditary syndromes as multiple endocrine neoplasia (MEN) 2A, MEN 2B and medullary thyroid carcinoma (Mulligan et al., 1993; Eng, 1996; Eng et al., 1996). Although the constitutive activation of Ret in MEN 2A is due to a mutation in a cysteine (Cys634Arg) which leads to dimerization, its activation, as well as a change in substrate specificity, MEN 2B results from a mutation in the catalytic domain (Met918Thr).

As might be expected, the converse type of mutation in components of the *ras*/ERK pathway can lead to resistance to activation. Mutations in the promoter of the downstream target of this signaling cascade, c-*fos*, inhibit binding of the *ras*/ERK–activated regulatory factors Elk-1 and SAP-1 and thereby prevent c-*fos* from being activated by growth factors and mitogens or by intracellular activators of the pathway such as v-*raf* (Graham and Gilman, 1991; Hill and Treisman, 1995). Similarly, a kinase-defective mutant of ERK 2 inhibits v-*raf*–dependant c-*fos* expression (Kortenjann et al., 1994). The inability to activate a growth-promoting transcriptional factor such as c-*fos* is anticipated to confer resistance to cellular transformation by normal activators of this oncogene. Accordingly, the mutant ERK 2 also inhibits v-*raf*–dependent transformation.

Tyrosine Kinase–Associated Receptors/Nonreceptor Tyrosine Kinases. The cellular responses to cytokines such as growth hormone, prolactin, erythropoietin, interleukin-2 (IL-2), IL-3, IL-4, IL-6, IL-7, granulocyte colony-stimulating factor (CSF), granulocyte-macrophage CSF, interferon-α (INF-α), and interferon-γ (INF-γ) are mediated by a signaling system in which protein phosphorylation depends on nonreceptor tyrosine kinases (Taniguchi, 1995; Fenton and Longo, 1998). The receptor in such cases consists of multiple subunits which form heteromers or homodimers but which lack intrinsic tyrosine kinase activity. The ability of these receptors to transmit proliferative signals to the cell on engagement of ligand depends on their recruitment of ancillary molecules necessary for signal transmission; thus, their designation as tyrosine kinase–associated receptors. Three families of kinases are associated with this class of receptors and function in such an ancillary capacity to transduce the receptor-initiated signal into a cascade of phosphorylation: Src family, Syk family, and Janus family kinases. The Src family kinases (Src, Yes, Fyn, Lyn, Lck, Blk, Hck, Fgr, Yrk) can associate with receptor tyrosine kinases as well as with tyrosine kinase–associated receptors, both leading to signaling via similar cascades. Lck, for example, is physically associated with the interleukin-2 receptor (IL-2R) βc chain in the absence of IL-2 stimulation but is rapidly activated on ligand binding to the IL-2R, priming it to initiate a signaling cascade which culminates in the induction of the c-*fos* and c-*jun* genes (Taniguchi, 1995). The Syk family (includes Syk, ZAP-70) kinase, Syk, also interacts with the IL-2R, but signals initiated by receptor engagement in this case lead to the induction of the c-*myc* oncogene rather than c-*fos* and c-*jun*. Finally, the Janus kinase (JAK) family members (Jak1, Jak2, Jak3, Tyk2, hopscotch [*Drosophila*]) are involved in signaling from cytokine receptors. Each JAK family member associates selectively with specific cytokine receptors, such as IL-2R (Hill and Treisman, 1995; Ihle, 1995; Taniguchi, 1995). Following ligand binding, receptor molecules aggregate, causing concomitant aggregation of homotypic or heterotypic JAKs, resulting in their activation by cross phosphorylation. These activated JAKs in turn activate the STAT (signal transducers and activators of transcription) class of transcription factors which, once phosphorylated, complex with a DNA-binding protein and move to the nucleus where they initiate transcription from specific target genes. The prototypic example of a JAK/STAT pathway is IFN-regulated gene expression in which engagement of the type I IFN (IFN-α and INF-β) receptor by ligand INF-α or INF-β elicits formation of a STAT 1 and 2/DNA–binding protein p48 complex which targets genes bearing the interferon-response element (ISRE) in their promoters.

Mutations have been observed in the JAK/STAT signaling cascade. Inactivation of the IL-2R has been traced to deletions or mutations in its γ_c chain that disrupt its association with Jak3, leading to X-linked severe combined immunodeficiency in humans (Ihle, 1995). Similarly, a Jak2 mutant lacking kinase activity dominantly disrupts the cellular response to erythropoietin or IL-6. Transformation has been shown to result from JAK mutations in *Drosophila* as well as from mutations leading to constitutive dimerization of cytokine receptors with resulting constitutive JAK activation. However, thus far, JAKs have not been shown to transform mammalian cells.

Serine–Threonine Kinase Receptors.   Among this class of receptors are those that recognize TGF-β, a molecule which induces fibroblast proliferation but inhibits the proliferation of most cell types (Hill and Treisman, 1995; Fenton and Longo, 1998). Tumor growth factor-β mutations that result in the loss of expression or function have been detected in tumors of colon cancer and lymphomas (Markowitz et al., 1995; Parsons et al., 1995).

Tyrosine Phosphatase Receptors.   The prototypical example of a tyrosine phosphatase receptor is the T-cell antigen CD45 which, on activation by an unknown ligand, removes phosphate from an inhibitory site on Lck, a Src family kinase. The dephosphorylation of Lck then permits signal transduction through the T-cell antigen receptor. Mutations in tyrosine phosphatase receptors are not yet known to contribute to carcinogenesis.

Guanylyl Cyclase Receptors.   The atrial natriuretic peptide receptor is a guanylyl cyclase receptor. Some evidence points to a role for this receptor in the paraneoplastic manifestation of hyponatremia in small-cell lung cancer (Johnson et al., 1997), but a direct role in tumorigenesis has not yet been documented for this molecule.

C. Cell Adhesion

Adhesion between normal epithelial cells, the cell of origin for carcinomas, is generally strong and stable. In contrast, cell–cell association often becomes disorganized in tumors, a feature that may contribute to their unregulated growth, resulting in invasion and metastasis (Takeichi, 1993). The loss or inactivation of the molecules that mediate normal cell adhesion may underlie the cellular dissociation observed in tumors.

The integrins, which are transmembrane receptors, constitute one such family of cell adhesion molecules (CAMs) (Wagner, 1995). In a manner analogous to the receptors just described, which are stimulated by binding to soluble ligands, the integrins function as receptors, but they are activated by ligands that are contained in the extracellular matrix (ECM) (such as proteins or glycoseaminoglycans) or on the surface of neighboring cells (Ruoslahti, 1997). In addition to providing a mechanical link between the cell surface and the ECM, integrins link the external ECM ''cytoskeleton'' to the intracellular actin cytoskeleton at specialized membrane structures called focal adhesions, which contain many accessory cytoskeletal proteins as well as signaling molecules. Thus, the integrins also trigger several signaling pathways. By transducing extracellular messages from the ECM and from other cells into internal signaling pathways, the integrins regulate cellular processes pertaining to shape, movement, cell–cell and cell–ECM adhesion. The focal adhesion kinase (FAK) pathway, for example, plays a role in the control of anchorage dependence, the dependence of cell growth and survival on substrate attachment. A form of FAK that does not require integrins and cell attachment for activation can lead to anchorage-independent cell growth, a characteristic of cancer cells.

Of the CAM families, only the integrins and the cadherins require calcium to carry out their adhesion function. The extracellular portion of cadherins mediates their adhesive activity by homophilic binding to similar cadherins, whereas the short cytoplasmic tail is anchored to the cytoskeletal actin microfilaments through proteins called catenins. The catenins in turn carry out dual functions. In addition to its role in promoting cell adhesion via mediation of an interaction between cadherins and the cytoskeleton, β-catenin performs a signaling function as part of the Wnt signaling pathway (Hunter, 1997). The gene *wnt1*, originally identified as an oncogene activated by proviral insertion in MMTV (mouse mammary tumor virus)–induced mouse mammary carcinomas, produces a secreted protein, Wnt1, that binds to the G protein–linked receptor Frizzled. In this manner, Wnt1 activates a signaling pathway that involves a complex interplay among several proteins: GSK3 (glycogen synthase kinase 3), APC (adenomatous polyposis coli), and β-catenin (see Fig. 2). Free β-catenin associates with a number of transcription factors to drive transcription and presumably cell proliferation. To counter this, APC, phosphorylated by GSK3, associates with and sequesters α- and β-catenin and triggers degradation of free β-catenin, thereby causing downregulation of transcription. On the other hand, *wnt1* signaling leads to inactivation of GSK3, and thus APC, allowing release and stabilization of β-catenin with resulting upregulation of transcription.

The intertwining pathways just described have multiple vulnerable points at which alteration of function may lead to cancer. For instance, in most vertebrates, expression of at least one cadherin and the presence of Ca^{2+} are required to form solid tissue. Thus, the loss of epithelial cadherin (E-cadherin) expression has been shown to correlate with the invasive potential of tumor cells (Takeichi, 1993; Overduin et al., 1995). The free pool of β-catenin is expected to increase following Wnt activation or APC inactivation or loss, with a resultant increase in transcription and cell growth. In fact, the oncogenic potential of activated *wnt* alleles in virus-induced tumors is paralleled by the mammary hyperplasia and tumorigenesis that occurs in *wnt* (particularly *wnt1* and *wnt3*) transgenic mice (Nusse and Varmus, 1992). Similarly, truncating APC mutations, found in the germline DNA of individuals with the inherited disease familial adenomatous polyposis as well as in the somatic DNA of the majority of sporadic colorectal carcinomas, release enough β-catenin to upregulate transcription in colon cancer cell lines, a feature that may well underlie tumorigenesis. The APC gene has thus been attributed a ''gatekeeper'' function in that it is responsible for maintaining a constant cell number in the colonic epithelium, ensuring appropriate responses to conditions requiring net cell growth (e.g., tissue damage), presumably by sequestering and only judiciously releasing β-catenin, a stimulus to cell growth (Kinzler and Vogelstein, 1996; Nusse, 1997).

D. Patterns of Gene Expression

As indicated above, signaling cascades frequently culminate downstream in the induction of transcription factors, proteins that directly control gene expression by binding to specific short DNA sequences in the promoter regions of their target genes. Three essential features characterize such factors: first, the ability to bind to specific short sequences (consensus sequences) of DNA; second, the subsequent interaction with other factors or with the RNA polymerase itself in order to regulate transcription either positively or negatively. Third, for factors that operate in response to particular stimuli or in a particular tissue, either the synthesis or activity of the factor must itself be appropriately controlled (Latchman, 1990). Each transcription factor contains specific amino acid sequences, or motifs, which cause it to assume a distinct three-dimensional conformation that mediates its interaction with DNA at its consensus sequence. An example of such a structural motif is the zinc finger, which is found in factors that regulate RNA polymerase III (TFIIIA, regulating 5S ribosomal RNA genes) and, in some cases, RNA polymerase II (e.g., Sp1, *Drosophila kruppel*, yeast ADR1). Other motifs, such as the leucine zipper, do not act directly on DNA binding but rather facilitate homo- or heterodimerization of transcription factor(s), which in turn results in the correct structure for DNA binding by the adjacent amino acid regions. The liver-specific transcription factor C/EBP and the proto-oncogene proteins Myc, Fos, and Jun, downstream targets in various signaling pathways, conform to this pattern.

The specific pattern of expression of a given factor with regard to timing and tissue type results at least in part from the particular combination of signaling pathways that regulate it. Additional features such as chromatin condensation make different regions of the genome available or unavailable for transcription. The organization of chromatin is largely based on histones, basic proteins that aggregate to form a core around which DNA is wound to form nucleosomes. Thus, the accessibility of transcription factors to promoter regions of target genes can be regulated by the reversible acetylation of lysine residues clustered near the NH_2-terminus of the histones (Taunton et al., 1996; Wolffe, 1996), with core histone acetylation promoting gene expression and histone deacetylation leading to transcriptional repression (Pazin and Kodonaga, 1997). Methylation of cytosine residues in critical cytosine- and guanosine-rich regions of a gene can inhibit transcription. Besides transcription, gene expression may be regulated at other levels. The proteins apoferritin and thymidylate synthase, for example, regulate the translation of their own messenger RNAs by binding to the message and preventing the initiation of protein synthesis.

In humans, changes in the expression of specific oncogenes that encode transcription factors leads to malignancy (Latchman, 1996). Increased expression may be due to translocation of the proto-oncogene to the vicinity of a promoter or enhancer region. Examples of resulting cancers include Burkitt's lymphoma in which the t(8;14) translocation juxtaposes the c-*myc* oncogene (chromosome 8) with the immunoglobulin heavy chain locus (Spencer and Groudine, 1991) and acute childhood leukemia in which the homeobox-containing gene *HOX-11* is activated by translocation to the T-cell receptor locus (Hatano et al., 1991). Translocation of transcription factors may result in oncogenic fusion proteins, as in the case of chronic myelomonocytic leukemia where the Ets transcription factor is fused to the receptor for platelet-derived growth factor. In other cases, fusion of the genes for two transcription factors results in an oncogenic fusion protein, such as that consisting of the retinoic acid receptor-α (a member of the steroid-thyroid receptor gene family) fused to the promyelocytic leukemia transcription factor in acute promyelocytic leukemia. In another example, a t(2;13) translocation fuses the PAX-2 and the FKHR transcription factors into a transcriptional activator that is stronger than either alone and results in alveolar rhabdomyosarcoma (Fredericks et al., 1995).

Apart from the aberrant expression of specific genes in cancer cells, there is evidence for a difference in the overall array of genes that are expressed in cancer versus normal cells. Application of new technological advances has made possible the elucidation of such differential expression between tumor and normal cells in comparisons of messenger RNA expression from colon tumors, for example, to messenger RNA from normal colon cell lines (Zhang et al., 1997).

E. Angiogenesis

The development and maintenance of normal tissues requires concurrent development, maintenance, and appropriate remodeling of a supportive vascular network. Two processes contribute to the construction of blood vessels: vasculogenesis, the appearance of new vessels, and angiogenesis, the sprouting of new vessels from preexisting vessels (Folkman, 1995; Sage, 1996; Hanahan, 1997). Normal angiogenesis depends on a balance between endogenous positive and negative regulatory molecules which act in a paracrine fashion to establish and remodel blood vessels (Hanahan, 1997; Maisonpierre et al., 1997). Disruption of this balance characterizes carcinogenesis, since dysregulated proliferation of the primary neoplastic cell type, at least in the clinically detectable stages, depends on accompanying neovascularization for support. A number of protein ligands have been shown to bind and modulate transmembrane receptor tyrosine kinases on endothelial cells. The ligand vascular endothelial growth factor (VEGF) (also called vascular permeability factor, VPF) interacts with the endothelial cell–selective receptor tyrosine kinases VEGF-R1 (Flt1) and VEGF-R2 (Flk1/KDR) to promote the components of vasculogenesis: cell birth, migration, and proliferation (VEGF-R1); and tube assembly and cell–cell interaction (VEGF-R2). The ligand Ang (angiopoietin) 1 binds to the Tie2 (Tek) receptor tyrosine kinase to mediate recruitment of and interaction with periendothelial support cells. Both Ang1 and a largely homologous Ang2 modulate a fourth endothelial cell–selective receptor tyrosine kinase, Tie1, to loosen periendothelial support by the loss of structure and matrix contacts, thereby allowing exposure of endothelial cells to activating signals from angiogenesis inducers, including VEGF. Ang1 and Ang2 act in an antithetical fashion, the former signaling Tie2 to recruit support cells, the latter inhibiting this activity via Tie1 signaling. Differential expression of these three ligands characterizes vascular morphogenesis (VEGF), maintenance (Ang1), remodeling (Ang2 and VEGF), and regression (Ang2). Other factors have been implicated in this balanced regulation of vasculogenesis and angiogenesis in the embryo as well as physiological and pathological angiogenesis in the adult. In addition to the receptor tyrosine kinases, G protein–linked receptors participate in the regulation of angiogenesis. For example, disruption of the gene encoding the α subunit of the heterotrimeric G_{13} protein in mice impairs the ability of endothelial cells to develop into an organized vascular system, resulting in intrauterine death (Offermanns et al., 1997). In another example, platelet-derived growth factor-β (PDGF-β), a high-affinity ligand for the receptor tyrosine kinases PDGFR-α and -β, appears to be necessary for the migration of pericytes to the capillary wall (Lindahl et al., 1997). PDGF-β–deficient mouse embryos lack microvascular pericytes and develop capillary microaneurysms as a result of mechanical instability of the wall.

There are at least two aspects of tumor neovascularization that are relevant to clinical oncology. On the one hand, the growth of solid tumors beyond a certain critical mass as well as the pathogenesis of metastases correlate with tumor vascularity. The density of microvessels in lymph node–negative breast cancer was shown to be a better predictor of metastasis than tumor grade, tumor size, estrogen receptor positivity, or other prognostic markers (Folkman, 1995). In other types of tumors as well, a positive correlation between tumor angiogenesis and the risk of metastasis, tumor recurrence, or death has been noted. A direct correlation has been noted between p53 accumulation, a manifestation of mutant p53, and microvessel count and between p53 accumulation and VEGF expression in non–small-cell lung cancer. These observations are consistent with the hypothesis that wild-type p53 regulates the angiogenic process via an angiogenesis inhibitor that acts on VEGF (Fontanini et al., 1997).

In view of such prognostic associations, therapeutic interventions aimed at the inhibition of angiogenesis are being studied in clinical trials as treatment for a variety of solid tumors, including breast, colon, lung, and prostate cancer. The second clinically pertinent issue is the somewhat paradoxical observation that neovascularization gradually reduces the accessibility of a tumor to chemotherapeutic drugs. Tumors are well perfused in the earliest stages of neovascularization. However, as tumors become clinically detectable, increased interstitial pressure from leaky vessels, exacerbated by the paucity of intratumor lymphatics, causes vascular compression and ultimately central necrosis. Antiangiogenic therapy offers a potential clinical approach to this obstacle of poor drug delivery, since studies in rodents have shown increased perfusion of tumor by chemotherapeutic drugs when they are administered concomitantly with antiangiogenic agents. Inhibitors of angiogenesis that have been studied in clinical trials in patients with advanced cancer include platelet factor-4, thalidomide, interleukin-12,and linomide. In some cases, the intracellular targets or effects of antiangiogenic agents have been demonstrated. Thus, fumagillin (AGM-1470) interacts with several cyclins (E, A) or their associated kinases (cdc2), resulting in the blockage of cells at the G1–S and/or G2–M interfaces (Sage, 1996). Platelet factor-4 also interacts with cyclins and/or cdk kinases to arrest endothelial cells in S phase. Finally, an antiangiogenic 16-kDa fragment of prolactin has been shown to inhibit the phosphorylation of two MAPKs by VEGF, with resultant suppression of VEGF-induced signal transduction. Finally, tailored therapies such as antisense targeting of basic fibroblast growth factor (bFGF) and fibroblast growth factor receptor-1 (FGFR-1) messenger RNAs have been shown to block growth of melanoma in mice at least in part by blocking angiogenesis (Wang and Becker, 1997).

III. MOLECULAR BIOLOGY OF CANCER AS IT RELATES TO THE AGING PROCESS

The preceding discussion centered on cellular and molecular processes which, when altered, may lead to cancer in humans in general. Yet, cancer is primarily a disease of older individuals. Over half of the cases of cancer are diagnosed in persons past age 65, and more than 50% of cancer deaths occur in this older group despite the fact that this group constitutes only 12% of the population (Anisimov, 1990; Kennedy, 1990). Although the literature on the molecular biology of cancer as it pertains to cancer in the elderly is limited, select areas of molecular biological and genetic research are of growing interest for cancer as part of the aging process both at the cellular and the organismal levels.

A number of potential age-related factors predisposing to cancer have been identified: prolonged exposure to multiple carcinogens; increased susceptibility of cells to carcinogens; decreased DNA repair, activation of oncogenes and inactivation of tumor suppressor genes, and decreased immune surveillance (Anisimov, 1990; Cohen, 1994). Two major theories of aging can be interpreted in terms of these cancer-causing factors to explain the increasing incidence of cancer with age (Reis and Slagboom 1989; Cohen, 1994; Afshari and Barrett, 1996). The damage, or error, theories hold that events occur over time to cause the accumulation of damage to vital areas of cellular or organ function, culminating in the phenotype regarded as the aging process. The damage to critical functions may be due to either the pleiotropic effects of mutations in certain key genes or to mutations in many individual genes occurring gradually over time in a stochastic manner; that is, on a more or less random basis (Reis and Slagboom, 1989). The multistep model of carcinogenesis (Vogelstein et al., 1988; Kinzler and Vogelstein, 1996) feeds directly into this theory, offering successive cancer-causing mutations as the specific damaging insults that accumulate during the aging process. The alternative, or program, theories view aging and senescence (the end stage of the aging process more proximal to death) as the latter phase of a genetic program that proceeds through embryogenesis, growth, development, and maturation. According to the program theories, during aging certain genes are shut down and others become expressed, with the latter presumably consisting of genes relating most directly to the senescence process. The molecular components of a number of general cellular processes, such as those discussed in Part II of this chapter, undergo modification as a result of this aging program. A merging of the two theories of aging can be envisioned at this point, with the programmed alteration of fundamental cellular processes (e.g., defective DNA repair, genetic instability, DNA hypomethylation, increased apoptosis, progressive telomere shortening) contributing to the accumulation of cancer-causing genetic mutations, or "errors," and the programmed compromise in other key cellular processes causing decreased surveillance of such oncogenic changes (alterations in the immune and endocrine systems).

A. Multistage Model of Carcinogenesis: Accumulation of Mutations

The classic model of multistage carcinogenesis involves first initiation, a rapid induction of permanent and irreversible alterations in the genome by a carcinogen called an initiator (Anisimov, 1990; Sugimura, 1992). The next step is promotion, which may elicit mitogenesis (induced cell division), requiring prolonged exposure to a carcinogen called a promoter, and which may be reversible. Recent evidence suggests that cell proliferation, in addition to providing increased raw material for subsequent genetic alterations (Dunn and Longo, 1996), may in and of itself play a dominant role in carcinogenesis, that is, mitogenesis increases mutagenesis (Ames and Gold, 1990; Cohen and Ellevein, 1990; Farber, 1995). Promotion involves the activation of a variety of enzymes that contribute to carcinogenesis. In the last step, progression, cells finally become malignant, may undergo clonal evolution, and metastasize. With the revelation in recent years of genetic changes that predispose to cancer (activated oncogenes, inactivated tumor suppressor genes, genetic instability), it has become clear that these genetic alterations are the building blocks of initiation, promotion, and progression, which are the actual events that contribute to tumorigenesis. The ultimate target of the tumor-promoting metabolic changes of initiation, promotion, and progression are the genes which in turn acquire mutations. Sequential alterations in key genes lead to the accumulation of a critical number of cancer-causing mutations, with each step causing the mutated cell to acquire a slightly greater growth advantage, leading to higher grades of neoplasia, culminating in frank invasive malignancy and finally metastases (Vogelstein et al., 1988; Kinzler and Vogelstein, 1996; Collins and Trent, 1998).

In accord with the first, or damage, theory of aging, the mere fact of longevity in the elderly allows more time over which tumorigenic insults have the opportunity to occur by virtue of prolonged exposure to carcinogenic insults (Cohen, 1994), both exogenous and endogenous (Ames and Gold, 1990). The second, or program, theory would hold that programmed changes make aging cells more susceptible to mutagenic insults. For instance, in addition to prolonged carcinogenic exposure, aging cells may be more vulnerable to a given amount of carcinogen. Any damage, once initiated, is more difficult to repair in older cells. Finally, changes in immune and endocrine functions may result in decreased surveillance of emerging malignant clones by an internal milieu that is less able to counteract the growth-promoting advantages acquired by the cell through successive mutations.

B. Changes in General Cellular Processes with Aging that Are Associated with Cancer

1. DNA Repair and Genetic Instability

a. DNA Repair

In accord with the gene-based model of multistep carcinogenesis, continually occurring DNA damage is the basis for 80–90% of human cancers (Sancar, 1994). Cells are usually able to eliminate DNA lesions by molecular DNA repair, a group of mechanisms for returning the DNA sequence to its original pattern. Each mechanism should be understood as a system, with a net activity that depends on the sequential and partly overlapping activities of several polypeptides that bind DNA and utilize the energy released from adenosine triphosphate (ATP) hydrolysis to deform it (kink and unwind) and to excise the lesion by dual incisions. Base excision repair involves first the excision of the damaged base and then the abasic sugar (AP site) by an AP endonuclease. On the other hand, nucleotide excision repair (NER) entails hydrolysis of a phosphodiester bond on either side of the lesion, with release of an oligonucleotide carrying the damage. The resulting gaps are then filled in and ligated to complete the repair reaction. The activity responsible for NER, which has been called an excinuclease, encompasses the activity of at least 17 polypeptides and, in some cases, has been linked to transcription, with preferential repair of the transcribed DNA strand in expressed genes, leading to its designation as transcription-coupled repair (Hanawalt, 1994). Base excision repair has a limited substrate range consisting of redundant information in the damaged DNA molecule. In contrast, the excinuclease of nucleotide excision repair, which is the sole enzyme system for removing bulky DNA adducts, has a much broader substrate spectrum, including mismatched nucleotides. However, in addressing this last type of error, the excinuclease is somewhat indiscriminate in that it cannot differentiate the ''right'' from the ''wrong'' strand and therefore may actually induce mutation rather than prevent it. In contrast, a third DNA repair system, the mismatch repair system, specializes in remedying mismatches and has a built-in mechanism to identify the strand with the correct sequence (Modrich, 1994). Mismatch repair defects are detected by identifying excessive replication infidelity in microsatellite DNA, short, repetitive DNA sequences that are dispersed throughout the genome, including within genes.

Mutations in the genes for components of the various DNA repair systems have been shown to underlie a number of disease states, including cancer (Hanawalt, 1994). Defects in transcription-coupled repair (NER) genes are found in three rare genetic disorders, xeroderma pigmentosum (XP), Cockayne's syndrome (CS), and trichothiodystrophy (TTD). Although the last two are developmental disorders, XP involves a predisposition to cancer in sun-exposed areas of skin, since the DNA repair defect prevents cells from appropriately remedying ultraviolet (UV) light–inflicted DNA damage (Hanawalt, 1994). Four genes for mismatch repair proteins, hMSH2, hMLH1, hPMS1, and hPMS2, have been proven to be defective in tumors associated with hereditary nonpolyposis colorectal cancer (HNPCC) (Fishel et al., 1993; Leach et al., 1993; Parsons et al., 1993). The genetic instability conferred by defective DNA repair on cells showing homozygous inactivation or loss of mismatch repair genes predisposes such cells to further genetic mutations, which, according to the multistage model of carcinogenesis, may accumulate until a critical number leads to uncontrolled cell growth and transformation. In some cases, the mutations that occur in mismatch repair-deficient tumor cells are consistent with replication errors, confirming the existence of a true mutator, or replication error (RER+), phenotype. The RER+ phenotype has been established primarily in HNPCC (Aaltonen et al., 1993; Liu et al., 1996). Nevertheless, colorectal carcinoma cell lines (Battacharyya et al., 1994) and cells from some sporadic colorectal cancers (Han et al., 1993; Ionov et al., 1993; Thibodeau et al., 1993) as well as other tumor types, such as chronic lymphocytic leukemias (7%) (Gartenhaus et al., 1996), primary gastric carcinomas (including 91% of the intestinal type) (Chung et al., 1996), advanced head and neck tumors (29%) (Nawroz et al., 1996), and small-cell lung carcinomas (76%) (Chen et al., 1996), exhibit microsatellite instability. In a few cases, specific target genes of mismatch repair have been identified. A tract of eight deoxyguanosine residues within the apoptosis-promoting *BAX* gene (see below) shows frameshift mutations in over 50% of human RER+ colon cancer cell lines (Rampino et al., 1997). A polyadenylate tract within the *TGF-β RII* gene shows mutations due to microsatellite instability in colon cancer cells from both sporadic (Markowitz, 1995; Akiyama, 1996) and HNPCC (Parsons et al., 1995) tumors and in a high percentage of gastric carcinomas (Chung et al., 1996), distinguishing this gene as a potential tumor suppressor gene.

b.   DNA Repair and Genetic Instability as They Relate to Aging

Evidence has long pointed to a positive correlation between the amount of DNA repair and the longevity of a given species (Kirkwood, 1989). A typical measurement has been the amount of unscheduled DNA synthesis induced by UV irradiation, which is considered to be a marker for DNA excision repair of pyrimidine dimers. Extrapolation of these observations on longevity as a function of DNA repair to the intraspecies level would be consistent with the idea that the ability of cells to repair DNA diminishes with age. The situation is more complex, however, since different repair processes vary in terms of their relationship to the relative longevity of species. Those repair processes that correlate more strongly with longevity should be better candidates for mechanisms that play an important role in regulating the duration of life.

Several indices of DNA repair and genetic instability have been shown to support a relationship between these parameters and age. For example, there is a near-exponential increase in the misincorporation of nucleotides during the life span of cultured human fibroblasts, indicating a progressive decrease in the fidelity of DNA polymerase-α (Murray and Holliday, 1981). In another example, not only do patients with ataxia telangiectasia (AT) exhibit premature aging, but cultured cells from such individuals have a decreased life span combined with multiple manifestations of deficient DNA repair, including increased sensitivity to ionizing radiation, a checkpoint defect in response to DNA damage and increased levels of chromosome instability (Friedberg et al., 1995; Greenwell et al., 1995). Among the chromosome aberrations found in AT cells are end-to-end attachments, a characteristic abnormality seen also in senescing human cells with short telomeres, as described below (Counter et al., 1992; Greenwell et al., 1995). There is a reduction in the activity of DNA polymerase-β, another DNA repair enzyme, in the brains of old as compared to young rats (Rao et al., 1994). Aging in humans is associated with a decreasing ability to process new UV-induced DNA damage, leading to an increase in DNA mutability and presumably contributing to the observed increased risk of skin cancer in older individuals (Moriwaki et al., 1996). DNA topoisomerase-I (Topo-I), an enzyme that plays a role in DNA repair by altering the coiling of DNA, is significantly less active in senescent diploid fibroblasts when compared to young (early passage) fibroblasts (Lee et al., 1997). Chemically induced DNA damage, such as benzo[a]pyrene–DNA adducts in mice (Boerrigter et al., 1995) and cisplatin-induced DNA interstrand crosslinks in human peripheral blood mononuclear cells (Rudd et al., 1995), are repaired and cleared less efficiently in older versus younger subjects.

Oxidative damage to DNA caused by exposure to reactive oxygen species (ROS) throughout life is repaired less efficiently in older individuals. This outcome is reflected in such parameters of oxidative DNA damage as the age-related increase in accumulation of 8-hydroxydeoxyguanosine (8-OH-dG), the hydroxyl radical adduct of deoxyguanosine (dG), a highly mutagenic lesion that results in GT transversions frequently found in tumor-relevant genes (Homma et al., 1994; Loft and Paulsen, 1996); the higher levels of the percentage of single-stranded DNA in lymphocytes from older individuals (Barnett and King, 1995); and age-related increases in deletions in mitochondrial DNA, a particularly vulnerable target because of its continual exposure to high levels of ROS and free radicals (Randerath et al., 1996; Wei et al., 1996). There is an especially rapid accumulation of somatic mitochondrial DNA (mtDNA) lesions late in life. This has been attributed to a vicious cycle of increasing numbers of deletion-inducing oxygen radicals (particularly 8-OH-dG adducts), leading to defects in mitochondrial respiratory chain enzymes which in turn promote further oxidative damage (Ozawa, 1997). The escalating course of oxidative damage–induced mutation is exacerbated by the inefficiency of mtDNA repair systems which are exemplified by the absence of a pyrimidine dimer repair mechanism in mammalian mitochondria. This age-related escalation in mtDNA mutations is specifically implicated in carcinogenesis in that the repair of mtDNA in tumor cells is more effective and complete than in normal cells, where repair of only 43% of UV-induced mtDNA lesions has been observed.

In summary, it should be kept in mind that the relationships between DNA repair and aging have been localized to specific regions of DNA, including active genes, telomeres, and mitochondria, emphasizing the connection between DNA repair and transcription (Bohr and Anson, 1995). Finally, as noted for a number of the parameters just discussed, a corresponding increase in mutation and/or cancer has been shown to accompany the decreased DNA repair that occurs with aging (Loft and Poulsen, 1996; Moriwaki et al., 1996).

2. Apoptosis

a. Apoptosis Background

The homeostasis that characterizes tissues in multicellular organisms depends on a balance between the generation of new cells and the death of old cells. When cells are no longer needed or become damaged, a genetically controlled cell "suicide" machinery leads to programmed cell death (PCD). Apoptosis is a morphologically distinct form of PCD whereby the cell responds to specific extracellular or intracellular signals by developing characteristic changes: DNA fragmentation due to the activation of nucleases that degrade the DNA at internucleosomal sites; condensation of the nucleus and cytoplasm; and fragmentation of the dying cell fragments into membrane-bound apoptotic bodies that are phagocytosed by macrophages (Steller, 1995; Thompson, 1995; Fraser and Evan, 1996; Manning and Patierno, 1996; Nagata, 1997; Fenton and Longo, 1998). For instance, apoptosis may be elicited extracellularly by signaling through ligand activation of the tumor necrosis factor receptor (TNFR) or a structurally related receptor Fas (also called APO-1 or CD95) (Cleveland and Ihle, 1995; Nagata, 1997) or intracellularly by activation of a number of genes (p53, c-*myc, RB, EIA, CCNDI* (cyclin DI locus), c-*fos, CDC2*), all of which may ultimately require p53 to implement an apoptotic response to cell damage (Steller, 1995). Signaling through either route leads to the activation of a series of cysteine proteases belonging to the family of interleukin-1β–converting enzyme (ICE)–related proteases which cleave their target proteins at specific residues, leading ultimately to apoptosis (Martin, 1995; Fraser and Evan, 1996).

The signals leading to apoptosis are counterbalanced by the activity of gene products that suppress cell death. The most prominent suppressor of apoptosis is *bcl2*, a proto-oncogene, discovered by virtue of its presence at the chromosome 18 breakpoint of the t(14;18)(q32;q21) translocation which characterizes 85% of follicular lymphomas (Korsmeyer, 1992; Yang, and Korsmeyer, 1996; Fenton and Longo, 1998). Deregulated expression of *bcl2* as a result of its juxtaposition with the immunoglobulin heavy chain locus (IgH) on chromosome 14 leads to suppression of cell death and lymphoid hyperplasia. Although *bcl2* overexpression itself does not induce malignant transformation, prolongation of lymphocyte survival lays the groundwork for subsequent oncogenic events (such as translocation of a *myc* gene) to induce a truly monoclonal malignancy. The *bcl2* proto-oncogene is a member of a family of genes whose products dimerize in various combinations to prevent (*bcl2, bcl-X$_L$*) or promote (e.g., *bax, bad, bak*) cell death. Although recent data suggest that Bcl2 and Bax can function independently to regulate cell death (Knudson, 1997), the general view is that heterodimerization of any death promoter with Bcl2 or Bcl-X$_L$ suppresses apoptosis in contrast to dimerization of death promoters among themselves, which leads to cell death. The relative amounts of the different Bcl2 family members create a dynamic balance of homo- and heterodimers that weights the net physiological outcome toward or against cell death. This is particularly true of death induced as a result of damage inflicted by reactive oxygen species, consistent with the localization of Bcl2 to the mitochondrial membrane (Hockenbery et al., 1990; Kluck et al., 1997; Yang et al., 1997).

The implication of *bcl2* for cancer extends beyond its deregulation in follicular lymphomas. Bcl2 expression is positively correlated with estrogen receptor and progesterone receptor positivity in breast carcinoma (Yang and Korsmeyer, 1996). In prostate cancer, high levels of Bcl2 are seen in androgen-independent tumors. Apoptosis, in addition to being an important physiological process, is also a mechanism of death for cells treated with various chemotherapeutic agents. Consistent with this fact, a poor response to chemotherapy has been shown to correlate with high Bcl2 expression. For many toxic agents (γ-irradiation, etoposide), wild-type p53 is required to induce apoptosis, whereas death induced by other agents (glucocorticoid, calcium) is p53-independent (Clarke et al., 1993). The requirement of a functional p53 for a response to many types of radiation and chemotherapy explains the resistance of many tumor cells to the cytotoxic effects of these agents. An alternate route to apoptosis that is active in tumor cells, but not in normal ones, involves a cytotoxic protein called TRAIL (Apo2L) and is independent of p53 (Pan et al., 1997; Sheridan et al., 1997). Both p53-dependent as well p53-independent mechanisms of cell death can be inhibited by Bcl2.

Although the *bcl2* family dominates the realm of antiapoptotic genes, recently discovered inhibitors of programmed cell death may contribute to prolonged cell longevity and ultimately to cancer. The novel antiapoptotic gene, *survivin*, for example, is highly expressed in transformed cell lines and in the common cancers of lung, colon, pancreas, prostate, and breast in vivo as well as 50% of high-grade non-Hodgkin's lymphomas (centroblastic, immunoblastic) but not in low-grade lymphomas (lymphocytic) (Ambrosini et al., 1997).

b. Apoptosis as It Relates to Aging

In a number of cell systems, there is an increased tendency to undergo apoptosis with aging. The apoptotic process is greatly amplified in activated T lymphocytes from aged individuals (Phelouzat et al., 1996), especially in their CD3$^+$ CD45RO$^-$ T-cell subset (Herndon et al., 1997). In contrast, no significant difference exists between older and younger adults in the CD3$^+$ CD45RO$^+$ T cells. The selective increase in apoptosis in the RO$^-$ subset leads to replacement of virgin T cells by memory T cells in older people (Miller, 1996), which in turn may account for the poor response of elderly individuals to novel immunological stimuli, contributing to the overall compromise in immune function in this population (see below). Apoptosis is also increased in the sensory hair cells as well as a variety of other cell types in the cochlea and saccules of the inner ear of aged mice, suggesting this as a mechanism for age-related hearing loss and dysequilibrium (Usami et al., 1997). A progressive increase in apoptosis with age has also been demonstrated in hepatocytes in rats (Higami et al., 1997). The enhanced propensity of senescent cells toward apoptotic cell death would seem in conflict with the predisposition to cancer in elderly individuals. A possible explanation for this paradox is that increased apoptosis in a cell population leads to selection for a mutated clone, perhaps carrying an activated antiapopotic gene such as *bcl2*, which is refractory to the normal signals for cell death (see below).

3. Telomerase and Senescence

The integrity of chromosomes is maintained in part by specialized structures that cap their ends, or telomeres. Telomeres protect eukaryotic chromosomes from degradation and terminal fusion, facilitate chromosome movement and organization, and regulate transcription of nearby genes by the process of telomere silencing. The telomere consists of a protein–DNA complex containing species-specific tandem repeats of short five to eight base pair (bp) guanine-rich DNA sequence. At birth, the DNA fragments that contain the telomeres (TRFs, or terminal restriction fragments) are about 10–12 kilobase (kb) pairs (Greider and Harley, 1996). Similarly, human germline cells have an average of 10 kb of the sequence TTAGGG at each chromosomal end (Blackburn, 1991). Because the ends of DNA molecules cannot be fully replicated by the conventional DNA polymerase (the ''end replication problem'' described in Watson, 1972; Harley, 1995), at each cell division there is a loss of DNA such that the mean telomere (i.e., TRF) length gradually decreases with the number of cell divisions in culture and as a function of donor age in vivo in human somatic cells but not in germline or cancer cells. The rate of telomere loss in cultured fibroblasts ranges from 50 to 200 bp per population doubling in contrast to a rate of loss of 15–50 bp per year in renewing tissues in vivo over the age range of 4–80 years (Martin, 1994; Harley, 1995). To prevent such loss, telomerase, a ribonucleoprotein enzyme complex with RNA-dependent DNA polymerase activity, reiteratively directs the synthesis of the species-specific telomere repeat sequence onto the 3'-end of existing telomeres (Blackburn, 1991, 1994; Greider and Harley, 1996). In normal human somatic cells, telomerase activity is stringently repressed in contrast to its detectable levels in immortal cell populations in culture, some human tumors in vivo, and select normal in vivo tissues such as testes. With regard to human tumors, although its RNA component is upregulated in early-stage tumors, activation of telomerase is observed only in late-stage tumors, reflecting a progression through the multistep process of tumorigenesis (Blasco et al., 1996). The implication is that there is a correlation between indefinite replicative capacity and measurable telomerase and, conversely, between a mortal phenotype and lack of telomerase (Harley et al., 1994). The association of telomerase expression with cancer has led to investigations into correlations between the telomerase level and tumor phenotype, potentially as a prognostic or risk factor, as well as proposals to focus on telomerase as a target for anticancer therapy.

Young, normal (untransformed) human somatic cells have a limited replicative capacity, approximately 50–100 divisions in culture, a characteristic known as replicative senescence (Goldstein, 1990; Harley et al., 1994; Smith and Pereira-Smith, 1996). Mutations occurring before or near this limit, or mortality phase 1 (M1, or Hayflick limit), allow cells to escape this block in proliferation. An extended life span of 20–30 doublings brings the cell population to a mortality phase 2 (M2), at which time the population as a whole undergoes crisis. An occasional mutation at or near crisis leads to a rare clone that escapes M2 and yields an immortal cell population. Placing these observations in the context of the multistep model of tumorigenesis, studies have shown that no known combination of activated oncogenes or mutated tumor suppressor genes can directly immortalize normal human somatic cells in vitro. Rather these mutations constitute early steps in tumorigenesis leading to transformation of cells with an increased, but still finite, proliferative capacity corresponding to escape from M1 (Counter et al., 1992; Harley et al., 1994). As an example, a key tumor-suppressive function of wild-type p53 and pRB is believed to be growth arrest at M1, since inactivation of both of these proteins is required to extend the proliferative life span of human diploid fibroblasts by approximately 17 population doublings (Shay et al., 1991; Bond et al., 1994). In contrast to M1, the ability to bypass crisis at M2 and achieve immortalization derives from a different set of cellular processes—those involving chromosomal stability.

The association of the lack of telomerase with a mortal cell phenotype, together with decreasing telomere length in aging tissues, has led to the telomeric hypothesis of cellular aging (Harley, 1991). This hypothesis states that replicative senescence is due to the gradual loss of chromosomal ends (telomeres). Accordingly, the growth arrest induced at M1 by tumor suppressor gene products such as p53 and pRB is a response to a specific, advanced degree of telomere shortening. If the life span is extended beyond M1, ongoing erosion of chromosomal telomeres leads to a critical stage at which the chromosome ends become "recombinogenic" (Counter et al., 1992; Bond et al., 1994). In the terminal passages preceding the crisis, there is a rapid increase in the frequency of chromosomal aberrations, particularly telomeric associations, and ultimately cell death. At this point, there is a strong selection for mutations conferring chromosomal stability and allowing continued cell growth. Thus, in contrast to the progressive decline in the telomere length which occurs in the normally aging cell, an aging cell that bypasses crisis and becomes immortalized, corresponding to an advanced malignant phenotype, is expected to have stabilization of the telomere length owing to increased expression of telomerase. In fact, telomeres do shorten during tumorigenesis, since tumors from many types of cancer have been shown to contain telomeres that are shorter than those in control tissues. In addition, there is a trend toward decreasing the telomere length with increasing disease severity in several cancers, with some cancers possessing critically short telomeres (Harley et al., 1994; Bacchetti and Counter, 1995). Finally, longitudinal studies in ovarian cancer (Counter et al., 1994) demonstrate in vivo maintenance of short telomeres. Together these observations on telomeres and telomerase in the context of replicative senescence suggest that at the point when telomeres have shortened to a critical length, that is, at crisis, there is selection for mutations that activate telomerase, preventing death and supporting immortalization.

Strong support for a causal relationship between telomere shortening and the senescence of human cells comes from recent experiments in which telomerase expression was activated in three different primary cell types by transfection with the human telomerase reverse transcriptase subunit (hTRT) (Bodnar et al., 1998). Telomerase-negative control cells exhibit telomere shortening and senesce after a well-defined number of cell divisions. In contrast to their telomerase-negative counterparts, the telomerase-expressing cells have elongated telomeres, a normal karyotype, and divide vigorously, exceeding their normal life span by at least 20 doublings, and show reduced staining for β-galactosidase, a biomarker for senescence.

A recently disclosed interplay between the cell cycle and senescence involves the product of the p21$^{CIP1/WAF1}$ gene, an inhibitor of cyclin-dependent kinases (CDKs) (see above). *CIP1* is induced by p53 in response to cell damage and in turn inhibits CDKs, causing cell cycle arrest. Inactivation of *CIP1* is sufficient to bypass senescence in normal diploid human fibroblasts, which is consistent with a failure to arrest the cell cycle in response to normal physiological cues for cessation of cell division (Brown et al., 1997). Extension of the life span of normal cells in response to *CIP1* inactivation points to this gene as a major player in the programmed induction of replicative senescence.

4. Immune Suppression

In the presence of an intact immune system, even frankly malignant cells may experience a biological challenge on behalf of host defense. The presentation of cell surface antigens unique to a malignant cell type may elicit an appropriate cytotoxic T-cell response (Guinan et al., 1994). Since functional compromise in both humoral and cell-mediated immune responses is a cardinal feature of the aging organism (Bell and High, 1997; Meydani et al., 1997), such weapons for fighting malignancy may fail, allowing progression of a tumor that would otherwise be thwarted at an early stage. In particular, a variety of changes in T-cell–mediated immunity may predispose to malignancy. There is a shift from naive T-cell subpopulations to those associated with activated or memory T cells (Miller, 1996), which may have implications for resulting cytokine production (Weigle, 1993). There is also an accumulation of cells with signal transduction defects (Miller, 1996). Rather dramatic changes have been noted in T-cell and natural killer cell (NK) subtypes in the elderly, with a decline in the number of mature effector (CD8$^+$) T cells in contrast to a stable number of helper (CD4$^+$) T cells (Lesourd and Meaume, 1994). In a longitudinal, observational cohort study of healthy elderly individuals, designed to avoid the pitfall of confounding immunological effects due to comorbidities, no differences were seen in the number of circulating CD3$^+$ or CD4$^+$ T lymphocytes and only a slight decline in CD8$^+$ T lymphocytes was noted, whereas marked elevations were observed in the number of circulating NK cells (CD56$^+$, CD2$^+$ CD3$^-$) (Lesourd and Meaume, 1994).

The most obvious change in immune function is the impairment of lymphocyte proliferative responses in the elderly, a natural culmination of the gradual decline that occurs throughout life (Weigle, 1993; Lesourd and Meaume, 1994). Accompanying this decrease in responsiveness to antigenic stimulation is an age-associated decrease in levels of expression of the costimulus receptor, CD28 (Pawelec et al., 1997). The expression of IL-2 receptors in lymphocytes is also decreased, which is a possible reflection of impaired signal processing in aged lymphocytes, poor mobilization of Ca^{2+}, or changes in the lymphocyte membrane. In addition, resting T cells fail to downregulate p27 expression during activation resulting in cells arresting in G1 (Kwon et al., 1996, 1997). Increased proportions of cholesterol and phospholipids in the membranes of T cells in the elderly lead to changes in viscosity that may alter cytokine access to membrane-bound receptors. Sera obtained from the elderly, which is high in very low density lipoproteins (VLDLs) and low-density lipoproteins (LDLs), inhibits IL-2–dependent proliferation of T cells. Furthermore, changes in cytokine production occur in the elderly that may compromise cell-mediated immunity (Weigle, 1993). There is a shift in the balance of T-cell responses from Th-1– to Th-2–type responses (Cakman et al., 1996). A Th-1 response, characterized by secretion of IL-2 and interferon-γ, is associated with cell-mediated immunity, in contrast to a Th-2 response, with secretion of IL-4, IL-5, and IL-10, which generally favors the production of humoral, or antibody-based, immunity (Mosmann and Sad, 1996). T-cell responses may be further compromised because of abnormalities in T-cell interaction with macrophages. Prostaglandin E$_2$ (PGE$_2$) secretion by macrophages may be increased in elderly subjects, whereas the elderly T cells show exaggerated sensitivity to inhibition by PGE$_2$. Finally, the lymphocytes in aging individuals are less capable of mounting an allogenic response to foreign major histocompatibility complex (MHC) molecules (Russo et al., 1993; Pawelec et al., 1997).

An interesting and potentially antithetical role of the aging immune system in cancer has been proposed to explain the observation that tumor growth and progression tend to proceed at a slower rate in the older host (Cohen and Ellwein, 1994). Decreased activity of those cells in the host's immune system that normally produce tumor-enhancing factors (such as angiogenesis-promoting factors) in response to stimulation by tumors may result in the paradoxical effect of diminished tumor growth.

As a final comment, it should be noted that the role that the immune compromise seen in the elderly plays in carcinogenesis is controversial. Depressed cell-mediated immunity has been shown to correlate with all-cause mortality, but an association between anergy and cancer mortality, although present, is not statistically significant (Wayne et al., 1990). Although relevant to certain tumor types such as lymphoid malignancies, immune dysfunction may not play as important a role in solid tumors (Cohen and Ellwein, 1994).

C. Genetics of Aging and Age-Associated Changes in Specific Biological Markers Related to Cancer

The actual role of the genes in the aging process remains to be established (Finch, 1997). On the one hand, program theories of aging (Reis and Slagboom, 1989; Cohen and Ellwein, 1994), which hold that senescence evolved as an active genetic program in an adaptive response to the forces of natural selection, is supported by the identification of a number of genes that appear to regulate the aging process directly. The alternative damage, or error, theories emphasize the nonadaptive nature of cumulative genetic errors over time which in the aggregate contribute to the aging phenotype.

Support for a predetermined program of aging comes from the nematode worm *Caenorhabditis elegans* in which at least two series of genes (the *clk-1, clk-2, clk-3, gro-1* series and the *daf* series, including *daf-2, daf-23, daf-16*) operate through separate pathways to determine both the duration of development and the life span (Johnson et al., 1996; Lakowski and Hekimi,). Recently, *daf-2* has been shown to encode a member of the insulin receptor family which causes an increase in life span when its signaling is decreased owing to mutation (Kimura et al., 1997). The data from *C. elegans* coincide with the evidence in humans for specific genes that regulate an aging program (Jazwinski, 1996). Although aging in higher organisms appears to be multifactorial, a few syndromes of premature aging have served as models for the genetic programming of the aging process (Greenwell et al., 1995; Jazwinski, 1996). Furthermore, there has been controversy as to whether these syndromes actually simulate the normal aging process (Jazwinski, 1996; Martin, 1997). Although affected individuals exhibit some or many features of aging at an accelerated rate, in none of the syndromes do patients present with all the characteristics of normal aging, which accounts for the appellation ''segmental'' progeroid syndromes. Nevertheless, such medical disorders are useful in providing a framework within which elements of aging, such as the propensity to cancer, can be understood. Three of these disorders, Werner's syndrome, Cockayne's syndrome, and ataxia telangiectasia (AT), are related in a number of ways.

Werner's syndrome (WS) is a rare autosomal recessive disorder encompassing multiple facets of aging (Yu et al., 1996; Martin, 1997; Matsumoto et al., 1997). Patients prematurely develop several forms of atherosclerosis, malignant neoplasms, type II diabetes mellitus, osteoporosis, and ocular cataracts. They also manifest early graying and hair loss, skin atrophy, and a generally aged appearance. Retardation of growth occurs due to a failure of the usual adolescent growth spurt. Death typically takes place in the late 40s due to atherosclerosis or cancer. In contrast to Alzheimer's disease, another disorder of premature aging, brain function is not affected. At the cellular level, there are parallels between WS and aging in that the replicative life span of fibroblasts is reduced and is similar to that of fibroblasts taken from elderly individuals. Cells display genetic instability in the form of chromosomal deletions, inversions, and reciprocal translocations, as well as intragenic mutations, primarily deletions (Weirich-Schwaiger et al., 1994). Telomeres in cells from a patient with WS were observed to be shorter than those in fibroblasts from a normally aging individual (Kruk et al., 1995). The WS gene (*WRN*) is located on chromosome 18p12 and encodes a 1432–amino acid protein with homology to a specific type of helicase. DNA helicases unwind duplex DNA, as required for replication, recombination, repair, or transcription, explaining the chromosome instability that characterizes helicase-associated diseases. Most mutations in the *WRN* gene result in premature termination of its protein product leading to impaired nuclear localization and, consistent with its presumed function as a helicase, genetic instability (Matsumoto et al., 1997). The WS protein has, in fact, been reported to catalyze DNA unwinding (Gray et al., 1997).

The tumors in Werner's syndrome are divided equally between those of mesenchymal and epithelial origin (Martin, 1997). Meningiomas, fibromas, and sarcomas are common and patients are particularly susceptible to acrolentiginous melanoma. In contrast, normally aging individuals are 10 times more likely to develop tumors of epithelial origin, such as prostatic or colorectal carcinoma. Therefore, WS offers a scenario in which an abnormality in DNA replication precipitates both the physiological changes characteristic of normal aging (skin, hair) and disease-related aging (tumorigenesis), suggesting once again that the mechanistic underpinnings of the aging process may contribute to the development of cancer in the elderly. Yet, the skewed distribution of tumor types seen in WS should caution against adopting this disorder as a comprehensive model for the interrelationship between aging and carcinogenesis.

Besides WS, other phenotypically distinct disorders that are caused by different mutations in helicases include Cockayne's syndrome (CS), Bloom's syndrome, xeroderma pigmentosum, and trichothiodystrophy (Epstein and Motulsky, 1996). Cockayne's syndrome is a disorder involving skeletal abnormalities and neurological dysfunction. Cells from patients with CS are defective in the preferential removal of lesions from transcribed strands of active genes by a transcription-coupled repair process (TCR), a subtype of nuclear excision repair (NER) (Evans and Bohr, 1994; Cooper et al., 1997). The genetic bases for CS are mutations in helicases encoded by the *ERCC-6* or the *ERCC-3* gene (Jazwinski, 1996). The genetic basis for another disorder of premature aging, AT, is a mutation of the *ATM* gene. *ATM* encodes a protein that is homologous to the yeast *TEL1* gene, a participant in telomere metabolism (Morrow et al., 1995). Other homologues of *ATM* include phosphatidylinositol-

3 kinase, a DNA-dependent protein kinase, and *MEC1*, a yeast checkpoint control gene (Keith and Schreiber, 1995), supporting a role for *ATM* in the regulation of DNA repair.

Recent data in yeast suggest that the molecular mechanisms influencing aging in this organism bear a resemblance to those involved in the premature aging syndromes of humans (Kennedy et al., 1997). SIR4 is one of several proteins that normally operate to silence transcription of genes at yeast telomeres. A SIR4 mutant truncated at its carboxyl terminus (SIR4-42) can no longer bind to the telomere and relocates from the telomere to a second locus, *AGE*, where it functions to delay the aging process. An analogous redistribution of SIR protein complexes to the *AGE* locus occurs in old cells to forestall senescence. Additional evidence points to the *AGE* locus as the nucleolus, the site of ribosomal DNA (rDNA). Relocation of the SIR-silencing complex to the *AGE* locus influences the rates of recombination in the rDNA. Furthermore, mammalian cells exhibit a decreased nucleolar volume, reduced synthesis of nucleolar RNA, and progressive decreases in the number of rDNA copies with age. Another yeast gene, *SGS1*, when deleted, leads to a large increase in the rDNA recombination rate, with profound enlargement and fragmentation of the nucleolus, as well as premature aging and redistribution of the SIR protein–silencing complex from telomeres to the nucleolus (Sinclair et al., 1997). The nucleolar changes are probably due to the accumulation of extrachromosomal rDNA circles (ERCs) in old cells. These ERCs in turn appear to cause aging manifested by a shortened life span and accelerated onset of sterility (Sinclair and Guarante, 1997). Mutants of *SGS1* accumulate ERCs more rapidly, resulting in premature aging and a shorter life span. *SGS1* bears homology to the DNA helicase product of the *WRN* gene of WS. These observations bring together a role for telomere silencing proteins, DNA helicases, and rDNA recombination in the aging process. Another recently identified gene in yeast, MORF4 (*mor*tality *f*actor from chromosome 4), imparts immortality to some types of cells when it is mutated (Ehrenstein, 1998).

Finally, in the mouse, a newly identified gene, *klotho*, encodes a membrane protein with sequence similarity to the β-glucosidase enzymes. A defect in *klotho* gene expression results in a syndrome with similarities to human aging, including a short life span, infertility, atherosclerosis, skin atrophy, osteoporosis, and emphysema (Kuro-o et al., 1997).

1. Biomarkers of Aging and Cancer

As discussed in Part II of this chapter, there are multiple key cellular processes that depend on the activity of molecules that are frequently altered in tumors. Some of these oncogenic changes parallel alterations that are characteristic of cellular senescence, suggesting a commonality in causation of the processes of carcinogenesis and aging. When expression of a particular gene is consistently observed within a given context such as carcinogenesis or aging, in contradistinction to the absence of expression in the reciprocal setting of normal or young tissue, this gene can be used as a biomarker of the associated process. The proposed biomarker must be validated by demonstrating its ability to be assayed reliably and quantitatively, measured easily, and correlated with the incidence of the process in question—cancer or aging (ASCO, 1996; Hayes et al., 1996; Hayes, 1997; Kelloff et al., 1996). The biomarker should reflect the biological process with which it is putatively associated; that is, it should be on or linked to the causal pathway of this process, cancer or senescence. Reference to appropriate biomarkers of a given biological process provides an efficient index by which risk cohorts can be identified for clinical trials, and modulation of the process, either ''disease''-causing (oncogenic, aging) or therapeutic, can be evaluated. A few of the genes whose expression have potential to serve as biomarkers of oncogenesis within the context of aging are discussed here.

a. CDK Inhibitors: Increased Expression with Age

The CDK inhibitor p16$^{INK1a/CDKN2}$, which inhibits cyclin-dependent kinases CDK4 and CDK6, facilitators of the cell cycle G1-to-S transition, is expressed at very low levels in primary human fibroblasts. In contrast, both p16 RNA and protein accumulate in late-passage, senescent cells (Hara et al., 1996). This rise in p16 is consistent with a role for this protein in cellular senescence, although its elevation in this setting is also compatible with an inducible role in surveillance. Interestingly, high levels of p16 are also observed in human tumor cell lines lacking a functional *RB* gene, suggesting a negative-feedback loop by which pRB might regulate p16 expression in late G1 (Sherr, 1996). The CDK inhibitor induced by p53 in response to cell damage, p21, is also elevated in senescent cells (El-Deiry et al., 1993; Harper et al., 1993). Furthermore, senescent human diploid fibroblasts contain the unphosphorylated form of pRB. Together these observations can be interpreted in terms of a model which points to the impairment of pRB phosphorylation in response to G1 cyclin–CDK inhibition as the basis for failure to activate many cell proliferation genes (Smith and Pereira-Smith 1996). Thus, the failure to phosphorylate pRB, due to elevated levels of p16 and p21, may be an immediate cause of the failure to enter S phase in senescent fibroblasts (Stein et al., 1990).

b. Oncogene Activation

DNA Methylation.   Up to 5% of all cytosine (C) residues in mammalian DNA are methylated at the 5' position to form 5-methylcytosine (5-mC). Methylated C residues are always flanked by a guanine (G) residue on the 3' side and the methylation occurs in both strands such that it is symmetrical (Catania and Fairweather, 1991). A large body of evidence points to the methylation of certain genes as a mechanism to regulate their expression negatively. As an example, highly repetitive segments of DNA, which are generally not transcribed, are highly methylated, in contrast to other repetitive regions, ''CpG islands,'' which are undermethylated in many housekeeping genes that are expressed in every cell (Antequera et al., 1990). Methylation patterns change in both aging and carcinogenesis. There is an overall trend toward demethylation during both processes, which is consistent with the hypothesis that increases in oncogene expression might be related to the age-dependent increase in the incidence of cancer (Semsai et al., 1989; Goldstein, 1990; Cohen, 1994). However, inconsistencies with these tendencies abound and must be incorporated into any interpretation of this hypothesis in order to gain real insight into the role of methylation in the development of cancer in the elderly.

A general age-dependent decrease in the genomic content of 5-mC in various tissues of mice and humans has been demonstrated (Wilson et al., 1987; Semsai et al., 1989). Levels of 5-mC fall during in vitro aging of human diploid fibroblasts, with the rate of decline being related to the in vitro life span (Catania and Fairweather, 1991). The loss of methylation during replication varies among clones of fibroblasts in culture as well as among different genetic loci and genetic domains within a single clone (Goldstein, 1990). In parallel with this progressive, apparently sporadic, demethylation, gene regulation becomes less efficient, leading to age-related gene derepression (Catania and Fairweather, 1991). Human lymphocytes from old (mean age 75) as opposed to young (mean age 25) individuals show significantly lower levels of 5-mC in all areas of the genomic DNA whereas, in both groups, the transcriptionally active DNA contains 10% less 5-mC than DNA from which transcriptionally active sequences are removed (Drinkwater et al., 1989). Support for a correlation between age-related demethylation and gene derepression comes from mouse studies showing that genes repressed by translocation to the highly methylated inactivated X chromosome become reactivated after a period of time.

There is also an association between decreased methylation and carcinogenesis. Not only have primary tumors been shown to be undermethylated (Nyce et al., 1983), but reduced levels of 5-mC have been demonstrated in carcinogen-treated tissues and carcinogen-induced tumors (Catania and Fairweather, 1991). The extrapolation from demethylation to upregulation of gene expression as a correlate and possible contributor to tumorigenesis directs the focus to genes that promote growth; that is, for example, oncogenes coding for growth factors and signal transduction components. Yet, some cancer-causing genes, namely, the tumor suppressor, or anti-oncogenes, exert their tumorigenic effects by virtue of being inactivated. In fact, CpG islands in the core promoter of the retinoblastoma (RB) tumor suppressor gene are hypermethylated in retinoblastoma tumor tissue, although the methylation pattern varies among different tumor samples (Stirzaker et al., 1997). Other instances that show an association between increased methylation and cancer involve cells in culture. Increased DNA methyltransferase activity, which results in a marked increase in overall DNA methylation, is accompanied by tumorigenic transformation of NIH3T3 cells (Wu et al., 1993). In fact, NIH3T3 cells show stable methylation. Furthermore, in contrast to the methylation patterns seen during normal in vitro aging of human diploid fibroblasts, described above, these same cells transformed and immortalized with the SV40 virus (simian virus 40) show stable methylation over 700 divisions (Catania and Fairweather, 1991). Together these observations suggest that methylation is a feature of immortality and not merely of the transformation of cells. The relationship between methylation of DNA and cancer is therefore complex and must be analyzed in terms of the specific tissues, genes, regions of DNA, and stage of carcinogenesis of the tissues or cells being examined.

Activated Oncogenes as Biomarkers. As expected from the preceding arguments, the identification of specific genes exhibiting age-related methylation changes that are associated with oncogenesis has appropriately centered on known oncogenes. Serum stimulation of senescent human diploid fibroblasts does not induce transcription of c-*fos*, in contrast to c-*myc*, c-H-*ras*, ornithine decarboxylase, and actin, suggesting that c-*fos* is under specific transcriptional repression (Goldstein, 1990; Seshadri and Campisi, 1990), perhaps via methylation. Overexpression of a transfected c-*fos* gene in senescent human diploid fibroblast cells restores the DNA replicative potential at least transiently, suggesting that the senescent state in these fibroblasts is a result not only of replicative arrest but also of anti–oncogenesis.

The c-*myc* proto-oncogene is involved in the G0 to G1 transition from quiescence to proliferation in the cell cycle and appears to be required for cellular proliferation (Spencer and Groudine, 1991; Evan and Littlewood, 1993). In many tumor types, including Burkitt's lymphoma, B-cell acute lymphocytic leukemia, small-cell lung carcinomas, breast and colorectal cancers (DePinho et al., 1991; Fearon and Cho, 1996), c-*myc* is overexpressed. In addition, an overall age-dependent increase in the expression of c-*myc* has been observed in mice, with the highest expression being noted in spleen and liver (Semsei et al., 1989). These two sets of observations support a model in which the age-related upregulation of c-*myc* may predispose to tumorigenesis. However, the actual situation is more complex. Attempts to correlate the methylation pattern of c-*myc* with expression during aging reveal inconsistencies among and within studies that may, in part, be attributed to tissue, and possibly species, specificity. Although spleen DNA undergoes hypomethylation as mice age, liver DNA experiences hypermethylation (Ono et al., 1986). The corresponding changes in c-*myc* expression are not entirely clear-cut, however, with the liver in these studies exhibiting a marked decrease in the steady-state level of c-*myc* messenger RNA with aging, as expected according to the hypermethylation pattern, but with the spleen showing very little change in messenger RNA (Ono et al., 1989). In rat liver, on the other hand, c-*myc* messenger RNA transcript levels rise dramatically with age in contrast to messenger RNA transcripts of other oncogenes like c-*sis* and c-*src* and in contrast to c-*myc* levels in aging brain, which show no substantial change (Matocha et al., 1987). Finally, c-*myc* is fully expressed in senescent human diploid fibroblast cells, as is another proto-oncogene, c-H-*ras* (Goldstein, 1990).

Studies reveal that the activity of members of the NF-κB/Rel family of transcription factors varies with aging (Papaconstantinou et al., 1996). NF-κB DNA-binding activity is increased in liver of aged mice. In addition, messenger RNA expression from the angiotensinogen gene, which is regulated by NF-κB, is induced to higher levels in aged mice in response to mitogenic stimulation. Thus, both the constitutive and the stimulated levels of NF-κB transcription factor appear to increase with aging. The implication of these examples of age-related increases in transcription factor expression is that the resulting upregulation of their target genes may predispose to cellular proliferation and oncogenesis.

D. Other Markers of Aging

The translation of messenger RNA into protein is implemented by soluble protein factors that control the three basic steps of initiation, elongation, and termination. Levels of the elongation factor 1α (EF-1$_\alpha$), which helps to bind charged transfer RNA molecules to the ribosome, are 45% lower in late-passage senescent human fibroblasts (Lee et al., 1996). Yet, levels of EF-1$_\alpha$ messenger RNA show no significant change during the adult life span in the rat, suggesting that age-related regulation of EF-1$_\alpha$ is not at the transcriptional level. Both transformed cells in culture and tumor cells in vivo accumulate higher levels of EF-1$_\alpha$ messenger RNA than cells in normal tissues, implicating upregulated EF-1$_\alpha$ expression as a correlate of tumorigenesis. Furthermore, different isotypes of EF-1$_\alpha$ are normally expressed in terminally differentiated (S1 isotype) versus transformed cells (EF-1$_\alpha$ isotype). The reciprocal relationship that EF-1$_\alpha$ levels bear to aging versus cancer, together with the expression of different EF-1$_\alpha$ isotypes in the two settings, suggest that the normal state of aging cells with regard to this growth-associated factor does not directly predispose toward malignancy but rather allows selection of mutations which defy the winding down of protein synthesis in senescent cells.

IV. CONCLUSIONS

The salient point to be gleaned from this discussion is that both aging and cancer are strongly associated with genetic instability, at the chromosomal, gene, and nucleotide levels. The common denominator underlying these genetic aberrations is dysregulation of a basic cellular process such as cell cycle control, signal transduction, RNA transcription, or DNA replication. The dysregulation in both cancer and aging evolves from the accumulation of alterations in genes encoding components of these cellular processes. The resulting genetic instability may in the end be self-perpetuating, with initial alterations leading to further genetic changes, culminating in an exponential increase in associated physiological changes that define progressive aging or carcinogenesis.

In view of many of the cellular processes discussed, the conclusion that changes associated with aging predispose to malignancy may sometimes appear counterintuitive. Thus, the fact that many of the cellular processes that occur with aging are consistent with a general decrease in proliferative capacity (telomere shortening, predisposition to apoptosis, increased p16$^{INK1a/CDKN2}$), with senescence actually being described as ''an antineoplastic mechanism designed to limit the proliferative potential of cell clones in the body'' (Weinberg, 1995), may seem antithetical to the growth-promoting alterations that characterize carcinogenesis. Yet, some processes that typify aging involve increased growth (prostatic hypertrophy, increase in the activation of certain oncogenes with the potential for attendant increased cellular proliferation). It is even possible to view the apparently contradictory tendencies of decreased cell growth with aging and carcinogenesis as collaborating to predispose the elderly individual to develop cancer. A given growth-inhibitory feature of the aging cell program may actually provide a setup for emergence of a counteracting growth-promoting attribute that contributes to malignant transformation. For instance, a decline in telomere size to a critical point places a selective pressure on a cell population, allowing for the emergence of a rare clone with increased telomerase levels, leading to telomere stabilization and the potential for immortalization. Similarly, the tendency of aging cells to undergo apoptosis might select at a population level for a single cell in which the cell death program is inhibited, perhaps due to upregulation of *bcl2*. Clearly, the net tendency to succumb to malignant transformation will derive from a balance between these opposing sets of factors. In summary, one view that has evolved in response to this dilemma is that a major characteristic of aging is an aberration in proliferative homeostasis, a failure in growth control mechanisms that leads to an overall dysregulation of growth control, both positive and negative (Cohen, 1994). One important outcome of this dysregulation is the development of cancer.

REFERENCES

Aaltonen LA, Peltomaki P, Leach FS, et al. Clues to the pathogenesis of familial colorectal cancer. Science 260:812–816 (1993).

Afshari CA, Barrett JC. Molecular genetics of in vitro cellular senescence. In: NJ Holbrook, GR Martin, RA Lockshin, eds. Cellular Aging and Cell Death. New York: Wiley-Liss, 1996, pp 109–121.

Aguilar F, Harris CC, Sun T, et al. Geographic variation of p53 mutational profile in nonmalignant human liver. Science 1994; 264:1317–1319.

Akiyama R, Iwanaga R, Ishikawa T, et al. Mutations of the transforming growth factor-beta type II receptor gene are strongly related to sporadic proximal colon carcinomas with microsatellite instability. Cancer 1996; 78:2478–2484.

Ambrosini G, Adida C, Altieri DC. A novel anti-apoptosis gene, survivin, expressed in cancer and lymphoma. Nature Med 1997; 3:917–921.

Ames BN, Gold LS. Too many rodent carcinogens: mitogenesis increases mutagenesis. Science 1990; 249:970–971.

Anisimov VN. Chapter 6: Age as a factor of risk in multistage carcinogenesis. In FI Caird, T Brewin, eds. Cancer in the Elderly. London: Butterworths 1990, pp 53–59.

Antequera F, Boyes J, Bird A. High levels of de novo methylation and altered chromatin structure at CpG islands in cell lines. Cell 1990; 62:503–514.

Arnold A, Staunton CE, Kim HG, et al. N Engl J Med 1988; 318:658–662.

ASCO (American Society of Clinical Oncologists) Expert Panel T. Clinical practice guidelines for the use of tumor markers in breast and colorectal cancer: report of the American Society of Clinical Oncology Expert Panel. J Clin Oncol 1996; 14:2843–2877.

Auphan N, DiDonato JA, Rosette C, et al. Immunosuppression by glucocorticoids: inhibition of NF-κB activity through induction of IκB synthesis. Science 1995; 270:286–290.

Bacchetti S, Counter CM. Telomeres and telomerase in human cancer (review). Int J Oncol 1995; 7:423–432.

Barnett YA, King CM. An investigation of antioxidant status, DNA repair capacity and mutation as a function of age in humans. Mutat Res 1995; 338:115–128.

Basu TN, Gutmann DH, Fletcher JA, et al. Aberrant regulation of ras proteins in malignant tumour cells from type 1 neurofibromatosis patients. Nature 1992; 356:713–715.

Battacharyya NP, Skandalis A, Ganesh A, et al. Mutator phenotypes in human colorectal carcinoma cell lines. Proc Natl Acad Sci USA 1994; 91:6319–6323.

Beach D. Cyclins, cell cycle control, and neoplasia. Adv Oncol 1994; 10:3–9.

Beg AA, Baldwin AS Jr. The IκB proteins: mutifunctional regulators of Rel/NF-κB transcription factors. Genes Dev 1993; 7:2064–2070.

Bell RA, High KP. Aterations of immune defense mechanisms in the elderly: The role of nutrition. Infect Med May 1997; 415–424.

Berridge MJ. Calcium signalling and cell proliferation. Bioessays 1995; 17:491–500.

Blackburn EH. Structure and function of telomeres. Nature 1991; 350:569–573.

Blackburn EH. Telomeres: no end in sight. Cell 1994; 77:621–623.

Blasco MA, Rizen M, Greider CW, Hanahan D. Differential regulation of telomerase activity and telomerase RNA during multi-stage tumorigenesis. Nature Genet 1996; 12:200–204.

Bodnar AG, Ouellette M, Frolkis M, et al. Extention of life-span by introduction of telomerase into normal human cells. Science 1998; 279:349–342.

Boerrigter ME, Wei JY, Vijg J. Induction and repair of benzo[a]pyrene-DNA adducts in C57BL/6 and BALB/c mice: association with aging and longevity. Mech Aging Dev 1995; 82:31–50.

Bohr VA, Anson RM. DNA damage, mutation and fine structure DNA repair in aging. Mutat Res 1995; 338:25–34.

Bond JA, Wyllie FS, Wynford-Thomas D. Escape from senescence in human diploid fibroblasts induced directly by mutant p53. Oncogene 1994; 9:1885–1889.

Brown K, Gerstberger S, Carlson L, et al. Control of IκB-α proteolysis by site-specific, signal-induced phosphorylation. Science 1995; 267:1485–1488.

Brown J, Wei W, Sedivy JM. Bypass of senescence after disruption of p21[CIP1/WAF1] gene in normal diploid human fibroblasts. Science 1997; 288:831–834.

Cairns P, Polascik TJ, Eby Y, et al. Frequency of homozygous deletion at p16/CKDN2 in primary human tumors. Nature Genet 1995; 11:210–212.

Cakman I, Rhwer J, Schutz RM, et al. Dysregulation between TH1 and TH2 T cell subpopulations in the elderly. Mech Aging Dev 1996; 87:197–209.

Cannon-Albright LA, Goldgar DE, Meyer LJ, et al. Assignment of a locus for familial melanoma, MLM, to chromosome 9p13-p22. Science 1992; 258:1148–1152.

Cano E, Mahadevan LC. Parallel signal processing among mammalian MAPKs. Trends Biochem Sci 1995; 20:117–122.

Carey LA, Davidson NE. Tumor markers in breast cancer: utility and limitations. Adv Oncol 1997; 13:21–29.

Casey PJ. Protein lipidation in cell signaling. Science 1995; 268:2221–225.

Catania J, Fairweather DS. DNA methylation and cellular ageing. Mutat Res 1991; 256:283–293.

Chen XQ, Stroun M, Magnenat JL, et al. Microsatellite alterations in plasma DNA of small cell lung cancer patients. Nature Med 1996; 2:1033–1035.

Chung YJ, Song JM, Lee JY, et al. Microsatellite instability-associated mutations associate preferentially with the intestinal type of primary gastric carcinomas in a high-risk population. Cancer Res 1996; 56:4662–4665.

Clarke AR, Purdie CA, Harrison DJ, et al. Thymocyte apoptosis induced by p53-dependent and independent pathways. Nature 1993; 362:849–852.

Cleveland JL, Ihle JN. Contenders in FasL/TNF death signaling. Cell 1995; 81:479–482.

Cohen H. Biology of aging as related to cancer. Cancer 1994; 74(Suppl. 7):2092–2100.

Cohen SM, Ellwein LB. Cell proliferation in carcinogenesis. Science 1990; 249:1007–1011.

Collins F, Trent J. Cancer genetics. In: AS Fauci, E Braunwald, KJ Isselbacher, et al., eds. Harrison's Principals of Internal Medicine. Philadelphia: Lippincott, 1998, pp 120–128.

Cooper PK, Nouspikel T, Clarkson SG, Leadon SA. Defective transcription-coupled repair of oxidative base damage in Cockayne syndrome patients from XP group G. Science 1997; 275:990–993.

Counter CM, Avilion AA, LeFeuvre CE, et al. Telomere shortening associated with chromosome instability is arrested in immortal cells which express telomerase activity. EMBO 1996; 11:1921–1929.

Counter CM, Hirte HW, Bacchetti S, Harley CB. Telomerase activity in human ovarian carcinoma. Proc Natl Acad Sci USA 1994; 91:2900–2904.

Cross SM, Sanchez CA, Morgan CA, et al. A p53-dependent mouse spindle checkpoint. Science 1995; 267:1353–1356.

Cryns VL, Thor A, Xu HJ, et al. Loss of the retinoblastoma tumor-suppressor gene in parathyroid carcinoma. N Engl J Med 1994; 330:757–761.

Del Sal GD, Ruaro EM, Utrera R. Gas1-induced growth suppression requires a transactivation-independent p53 function. Mol Cell Biol 1995; 15:7152–7160.

DePinho R, Schreiber-Agus N, Alt FW. myc family oncogenes in the development of normal and neoplastic cells. Adv Cancer Res 1991; 57:1–46.

Dickson RB, Lippman ME. Growth factors in breast cancer. Endocrine Rev 1995; 16:559–589.

Drinkwater RD, Blake TJ, Morley AA, Turner DR. Human lymphcytes aged in vivo have reduced levels of methylation in transcriptionally active and inactive DNA. Mutat Res 1989; 219:29–37.

Dunn BK, Longo DL. Lymphoma occurring in association with other diseases. In: PH Wiernik, RA Kyle, JP Dutcher, eds. Neoplastic Diseases of the Blood. New York: Churchill-Livingstone, 1996; pp 963–997.

Ehrenstein D. Immortality gene discovered. Science (News) 1998; 279:177.

El-Deiry WS, Tokino R, Velculescu VE, et al. WAF1, a potential mediator of p53 tumor suppression. Cell 1993; 75:817–825.

Elledge S. Cell cycle checkpoints: preventing an identity crisis. Science 1996; 274:1664–1672.

Eng C. The RET proto-oncogene in multiple endocrine neoplasia type 2 and Hirschprung's disease. N Engl J Med 1996; 335:943–951.

Eng C, Clayton D, Schuffenecker I, et al. The relationship between specific RET proto-oncogene mutations and disease phenotype in multiple endocrine neoplasia type 2. JAMA 1996; 276:1575–1579.

Epstein CJ, Motulsky AG. Werner syndrome: entering the helicase era. Bioessays 1996; 18: 1025–1027.

Evan GI, Littlewood TD. The role of c-myc in cell growth. Curr Opin Genet Dev 1993; 3: 44–49.

Evans MK, Bohr VA. Gene-specific DNA repair of μv-induced cyclobutane pyrimidine dimers in some cancer-prone and premature-aging human syndromes. Mutat Res 1994; 314:221–231.

Farber E. Cell proliferation as a major risk factor for cancer: a concept of doubtful validity. Cancer Res 1995; 55:3759–3762.

Fearon ER, Cho KR. The molecular biology of cancer. In R Emery, ed., Principles and Practice of Medical Genetics. New York: Churchill-Livingstone, 1996, pp 405–438.

Fenton RG, Longo DL. Cell biology of cancer. In: AS Fauci, E Braunwald, KJ Isselbacher, et al., eds. Harrison's Principals of Internal Medicine, Philadelphia: Lippincott, 1998, pp 113–120.

Finch CE, Tanzi RE. Genetics of aging. Science 1997; 278:407–411.

Fishel R, Lescoe MK, Rao MRS, et al. The human mutator gene homolog MSH2 and its association with hereditary nonpolyposis colon cancer. Cell 1993; 75:1027–1038.

FitzGerald MG, Bean JM, Hegde SR, et al. Heterozygous ATM mutations do not contribue to early onset of breast cancer. 1997; Nature Genet 15:307–310.

Folkman J. Clinical applications of research on angiogenesis. N Engl J Med 1995; 333:1757–1763.

Fontanini G, Vignati S, Lucchi M, et al. Neoangiogenesis and p53 protein in lung cancer: their prognostic role and their relation with vascular endothelial growth factor (VEGF) expression. Br J Cancer 1997; 75:1295–1301.

Fraser A, Evan G. A license to kill. 1996; Cell 85:781–784.

Fredericks WJ, Galili N, Mukhopadhyay S, et al. The PAX3-FKHR fusion protein created by the (2;13) translocation in alveolar rhabdomyosarcomas is a more potent transcriptional activator than PAX3. Mol Cel Biol 1995; 15:1522–1535.

Friedberg EC, Walker GC, Siede W. Human hereditary diseases with defective processing of DNA damage. In: DNA Repair and Mutagenesis. Washington, DC, American Society for Microbiology 1995, pp. 662–669.

Fujimoto J, Shiota M, Iwahara T, et al. Characterization of the transforming activity of p80, a hyperphosphorylated protein in a Ki-1 lymphoma cell line with chromosomal translocation t(2;5). Proc Natl Acad Sci USA 1996; 93:4181–4186.

Furnari B, Rhind N, Russell P. Cdc25 mitotic inducer targeted by chkl DNA damage checkpoint kinase. Science 277:1495–1497, 1997.

Gallie BL. Retinoblastoma gene mutations in human cancer. N Engl J Med 1994; 330:786–787.

Gartenhaus R, Johns III MM, Wang P, et al. Mutator phenotype in a subset of chronic lymphocytic leukemia. Blood 1996; 87:38–41.

Geradts J, Kratzke RA, Niehans GA, Lincoln CE. Immunohistochemical detection of the cyclin-dependent kinase inhibitor 2/multiple tumor suppressor gene 1 (CDKN2/

MTS1) product p16[INK4A] in archival human solid tumors: correlation with retinoblastoma protein expression. Cancer Res 1995; 55:6006–6011.

Ghosh A, Greenberg ME. Calcium signaling in neurons: molecular mechanisms and cellular consequences. Science 1995; 268:239–247.

Goldstein S. Replicative senescence: the human fibroblast comes of age. Science 1990; 249: 1129–1133.

Graham R, Gilman M. Distinct protein targets for signals acting at the c-fos serum response clement. Science 1991; 251:189–192.

Gray MD, Shen JC, Kamath-Loeb AS, et al. The Werner syndrome protein is a DNA helicase. Nature Genet 1997; 17:100–103.

Greco A, Pierotti MA, Bongarzone I, et al. Trk-t1 is a novel oncogene formed by the fusion of tpr and trk genes in human papillary thyroid carcinomas. Oncogene 1992; 78:237–242.

Greenwell PW, Kronmal S, Porter SE, et al. TEL1, a gene involved in controlling telomere length in S. cerevisiae, is homologous to the human ataxia telangiectasia gene. Cell 1995; 82:823–829.

Greider CW, Harley CB. Telomeres and telomerase in cell senescence and immortalization. In: NJ Holbrook, GR Martin, RA Lockshin, eds. Cellular Aging and Cell Death, New York: Wiley-Liss; 1996, pp. 123–138.

Guinan EC, Gribben JG, Boussiotis VA, et al. Pivotal role of the B4:CD28 pathway in transplantation tolerance and tumor immunity. Blood 1994; 84:3261–3282.

Gutmann DH, Aylsworth A, Carey JC. The diagnostic evaluation and multidisciplinary management of neurofibromatosis 1 and neurofibromatosis 2. JAMA 1997; 278:51–57.

Hall M, Peters G. Genetic alterations of cyclins, cyclin-dependent kinases, and Cdk inhibitors in human cancers. Adv Cancer Res 1996; 68:67.

Han HJ, Yanagisawa A, Kato Y, et al., Genetic instability in pancreatic cancer and poorly differentiated type of gastric cancer. Cancer Res 1993; 53:5087–5089.

Hanahan D. Signaling vascular morphogenesis and maintenance. Science 1997; 277:48–50.

Hanawalt PC. Transcription-coupled repair and human disease. Science 1994; 266:1957–1958.

Hara E, Smith R, Parry D, et al. Regulation of p16[CDKN2] expression and its implications for cell immortalization and senescence. Mol Cel Biol 1996; 16:859–867.

Harley CB. Telomere loss: mitotic clock or genetic time bomb? Mutat Res 1991; 256:271–282.

Harley CB. Telomeres and aging: fact, fancy, and the future. J NIH Res 1995; 7:64–68.

Harley CB, Kim NW, Prowse KR, et al. Telomerase, cell immortality, and cancer. Cold Spring Harb Symp Quant Biol 1994; 59:307–315.

Harper MW, Adami GR, Wei N, et al. The p21 Cdk-interacting protein Cip1 is a potent inhibitor of G1 cyclin-dependent kinases. Cell 1993; 75:805–816.

Harris CC, Hollstein M. Clinical implications of the p53 tumor-suppressor gene. N Engl J Med 1993; 329:1318–1327.

Hartwell LH, Kastan MB. Cell cycle control and cancer. Science 266:1821–1828, 1994.

Hatada EN, Nieters A, Wulczyn FG, et al. The ankyrin repeat domains of the NF-κB precursor p105 and the proto-oncogene bcl-3 act as specific inhibitors of NF-κB DNA binding. Proc Natl Acad Sci USA 1992; 89:2489–2493.

Hatano M, Roberts CWM, Minden M, et al. Deregulation of a homeobox gene, HOX11, by the (10;14) in T cell leukemia. Science 1991; 253:79–82 (1991).

Hayes DF. When is a tumor marker ready for prime time? The tumor marker utility grading scale. ASCO Educational Book, Thirty-third Annual Meeting, 1997, pp 206–212.

Hayes DF, Bast R, Desch CE, et al. A tumor marker utility grading system (TMUGS): a framework to evaluate clinical utility of tumor markers. J Natl Cancer Inst 1996; 88: 1456–1466.

Heidin CH. Dimerization of cell surface receptors in signal transduction. Cell 1995; 80:213–223.

Hengst L, Reed SI. Translational control of p27[Kip1] accumulation during the cell cycle. Science 1996; 271:1861–1864.

Herndon FJ, Hsu HC, Mountz JD. Increased apoptosis of CD45RO−T cells with aging. Mech Aging Dev 1997; 94:123–34.

Higami Y, Shimokawa I, Okimoto T, et al. Effect of aging and dietary restriction on hepatocyte proliferation and death in male F344 rats. Cell Tissue Res 1997; 288:69–77.

Hill CS, Treisman R. Transcriptional regulation by extracellular signals: mechanisms and specificity. Cell 1995; 80:199–211.

Hockenbery D, Nunez G, Milliman C, et al. Bcl-2 is an inner mitochondrial membrane protein that blocks programmed cell death. Nature 1990; 348:334–336.

Hollstein M, Sidransky D, Vogelstein B, Harris CC. p53 Mutations in human cancers. Science 1991; 253:49–58.

Homma Y, Tsunoda M, Kasai H. Evidence for the accumulation of oxidative stress during cellular aging of human diploid fibroblasts. Biochem Biophys Res Commun 1994; 203: 1063–1068.

Hunter T. Oncoprotein networks. Cell 1997; 88:333–346.

Hunter T, Pines J. Cyclins and cancer II: cyclin D and CDK inhibitors come of age. Cell 1994; 79:573–582.

Hussussian CJ, Struewing JP, Goldstein AM, et al. Germline p16 mutations in familial melanoma. Nature Genet 1994; 8:15–21.

Ichikawa A, Kinoshita T, Watanabe T, et al. Mutations of the p53 gene as a prognostic factor in aggressive B-cell lymphoma. N Engl J Med 1997; 337:529–534.

Ihle JN. Cytokine receptor signalling. Nature 1995; 377:591–594.

Ionov Y, Peinado MA, Malkhosyan S, et al. Ubiquitous somatic mutations in simple repeated sequences reveal a new mechanism for colonic carcinogenesis. Nature 1993; 363:558–561.

Iyengar R. There are GAPS and there are GAPS. Science 1997; 275:42–43.

Jabbar SA, Hoffbrand AV, Wickremasinghe RG. Defects in signal transduction pathways in chronic B lymphocytic leukemia cells. Leuk Lymphoma 1995; 18:163–170.

Jazwinski SM. Longevity, genes, and aging. Science 1996; 273:54–59.

Johnson TE, Lithgow GJ, Murakami S, et al. Genetics of aging and longevity in lower organisms. In: NJ Holbrook, GR Martin, RA Lockshin, eds. Cellular Aging and Cell Death. New York: Wiley-Liss, 1996, pp 1–17.

Johnson BE, Damodaran A, Rushin J, et al. Ectopic production and processing of atrial natriuretic peptide in a small cell lung carcinoma cell line and tumor from a patient with hyponatremia. Cancer 1997; 79:35–44.

Kaelin WG. Recent insights into the functions of the retinoblastoma susceptibility gene product. Cancer Invest 1997; 15:243–254.

Kamb A, Gruis NA, Weaver-Feldhaus J, et al. A cell cycle regulator potentially involved in genesis of many tumor types. Science 1994; 264:436–440.

Karin M, Zg L, Zandi E. AP-1 function and regulation. Curr Opin Cell Biol 1997; 9:240–246.

Kastan M. Clinical implications of basic research. Ataxia-telangiectasia—broad implications for a rare disorder. N Engl J Med 1995; 333:662–663.

Kastner P, Mark M, Chambon P. Nonsteroid nuclear receptors: What are genetic studies telling us about their role in real life? Cell 1995; 83:859–869.

Keith CT, Schreiber SL. PIK-related kinases: DNA repair, recombination, and cell cycle checkpoints. Science 1995; 270:50–51.

Kelloff GJ, Boone CW, Crowell JA. et al. Risk biomarkers and current strategies for cancer chemoprevention. J Cell Biochem 1996; 25(Suppl):1–14.

Kennedy BJ. Aging and cancer. C 1 In: FI Caird, T Brewin, eds. Cancer in the Elderly. London: Butterworths, 1990, pp. 3–7.

Kennedy BJ, Gotta M, Sinclair DA, et al. Redistribution of silencing proteins from telomeres to the nucleolus is associated with extension of life span in S. cerevisiae. Cell 1997; 89:381–391.

Kimura KD, Tissenbaum HA, Liu Y, Ruvkun G. daf-2, an insulin receptor-like gene that regulates longevity and diapause in Caenorhabditis elegans. Science 1997; 277:942–946.

Kinzler K, Vogelstein B. Lessons from hereditary colorectal cancer. Cell 1996; 87:159–170.

Kirkwood TBL. DNA, mutations and aging. Muta Res 1989; 219:1–7.

Kluck RM, Bossy-Wetzel E, Green DR, Newmeyer DD. The release of cytochrome c from mitochondria: A primary site for Bcl-2 regulation of apoptosis. Science 1997; 275:1132–1136.

Knudson AG. Antioncogenes and human cancer. Proc Natl Acad Sci USA 1993; 90:10914–10921.

Knudson CM, Korsmeyer SJ. Bcl-2 and Bax function independently to regulate cell death. Nature Genet 1997; 16:358–363.

Komatsu H, Iida S, Yamamoto K, et al. A variant chromosome translocation at 11q13 identifying PRAD1/Cyclin D1 as the BCL-1 gene. Blood 1994; 84:1226–1231.

Korsmeyer SJ. Bcl-2 initiates a new category of oncogenes: regulators of cell death. Blood 1992; 60:879–886.

Kortenjann M, Thomae E, Shaw PE. Inhibition of v-raf-dependent c-fos expression and transformation by a kinase-defective mutant of the mitogen-activated protein kinase Erk 2. Mol Cell Biol 1994; 14:4815–4824.

Kruk PA, Rampino NJ, Bohr VA. DNA damage and repair in telomeres: relation to aging. Proc Natl Acad Sci USA 1995; 92:258–262.

Kuro-o M, Matsumura Y, Aizawa H, et al. Mutation of the mouse klotho gene leads to a syndrome resembling aging. Nature 1997; 390:45–51.

Kwon TK, Nagel JE, Buchholz MA, Nordin AA. Characterization of the murine cyclin-dependent kinase inhibitor gene p27Kip1. Gene 1996; 180:113–120.

Kwon TK, Buchholz MA, Ponsalle P, et al. The regulation of p27Kip1 expression following the polyclonal activation of murine 60 T cells. J Immunol 1997; 158:5642–5648.

Lakowski B, Hekimi S. Determination of life-span in Caenorhabditis elegans by four clock genes. Science 1996; 272:1010–1013.

Latchman DS. Eukaryotic transcription factors. J Biochem 1990; 270:281–289.

Latchman DS. Transcription-factor mutations and disease. N Engl J Med 1996; 334:28–33.

Leach FS, Nicolaides NC, Papadopoulos N, et al. Mutations of mutS homolog in hereditary nonpolyposis colorectal cancer. Cell 1993; 75:1215–1225.

Lee S, Duttaroy A, Wang E. EF-1$_\alpha$-S1 gene family and regulation of protein synthesis during aging. In: NJ Holbrook, GR Martin, RA Lockshin, eds. Cellular Aging and Cell Death, New York: Wiley-Liss, 1996; pp 130–151.

Lee SW, Fukunaga N, Rigney DR, et al. Downregulation of DNA topoisomerase I in old versus young human diploid fibroblasts. Mutat Res 1997; 373:179–184.

Lesourd BM, Meaume S. Cell mediated immunity changes in ageing, relative importance of cell subpopulation switches and of nutritional factors. Immunol Lett 1994; 40:235–242.

Levine AJ. p53, the cellular gatekeeper growth and division. Cell 1997; 88:323–331.

Levitzki A. From epinephrine to cyclic AMP. Science 1988; 241:800–806.

Lindahl P, Johansson BR, Leveen P, Betsholtz C. Pericyte loss and microaneurysm formation in PDGF-B-deficient mice. Science 1997; 277:242–245.

Liu B, Parsons R, Papadopoulos N, et al. Analysis of mismatch repair genes in hereditary non-polyposis colorectal cancer patients. Nature Med 1996; 2:169–174.

Loft S, Poulsen HE. Cancer risk and oxidative DNA damage in man. J Mol Med 1996; 74: 297–312.

Lyons J, Landis CA, Harsh G, et al. Two G protein oncogenes in human endocrine tumors. Science 1990; 249:655–659.

Maisonpierre PC, Suri C, Jones PF, et al. Angiopoietin-2, a natural antagonist for Tie2 that disrupts in vivo angiogenesis. Science 1997; 277:55–60.

Malkin D, Li FP, Strong LC, et al. Germ line p53 mutations in a familial syndrome of breast cancer, sarcomas, and other neoplasms. Science 1990; 250:1233–1238.

Mangelsdorf DJ, Thummel C, Beato M, et al. The nuclear receptor superfamily: the second decade. Cell 1995; 83:835–839.

Manning FCR, Patierno SR. Apoptosis: Inhibitor or instigator of carcinogenesis? Cancer Invest 1996; 14:455–565.

Markowitz S, Wang J, Myeroff L, Parsons R, et al. Inactivation of the type II TGF-β receptor in colon cancer cells with microsatellite instability. Science 1995; 268:1336–1338.

Martin GM. Genetic modulation of telomeric terminal restriction-fragment length: relevance for clonal aging and late-life disease (invited editorial). Am J Hum Genet 1994; 55: 866–869.

Martin GM. Molecular genetics in clinical practice II: The genetics of aging. Hosp Pract 1997; 32:47–75.

Martin SJ, Green DR. Protease activation during apoptosis: Death by a thousand cuts? Cell 1995; 82:349–352.

Matocha MF, Cosgrove JW, Atack JR, Rapoport SI. Selective elevation of c-myc transcript levels in the liver of the aging Fischer-344 rat. Biochem Biophys Res Commun 1987; 147:1–7.

Matsumoto T, Shimamoto A, Goto M, Furuichi Y. Impaired nuclear localization of defective DNA helicases in Werner's syndrome. Nature Genet 1997; 16:335–336.

Meydani SN, Meydani M, Blumberg JB, et al. Vitamin E supplementation and in vivo immune response in healthy elderly subjects: a randomized controlled trial. JAMA 1997; 277:1380–1386.

Meyn MS. Ataxia-telangiectasia and cellular responses to DNA damage. Cancer Res 1995; 55:5991–6001.

Miller RA. The aging immune system: primer and prospectus. Science 1996; 273:70–74.

Millman JS, Andrews DA. Switching the model: a concerted mechanism for GTPases in protein targeting. Cell 1997; 89:673–676.

Mochly-Rosen D. Localization of protein kinases by anchoring proteins: a theme in signal transduction. Science 1995; 268:247–251.

Modrich P. Mismatch repair, genetic stability, and cancer. Science 1994; 266:1959–1960.

Moriwaki S, Ray S, Tarone RE, et al. The effect of donor age on the processing of μv-damaged DNA by cultured human cells: reduced DNA repair capacity and increased DNA mutability. Mutat Res 1996; 364:117–123.

Morrow DM, Tagle DA, Shiloh Y, et al. TEL1, an S. cerevisiae homolog of the human gene mutated in ataxia telangiectasia, is functionally related to the yeast checkpoint gene MEC1. Cell 1995; 82:831–840.

Mosmann TR, Sad S. The expanding universe of T-cell subsets: Th1 Th2 and more. Immunol Today 1996; 17:138–146.

Motokura T, Bloom T, Kim HG, et al. A novel cyclin encoded by a bcl1-linked candidate oncogene. Nature 1991; 350:512–515 (1991).

Mulligan LM, Kwok JB, Healey CS, et al. Germ-line mutations of the RET proto-oncogene in multiple endocrine neoplasia type 2A. Nature 1993; 363:458–460.

Murray V, Holliday R. Increased error frequency of DNA polymerases from senescent human fibroblasts. J Mol Biol 1981; 146:55–76.

Nagata S. Apoptosis by death factor. Cell 1997; 88:355–365.

Nasmyth K. Viewpoint: putting the cell cycle in order. Science 1996; 274:1643–1645.

Nawroz H, Koch W, Anker P, et al. Microsatellite alterations in serum DNA of head and neck cancer patients. Nature Med 1996; 2:1035–1037.

Nevins JR. E2F: a link between the Rb tumor suppressor protein and viral oncoproteins. Science 1992; 258:424–429.

Nishizuka Y. Intracellular signaling by hydrolysis of phospholipids and activation of protein kinase C. Science 1992; 258:607–614.

Nusse R. A versatile transcriptional effector of wingless signaling. Cell 1997; 89:321–323.

Nusse R, Varmus HE. Wnt genes. Cell 1992; 69:1073–1087.

Nyce J, Weinhouse S, Magee PN. 5-Methylcytosine depletion during tumor development: an extension of the miscoding concept. Br J Cancer 1983; 48:463–475.

Offermanns S, Mancino V, Revel JP, Simon MI. Vascular system defects and impaired cell chemokinesis as a result of $G\alpha_{13}$ deficiency. Science 1997; 275:533–536.

Ohno H, Takimoto G, McKeithan TW. The candidate proto-oncogene bcl-3 is related to genes implicated in cell lineage determination and cell cycle control. Cell 1990; 60:991–997.

Okamoto A, Demetrick DJ, Spillare EA, et al. Mutations and altered expression of p16[INK4] in human cancer. Proc Natl Acad Sci USA 1994; 91:11045–11049.

Ono T, Tawa R, Shinya K, et al. Methylation of the c-myc gene changes during aging process of mice. Biochem Biophys Res Commun 1986; 139:1299–1304.

Ono T, Takahashi N, Okada S. Age-associated changes in DNA methylation and mRNA level of the c-myc gene in spleen and liver of mice. Mutat Res 1989; 219:39–50.

Otterson GA, Kratzke RA, Coxon A, et al. Absence of p16[INK4] protein is restricted to the subset of lung cancer lines that retains wildtype RB. Oncogene 1994; 9:3375–3378.

Overduin M, Harvey TS, Bagby S, et al. Solution structure of the epithelial cadherin domain responsible for selective cell adhesion. Science 1995; 267:386–389.

Ozawa T. Genetic and functional changes in mitochondria associated with aging. Physiol Rev 1997; 77:425–464.

Pagano M, Tam SW, Theodoras AM, et al. Role of the ubiquitin-proteasome pathway in regulating abundance of the cyclin-dependent kinase inhibitor p27. Science 1995; 269: 682–685.

Pan G, Ni J, Wei YF, et al. An antagonist decoy receptor and a death domain-containing receptor for TRAIL. Science 1997; 277:815–818.

Papaconstantinou J, Reisner PD, Liu L, Kuninger DT. Mechanisms of altered gene expression with aging. In: EL Schneider, JW Rowe, eds. Handbook of the Biology of Aging. San Diego: Academic Press, 1996, pp 150–183.

Parsons R, Li GM, Longley MJ, et al. Hypermutability and mismatch repair deficiency in RER+ tumor cells. Cell 1993; 75:1227–1236.

Parsons R, Myeroff LL, Liu B, et al. Microsatellite instability and mutation of the transforming growth factor β type II receptor gene in colorectal cancer. Cancer Res 1995; 55:5548–5550.

Paulovich AG, Toczyski DP, Hartwell LH. When checkpoints fail. Cell 88:315–321, 1997.

Pawelec G, Adibzadeh M, Solana R, Beckman I. The T cell in the ageing individual. Mech Aging Dev 1997; 93:35–45.

Pazin MJ, Kadonaga JT. What's up and down with histone deacetylation and transcription? Cell 1997; 89:326–328.

Peng CY, et al. (5). Mitotic and G2 checkpoint control: Regulation of 14-3-3 protein binding by phosphorylation of Cdc25C on serine-216. Science 277:1501–1505, 1997.

Phelouzat MA, Arbogast A, Laforge T, et al. Excessive apoptosis of mature T lymphocytes is a characteristic feature of human immune senescence. Mech Aging Dev 1996; 88: 25–38.

Rampino N, Yamamoto Y, Ionov Y, et al. Somatic frameshift mutations in the BAX gene in colon cancers of the microsatellite mutator phenotype. Science 1997; 275:967–969.

Randerath K, Randerath E, Filburn C. Genomic and mitochondrial DNA alterations with aging. In: EL Schneider, JW Rose, eds. Handbook of the Biology of Aging. San Diego: Academic Press, 1996, pp 198–214.

Rao KS, Vinay Kumar D, Bhaskar MS, Sripad G. On the 'active' molecules of DNA-polymerase beta in aging rat brain. Biochem Mol Biol Int 1994; 34:287–294.

Reis RJS, Slagboom PE. Genetics of aging: longevity- and senescence-determining genes. A symposium report on the XVIth International Congress of Genetics, Toronto, August 1988. Mutat Res 1989; 219:135–137.

Rodrigues GA, Park M. Dimerization mediated through a leucine zipper activates the oncogenic potential of the *met* receptor tyrosine kinase. Mol Cell Biol 1993; 13:6711–6722.

Rudd GN, Hartley JA, Souhami RL. Persistence of cisplatin-induced DNA interstrand crosslinking in peripheral blood mononuclear cells from elderly and young individuals. Cancer Chemother Pharmacol 1995; 35:323–326.

Ruoslahti E. Stretching is good for a cell. Science 1997; 276:1345–1346.

Russo C, Cherniack EP, Wali A, et al. Age-dependent appearance of non-major histocompatibility complex-restricted helper T cells. Proc Natl Acad Sci USA 1993; 90:11718–11722.

Sage EH. Angiogenesis inhibition in the context of endothelial cell biology. Adv Oncol 1996; 12:17–29.

Sancar A. Mechanisms of DNA excision repair. Science 1994; 266:1954–1956.

Sanchez Y, et al. (6). Conservation of the Chk1 checkpoint pathway in mammals: Linkage of DNA damage to Cdk regulation through Cdc25. Science 277:1497–1501, 1997.

Sausville EA, Longo DL. Growth factors and growth factor inhibitors. In: BA Teicher, ed. The Cancer Therapeutics Handbook. Totowa, NJ: Humana Press, 1997: pp 337–370.

Savitsky K, Bar-Shira A, Gilad S, et al. A single ataxia telangiectasia gene with a product similar to PI-3 kinase. Science 1995; 268:1749–1753 (1995).

Scheffzek K, Ahmadian MR, Kabsch W, et al. The Ras-RasGAP complex: Structural basis for GTPase activation and its loss in oncogenic Ras mutants. Science 1997; 277:333–338.

Scheinman RI, Cogswell PC, Lofquist AK, Baldwin AS Jr. Role of transcriptional activation of IκBα in mediation of immunosuppression by glucocorticoids. Science 1995; 270: 283–286.

Schmidt L, Duh FM, Chen F, Kishida T, et al. Germline and somatic mutations in the tyrosine kinase domain of the MET proto-oncogene in papillary renal carcinomas. Nature Genet 1997; 16:68–73.

Semsai I, Ma S, Cutler RG. Tissue and age specific expression of the myc proto-oncogene family throughout the life span of the C57BL/6J mouse strain. Oncogene 1989; 4: 465–470.

Serrano M, Gomez-Lahoz E, DePinho RA, et al. Inhibition of Ras-induced proliferation and cellular transformation by p16[INK4]. Science 1995; 267:249–252.

Serrano M, Lee HW, Chin L, et al. Role of INK4a locus in tumor suppression and cell mortality. Cell 1996; 85:27.

Seshadri T, Campisi J. Repression of c-fos transcription and an altered genetic program in senescent human fibroblasts. Science 1990; 247:205–209.

Seto BM, Yamamoto K, Iida S, et al. Gene rearrangement and overexpression of PRAD1 in lymphoid malignancy with t(11;14)(q13;q32) translocation. Oncogene 1992; 7:1401–1406.

Shay JW, Pereira-Smith OM, Wright WE. A role for both RB and p53 in the regulation of human cellular senescence. Exp Cell Res 1991; 196:33–39.

Sheridan JP, Marsters SA, Pitti RM, et al. Control of TRAIL-induced apoptosis by a family of signaling and decoy receptors. Science 1997; 277:818–821.

Sherr D. Cancer cell cycles. Science 1996; 274:1672–1677.

Side L, Taylor B, Cayouette M, et al. Homozygous inactivation of the NF1 gene in bone marrow cells from children with neurofibromatosis type 1 and malignant myeloid disorders. N Engl J Med 1997; 336:1713–1720.

Sinclair DA, Guarente L. Extrachromosomal rDNA circles–A cause of aging in yeast. Cell 1997; 91:1033–1042.

Sinclair DA, Mills K, Guarente L. Accelerated aging and nucleolar fragmentation in yeast sgs1 mutants. Science 1997; 277:1313–1316.

Smith JR, Pereira-Smith O. Replicative senescence: Implications for in vivo aging and tumor suppression. Science 1996; 273:63–67.

Spencer CA, Groudine M. Control of c-myc regulation in normal and neoplastic cells. Adv Cancer Res 1991; 56:1–48.

Sprang SR. GAP into the breach. Science 1997; 277:329–330.

Steller H. Mechanisms and genes of cellular suicide. Science 1995; 267:1445–1449.

Stein GH, Beeson M, Gordon L. Failure to phosphorylate the retinoblastoma gene product in senescent human fibroblasts. Science 1990; 249:666–669.

Stillman B. Cell cycle control of DNA replication. Science 1996; 274:1659–1664.

Stirzaker C, Millar DM, Paul CL, et al. Extensive DNA methylation spanning the Rb promoter in retinoblastoma tumors. Cancer Res 1997; 57:2229–2237.

Sugimura T. Multistep carcinogenesis: a 1992 perspective. Science 1992; 258:603–607.

Swift M, Reitnauer PJ, Morrell D, Chase CL. Breast and other cancers in families with ataxia-telangiectasia. N Engl J Med 1987; 316:1289–1294.

Swift M, Morrell D, Massey RB, Chase CL. Incidence of cancer in 161 families affected by ataxia-telangiectasia. N Engl J Med 1991; 325:1831–1836.

Takeichi M. Cadherins in cancer: Implications for invasion and metastasis. Curr Opin Cell Biol 1993; 5:806–811.

Taniguchi T. Cytokine signaling through nonreceptor protein tyrosine kinases. Science 1995; 268:251–255.

Taunton J, Hassig CA, Schreiber SL. A mammalian histone deacetylase related to the yeast transcriptional regulator Rpd3p. Science 1996; 272:408–411.

Taylor AMR, Metcalfe JA, Thick J, Mak YF. Leukemia and lymhoma in ataxia telangiectasia. Blood 1996; 87:423–438.

Thibodeau SN, Bren G, Schaid D. Microsatellite instability in cancer of the proximal colon. Science 1993; 260:816–819.

Thompson CB. Apoptosis in the pathogenesis and treatment of disease. Science 1995; 267: 1456–1462.

Umemori H, Inoue T, Kume S, et al. Activation of the G protein Gq/11 through tyrosine phosphorylation of the α subunit. Science 1997; 276:1878–1879.

Usami S, Takumi Y, Fujita S, et al. Cell death in the inner ear associated with aging is apoptosis? Brain Res 1997; 747:147–150.

Vogelstein B, Fearon ER, Hamilton SR, et al. Genetic alterations during development. N Engl J Med 1988; 319:525–532.

Wagner G. E-cadherin: a distant member of the immunoglobulin superfamily. Science 1995; 267:342–343.

Wang Y, Becker D. Antisense targeting of basic fibroblast growth factor and fibroblast growth factor receptor-1 in human melanoma blocks intratumoral angiogenesis and tumor growth. Nature Med 1997; 3:887–893.

Warrell RP, De The H, Wang Z, Degos L. Acute promyelocytic leukemia. N Engl J Med 1993; 329:177–189.

Watson JD. Origin of concatemeric T7 DNA. Nature New Biol 1972; 239:197–201.

Wayne SJ, Rhyne RL, Garry PJ, Goodwin JS. Cell-mediated immunity as a predictor of morbidity and mortality in subjects over 60. J Gerontol. 1990; 45:M45–48.

Wei YH, Kao SH, Lee HC. Simultaneous increase of mitochondrial DNA deletions and lipid peroxidation in human aging. Ann NY Acad Sci 1996; 786:24–43.

Weigle WO. The effect of aging on cytokine release and associated immunologic functions. Immunol Allergy Clin North Am 1993; 13:551–569.

Weinberg RA. The retinoblastoma protein and cell cycle control. Cell 1995; 81:323–330.

Weinert T. Yeast checkpoint controls and relevance to cancer. Cancer Surv:109–132, 1997.

Weirich-Schwaiger H, Weirich HG, Gruber B, et al. Correlation between senescence and DNA repair in cells from young and old individuals and in premature aging syndromes. Mutat Res 1994; 316:37–48.

Whitmarsh AJ, Davis RJ. Transcription factor AP-1 regulation by mitogen-activated protein kinase signal transduction pathways. J Mol Med 1996; 74:589–607.

Williams M, Swerdlow SH, Rosenberg CL, Arnold A. Centrocytic lymphoma: a B-cell non-Hodgkin's lymphoma characterized by chromosome 11BCL-1 and PRAD 1 rearrangements. Curr Top Microbiol Immunol 1992; 182:325–329.

Wilson VL, Smith RA, Ma S, Cutler RG. Genomic 5-methyldeoxycytidine decreases with age. J Biol Chem 1987; 262:9948–9951.

Wolffe AP. Histone deacetylase: a regulator of transcription. Science 1996; 272:371–372.

Wu J, Issa JP, Herman J, et al. Expression of an exogenous eukaryotic DNA methyltransferase gene induces transformation of NIH 3T3 cells. Proc Natl Acad Sci USA 1993; 90: 8891–8895.

Yang E, Korsmeyer SJ. Molecular thanatopsis: a discourse on the BCL2 family and cell death. Blood 1996; 88:386–401.

Yang J, Liu X, Bhalla K, et al. Prevention of apoptosis by Bcl-2: Release of cytochrome c from mitochondria blocked. Science 1997; 275:1129–1132.

Yu CE, Oshima J, Fu YH, et al. Positional cloning of the Werner's syndrome gene. Science 1996; 272:258–267.

Zhang L, Zhou W, Velculescu VE, et al. Gene expression profiles in normal and cancer cells. Science 1997; 276:1268–1272.

7
Inherited Susceptibility to Cancer

Hanlee P. Ji and Robin L. Bennett
University of Washington
Seattle, Washington

Wylie Burke
University of Washington and
Fred Hutchinson Cancer Research Center
Seattle, Washington

I. INTRODUCTION

The identification of patients with a genetic predisposition to cancer is emerging as an important component of medical practice. Essential clues to the presence of an inherited cancer predisposition lie in characteristics of the family history, including the proportion of family members affected with cancer, the type of cancer, and the age of onset in those affected. Genetic cancer traits are distinguished by the dramatic clustering of cancers within an affected family. The greater the number of affected relatives and the more closely related they are, the greater the likelihood that an individual may carry an inherited predisposition to cancer. Familial clustering of cancers such as those of breast, ovary, and colon have been recognized as following Mendelian patterns of inheritance in some families. With molecular genetic analysis, the responsible genes for many of these cancer syndromes have been identified.

The early clinical studies for many genetic cancer traits were restricted to site-specific malignancies like colon or breast cancer. These cancer syndromes were first recognized because of the significantly younger age at which affected individuals developed cancer, but there is growing realization that the clinical spectrum of these syndromes extends to an older population as well. With the identification of the genetic mutations underlying these familial cancer syndromes, their clinical spectrum has expanded, and it is now recognized that many genetic cancer syndromes place individuals at increased risk for a broad variety of malignancies.

Familial cancers traits can be categorized based on the prevalence of their associated cancers (Table 1). One category includes cancer syndromes such as von Hippel–Lindau syndrome, multiple endocrine neoplasia, and Li–Fraumeni syndrome. These are rare clinical entities, usually associated with less common cancers and frequently involving multiple types of malignancies. The other category is inherited susceptibility to common malignancies like carcinoma of the breast, ovaries, or colon. An example is familial breast and ovarian cancer associated with mutations in the BRCA1 or BRCA2 genes. In this chapter, we review the rare cancer syndromes causing adult-onset cancers and the genetics of colon, breast, ovarian and prostatic cancers.

Genetic tests are now available to identify individuals with a predisposition to breast, ovarian, and colon cancers and to diagnose several other rare cancer syndromes. Additional testing options will continue to emerge with the discovery of new cancer-susceptibility genes. These technical advances challenge clinicians to identify appropriate candidates for genetic testing, without raising unnecessary anxiety in those unlikely to carry genetic susceptibilities, and to counsel individuals about cancer risk and testing options in a manner that allows informed decision making and optimal health outcomes.

A. Inheritance of Familial Cancer Traits

Familial cancers are attributed to genetic changes which occur in the germline. Most of the familial cancers so far described are autosomal dominant; that is, the genetic

Table 1 List of Autosomal Dominant Familial Cancer Traits and Their Associated Genes.

Cancer trait	Gene	Locus	Commercial testing
Rare cancer syndromes causing adult-onset cancer			
von–Hippel Lindau	VHL	3p25-26	Yes
MEN type I	MEN1	11q13	No
MEN type II	RET	10q11.2	Yes
Li–Fraumeni	p53	17p13.1	Yes
Cowden's	PTEN	10q23.3	No
Common cancer genetic susceptibilities			
Colon cancer			
Familial adenomatous polyposis	APC	5q21-22	Yes
Hereditary nonpolyposis colorectal cancer	MSH1	2p22-p21	Yes
	MLH1	3p21.3	Yes
	PMS1	2q31-q33	No
	PMS2	p22	No
Breast/ovarian cancer			
Familial breast cancer	BRCA1	17q21	Yes
	BRCA2	13q12.3	Yes

susceptibility is conferred by the presence of a mutation in one of the two copies of a gene, with vertical transmission of a cancer susceptibility mutation from parent to child. Mutation carriers are *heterozygotes*—the genetic term used to indicate individuals who carry one normal and one altered copy of a given gene.

Inherited (or germline) mutations account for only 5–10% of all cancers in the general population. Most cancers are sporadic and attributable to factors such as environmental exposure or dietary patterns or are without known cause. However, familial cancers and sporadic cancers are related, since the germline genetic changes identified in familial cancers frequently occur in the cells of sporadic cancers as well. As a result, identification of the mutations responsible for inherited cancer traits has been critical to increasing our understanding of the molecular basis of cancer in general, and it is likely to be an important step in developing new approaches to cancer treatment and prevention.

Most autosomal dominant cancer susceptibilities are known or assumed to be caused by alterations in tumor suppressor functions. As described by the Knudsen's two-hit hypothesis, individuals carrying a mutation that results in the loss of function of one copy of a tumor suppressor gene have a higher risk of developing a cancer because of their risk of losing the remaining functional copy of the gene through a somatic mutation event. Loss of both copies of a tumor suppressor gene leads to tumorogenesis. By contrast, a person with two functional copies of the tumor suppressor gene would require two separate somatic mutation events to lose the tumor suppressor function.

The children of an individual with an autosomal dominant trait have a 50% risk of inheriting the same germline mutation. However, even when the mutation is inherited, the occurrence of cancer is dependent on *penetrance* and *expressivity*. Penetrance refers to the likelihood that the distinctive clinical signs associated with a mutation will appear in the individual carrying the mutation. It is often given as a percentage, indicating the probability that clinical disease will occur in a carrier in his or her lifetime. Expressivity refers to the variable severity of the clinical presentation in an affected individual. In the case of inherited cancer syndromes, the issue of penetrance is particularly important. Most cancer-susceptibility mutations do not result in the inevitable development of cancer but rather produce an increased lifetime risk in comparison to average risk. Expressivity is also variable: Some familial cancer traits result in increased risk for different types of cancer. The age of onset of cancer may also vary. Given the average lifetime risk for developing a malignancy of 25–30%, an accurate estimate of the increased risk conferred by an inherited cancer trait is an important issue for individuals with a family history of cancer.

B. Recognition of a Familial Cancer Trait

Recording a pedigree is the simplest, most efficient way of recognizing a family with a potential inherited cancer trait. Pedigrees suggestive of a familial cancer susceptibility include multiple individuals affected in more than one generation; cancers at an early age (e.g., premenopausal breast cancer or colon cancer below age 50 years); "rare cancers" (e.g., male breast cancer, lung cancer in a nonsmoker); and multiple primary cancers in the same individual (Table 2).

Family history information should ideally be obtained for the two generations before the patient and for all subsequent descendants (i.e., parents, siblings, children, grandparents, aunts and uncles, nieces and nephews) (1). If cancer is present in the family, the pedigree should extend back as far as possible. For each relative, birthdate, age at death, cause of death, and any cancer diagnosis should be sought. If a relative has cancer, then it is appropriate to record the age of diagnosis, the primary site of cancer, whether the cancer was unilateral or bilateral, any cancer-related surgeries (e.g., mastectomy), and any known carcinogenic exposures. Obtaining medical records is a vital part of the evaluation, because a patient's historical reports are frequently inaccurate. Recording ethnicity is also crucial, since some cancer-susceptibility mutations are more easily identified in certain ethnic groups (e.g., breast cancer mutations among individuals of Jewish descent). Standard symbols used in recording pedigree data are shown in Table 3. (For a more extensive review of these symbols, see Ref. 1.)

C. Molecular Testing—Polymorphisms Versus Mutations

Genetic traits can be classified as *polymorphisms* or *mutations*. The difference is important both scientifically and clinically. A polymorphism is a normal variant in the DNA sequence that is present in 1% or more of the population. Usually, polymorphisms do not significantly alter the protein coded by the gene, but they may result in subtle structural changes associated with small differences in protein function. They tend to be clinically neutral, but they may sometimes result in small differences in cancer susceptibility. Mutations are rare changes in the DNA sequence of the gene. The mutations that have come to medical attention usually alter the function of the gene in a significant way. The majority of mutations that produce an inherited cancer susceptibility lead to inactivation of the gene or its protein product. The significance of a given mutation is immediately apparent when the mutation leads to deletion of some portion of the gene product, as in a protein truncation, or

Table 2 Important Aspects of Recognizing a Familial Cancer Trait

---

Multiple affected individuals
Two or more generations affected
Cancers at an early age
Rare cancers (i.e., male breast cancer)
Individual(s) with multiple primary cancers

Source: Ref. 123.

Table 3 List of Common Pedigree Symbols

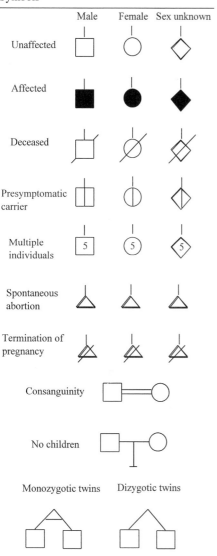

Source: Ref. 1.

changes the structure of a region that is known to have functional significance. However, for some mutations, the functional significance of the changes in the DNA sequence is not immediately apparent. These may involve regulatory functions affecting transcription or translation of the gene.

When DNA sequence analysis is used for genetic testing, some DNA base pair changes of uncertain clinical significance may be identified. In the initial identification of putative mutations within cancer-prone families, researchers look for the presence of a consistent linkage between the DNA sequence change and the disease state. The absence of such a correlation may argue that a given base pair change is a "benign" polymorphism rather than a disease-causing mutation.

The DNA-based testing currently available does not, always identify a mutation in people with a clinical diagnosis of a genetic cancer trait; that is, people whose personal and family history of cancer indicate an autosomal dominant inheritance of cancer susceptibility. The most likely explanation for this limitation is that there are additional cancer-related mutations yet to be identified. As a result, genetic testing for cancer susceptibility has limited sensitivity, which is an important factor to address in counseling for those who are considering testing. When a mutation can be identified in an affected individual from a cancer-prone family, however, an accurate test for inheritance of the family's cancer predisposition can be offered to other unaffected relatives.

With the growing availability of commercial DNA testing for genetic cancer syndromes, issues of medical management have become increasingly important for individuals with inherited susceptibilities. Indications for DNA testing include clarification of the diagnosis or treatment decisions, risk assessment, initiation of surveillance, prognosis, reduction of uncertainty and anxiety, and genetic counseling regarding future children's risk of inheriting an increased susceptibility to cancer. Given numerous ethical concerns, special attention must be paid to unaffected individuals who request or have strong indications for the genetic testing for a familial cancer trait.

II. RARE CANCER SYNDROMES

A. Von Hippel–Lindau Syndrome

Von Hippel–Lindau (VHL) syndrome is an autosomal dominant disorder which involves benign tumors in multiple organ systems. It is also a cancer-susceptibility syndrome, with renal cell carcinoma being the predominant malignancy. One study estimated a penetrance of 90% by the age of 65 years (2). Another found that approximately 4% of gene mutation carriers are free of any clinical manifestations (3). The age range at which diagnosis occurs is broad and has been reported from infancy into the 70s, but typically the mean age of onset of symptoms is in the mid-20s (4). There is extensive clinical heterogeneity in clinical findings even among affected members of the same family.

The major clinical findings in VHL are cysts, vascular tumors, and solid tumors (4). Specifically, these include renal cysts that are often bilateral, pancreatic cysts, epipdidymal cysts, retinal angiomas, cerebellar and spinal hemangioblastomas, pheochromocytomas, endolymphatic sac tumors, and renal cell carcinomas (4). The cumulative risk of a retinal hemangioblastoma, cerebellar hemangioblastoma, or renal cell carcinoma by the age of 60 years is estimated to exceed 70% (4). Retinal angiomatosis is one of the earliest manifestations and among one of the most frequent complications. Left untreated, blindness can result (5). Retinal hemangioblastomas have been reported in infants (4). Another frequent finding is cerebellar and spinal hemangioblastomas.

The malignancies that occur most frequently in VHL are renal cell carcinomas and pheochromocytomas (4). In one case report, 24–28% of patients with VHL developed renal cell carcinomas and 7–9% developed pheochromocytomas (4, 6). Renal cell carcinomas are usually of the clear cell type and are associated with cysts, but the exact nature of the relationship between renal cysts and cancer is not understood at this time (4, 7). Renal cell carcinomas are the major cause of death in VHL patients. It is estimated that the majority of patients with VHL will develop renal cell carcinoma if they live long enough (4).

The VHL gene has been cloned and commercial molecular testing is available (8, 9). The gene's cellular function does not show a relationship to any known gene. Detection of mutations in the VHL gene in clinically diagnosed individuals varies from 36 to 82% depending on the technique used (10). In general, greater than 70% of all VHL gene mutation can be detected (8). The incidence of de novo mutations may be as low as 5% (3, 11). Some evidence exists that certain type of mutations in the VHL gene may predispose individuals to the development of pheochromocytomas (12).

Lifelong screening for adults involves annual neurological physical examinations, magnetic resonance imaging (MRI) scans of the head and spinal cord, computed tomographic (CT) scans of the abdomen, 24-hour urine test for elevated catecholamines, and retinal examinations (13–15).

B. Multiple Endocrine Neoplasia Type I

Multiple endocrine neoplasia type I (MEN-I) is an autosomal dominant syndrome associated with hyperparathyroidism, tumors of the endocrine pancreas, carcinoid tumors, pituitary adenomas, and benign adrenal tumors (16, 17). Penetrance is as high as 80% (17). Hyperparathyroidism is the most frequent clinical manifestation and can be detected as early as 12 years of age, with the average age being 19 years (16, 17). The pituitary tumors seen in MEN-I include gastrinomas, insulinomas, and glucagonomas.

In affected individuals with MEN-I, pancreatic microadenomas and macroadenomas occur in approximately 30–75% of affected individuals (17). Malignant progression is seen in approximately 50% of patients with pancreatic involvement. The most frequent carcinoid syndromes associated with MEN-I are Zollinger–Ellison syndrome due to gastrinoma-related hypergastrinemia and hypoglycemic syndrome due to insulinomas. Some studies have indicated that as many as 30% of sporadic gastrinomas are an initial manifestation of MEN-I (17). Insulinomas are less frequent and are seen in 4–10% of affected individuals (17).

Screening for MEN-I relies on hormonal levels associated with the various pancreatic tumors (18). These include basal serum gastrin levels for detection of gastrinomas, combined measurement of serum glucose, insulin and peptide C levels, and measurement of other associated hormones when there is a clinical indication (17). The MEN-I gene has been cloned, but commercial DNA testing is not available (19). The gene's function is not known and it does not show similarity to previously cloned genes.

C. Multiple Endocrine Neoplasia Type II

Multiple endocrine neoplasia type II (MEN-II) is another autosomal dominant cancer syndrome associated with several endocrine tumors including medullary thyroid carcinoma, pheochromocytoma, and primary hyperparathyroidism (20, 21). Within MEN-II there are several subtypes of the syndrome. MEN-IIA manifests with the previously mentioned tumors. Familial medullary thyroid carcinoma is not associated with any of the other tumors seen in MEN-II. MEN-IIB is associated with medullary thyroid carcinoma, pheochromocytomas, mucosal neuromas, and skeletal abnormalities that resemble Marfan's syndrome.

Medullary thyroid carcinoma (MTC) is the most common cancer seen in MEN-II and has a penetrance of nearly 90% (20,21). It is more aggressive in MEN-IIB than in IIA (20). Pheochromocytomas are typically bilateral in 67.8% of the cases (22, 23). In both MEN-IIA and IIB, the penetrance of pheochromocytomas is approximately 50% (20).

MEN-II is caused by mutations in the *RET* gene, a member of the tyrosine kinase receptor gene family and a receptor for a growth factor called glial cell line–derived neurotrophic factor (21). Different *RET* mutations are seen in MEN-IIA, MEN-IIB, and familial medullary carcinoma. In MEN-IIA, 95% of the patients have mutations in exons 10 and 11 (21). Familial MTC has a distinct set of mutations in exons 10 and 11 as well (24). In MEN-IIB, a mutation in exon 16 of the gene has been identified in 97% of patients (25). The specificity of certain mutations not only differentiates variant forms of MEN-II but also predicts the aggressiveness of MTC (24). Commercial DNA testing is available for mutations in the *RET* gene.

With confirmation of an individual's carrier status for a *RET* gene mutation, appropriate screening for the development of associated tumors can be offered (20). Elevated levels of calcitonin are the most sensitive marker for diagnosis and monitoring of MTC. Surveillance for pheochromocytomas requires a 24-h urine collection for urine catecholamines. Hyperparathyroidism can be detected with an oral calcium load test. Surgical resection is indicated after detection of any of these endocrine malignancies.

D. Li–Fraumeni Syndrome

Li–Fraumeni syndrome is a rare familial cancer syndrome characterized by variety of different tumors. The syndrome was originally described as a distinct aggregation of cancers including early-onset sarcomas, brain tumors, breast cancer, leukemia, and adrenal cortical carcinoma (27). Individuals with the syndrome are also at higher risk for developing metachronous malignancies; that is, multiple primary tumors over time. Li–Fraumeni syndrome is inherited in an autosomal dominant pattern. Approximately 50% of cancers reported in Li–Fraumeni families occur before the age of 30 years (28). The frequency of cancers among carriers approaches 90% by the ages of 60–70 years (28).

The clinical criteria that define the syndrome are (a) an individual with a sarcoma diagnosed before the age of 45 years; (b) a first-degree relative with cancer before age 45 years; and (c) another first- or second-degree relative with a sarcoma diagnosed at any age or any cancer diagnosed under the age of 45 years (27, 28).

Among adult women with Li–Fraumeni syndrome, breast cancer is the predominant cancer. In a longitudinal study, 36 members of 16 families developed breast carcinoma as the first cancer (29). The majority were affected before the age of 45 years. Ten of the patients had bilateral metachronous breast cancers with a median age of 33 years. Information about the specific type of breast carcinoma is scattered, but in one study, infiltrating ductal carcinoma was the most frequent type diagnosed.

The most frequent soft-tissue sarcomas seen in Li–Fraumeni syndrome are rhabdomyosarcomas, leiomyosarcomas, liposarcomas, fibrous histiocytomas, and fibrosarcomas (28, 30). The sarcomas tend to occur most frequently in childhood, but individuals with Li–Fraumeni syndrome are still at risk for developing sarcomas in adulthood. The relative risk of any of the associated sarcomas is 27.8 before the age of 45 years but drops dramatically to 1.8 in individuals older than the age 45 years (29). Li–Fraumeni patients are at higher risk for osteosarcomas as well.

Leukemias are seen with increased frequency in Li–Fraumeni syndrome. The types of leukemias include acute lymphocytic leukemia, acute myelocytic leukemia, and chronic myelocytic leukemia (28). Before the age of 45 years, the relative risk of developing leukemia in Li–Fraumeni patients is 13.1 (29). After the age of 45 years, the risk decreases to 3.9. Brain tumors seen in Li–Fraumeni syndrome include gliomas, medulloblastomas, astrocytomas, ependymomas, spongioblastomas, and choroid plexus tumors (28, 29). The relative risk of brain tumors before the age of 45 years is 25.5. The age of diagnosis shows a bimodal distribution with peaks in the younger preteen age and in the 30s (30).

Germline mutations of the p53 tumor suppressor gene have been found to be a cause of Li–Fraumeni syndrome, and the finding of such a mutation can be useful as a marker of increased susceptibility to the tumor spectrum of the syndrome (31–33). Approximately 50% of Li–Fraumeni families are estimated to have germline p53 mutations (34). Another gene may account for families without detectable germline p53 mutations. The p53 tumor suppressor gene has multiple functions, including controlling cell cycle progression and regulation of the cellular response to DNA damage among many other functions (35).

Commercial genetic tests are based on sequence analysis in the exons 5–9 in which 95% of the mutations occur. The contribution of germline p53 mutations to isolated cases of breast cancer is small. The appearance of germline p53 mutations in women with breast cancers appears to be less than 1% (36). Currently, there is little in the medical literature regarding guidelines for surveillance of patients with Li–Fraumeni syndrome, but early initiation of breast cancer screening in women with a germline p53 mutation is recommended (37).

E. Cowden's Syndrome

Cowden's syndrome is an autosomal dominant familial cancer syndrome with involvement of multiple organ systems (38). The penetrance is unknown, but it is believed to be as high as 90% over a lifetime (39). Traditionally, the diagnosis has been established through recognition of distinct skin lesions, including acral keratosis, papillomatous papules, and facial trichilemmomas. Other features of the syndrome include macrocephaly; mental retardation; breast lesions, including fibroadenomas which occur in as many as 76% of those affected (40); thyroid gland lesions, including goiter, benign adenomas, fetal adenomas, and thyroglossal duct cysts; and multiple hamartomatous polyps in the gastrointestinal tract (38). Genitourinary abnormalities can also be seen, including benign ovarian cysts and leiomyomas.

The cancers that occur most frequently in Cowden's syndrome include ductal adenocarcinoma of the breast, thyroid follicular adenocarcinomas, and meningiomas (38). Breast cancers develop in approximately 30–50% of affected women and thyroid cancer in 10% of affected individuals (38, 39, 41). Other cancers documented in individuals with Cowden's syndrome include glioblastomas, colon carcinomas, uterine adenocarcinomas, and cervical carcinomas. (38). Whether these other tumors form part of the syndrome has not been determined.

A candidate tumor suppressor gene for Cowden's syndrome has recently been identified on chromosome 10, and it has been designated *PTEN*, or *MMAC1* (42). Interestingly, *PTEN* was also cloned through a molecular genetic analysis of sporadic glioblastomas. The *PTEN* gene is a phosphatase as well as having homology to cellular structural proteins, but its exact function is not known. (43). Commercial testing for *PTEN* mutations is not currently available.

Given the high risk of developing breast cancer at an early age, current recommendations for women with Cowden's syndrome include routine mamograms starting in the mid-20's (39). Regular testing of thyroid function tests is also recommended as part of a screening protocol.

III. INHERITED SUSCEPTIBILITY TO COMMON CANCERS

A. Colon Cancer

1. Familial Adenomatous Polyposis

Familial adenomatous polyposis (FAP) is an autosomal dominant familial cancer syndrome characterized by dramatic polyp formation within the colon (44, 45). It is thought to account for less than 1% of all colorectal cancers.

The polyposis in FAP manifests itself with hundreds to thousands of adenomatous polyps throughout the colon (45). The condition is defined clinically by the presence of greater than 150 polyps (45). Polyps can also exist in other regions of the gastrointestinal tract, including the stomach and small intestines. The adenomatous nature of these polyps is what places individuals at a high risk for developing colon cancer. The average age of onset for polyps is 25 years, the average onset of symptoms is 33 years, and the average age of diagnosis of colon cancer is 42 years. Familial adenomatous polyposis is 100% penetrant, with nearly all affected individuals developing colon cancer by their 40s (44).

Familial adenomatous polyposis is caused by mutations in the *APC* gene, an abbreviation for adenomatous polyposis coli. The function of the gene is not fully understood, but it appears to be involved in epithelial cell adhesion and cellular morphology (46, 47). The majority of mutations in the *APC* gene cause a truncation of the APC protein (48). Taking advantage of this fact, assays have been developed which detect the truncated APC protein as the basis for a mutation detection. Current testing with one such assay was successful in detecting mutations in 82% of the cases tested (48). APC testing is commercially available, using either the protein truncation test or DNA sequencing. Familial adenomatous polyposis also occurs as isolated cases in nearly 20% of patients. This presentation suggests de novo mutation of the *APC* gene in these individuals (44, 45).

Given the certainty of developing colon cancer in FAP, current management involves prophylactic colectomy in the mid-20s (44). Surgical therapy is the only option for patients with FAP after colonic polyps have been detected, since colonoscopy screening with polypectomy is impractical because of the number of polyps. Medical therapy with nonsteroidal anti-inflammatories like clinoril appears to produce regression of polyps, but the long-term effectiveness of this therapy is not known (49).

A number of other related syndromes with extracolonic findings, polyposis, and increased risk for colon cancer are caused by mutations in the *APC* gene. These syndromes were once thought to be independent entities, but cloning of the *APC* gene has shown that they are caused by different mutations in the same gene.

Gardner's syndrome is a variant of FAP with polyposis and a number of clinically benign findings, including mandibular osteomas, epidermoid cysts, soft-tissue tumors including desmoid tumors, and congenital hypertrophy of the retinal pigment epithelium (CHRPE) (45). Gardner's syndrome is caused by mutations in exons 9–15 of the *APC* gene (50). The eye findings associated with this syndrome are associated with a specific set of mutations in the *APC* gene (51).

Attenuated adenomatous coli is a less severe form of FAP; affected individuals have fewer than 150 polyps. There is evidence that attenuated adenomatous polyposis coli is attributable to mutations in the 5′ region of the *APC* gene (52).

Turcot's syndrome, a rare variant of FAP, is characterized by colonic and rectal polyposis and malignant brain tumors (53).

Another colon cancer–susceptibility trait related to a unique APC mutation has been identified in people of Ashkenazi Jewish descent (54). This mutation has been found in 28% of Ashkenazi Jews with a family history of colorectal cancer. The mutation is unique in that it does not significantly alter the gene product but may make it more susceptible to additional mutations in other regions. Patients with this mutation do not present with the dramatic polyposis of FAP. The degree of risk conferred by this mutation is unknown.

2. Hereditary Nonpolyposis Colorectal Cancer

Hereditary nonpolyposis colorectal cancer (HNPCC) is an autosomal dominant trait conferring an increased risk for colon and other cancers. It was first recognized in the familial clustering of early-onset colon cancer. Further characterization of affected families showed a predominance of proximal colorectal cancer, often with multiple primary tumors presenting concurrently (synchronous) or over time (metachronous) in the same individual. In addition, specific types of extracolonic cancers have been observed, including endometrial carcinomas, small intestinal adenocarcinomas, ureteral cancers, hepatobiliary cancer, gastric cancers, and ovarian carcinomas (55, 56). Of all colon cancers (57, 58), HNPCC probably accounts for at least 5%.

The International Collaborative Group (ICG, Amsterdam) established a list of criteria to define HNPCC (59). Excluding cases of familial adenomatous polyposis, the criteria include (a) at least three relatives with histologically verified colorectal cancer, with one a first-degree relative of the other two; (b) at least two successive generations affected; and (c) colorectal cancer diagnosed in at least one family member before the age of 50 years. These criteria were defined to aid in the genetic mapping of the syndrome but are restrictive in their scope, because they do not account for other types of malignancies seen in HNPCC.

Patients with HNPCC have a propensity to develop colorectal cancer before the age of 50 years (60). Cases as young as 13 years old have been reported (61). The lifetime risk colorectal cancer in HNPCC is estimated to be 68–75% (61–63). In HNPCC-affected individuals who develop cancer, the 10-year cumulative incidence of metachronous cancer is 40% if the first cancer is treated with a less extensive procedure than a total colectomy (60). The syndrome occurs more frequently in the right than left colon; approximately 70% of colon cancers in HNPCC are located proximal to the splenic flexure. No specific histological findings have been identified with HNPCC, but premalignant adenomas occur, as is the case with sporadic cancers (62).

A related group of four genes involved in DNA damage repair are the genetic basis for HNPCC: *MLH1*, *MSH2*, *PMS1*, and *PMS2*. The genes are involved in the repair of specific DNA lesions, called mismatches, that occur during DNA replication. Defects in these genes lead to genetic instability in which short repeated sequences are altered. This instability is believed to result in a rapid accumulation of somatic mutations in other genes that contribute to tumorogenesis. The majority of germline HNPCC mutations are found in the *MSH2* and *MLH1* genes (64, 65). Only a few families have been noted to have mutations in the *PMS1* and *PMS2* genes. Current mutation screening data suggest that mutations in *MSH2* account for 50% and mutations in *MLH* for 30% of all HNPCC families (64, 65). Commercial testing is available for both *MSH2* and *MLH1* mutations.

Recommendations for cancer surveillance in HNPCC-affected individuals include colonoscopy and enometrial cancer screening with endometrial aspirate or vaginal ultrasound (66). Screening for other extracolonic cancers, such as ovarian and ureteral cancers, is recommended when these cancers have been observed in the family history (56, 66–68).

B. Breast and Ovarian Cancers

Among families with multiple cases of breast or ovarian cancer, two clinical patterns have been seen: (a) Families with ''site-specific'' breast or ovarian cancer; that is, families in which all affected family members have one type of cancer; and (b) families in which both breast and ovarian cancers are seen. As with colon cancer, inheritance of cancer susceptibility occurs as an autosomal dominant trait. The study of such families led to the discovery of the BRCA1 and BRCA2 genes (69, 70).

Based on families participating in the initial linkage studies that led to gene discovery, BRCA1 mutations have been estimated to account for half of site-specific breast cancer families and 75% of families in which both breast and ovarian cancers are present (71, 72). In clinical series, however, mutations are identified less frequently. For example, among families with both breast and ovarian cancers at a clinical referral center, only 16% were found to carry BRCA1 mutations (73). The frequency was higher when breast cancer occurred early—at least 44% of families had BRCA1 mutations when the mean breast cancer diagnosis was under age 40 years—and even higher when at least one family member had both breast and ovarian cancers (73).

BRCA2 mutations are estimated to account for a small proportion of site-specific breast cancer families (74–76), and they appear to be associated with an overall lower risk of ovarian cancer than BRCA1 mutations (74). However, some BRCA2 families with high frequencies of ovarian cancer have been reported (77).

Multiple mutations occur in both genes (78, 79), and additional genes are likely to be discovered. In a summary of international studies of families with three or more cases of breast and/or ovarian cancers—many using less stringent criteria for high risk than the initial mapping studies—BRCA1 mutations were identified in only 23% of families and BRCA2 mutations in only 14% (79). Some families without mutations could represent a coincidental familial aggregation of cancer or a multifactorial etiology of cancer involving interactions between polymorphisms and the environment (see Multifactorial Cancer Susceptibility below). However, it is likely that at least a proportion of these families carry cancer-predisposing mutations that have not yet been identified.

1. Cancer Risk in BRCA1 Mutation Carriers

Initial estimates of cancer risk among BRCA1 mutation carriers were based on observation of families participating in BRCA1 mapping studies. Because these families were selected for the presence of multiple individuals affected with cancer at an early age, the risk estimates are likely to overestimate the average risk and may underestimate the likelihood of cancer at older ages. The cumulative risk of breast cancer was estimated to be 3.2% by age 30 years, 19.1% by age 40 years, 50.8% by age 50 years, 54.2% by age 60 years, and 85% by age 70 years (80). The median age at diagnosis ranged from 36 to 42 years in a study of 61 families carrying one of 6 BRCA1 mutations (81). Those who developed breast cancer were estimated to have a 64% risk of a contralateral breast cancer by age 70 years (82). Male breast cancer was found in 1990 of high risk families segregating a BRCA1 mutation (83).

The cumulative risk of ovarian cancer also appears to be variable and is presumed to differ with the mutation inherited (84). One model estimates a cumulative risk of 26% by age 70 years for the majority of mutation carriers, with a small subset carrying a much higher risk of 85% (80). A second genetic trait may be involved: Risk of ovarian cancer was twofold higher in BRCA1 mutation carriers who also carried one or two rare alleles of the HRAS1 VNTR locus (84). For those who have had breast cancer, the cumulative risk of ovarian cancer is estimated to be 44% by age 70 years (82).

The risk of prostate cancer is estimated to be threefold higher in men who carry the BRCA1 mutation than in the general population, with a cumulative risk of 8% by age 70 (82). The risk of colon cancer may be fourfold higher, with an estimated cumulative risk of 6% by age 70 (82). The onset of these cancers does not appear to occur earlier than in sporadic cases (82).

No population-based risk estimates for BRCA1 mutations are yet available. However, several studies suggest that breast and other cancer risks are variable and often lower than the initial estimates would suggest. A number of mutation carriers have now been described with an initial cancer diagnosis after age 60 years or a minimal family history (86–90). In addition, lower lifetime breast cancer risk estimates ranging from 36% to 74% (as opposed to 85%) have been derived from two clinical series (87, 88), a survey (91), and population-based ovarian cancer incidence rates (92).

2. Cancer Risk in BRCA2 Mutation Carriers

Female carriers of BRCA2 mutations appear to have a breast cancer risk similar to that of BRCA1 mutation carriers (83, 93, 94), although current estimates, as with BRCA1, are based on observations from a small number of high-risk families participating in research. The age at which cancer occurs may be later on average than for BRCA1. For example, BRCA2 mutations were found in only 2 of 73 (2.7%) of a clinical series of breast cancer patients diagnosed by age 32 years, whereas the figure for BRCA1 was 12% (75). Male breast cancer has been observed in BRCA2 families, and BRCA2 pedigrees with multiple cases of male breast cancer and no female breast cancer have been reported (83, 94–96).

The cumulative risk of ovarian cancer is estimated to be 2–4% by age 70 years (83). However, ovarian cancer has been seen in a substantial minority of BRCA2 families, ranging from 12 to 48% (77, 95, 97). As with BRCA1, the risk of ovarian cancer appears to be higher with some BRCA2 mutations than with others (98). Family data also suggest an increased risk for prostate cancer and pancreatic cancer in BRCA2 mutations carriers (98, 99), and laryngeal, esophageal, colon, and hematopoietic cancers have been observed in BRCA2 families (99). BRCA2 mutations have also been identified in 7% of apparently sporadic pancreatic cancers (102).

3. Mutations in Specific Ethnic Populations

The frequency of specific BRCA1 and BRCA2 mutations differs in different racial and ethnic groups. The most significant of these differences to date are the increased frequency of a BRCA2 mutation in the Icelandic population and the increased frequency of two BRCA1 mutations and one BRCA2 mutation in individuals of Jewish descent.

a. Icelandic Individuals

A single BRCA2 mutation, termed 999del5, occurs in 0.6% of the Icelandic population and in 7.7% of female and 40% of male Icelandic breast cancer patients (93, 94, 96). The mutation was more frequent (17%) in women diagnosed with breast cancer by the age of 50 years, but it was also seen in 4% of women diagnosed at later ages. Among mutation carriers, 17 of 44 (39%) had no first- or second-degree relatives with cancer, suggesting incomplete penetrance of the mutation (96). When the age of onset of cancer was compared in affected mother-daughter pairs, the mean age of onset was lower in daughters, suggesting a possible new environmental modifier of risk (96). A population-based study of the 999del5 mutation suggests that the breast cancer risk associated with this mutation is 37% by age 70 (94).

b. Individuals of Jewish Descent

Two mutations, the 185delAG mutation in BRCA1 and the 6174delT mutation in BRCA2, occur with a frequency of about 1% in individuals of Jewish descent (91, 101–103). Another BRCA1 mutation, 5382insC, has an estimated prevalence of 0.1–0.15%. All were initially observed in high-risk families. The 185delAG and 6174delT mutations have subsequently been found in 20–30% of clinical populations of Jewish women diagnosed with early breast cancer (85, 104) and in 45–60% of Jewish women diagnosed with ovarian cancer (85, 87). The frequency of both 185delAG and 6174delT is higher among individuals with a family history of cancer (87, 105), but mutation carriers with little or no family history of cancer have been identified (86–90, 105). Among Jewish women with breast cancer and a family history of breast cancer, the 185delAG mutation was seen four times more frequently than the 6174delT mutation (103). Because the two mutations occur with equal frequency in the population, this finding suggests a lower cumulative risk for 6174delT compared to 185delAG (103). Similarly, among a consecutive series of women with ovarian cancer, the mean age of cancer diagnosis was higher for 6174delT mutation carriers (68 years) than for 185delAG mutation carriers (50 years) (87).

These observations illustrate the value of genetic studies within relatively homogeneous groups. Because of the relatively high prevalence of specific mutations within these two defined populations, multiple individuals carrying the same mutation could be identified and compared. These data from Icelandic and Jewish populations provide strong support for the incomplete penetrance and variable expressivity of BRCA1 and BRCA2 mutations.

C. Prostatic Cancer

Given the high prevalence of sporadic prostatic cancer, identification of a susceptibility gene has been difficult. However, a number of studies have shown evidence for familial clustering of prostatic cancer, thus suggesting a genetic component in additions to the risk associated with BRCA1 and BRCA2 mutations (106). More refined analysis has pointed to the existence of a possible autosomal dominant mutation that contributes to increased susceptibility to prostatic cancer, and this may account for as much as 9% of all prostatic cancers and 40% of early-onset disease (107). The recent identification of a locus on chromosome 1 that appears linked to an increased predisposition to prostatic cancer is the strongest evidence yet pointing toward a prostate cancer gene (108).

D. Multifactorial Cancer Susceptibility

Some inherited cancer susceptibility is likely to be due to polymorphisms or muta-tions with mild functional effects that produce modest increases in cancer risk. There is evidence for such traits in both breast and colon cancers, and evidence from other clinical areas, such as cardiovascular disease, that suggests the genetic contribution to common diseases is typically complex. For example, several polymorphisms affect cholesterol levels, and genetic factors also contribute to the risk of hyperten-sion. The same involvement of multiple genes is likely to be true for cancer. These genetic traits may have an additive effects if more than one trait is present, and many may interact with environmental risk factors. The term *multifactorial* is used to describe this interaction.

Genetic traits involved in multifactorial cancer risk are hard to identify, be-cause they do not produce Mendelian patterns of inheritance. They are likely to contribute to cases of sporadic cancer and may also produce familial aggregation that is less dramatic than that seen in families carrying the mutations in the BRCA1, BRCA2, or HNPCC-associated genes. To identify these genetic traits, research stud-ies must combine genetic assessment with epidemiological evaluation of environ-mental risk factors.

1. Multifactorial Breast Cancer Risk

Several genetic traits have been identified as potential contributors to multifactorial breast cancer risk. One of these is the carrier state for ataxia telangiectasia (AT), a rare autosomal recessive disease causing neurological problems, skin changes, mild immune deficiency, and increased susceptibility to several childhood cancers. Cell studies document radiosensitivity in AT (109, 110). Carriers for AT, who are hetero-zygous for the AT mutation, are not affected. However, epidemiological studies of families in which AT has occurred suggest that women who are AT carriers may have a two- to five-fold higher risk for breast cancer than women from the general population (111–113). Further, in vitro studies indicate that AT carriers have in-creased sensitivity to radiation damage (114). The radiosensitivity seen in the carrier state is far less than that seen in AT, but it has been postulated to be the mechanism for the increased cancer risk in AT carriers.

Genetic studies have failed to identify a linkage between the *AT* gene locus and familial breast cancer (115) or to identify AT mutations in patients with early-onset breast cancer (116), but such findings would not necessarily be expected if the risk associated with the genetic trait is mediated by environmental exposures (116). Thus, although molecular studies have not yet confirmed this potential risk factor, it remains a plausible mechanism for gene–environment interaction produc-ing cancer risk (113).

A similar example is suggested by a recent study of N-acetyl transferase 2 (NAT2) polymorphisms and breast cancer (117). A case-control study of women with and without breast cancer found that neither NAT2 status (i.e., whether or not the subject had an *NAT2* polymorphism that produced a rapid acetylation phenotype) nor smoking was independently associated with breast cancer risk. However, among slow acetylators who smoked, the breast cancer risk was significantly increased.

Another polymorphism found in the *CYP17* gene may provide a protective effect (118). *CYP17* codes for a cytochrome P450 enzyme. In a population-based study, one polymorphism of this gene, when present in the homozygous state (A1/A1), was associated with a late menarche and a reduced risk of advanced postmenopausal breast cancer (i.e., breast cancer with regional or metastatic spread). The A1/A1 genotype was found in about one third of the study subjects, who were Asian, African-American, and Latino, and thus could have a significant impact on population risk.

Further population-based studies will be needed to confirm these genetic traits as contributors to multifactorial cancer risk. Such studies are likely to be an important area of research in the future. As the examples demonstrate, polymorphisms and mutations with mild functional effects are likely to be considerably more common than high-risk mutations, and as a result may have a larger effect on the overall population risk. In addition, an understanding of the environmental modifiers that interact with these genetic traits will provide important clues to strategies for cancer risk reduction.

E. Testing and Counseling

1. Molecular Testing as a Clinical Tool

The identification of specific mutations as the cause of an inherited cancer predisposition makes genetic testing possible. In some cases, this testing can be considered to be presymptomatic. For example, individuals with a mutation for familial adenomatous polyposis have virtually a 100% chance of developing colon cancer by the age of 50 years. In contrast, many recently discovered mutations produce increased susceptibility to cancer, but cancer is not inevitable. For example, a woman with a mutation in *BRCA1* has an increased susceptibility to develop breast and ovarian cancer over her lifetime, but the risk is less than 100%. Likewise, a man who carries a *BRCA2* mutation has an estimated 8% lifetime risk of breast cancer, which is much higher risk than that of the average man, yet this absolute risk overall is relatively low.

Genetic testing for known familial cancer traits provides information about future cancer risk. This information is potentially of great value to individuals from high-risk families and their health care providers. Individuals with positive test results can be offered intensive screening or other measures to reduce risk. Testing can also identify some individuals who have not inherited the cancer-predisposing trait and can be counseled accordingly. In approaching this testing process, however, many uncertainties and potential risks need to be considered.

2. False-Negative Results

Genetic testing must be interpreted in the context of a thorough clinical evaluation and comprehensive family history information. For example, if an individual has a strong family history of breast and ovarian cancers, but testing fails to identify a mutation in BRCA1 or BRCA2, a familial cancer syndrome is still likely, and family members should be counseled and managed accordingly. Molecular testing for familial cancer traits is still in its infancy, and a negative screening test for a specific DNA mutation does not necessarily imply that a genetic cancer syndrome is not present. Patients and physicians may have difficulty understanding this aspect of genetic testing, and a false sense of security derived from a negative test may lead to failure to participate in recommended cancer screening. A striking example of this potential misunderstanding was demonstrated in a recent study looking at indications for APC gene testing in patients with the clinical features of familial adenomatous polyposis (119). In this study, only 18.6% of the patients received genetic counseling before the testing. Nearly 20% of tests were ordered for unconventional indications and had a low yield for positives. In 31.6% of cases, test results were misinterpreted, primarily because ordering physicians did not appreciate the potential for a false-negative result (119).

3. Potential Risks of Genetic Testing

With the identification of a familial cancer syndrome, guilt may occur. Despite the fact that we have no control over the genes we receive from our parents or pass to our children, a parent can have overwhelming feelings of guilt that he or she has passed the specter of cancer to generations to come. Guilt can also be seen in the form of "survivor guilt." For example, if three sisters are tested for a breast/ovarian cancer susceptibility mutation and two have the mutation and one does not, the "surviving sister" may feel guilty for having "escaped."

Other repercussions from being diagnosed with a genetic cancer trait include fear of stigmatization and discrimination stemming from multiple sources. Although legislation may soon protect individuals from medical discrimination, a person with a genetic susceptibility to cancer may have difficulty obtaining life or disability insurance. Overt discrimination by employers may be illegal under the Americans With Disability Act but subtler forms of discrimination can occur. For example, a person may not be hired because of fears of medical-related absences from work, although this would not be stated as a reason for denial of employment.

The long-term psychological consequences of providing presymptomatic and presusceptibility genetic testing for cancer are unknown (120). Psychological studies to date have focused on members of families participating in research. Limited psychosocial studies have been conducted, and these studies have been done on individuals who have received genetic education and counseling from counselors highly specialized in providing this complex risk-assessment information. The impact of the information has focused on the individuals tested and not on their relationships and families. Until the long-term consequences of presymptomatic and presuscepti-bility testing for cancer are known, offering such testing as a clinical service should be approached with caution.

4. Uncertainty in Prognosis

Oftentimes, the results of DNA testing provide little information about clinical sever-ity or prognosis. So far, only families with a high frequency of cancer have been studied by researchers; this ascertainment is likely to have biased what we know of the natural history of genetic cancer traits. Little is known about the clinical manifestations of individuals who carry cancer-predisposing mutations but lack a family history of cancer. The fact that penetrance is less than 100% for many muta-tions, even within families ascertained because of multiple cases of cancer, indicates the presence of modifying factors. Information about lifestyle risk factors and modi-fying genes in tumorigenesis, as they relate to inherited cancer syndromes, will play increasingly important roles in providing accurate prognostic information and coun-seling in the future.

5. Uncertainties in Surveillance

Recommendations for surveillance and clinical management of individuals with an inherited susceptibility to cancer are largely based on expert opinions and reflect potential but undocumented benefits of various interventions (66, 121). Some ex-perts have suggested that the age of onset of cancer or the spectrum of cancers seen in an individual's family be used in determining the timing and scope of surveillance; however, there are only limited data on interfamilial variation in cancer risk to sup-port this approach (81). For many cancers, for example, ovarian cancer, pancreatic cancer, urinary tract cancers, and most rare cancers, there are no proven screening tools available. When effective tools are available, for example, mammography or colonscopy, there are uncertainties in the optimal timing and intensity of surveil-lance.

6. Importance of Genetic Counseling and Informed Consent

Given the potential risks of genetic testing and the uncertainties in risk estimates and management strategies, groups such as the Institute of Medicine (122), the American Society of Clinical Oncologists (ASCO) (123), and the National Society of Genetic Counselors (126) have issued statements about the importance of pretest education and informed consent in the provision of genetic counseling and testing for adult-onset disorders. The minimum elements of informed consent for germline DNA testing as outlined by ASCO (123) are reviewed in Table 4. ASCO recommends that cancer predisposition testing be offered only when the personal or family history is highly suggestive of a genetic cancer syndrome, the test can be adequately inter-preted, and the result will influence the medical management of the patient or other

Table 4   Minimal Elements of Informed Consent for DNA Testing for Cancer Susceptibility

---

Give information on the specific genetic test(s) being performed
What are the implications of both positive and negative results?
What is the possibility that the test will be uninformative?
What options are available besides genetic testing?
What are the risks of passing the mutation (condition) on to offspring?
How accurate is the testing?
What are the fees involved with the testing and counseling?
Are there risks for psychological distress?
What are the potential risks of insurance and/or employer discrimination?
How will the testing information be kept confidential?
What options are available for medical surveillance and screening before and following
    testing, and what are their limitations?

Source: Adapted from Ref. 123.

family members. The components of genetic assessment and pre- and posttest education should include pedigree analysis and risk assessment; review of the natural history of the potential genetic cancer syndrome (including the role of nongenetic factors in the development of cancer); the predictive value of genetic testing, the risks benefits, limitations, and costs of testing; discussion of the patient's motivations for testing; the potential impact the test will have on other family members, friends, and coworkers; discussion of confidentiality issues; review of medical surveillance options in the presence or absence of DNA testing; and adequate emotional support after follow-up. A comprehensive written summary to the patient, using easily interpretable language, provides the patient with documentation of the counseling session(s) (124).

Genetic counseling involves the psychological, medical, and genetic issues associated with the occurrence or risk of a genetic disorder within a family. Since genetic information carries unique personal, family, and social burdens, an individual considering testing may weigh risks and benefits differently than his or her health care providers. A nondirective, nonjudgmental, client-centered approach to counseling is generally used to protect the client's right to make autonomous decisions. Genetic counseling does not end with the identification of a syndrome and the provision of risk information; supportive counseling concerning the implications of the information is also imperative.

Because of the complex nature of testing for genetic cancer susceptibility, a multidisciplinary approach to providing genetic counseling and testing to high-risk individuals and familites is appropriate. Members of the team may include masters level certified genetic counselors, medical geneticists, nurse specialists, oncologists, surgeons, psychologists, and primary care providers. If prophylactic surgery is being considered (i.e. oophorectomy, mastectomy), the inclusion of a psychiatrist or psychologist is often beneficial for patients because of the personal implications of this kind of treatment.

If genetic testing is ordered, an important and often overlooked component is planning how the results will be presented. This is usually best done in person with a support person present. The results of genetic testing have profound implications for the person, and many questions are usually generated around the interpretation of the test result.

7. Counseling May Result in the Decision Not to Test

A reasonable outcome of genetic counseling is the decision not to pursue testing even if a genetic test is available. Germline molecular testing can be expensive, and the results of the testing may not alter the medical management of the patient or other family members. An alternative for individuals who choose to postpone genetic testing is DNA banking. There are multiple commercial laboratories and university medical centers that provide DNA banking. DNA banking involves extracting blood and using the sample to save DNA for future availability for other family members in the event of that person's death. In this way, people who may carry mutations associated with cancer risk can feel that they are helping future generations without undergoing genetic testing of doubtful personal value.

8. Psychological Implications of a Diagnosis of an Inherited Cancer Trait

There are unique psychological consequences of making a genetic diagnosis of a cancer trait versus a cancer of sporadic etiology (120). By definition, a genetic diagnosis implies a familial problem. The diagnosis of a cancer syndrome affects multiple family members; children, siblings, and parents may now be at risk. Making a diagnosis of a cancer genetic trait requires obtaining information on multiple family members, including personal information about their health and lifestyles. For example, information about the age of diagnosis of cancer is important as well as information about exposure to risk factors of the affected individuals (i.e., smoking history in someone with lung cancer; drinking history in someone with liver cancer). The involvement of the family often extends to contacting appropriate relatives to obtain their medical records or even requesting that an affected member participate in DNA testing.

The diagnosis of an inherited cancer syndrome can affect an individual's very concept of self. The person is no longer a person who happens to have cancer but, for example, a "BRCA1 patient" or a "Li–Fraumeni patient." The patient may see him or herself as "mutant," "flawed," or "abnormal." Instead of seeing that the cancer is limited to a particular organ, such as the breast or colon, the person may feel that cancer is in every cell of the body given the presence of a cancer-susceptibility gene mutation. The power of words in communicating with individuals and families with a genetic cancer syndrome should not be underestimated.

IV. CONCLUSIONS

The rapid growth of knowledge about cancer genetics is encouraging, because it represents the first step toward a better understanding of cancer biology and lays the groundwork for new approaches to treatment and prevention. Currently, however, this knowledge serves primarily to enable clinicians to identify an increasing number of people with inherited cancer susceptibilities. Such diagnoses provide the opportunity for increased cancer surveillance and for aggressive treatment when cancer is found. However, much is still to be learned about the risks associated with known cancer-predisposing mutations and about the optimal clinical management of people who carry them. In addition, identifying a person as genetically susceptible to cancer may cause psychological and social harm. These uncertainties provide an ongoing challenge for clinicians, consumers, and researchers.

REFERENCES

1. Bennett R, Steinhaus K, Uhrich S, et al. Recommendations for standardized human pedigree nomenclature. Pedigree–Standardization Task Force of the National Society of Genetic Counselors. Am J Hum Genet 1995; 56:745–752.
2. Maher ER, Iselius L, Yates JR, et al. Von Hippel–Lindau disease: a genetic study. J Med Genet 1991; 28:443–447.
3. Maddock IR, Moran A, Maher ER, et al. A genetic register for von Hippel–Lindau disease. J Med Genet 1996; 33:120–127.
4. Maher ER, Yates JR, Harries R, et al. Clinical features and natural history of von Hippel–Lindau disease. Q J Med 1990; 77:1151–1163.
5. Hardwig P, Robertson DM. von Hippel–Lindau disease: a familial, often lethal, multisystem phakomatosis. Ophthalmology 1984; 91:263–270.
6. Maher ER. Von Hippel–Lindau disease. Eur J Cancer 1994; 30A:1987–1990.
7. Decker HJ, Weidt EJ, Brieger J. The von Hippel–Lindau tumor suppressor gene. A rare and intriguing disease opening new insight into basic mechanisms of carcinogenesis. Cancer Genet Cytogenet 1997; 93:74–83.
8. Maher ER, Bentley E, Yates JR, et al. Mapping of the von Hippel–Lindau disease locus to a small region of chromosome 3p by genetic linkage analysis. Genomics 1991; 10:957–960.
9. Latif F, Tory K, Gnarra J, et al. Identification of the von Hippel–Landau disease tumor suppressor gene. Science 1993; 260:1317–1320.
10. Glavac D, Neumann HP, Wittke C, et al. Mutations in the VHL tumor suppressor gene and associated lesions in families with von Hippel–Lindau disease from central Eur Hum Genet 1996; 98:271–280.
11. Davies DR, Norman AM, Whitehouse RW, Evans DG. Non-expression of von Hippel–Lindau phenotype in an obligate gene carrier. Clin Genet 1994; 45:104–106.
12. Chen F, Kishida T, Yao M, et al. Germline mutations in the von Hippel–Lindau disease tumor suppressor gene: correlations with phenotype. Hum Mutat 1995; 5:66–75.

13. Foulkes WD, Narod SA. Screening for cancer in high-risk families. Cancer Treat Res 1996; 86:165–182.

14. Harries RW. A rational approach to radiological screening in von Hippel–Lindau disease. J Med Screen 1994; 1:88–95.

15. Karsdorp N, Elderson A, Wittebol-Post D, et al. Von Hippel–Lindau disease: new strategies in early detection and treatment. Am J Med 1994; 97:158–168.

16. Skogseid B. Multiple endocrine neoplasia type I. Clinical genetics and diagnosis. Cancer Treat Res 1997; 89:383–406.

17. Chanson P, Cadiot G, Murat A. Management of patients and subjects at risk for multiple endocrine neoplasia type 1: MEN 1. GENEM 1. Groupe d'Etude des Neoplasies Endocriniennes Multiples de type 1. Hormone Res 1997; 47:211–220.

18. Skogseid B, Oberg K. Prospective screening in multiple endocrine neoplasia type 1. Henry Ford Hosp Med J 1992; 40:167–170.

19. Chandrasekharappa SC, Guru SC, Manickam P, et al. Positional cloning of the gene for multiple endocrine neoplasia-type 1. Science 1997; 276:404–407.

20. Conte-Devolx B, Schuffenecker I, Niccoli P, et al. Multiple endocrine neoplasia type 2: management of patients and subjects at risk. French Study Group on Calcitonin-Secreting Tumors (GETC). Hormone Res 1997; 47:221–226.

21. Gagel RF. Multiple endocrine neoplasia type II and familial medullary thyroid carcinoma. Impact of genetic screening on management. Cancer Treat Res 1997; 89:421–441.

22. Modigliani E, Vasen HM, Raue K, et al. Pheochromocytoma in multiple endocrine neoplasia type 2: European study. The Euromen Study Group. J Intern Med 1995; 238:363–367.

23. Casanova S, Rosenberg-Bourgin M, Farkas D, et al. Phaeochromocytoma in multiple endocrine neoplasia type 2 A: survey of 100 cases. Clin Endocrinol 1993; 38:531–537.

24. Eng C, Clayton D, Schuffenecker I, et al. The relationship between specific RET proto-oncogene mutations and disease phenotype in multiple endocrine neoplasia type 2. International RET mutation consortium analysis. JAMA 1996; 276:1575–1579.

25. Eng C. The RET proto-oncogene in multiple endocrine neoplasia type 2 and Hirschsprung's disease. N Engl J Med 1996; 335:943–951.

26. Eng C, Crossey PA, Mulligan LM, et al. Mutations in the RET proto-oncogene and the von Hippel–Lindau disease tumour suppressor gene in sporadic and syndromic phaeochromocytomas. J Med Genet 1995; 32:934–937.

27. Li FP, Fraumeni JF Jr. Prospective study of a family cancer syndrome. JAMA 1982; 247:2692–2694.

28. Li FP, Fraumeni JF Jr, Mulvihill JJ, et al. A cancer family syndrome in twenty-four kindreds. Cancer Res 1988; 48:5358–5362.

29. Garber JE, Goldstein AM, Kantor AF, et al. Follow-up study of twenty-four families with Li–Fraumeni syndrome. Cancer Res 1991; 51:6094–6097.

30. Kleihues P, Schauble B, zur Hausen A, et al. Tumors associated with p53 germline mutations: a synopsis of 91 families. Am J Pathol 1997; 150:1–13.

31. Malkin D, Li FP, Strong LC, et al. Germ line p53 mutations in a familial syndrome of breast cancer, sarcomas, and other neoplasms. Science 1990; 250:1233–1238.

32. Srivastava S, Zou ZQ, Pirollo K, et al. Germ-line transmission of a mutated p53 gene in a cancer-prone family with Li–Fraumeni syndrome. Nature 1990; 348:747–749.

33. Li FP, Correa P, Fraumeni JF Jr. Testing for germ line p53 mutations in cancer families. Cancer Epidemiol Biomarkers Preven 1991; 1:91–94.

34. Birch J. Li–Fraumeni syndrome. Eur J Cancer 1994; 30A:1935–1941.

35. Levine A. p53, The cellular gatekeeper for growth and division. Cell 1997; 88:323–331.

36. Sidransky D, Tokino T, Helzlsouer K, et al. Inherited p53 gene mutations in breast cancer. Cancer Res 1992; 52:2984–2986.

37. Hoskins KF, Stopfer JE, Calzone KA, et al. Assessment and counseling for women with a family history of breast cancer. A guide for clinicians. JAMA 1995; 273:577–785.

38. Starink TM, van der Veen JP, Arwert F, et al. The Cowden syndrome: a clinical and genetic study in 21 patients. Clin Genet 1986; 29:222–233.

39. Eng C. Cowden syndrome. J Genet Counsel 1997; 6:181–192.

40. Mallory SB. Cowden syndrome (multiple hamartoma syndrome). Dermatol Clin 1995; 13:27–31.

41. Carlson HE, Burns TW, Davenport SL, et al. Cowden disease: gene marker studies and measurements of epidermal growth factor. Am J Hum Genet 1986; 38:908–917.

42. Liaw D, Marsh DJ, Li J, et al. Germline mutations of the PTEN gene in Cowden disease, an inherited breast and thyroid cancer syndrome. Nature Genet 1997; 16:64–67.

43. Li DM, Sun H. TEP1, encoded by a candidate tumor suppressor locus, is a novel protein tyrosine phosphatase regulated by transforming growth factor beta. Cancer Res 1997; 57:2124–2129.

44. Rustgi A. Hereditary gastrointestinal polyposis and nonpolyposis syndromes. N Engl J Med 1994; 331:1694–1702.

45. Haggitt R, Reid B. Hereditary gastrointestinal polyposis syndromes. Am J Surg Pathol 1986; 10:871–887.

46. Fearon ER. Molecular genetics of colorectal cancer. Ann NY Acad Sci 1995; 768:101–110.

47. Powell SM. Familial polyposis syndromes. Advances in molecular genetic characterization. Surg Oncol Clin North Am 1996; 5:569–587.

48. Powell SM, Petersen GM, Krush AJ, et al. Molecular diagnosis of familial adenomatous polyposis. N Engl J Med 1993; 329:1982–1987.

49. Sandler RS. Aspirin and other nonsteroidal anti-inflammatory agents in the prevention of colorectal cancer. Import Adv Oncol 1996:123–137.

50. Nishisho I, Nakamura Y, Miyoshi Y, et al. Mutations of chromosome 5q21 genes in FAP and colorectal cancer patients. Science 1991; 253:665–669.

51. Hodgson S, Bishop D, Jay B. Genetic heterogeneity of congenital hypertrophy of the retinal pigment epithelium (CHRPE) in families with familial adenomatous polyposis. J Med Genet 1994; 31:55–58.

52. Nagase H, Miyoshi Y, Horii A, et al. Correlation between the location of germline mutations in the APC gene and the number of colorectal polyps in familial adenomatous polyposis patients. Cancer Res 1992; 52:4055–4057.

53. Hamilton SR, Liu B, Parsons RE, et al. The molecular basis of Turcot's syndrome. N Engl J Med 1995; 332:839–847.

54. Laken SJ, Petersen GM, Gruber SB, et al. Familial colorectal cancer in Ashkenazim due to a hypermutable tract in APC. Nature Genet 1997; 17:79–83.

55. Watson P, Lynch HT. Extracolonic cancer in hereditary non-polyposis colorectal cancer. Cancer 1993; 71:677–685.

56. Lynch HT, Smyrk T, Lynch J. An update of HNPCC (Lynch syndrome). Cancer Genet Cytogenet 1997; 93:84–99.

57. Mecklin J-P. Frequency of hereditary colon cancer. Gastroenterology 1987; 93:1021–1025.

58. Lynch H. Frequency of hereditary nonpolyposis colorectal carcinoma. Gastroenterology 1986; 90:486–492.

59. Vasen H, Mecklin J-P, Meera KP, Lynch H. Hereditary non-polyposis colorectal cancer. Lancet 1991; 338:877.

60. Lynch HT, Smyrk T. Hereditary nonpolyposis colorectal cancer (Lynch syndrome). An updated review. Cancer 1996; 78:1149–67.

61. Aarnio M, Mecklin J-P, Aaltonen L, et al. Life-time risk of different cancers in hereditary non-polyposis colorectal cancer (HNPCC) syndrome. Int J Cancer 1995; 54:430–433.

62. Mecklin J, Jarvinen H. Clinical features of colorectal carcinoma in cancer family syndrome. Dis Colon Rectum 1986; 29:160–164.

63. Marra G, Boland C. Hereditary nonpolyposis colorectal cancer: the syndrome, the genes and historical perspectives. J Natl Cancer Inst 1995; 1995:160–164.

64. Liu B, Parsons RE, Hamilton SR, et al. hMsh2 Mutations in hereditary nonpolyposis colorectal cancer kindreds. Cancer Res 1994; 54:4590–4594.

65. Liu B, Parsons R, Papadopoulos N, et al. Analysis of mismatch repair genes in hereditary non-polyposis colorectal cancer patients. Nature Med 1996; 2:169–174.

66. Burke W, Petersen G, Lynch P, et al. Recommendations for follow-up care of individuals with an inherited predisposition to cancer. I. Hereditary nonpolyposis colon cancer. Cancer Genetics Studies Consortium. JAMA 1997; 277:915–919.

67. Lynch HT, Smyrk T, Lynch JF. Overview of natural history, pathology, molecular genetics and management of HNPCC (Lynch syndrome). Int J Cancer 1996; 69:38–43.

68. Lynch HT, Lynch J. Genetic counseling for hereditary cancer. Oncology 1996; 10:27–34.

69. Miki Y, Swensen J, Shattuck-Eidens D, et al. A strong candidate for the breast and ovarian cancer susceptibility gene BRCA1. Science 1994; 266:66–71.

70. Wooster R, Neuhausen SL, Mangion J, et al. Localization of a breast cancer susceptibility gene, BRCA2, to chromosome 13q12-13. Science 1994; 265:2088–2090.

71. Ford D, Easton DF. The genetics of breast and ovarian cancer. Br J Cancer 1995; 72:805–812.

72. Narod SA, Ford D, Devilee P, et al. An evaluation of genetic heterogeneity in 145 breast ovarian cancer families. Am J Hum Genet 1995; 56:254–264.

73. Couch FJ, DeShano ML, Blackwood MA, et al. BRCA1 mutations in women attending clinics that evaluate the risk of breast cancer. N Engl J Med 1997; 336:1409–1415.

74. Ford D, Easton DF. The genetics of breast and ovarian cancer. Br J Cancer 1995; 72:805–812.

75. Krainer M, Silva-Arrieta S, FitzGerald MG, et al. Differential contributions of BRCA1 and BRCA2 to early-onset breast cancer. N Engl J Med 1997; 336:1416–1421.

76. Schubert EL, Lee MK, Mefford HC, et al. BRCA2 in American families with four or more cases of breast or ovarian cancer: recurrent and novel mutations, variable expres-

sion, penetrance, and the possibility of families whose cancer is not attributable to BRCA1 or BRCA2. Am J Hum Genet 1997; 60:1031–1040.

77. Tavtigian SV, Simard J, Rommers J, et al. The complete BRCA2 gene and mutations in chromosome 13q-linked. Nature Genet 1996; 12:10–14.
78. Szabo CI, King MC. Inherited breast and ovarian cancer. Hum Mol Genet 1995; 4: 1811–1817.
79. Szabo C, King M-C. Population genetics of BRCA1 and BRCA2. Am J Hum Genet 1997; 60:1013–1020.
80. Easton DF, Ford D, Bishop DT, Constortium tBCL. Breast and ovarian cancer incidence in BRCA1-mutation carriers. Am J Hum Genet 1995; 56:265–271.
81. Neuhausen SL, Mazoyer S, Friedman L, et al. Haplotype and phenotype analysis of six recurrent BRCA1 mutations in 61 families: results of an international study. Am J Hum Genet 1996; 58:271–280.
82. Ford D, Easton DF, Bishop DT, et al. Risks of cancer in BRCA1-mutation carriers. Lancet 1994; 343:692–695.
83. Ford D, Easton DF, Stratton M, et al. Genetic heterogeneity and penetrance analysis of the BRCA1 and BRCA2 genes in breast cancer families. Am J Hum Genet 1998; 62:676–689.
84. Phelan CM, Rebbeck TR, Weber BL, et al. Ovarian cancer risk in BRCA1 carriers is modified by HRAS1 variable number of Farden repeat (VNTR) locus. Nature Genet 1996; 12:7–9.
85. Abeliovich D, Kaduri L, Lerer I, et al. The Founder mutations 185delAG and 5382insC in BRCA1 and 6174delT in BRCA2 appear in 60% of ovarian cancer and 30% of early-onset breast cancer patients among Ashkenazi women. Am J Hum Genet 1997; 60:505–514.
86. Langston AA, Malone KE, Thompson JD, et al. BRCA1 mutations in a population-based sample of young women with breast cancer. N Engl J Med 1996; 334:137–142.
87. Levy-Lahad E, Catane R, Eisenberg S, et al. Founder BRCA1 and BRCA2 mutations in Ashkenazi Jews in Israel: frequency and differential penetrance in ovarian cancer and in breast-ovarian cancer families. Am J Hum Genet 1997; 60:1059–1067.
88. Fodor FH, Weston A, Bleiweiss IJ, et al. Frequency and carrier risk associated common BRCA1 and BRCA2 mutations in Ashkenazi Jewish breast cancer patients. Am J Hum Genet 1998; 63:45–51.
89. Ozcelik H, Schmocker B, Di Nicola N, et al. Germline BRCA2 6174delT mutations in Ashkenazi Jewish pancreatic cancer patients. Nature Genet 1997; 16:17–18.
90. Richards CS, Ward PA, Roa BB, et al. Screening for 185delAG in the Ashkenazim. Am J Hum Genet 1997; 60:1085–1098.
91. Struewing JP, Hartge P, Wacholder S, et al. The risk of cancer associated with specific mutations of BRCA1 and BRCA2 among Ashkenazi Jews. N Engl J Med 1997; 336: 1401–1408.
92. Whittemore AS, Gong G, Itnyre J. Prevalence and contribution of BRCA1 mutations in breast cancer and ovarian cancer: results from three U.S. population-based case-control studies of ovarian cancer. Am J Hum Genet 1997; 60:496–504.
93. Thorlacius S, Sigurdsson S, Bjarnadottir H, et al. Study of a Single BRCA2 mutation with high carrier frequency in a small population. Am J Hum Genet 1997; 60:1079–1084.
94. Thorlacius S, Struewing JP, Hartge P, et al. Population-based study of risk of breast

cancer in carriers of BRCA2 mutation. Lancet 1998; 352:1337–1339.

95. Couch FJ, Farid LM, DeShano ML, et al. BRCA2 germline mutations in male breast cancer cases and breast cancer families. Nature Genet 1996; 13:123–125.

96. Thorlacius S, Olafsdottir G, Tryggvadottir L, et al. A single BRCA2 mutation in male and female breast cancer families from Iceland with varied cancer phenotypes. Nature Genet 1996; 13:117–119.

97. Thorlacius S, Tryggvadottir L, Olafsdottir GH, et al. Linkage of BRCA2 region in hereditary male cancer. Lancet 1995; 345:544–555.

98. Gayther SA, Mangion J, Russell P, et al. Variation of risks of breast and ovarian cancer associated with different germline mutations of the BRCA2 gene. Nature Genet 1997; 15:103–105.

99. Berman DB, Costalas J, Schultz DC, et al. A common mutation is BRCA2 predisposes to a variety of cancers is found in both Jewish Ashkenazi and non-Jewish individuals. Cancer Res 1996; 56:3409–3414.

100. Goggins M, Schutte M, Moskaluk CA, et al. Germline BRCA2 mutations in patients with apparently sporadic pancreatic carcinomas. Cancer Res 1996; 56:5360–5364.

101. Struewing JP, Abeliovich D, Peretz T, et al. The carrier frequency of the BRCA1 185delAG mutation is approximately 1 percent in Ashkenazi Jewish individuals. Nature Genet 1995; 11:198–120.

102. Roa BB, Boyd AA, Volcik K, Richards CS. Ashkenazi Jewish population frequencies for common mutations in BRCA1 and BRCA2. Nature Genet 1996; 14:185–187.

103. Oddoux C, Struewing JP, Clayton CM, et al. The carrier frequency of the BRCA2 6174delT mutation among Ashkenazi Jewish individuals is approximately 1%. Nature Genet 1996; 14:188–190.

104. Fitzgerald MG, MacDonald DJ, Krainer M, et al. Germ-line BRCA1 mutations in Jewish and non-Jewish women with early onset breast cancer. N Engl J Med 1996; 334:143–149.

105. Modan B, Gak E, Sade-Bruchim RB, et al. High frequency of BRCA1 185delAG mutation in ovarian cancer in Israel. JAMA 1996; 276:1823–1825.

106. Steinberg GD, Carter BS, Beaty TH, et al. Family history and the risk of prostate cancer. Prostate 1990; 17:337–347.

107. Carter BS, Beaty TH, Steinberg GD, et al. Mendelian inheritance of familial prostate cancer. Proc Natl Acad Sci USA 1992; 89:3367–3371.

108. Smith JR, Freije D, Carpten JD, et al. Major susceptibility locus for prostate cancer on chromosome 1 suggested by a genome-wide search. Science 1996; 274:1371–1374.

109. Scott D, Spreadboroug AR, Roberts SA. Radiation-induced G2 delay and spontaneous aberrations in ataxia telangiectasia. Int J Radiat Biol 1994; 66:S157–S163.

110. Murname JP, Kapp LN. A critical look at the association of human genetic syndromes with sensitivity to ionizing radiation. Cancer Biol 1993; 4:93–104.

111. Swift MD, Morrell D, Massey RB, Chase CL. Incidence of cancer in 161 families affected by ataxia telangiectasia. N Engl J Med 1991; 325:1831–1836.

112. Swift MD, Reitnauer PJ, Morrell D, Chase CL. Breast and other cancers in families with ataxia telangiectasia. N Engl J Med 1986; 316:1289–1294.

113. Easton DF. Cancer risks in AT heterozygotes. Int J Rad Biol 1994; 66:S177–S182.

114. Scott D, Spreadborough AR, Jones LA, et al. Chromosomal radiosensitivity in G2-phase lymphocytes as an indicator of cancer predisposition. Radiat Res 1996; 145:3–16.

115. Wooster R, Ford D, Mangion J, et al. Absence of linkage to the ataxia telangiectasia locus in familial breast cancer. Hum Gene 1993; 92:91–94.
116. Fitzgerald MG, Bean JM, Hegde SR, et al. Heterozygous ATM mutations do not contribute to early onset breast cancer. Nature Genet 1997; 15:307–310.
117. Ambrosone CB, Freudenheim JL, Graham S, et al. Cigarette smoking, N-Acetyltransferase 2 genetic polymorphisms and breast cancer risk. JAMA 1996; 276:1494–1501.
118. Feigelson HS, Coetzee GA, Kolonel LN, et al. A polymorphism in the CYP17 gene increases risk of early onset breast cancer. Cancer Res 1997; 57:1063–1065.
119. Giardiello FM, Brensinger JD, Petersen GM, et al. The use and interpretation of commercial APC gene testing for familial adenomatous polyposis. N Engl J Med 1997; 336:823–827.
120. Croyle T, Achilles J, Lerman C. Psychological aspects of cancer genetic testing. Cancer 1997; 80(suppl):569–575.
121. Burke W, Daly M, Garber J, et al. Recommendations for follow-up care of individuals With an inherited predisposition to cancer II.BRCA1 and BRCA2. JAMA 1997; 277: 997–1003.
122. Andrews L, Fullarton J, Holtzman N, Motulsky A. Assessing Genetic Risks. Implications for Health and Social Policy. Washington, DC: National Academy Press, 1994.
123. Statement of the American Society of Clinical Oncology: Genetic testing for cancer susceptibility. J Clin Oncol 1996; 14:1730–1736.
124. McKinnon W, Baty B, Bennett R, et al. Predisposition genetic testing for late-onset disorders in adults: a position paper of the National Society of Genetic Counselors. JAMA 1997; 278:1217–1220.

8

Surgery in the Elderly Oncology Patient

Erna Busch-Devereaux
Prohealth Care Associates
Lake Success, New York

Margaret M. Kemeny
SUNY Stony Brook
Stony Brook, New York

I. INTRODUCTION

Surgery is an important modality for cancer treatment regardless of age. It is needed for diagnosis, resection with curative intent, or palliation. The incidence of many solid cancers continues to rise with age. Since the population of the United States is not only growing but aging, the number of elderly patients with cancers requiring surgical intervention can be expected to rise.

Life expectancy is often underestimated for the elderly. According to the Metropolitan Life Insurance Tables, the life expectancy of a girl born in 1992 is 79.1 years and of a boy 72.2 years (1). Furthermore, the life expectancy of a person reaching the age of 65 years is an additional 17.5 years; and an 85-year-old has an additional 6 years. Inadequate initial therapy for someone diagnosed with cancer at an older age can result in recurrence or metastases and death from cancer; outcomes which may have been preventable or avoidable with correct treatment at the outset.

Surgery is the mainstay of treatment of the tumors most common in the elderly: colorectal, breast, gastric, and pancreatic cancers. Other tumors which are also seen requiring surgery for optimal therapy are melanoma and hepatobiliary tumors. What constitutes "adequate" or "appropriate" surgical therapy for the elderly is not accurately known. Whether it should be any different from the standard treatment provided to younger patients is also not known. Scientific data from ran-

153

domized studies are not available for the older population because of the exclusion of the elderly from most clinical trials in the past. Studies which are available are retrospective and often display considerable bias in the patients chosen for certain treatments, especially surgical procedures.

Many biases influence the selection of therapy in the elderly. Concerns stem from what is perceived as limited life expectancy, the presence of comorbid disease, decreased functional status, alterations in mental status, limitations in economic resources, and assumed inability to tolerate treatment. The influence of these biases may affect survival from cancer in the elderly.

In one study evaluating survival up to 10 years after the diagnosis of cancer in patients over 65 years of age with cancers of the colon, rectum, breast, and prostate, variable factors which influenced survival were health status (comorbidity, functional status, level of activity), socioeconomic status (income and education level), cognitive status, and availability of social support (2). Another important factor, not receiving definitive therapy for the cancer (with the exception of prostate), was associated with a threefold greater death rate. Inadequate treatment remained a significant factor even after controlling for stage at diagnosis, socioeconomic factors, comorbidity, and physical functioning. These factors should be taken into account in order to optimize therapy outcome, but they should not necessarily be used to withhold appropriate treatment.

Surgical procedures in particular have been viewed as carrying prohibitive risk in many elderly patients in the past. Numerous studies have indicated that surgical procedures can be performed safely in the elderly (3–12). The balance between operative risk and expected cure or palliation is important when treating any patient with cancer but especially in the elderly with cancer. The impact of treatment on the quality of life is also of prime importance. Many cancer operations are complex and extensive with significant morbidity and mortality when attempted for cure. In this chapter, we review the current knowledge on risk assessment, breast cancer, gastrointestinal cancers, melanoma, and laparoscopic surgery as it pertains to the elderly population.

II. RISK ASSESSMENT

The determination of operative risk in the elderly is fraught with imprecision. Studies of operative risk in the elderly are often retrospective and fail to include adequate matched younger controls for comparison. The assessment of risk involves the interaction of the underlying physiological status, including normal physiological changes of aging, in addition to physiological changes attributable to comorbidity, the disease process, the surgical procedure itself, and the anesthesia. Age alone should not be used as the sole criterion to assess risk or to make therapeutic decisions.

Normal physiological changes occur with aging in every major organ system and affect the response to surgical procedures (13). In the cardiovascular system, atherosclerotic disease, cardiac arrhythmias, and conduction disturbances are more common. There is also a generalized decrease in distensibility of the cardiac wall and greater dependence on preload to increase cardiac output. Therefore, volume depletion is not well tolerated. Large complicated cancer resections often involve significant fluid shifts which may be much more dangerous in this population.

It is well known that renal function decreases with age, with a gradual loss of renal mass, glomerular filtration rate, and creatinine clearance (13). Drugs are not cleared as well and acid-base, fluid and electrolyte regulation is not as efficient as in younger individuals. The kidneys are more sensitive to nephrotoxic and ischemic insults which may occur with anesthesia and major cancer operations.

Liver function is also changed, with a decrease in liver volume and weight, blood flow, and perfusion with advancing age (14). The existence of multisystem disorders, particularly congestive heart failure, can also affect liver function (15). Histological and metabolic changes occur which influence the ability of the liver to metabolize drugs resulting in an increased half-life of many drugs (15). Polypharmacy, common in the elderly, is known to increase the risk for adverse drug reactions based on both hepatic and renal dysfunction (15).

There are age-related changes in the respiratory tract as well. Pulmonary function shows alterations in compliance and critical lung volumes due in part to decreased muscle mass (13). These changes affect not only oxygenation and ventilation but also the ability to prevent atelectasis and clear secretions. This deficiency along with decreased ciliary function and impaired immunological functions increase the risk for pneumonia in the postoperative period. Decreased muscle mass contributes to a diminished ability to reach tidal volumes.

The nervous system is also affected by aging. The presence of dementia or depression can affect the ability to make informed treatment decisions and can increase postoperative morbidity and hospital stay and decrease functional recovery (16). A reduction in neurons, cerebral blood flow, metabolic oxygen consumption, and receptor sites for neurotransmittors contribute to an increased sensitivity in the elderly to drugs and leads to postoperative delirium (17). Anesthetic agents and postoperative analgesics in particular must be used with caution in order not only to avoid postoperative mental status changes and delirium but hypoventilation and anoxia.

Operative risk can be assessed in a number of ways. One of the most common scales still used today to grade operative risk from anesthesia is the American Society of Anesthesiologists' (ASA) general classification of Physical Status (18). This scale demonstrates a relationship between the mortality rate related to anesthesia and the physical status of the patient defined according to five groups (Table 1).

More accurate measures of specific organ system risk have also been developed. Cardiac events remain a primary cause of perioperative morbidity and mortality. A commonly reported statistic is that patients who have had an myocardial infarction (MI) within 3 months of surgery have a 30% risk of recurrent MI or cardiac death (19). The risk decreases to 15% after 3–6 months and to a constant

Table 1 ASA Classification

Class I: The patient has no organic, physiological, biochemical, or psychiatric disturbance. The pathological process for which the operation is to be performed is localized and does not entail a systemic disturbance.

Class II: Mild to moderate systemic disturbances caused by the condition to be surgically treated or the pathophysiological processes. The extremes of age are included here, the neonate or the octogenarian, even though no discernible systemic disease is present. Extreme obesity and chronic bronchitis also are included in this category.

Class III: Severe systemic disturbance or disease from whatever cause even though it may not be possible to define firmly the degree of disability.

Class IV: Indicative of the patient with severe systemic disorders that already are life threatening and not always correctable by an operation.

Class IV: The moribund patient who has little chance of survival but who has submitted to operation in desperation. Most of these patients require an operation as a resuscitative measure with little, if any, anesthesia.

Emergency Operation (E): Any patient in classes I through V who is operated on as an emergency is considered to be in poor physical condition. The letter "E" is placed beside the numerical classification.

5% thereafter. Attempts have been made to define cardiac risk more precisely. Nine factors were found to predict independently cardiac complications by multivariate analysis in patients undergoing noncardiac surgery (20). A discriminant-function coefficient was assigned to each factor and a point value derived (Table 2). Four risk categories were defined based on each patient's point total. The categories corre-

Table 2 Goldman Criteria for Predicting Postoperative Cardiac Complications

Criteria	Point value
1. S3 gallop or jugular vein distention on preoperative examination	11
2. Myocardial infarction in the preceding 6 months	10
3. Rhythm other than sinus or premature atrial contractions on preoperative electrocardiogram	7
4. >5 premature ventricular contractions/min documented at any time before operation	7
5. Age >70 years	5
6. Emergency operation	4
7. Important valvular aortic stenosis	3
8. Intraperitoneal, intrathoracic or aortic operation	3
9. Poor general medical condition[a]	3

[a]$Po_2 < 60$ or $Pco_2 > 50$ mm Hg; $K < 3.0$ or $Cr > 3.0$ mg/dL; abnormal SGOT; signs of chronic liver disease; or patient bedridden from noncardiac causes.

Table 3 Goldman Risk Categories for Predicting Postoperative Cardiac Complications

Class	Point total	No or only minor complication (%)	Life threatening complication (%)	Cardiac death (%)
I	0–5	99	0.7	0.2
II	6–12	93	5	2
III	13–25	86	11	2
IV	≥26	22	22	56

lated well with the risk for cardiac death (Table 3). An age of over 70 years does contribute to an increased risk for cardiac complications. These risk categories were not designed to be exclusionary but to increase the awareness for potential complications and ensure full preoperative evaluation and attempts to provide interventions to decrease the risk of surgery.

Invasive monitoring to evaluate and optimize hemodynamic function has been advocated in elderly patients prior to major surgery. In one study, 34 of 148 patients (23%) over the age of 65 years were found to have an unacceptable risk based on severe cardiopulmonary defects on invasive hemodynamic evaluation which did not improve with treatment (21). All of the eight patients who went on to have the originally planned surgery despite the findings died. However, invasive monitoring is not without risks. A Pulmonary Artery Consensus Conference concluded that routine perioperative pulmonary artery catheter monitoring is not appropriate based on age alone, and further research is needed to define the proper role in geriatric patients (22).

Measures of physiological risk have also been used to predict operative risk in an attempt to take into account multisystem influences aside from just cardiac factors. The APACHE II score originally developed and used for assessing risk in patients in the intensive care unit has been applied to assessing risk in the preoperative setting. Age is included as one of the 12 variables used in the APACHE II score. High preoperative APACHE II scores have been associated with an increase in the morbidity and mortality seen for patients undergoing major hepatic surgery, pancreatic surgery, and gastric resections (23, 24).

Others have attempted more specifically to evaluate the risk of major surgery in the elderly. In one review by Reiss of over 1000 major abdominal operations performed on patients over the age of 70 years, nearly half were performed for malignant conditions (12). The overall mortality rate was 14%, and five variables were found to be predictive of increased mortality. These included patient age; modified ASA class; elective versus emergency surgery; operation for benign, malignant, operable, or malignant inoperable disease; and major diagnostic group (Table 4). If a patient had two or more features associated with a poor prognosis, the mortality rate was over 50%.

Table 4 Variables Associated with
Increased Risk for Major Abdominal
Operations

Risk factor	Mortality rate (%)
ASA I	7.4
III	32.7
Age 70–74	8.4
75–79	18.9
≥80	23.3
Type of surgery	
Elective	9.7
Emergency	19.7
Condition	
Benign	9.1
Operable malignancy	13.4
Inoperable malignancy	31.4
Diagnosis	
Biliary	2.1
Appendicitis	2.9
Peptic	9.7
Malignant colorectal	12.3
Benign obstruction	22.9
Malignant stomach/esophageal	23.1
Malignant pancreatic	28.1

Another series from the Mayo Clinic evaluated outcomes of surgery in 795 patients over the age of 90 years (25). The 30-day operative mortality was 8.4%. ASA class and emergency surgery correlated well with postoperative morbidity and mortality within 48 hours. Gastrointestinal surgery was associated with an increase in the case fatality within 48 hours. Preoperative renal and biliary dysfunction were associated with increased early postoperative morbidity. However, the overall 5-year survival rate was comparable to the rate expected for matched peers.

In light of this information, what can be done to minimize the surgical risks in the elderly? Careful preoperative assessment of the physiological status and the state of coexisting diseases can be used to guide therapeutic interventions to optimize abnormal results prior to, during, or in the postoperative recovery period. Anticipating problems may help recognize certain events before they become irreversible. Morbidity and mortality is known to be increased when operating on patients with advanced disease states; and moreover, emergency surgery is clearly associated with an increased risk of morbidity and mortality (11, 12, 25). It has often reported that there is a delay in diagnosis in elderly patients with malignancies leading to more advanced cancers and emergency presentations. Early diagnosis and treatment in the elderly rather than waiting for complications of untreated cancers should be encouraged.

III. BREAST CANCER

The incidence of breast cancer rises with age. Nearly one third of breast cancers occur in women over the age of 70 years (26). One half the deaths are in women more than 65 years of age (27). Yet, many studies have demonstrated that breast self-examination, clinical examination by health care providers, and screening mammography are underutilized in the elderly (28–30).

The National Cancer Institute Breast Cancer Screening Consortium performed screening surveys in 1987 and 1991 in women between the ages of 65 and 74 years in five metropolitan areas (31). More mammograms were performed in 1991, but 17–38% of the women in this age group still had *never* had a mammogram. A lack of patient awareness of the value of mammograms and a lack of physicians recommending mammograms for their patients were the most common reasons cited. Clinical trials have shown a 30% reduction in breast cancer mortality in women over the age of 50 years undergoing mammographic screening (32, 33). However, the appropriate use and interval for screening in the elderly is not clearly known, since most trials did not include women over age 75 years. A Dutch study did look at a subset of women over 75 years of age and found no reduction in breast cancer mortality for screened women, whereas a relative mortality of 0.45 was seen for women between the ages of 65 and 74 years, although the number of women over 75 years old was small (34). The Swedish two-county trial also confirmed an advantage for women between the ages of 50 and 74 years (35). The relative risk was lower for women between the ages of 60 and 69 years (RR 0.6) than for women aged 70–74 years (RR 0.79). It seems reasonable that mammography should remain important in the elderly, because the incidence of breast cancer continues to rise with age, and since the breasts become less dense with aging, the sensitivity of mammography should be expected to improve. In one series, the positive predictive value of an abnormal mammogram was greater for women over 65 years of age than for women 50 – 64 years old (36). However, there may be as many as 7 years of delay in seeing a benefit, which must be considered in relation to life expectancy. By using a decision analysis model, a benefit was demonstrated to screening women over 65 years old and even over the age of 85 years and taking into account the presence of comorbidities (37).

There is a belief that breast cancers in the elderly may not be as aggressive as in younger women. However, tumor characteristics of breast cancer in the elderly are only slightly different than those in younger women. The upper outer quadrant of the breast is still the most frequent site and infiltrating ductal the most common histological type (38, 39). In situ carcinomas do tend to be less common in the elderly (38, 40). This may reflect an underutilization of mammography, since the overall incidence of in situ disease has increased dramatically in the last 20 years with the advent of routine mammography (38, 41). Some reports also indicate a lower incidence of medullary and inflammatory carcinomas and a higher incidence of lobular, mucinous, and papillary histologies in the elderly (39, 42). The elderly do have a higher incidence of estrogen receptor (ER)–positive and progesterone receptor (PR)–positive tumors (38, 43). In one large series of over 10,000 women, 63% younger than the age of 50 years had ER-positive tumors, whereas 83% of those older than 50 years were ER positive (44). Another series demonstrated an upregulation of the receptors and an increase in the actual level of positivity occurring with aging (45).

There has been a shift toward earlier stage disease in breast cancers diagnosed in recent years. It is commonly believed that the elderly present with more advanced disease primarily on the basis of delayed diagnosis. However, recent data from an American College of Surgeons Commission on Cancer survey showed no difference in stage at diagnosis in the elderly compared to younger patients (38). The lack of complete staging in up to 20% of elderly patients limits interpretation.

One of the greatest areas of controversy is whether breast cancer in the elderly should be managed any differently than in younger women. The fear of treatment morbidity and mortality sometimes prompts a minimalistic approach in the elderly, whereas at other times, mastectomy is offered with little consideration of the possible desire for breast preservation or reconstruction. The role of axillary dissection, radiation therapy, or adjuvant therapy is also not completely clear.

Randomized trials in both the United States and Europe have shown breast-conserving therapy (BCT) to be equivalent to mastectomy in terms of survival from early-stage breast cancer (46–49). The National Institutes of Health (NIH) consensus conference also found it to be the preferable method of treating early-stage disease (50). However, breast-conserving therapy is still underutilized for all ages and particularly in the elderly.

The majority of cancers in the elderly are still treated with modified radical mastectomy and very rarely is breast reconstruction performed (38, 51). When breast conservation is performed, it is often done without axillary dissection or the use of postoperative radiation, as would be the standard for younger women (38, 51). In one retrospective series, the survival of elderly women was found to be lower for those treated with less than standard procedures, although it was not clear what selection criteria were used for determining choice of procedure (51). A lower survival was not demonstrated in a randomized series when lumpectomy alone was performed, although differences in local control rates were clear (46).

There are many factors that influence the use of BCT, including geographical location, race, and hospital characteristics. In one analysis of Medicare patients, geographical variations were marked in the use of BCT (52). In another review of over 18,000 caucasian women in three age groups, younger than 65, 65–74 and older than 74 years, the lowest rate of breast-conserving surgery was in the 65- to

74-year age group (53). In areas of the country where BCT was common in the younger ages, it was less common in the older age group, whereas in areas where it was not commonly used in the younger group, it was more commonly used in the older group. It was postulated that disfiguring surgery was avoided in the younger group, whereas morbidity and mortality was avoided in the older group. But the morbidity and mortality for breast surgery in the elderly is very low (38). The elderly have also been found to have a lower rate of BCT in the treatment of ductal carcinoma in situ (DCIS) (41).

Although axillary dissection is part of the standard surgical therapy for invasive breast cancer, its role in the elderly is not completely clear. Axillary dissections are primarily done for staging and secondarily for local control. The value in preventing distant disease is more controversial, and the procedure does carry risks. But axillary dissections are often omitted in elderly patients with clinically negative axillas (54). Even when node dissections are performed, the number of nodes removed in the elderly is less (55). As more of the elderly are being considered candidates for adjuvant therapy, nodal status will become more important. On the other hand, it becomes less important if nodal status will not influence the decision for adjuvant therapy.

The risk for the development of local recurrence in the axilla is another consideration. From the National Surgical Adjuvant Breast and Bowel Project (NSABP) B-04 trial, 18% of women with clinically negative axillae went on to develop delayed axillary disease (56). Delaying the dissection potentially subjects the elderly to an increase in the risk for surgical complications when they are even older and possibly in a more debilitated state. Two randomized trials looked specifically at node dissection in the elderly. In a series of 321 patients over 70 years old with clinically negative axillae treated with surgery and tamoxifen without node dissection, an axillary recurrence rate of only 4.3% was found (57). In a smaller series, only one axillary recurrence was seen at 103 months after treating the axilla with radiation and no surgery (58). A prospective randomized trial is being conducted in Europe to address this question in more detail.

Radiation therapy to the breast after breast-conserving surgery for invasive cancer is considered standard therapy. Yet radiation is omitted in many elderly patients after breast-conserving surgery. In one series, even in areas where breast-conserving therapy was used frequently, only 41% of women over the age of 75 years had radiation in contrast to 90% of women younger than 65 years and 86% of women between the ages of 65 and 74 years (53). In another report, when surgical therapy was more aggressive and included axillary dissection in the elderly, the use of radiation was also more frequent (38). Concerns have been expressed about whether the elderly will tolerate radiation and whether they will have difficulty completing therapy because of physical restraints in getting to radiation facilities and whether long-term outcomes are the same as in younger patients. However, studies have provided evidence to refute these concerns (59, 60).

Disturbingly, local recurrence rates for breast cancer have been reported as high as 35% in the elderly when radiation is not given (61). However, several recent trials have suggested that the risk for local recurrence may in fact not be as high in the elderly as in younger patients (49, 62). One hypothesis is that tamoxifen, frequently used in this age group, may be protective against local recurrence of breast cancer. A randomized trial is being conducted by Cancer and Leukemia Group B (CALGB) to address this question. Women over 70 years old with ER-positive tumors less than 2 cm are being randomized to lumpectomy and tamoxifen versus lumpectomy and tamoxifen and radiation.

For the elderly with breast cancer who have other coexisting medical problems which preclude any form of surgical therapy and who have a limited life expectancy, it is not unreasonable to treat patients with tamoxifen alone. Two prospective randomized trials compared tamoxifen alone to surgery alone and found good initial response rates for tamoxifen, although local control rates were worse with tamoxifen than with surgery (61, 63).

It is a common belief that breast cancer has a more favorable course in the elderly. Some series show no difference in survival based on age, whereas others actually show a worse survival in the elderly even after correcting for death from other causes (38, 64, 65). Up to 60% of deaths in elderly breast cancer patients are due to other causes. (43). A more recent study concluded that survival was worse in elderly patients as a result of inadequate treatment (51).

In an attempt to better define why older women receive less than definitive therapy for breast cancer, one study looked at the extent to which patients' age, marital status, health status, tumor characteristics, and aspects of physician–patient interaction influenced the treatment received (66). The following factors, along with the percentage of patients citing them, were reported as being very important in their choice for therapy: minimizing possibility of recurrence, 100%; physician's recommendation, 96%; quality of life after treatment, 77%; their family's opinion, 52%; what they would have to pay over and above insurance, 28%; and problems they would experience after surgery, 22% (162). The following were found not to be important in the choice: effect of treatment on sexuality, 83%; difficulty getting to and from treatments, 65%; and effects of treatment on appearance, 63%. Patient age, marital status, and the number of times the breast cancer specialist discussed treatment options were independently and significantly associated with the receipt of definitive primary tumor therapy. Older women who were not married and women with whom treatment options were discussed less frequently were less likely to receive definitive primary tumor therapy. The conclusion of the investigators (66) was that older women might be better served if they are offered choices from among definitive therapies, since there is some clinical uncertainty about what is the most appropriate therapy.

Breast cancer in the elderly should be approached with the same guidelines as for younger patients until well-performed studies demonstrate it is safe to treat the elderly differently.

IV. COLORECTAL CANCER

Colorectal cancer ranks third in the incidence of all cancers in both men and women. Over 94,700 cases of colon cancer and 47,900 cases of rectal cancer are predicted for 1999 (162). According to the National Cancer Data Base in 1990, 55.5% of colon cancer and 46.4% of rectal cancer occurred in individuals over the age of 70 years (67).

Symptoms at presentation are reported to be similar in elderly compared to younger patients (68). Although some workers report the location of colon cancers to be similar in elderly and younger patients (69), others report a higher incidence of right-sided lesions and a lower incidence of rectal lesions in elderly patients (70–72). In one of these series, more of the elderly presented with anemia, whereas in the other, the incidence of anemia was the same as in younger patients despite the higher incidence of right-sided lesions (70, 71).

The elderly may present with a more advanced stage of colorectal disease, especially those over 80 years of age, and with less differentiated tumors, although it is difficult to document a time delay in diagnosis based on the duration of symptoms (70). Resectability rates are reported to be lower in patients over 80 years of age (70).

Surgical resection of the colon or rectum remains the mainstay of curative therapy for colorectal cancer. It is required in many cases even in the presence of disseminated disease to avoid or treat the inevitable complications of obstruction and bleeding. A number of retrospective series have looked at the influence of advanced age on the risk of surgical resection of colorectal cancer. The risk of perioperative complications is generally reported to be higher in the elderly than in younger patients. Cardiopulmonary complications were increased in one series from 1.8% in patients under 65 years old to 10.8% in patients 65–75 years old and 8.2% in patients over the age of 75 years (7). Anastomatic leak rates were also increased from 4.2% in patients less than 65 years old to 8.2% in those over 75 years old (7). Mortality rates are also reported to be higher; however, most series show that age is not an independent factor in predicting mortality (7, 73). The cause of death in older patients is systemic complications (mainly cardiopulmonary) in nearly two thirds of patients, whereas in the majority of younger patients, postoperative death is caused by anastomotic leakage and other local complications (7). Actual mortality rates for colorectal surgery in the elderly range from 4 to 21% for elective cases to up to 54% for emergency cases (Table 5). Emergency operations are clearly associated with an increased mortality rate.

Mortality rates are also high for palliative operations such as creation of a colostomy (6, 77). This procedure is often done as an emergency procedure in an end-stage patient; two factors known to contribute to an increased risk (6, 77). Although some workers report the stage at presentation and incidence of performing palliative surgery is the same in the elderly as in younger patients, others report

Table 5 Morbidity and Mortality Rates for Elderly Patients Undergoing Colorectal Surgery

Reference	Age	No. of points	Diagnosis	Total operative mortality (%)	Elective operative mortality (%)	Emergency operative mortality (%)
73	>70	141	70% cancer	8.5		
6	>70	163	63% cancer	10.4	7.5	23.3
74	>70	242	All cancer			38
		197			18	
69	>70	171	All cancer	6		
		140			4	
		31				16
9	>80	115	All cancer	20		
		93			18	
		22				27
7	>75	98	All cancer	8.2	8.2	
	65–75	139			5.8	5.8
75	>80	163	All cancer	15.3	7.4	53.5
76	>70	53	All cancer	7.5		
71	>70	219	All cancer	6	4	15
77	>80	103	All cancer		4.7	41

that a greater proportion of the elderly require emergency surgery or present as an emergency (69, 71, 74). Furthermore, patients presenting as emergencies also tend to have more advanced-stage disease (74). With the increase in mortality associated with emergency operation and advanced-disease stage, it seems advisable to intervene earlier on an elective basis to avoid such problems as bleeding, perforation, and obstruction and also to avoid colostomy.

The question of whether surgery is indicated in the setting of advanced disease in the elderly is often raised. One small retrospective study found no difference in morbidity or mortality between 43 elderly patients undergoing surgery for advanced disease (obstruction, perforation, hemorrhage, or metastases) compared to 39 patients with localized disease (78). Although surgery can be safely performed, one must also consider other factors such as impact on the quality of life.

The role for laparoscopy-assisted colon resection is presently being evaluated for patients with colon cancer. The advantages described from preliminary experience indicate laparoscopic colon resection may lead to a decrease in postoperative pain and ileus (79). A shorter hospital stay and a faster return to a normal lifestyle than with conventional colon resection might be expected. Minimally invasive colectomy (MIC) was performed successfully in 83 of 103 patients aged 65 years and older in one prospective study (80). The mean hospital stay was 5.3 days and a complication rate of 25% was reported. Two of the 81 patients died within 30 days of surgery. In another small series of elderly patients with disseminated or metastatic disease in ASA classes III and IV, laparoscopic colon resection was performed with minor morbidities and no mortality (81). The safety in terms of adequacy of resection for cancer treatment and staging remains to be answered by ongoing prospective randomized clinical trials. Of additional concern are documented port site recurrences. Thirty-five recurrences were reported over a 2-year period in one review of the literature (82).

Another potential option for palliative treatment and control of obstruction or hemorrhage in patients with advanced rectal cancer is the use of local intraluminal therapies such as electrofulguration, laser therapy, or cryotherapy (83). Laser therapy is effective for palliation in 85–95% of patients, and procedure-related morbidity and mortality rates are low (83).

The quality of life, although more difficult to measure, is an important outcome for any planned treatment. Creating a stoma must be viewed with caution, as it may be difficult for some elderly patients to manage not only physically but psychologically. One series examined how patients over 80 years old did after leaving the hospital after undergoing surgery for gastrointestinal tumor (9). Thirty-one percent of patients went home following surgery, 51% convalesced in a specialized home or medical recovery center, 10% went to a nursing home or specialized institution, and 4% required nursing assistance at home or went to a family's home. Overall, 83% returned to their homes without any change in their social environment.

Survival after curative resection for colon carcinoma has been reported to be lower for patients over the age of 70 (84). However, in one series, multivariate analysis demonstrated that the 3-year survival was influenced by disease stage and type of operation performed (resection vs palliation) but not age (older than 80 years vs younger than 80 years) (85). Hospital stay was longer for those over 80 years old, as was the cost (22% increased cost). Another series indicated although the physical status and operative mortality were worse in the elderly undergoing surgery for colorectal cancer, for those elderly who were fit for surgery, who underwent curative resection, and who survived over 30 days, the 5-year survival was as good as in younger patients by multivariate analysis (72).

A. Colorectal Liver Metastases

The optimal treatment for limited metastases to the liver from colorectal cancer when disease is confined to the liver is liver resection. Liver resection can lead to a 21–48% 5-year survival in selected patients (86–91). The safety for performing liver resections has greatly improved in recent years owing to improvements in techniques of resection and intraoperative and postoperative care. Liver resections can be performed with mortality rates of less than 5% (87, 88, 91).

Liver resections can also be performed safely in elderly patients. A number of series have looked at morbidity and mortality rates for older individuals. One reported on 90 patients ranging in age from 65 to 82 years old who underwent liver resection (92). The overall mortality rate was 11%, but it was unacceptably high in patients undergoing right trisegmentectomies (30.7%). This is reflected by 60% of deaths overall being due to hepatic failure. Cardiac complications were frequent (5/90 arrythmia, 4/90 congestive heart failure [CHF]) but were responsible for only one death. The investigators advised caution in performing extended resections in elderly patients until better assessments of hepatic reserve become available.

Several factors are believed to play a role in the lower tolerance of the elderly to liver resections. The liver is believed to have a lower regenerative capability and limited functional reserve. There is a decrease in the blood flow and decreased ability to clear drugs.

Another report from the same institution in 1995 reviewed liver resections for colorectal metastases in 128 patients over 70 years old (4). For patients over 70 years old, the perioperative mortality rate was lower than in the earlier report at 4% which was the same as for patients younger than age 70 years. Morbidity rates were 42 and 40%, respectively. Most of the complications in the elderly were cardiopulmonary. In multivariate analysis, three factors were found to be important in predicting complications. These were male sex (2.6×), resection of at least one lobe of the liver (2.4×), and an operating time of greater than 240 min (2.3×). Median hospital stay for patients aged 70 years and older was only 1 day longer than for patients less than 70 years old. Morbidity, mortality, and ICU admission rates were not statistically different from younger patients.

Long-term survival following liver resection for colorectal metastases is not clearly influenced by age. No statistically significant difference in survival was found between patients older or younger than 60 years in one report (93). In another report, the median survival time was 40 months and the overall 5-year survival was 35% for patients 70 years and older, and 44 months and 39%, respectively, for patients younger than 70 years, which was not significantly different (4). In another report, no significant difference was seen in the 5-year survival of patients under 70 years old and those over 70 years old at 39 and 36%, respectively ($P = .9$) (5). In the large registry data, age greater than 70 years was of borderline significance ($P < .05$) in predicting survival, but even these patients had a 5-year survival of 18% compared to an expected 0% for patients not undergoing resection (86).

Although it is not clear what selection criteria are used to chose elderly patients for the major operation of hepatic resection, it is possible to perform the procedure in the elderly with the anticipation they will survive the surgery and have the same chance of survival from the cancer as do younger individuals.

V. HEPATOCELLULAR CANCER

Hepatic resection also provides the only hope for cure of patients with hepatocellular cancer. However, many of these patients have underlying cirrhosis as an etiological

Table 6 Hepatic Resection for Hepatocellular Cancer in the Elderly

Reference	No. of patients	Age	Hepatic failure[a]	Operative mortality[a]	5-year survival (%)
94	39	>70	4 (10)	5	51.6
10	32	>70	2 (6.3)	4 (12.5)	17.6
95	27	≥65		11 (40.7)	
96	37	>65	1 (2.7)	2 (5)	18.1

[a]Numbers in parentheses are percentages.

factor which makes surgical resection more challenging and dangerous. The functional reserve problem encountered with liver resection in the elderly for colorectal metastases, where the liver is otherwise normal, is compounded by the presence of cirrhosis. Several small series have examined the outcome of hepatic resection for hepatocelluar cancer in the elderly (Table 6).

Postoperative complications do not vary appreciably from those encountered in younger patients (94). With the exception of one series, the mortality rates are quite acceptable and in keeping with the rates for younger patients (95). The majority of deaths in the one series with the poor outcome were sepsis related and potentially avoidable with improvements in monitoring and postoperative care (95). The presence and severity of cirrhosis as judged by Child's criteria (see Appendix, page 176) does seem to influence the rate of operative mortality, and it is advised that patients with advanced cirrhosis be regarded carefully prior to consideration for major hepatic resection (10). The 5-year survival, although somewhat limited, remains better than for any other therapeutic modality for this disease.

VI. PANCREATIC CANCER

The incidence of pancreatic cancer rises with age. Over two thirds of patients are over the age of 65 years at diagnosis (97). The overall survival of patients with pancreatic cancer is dismal with 5-year survivals of 4–5% (97, 98). This is attributed in part to the unfortunate fact that the majority of patients with pancreatic cancer are diagnosed late in the course of the disease when surgical resection is no longer feasible. Only 14% of the patients diagnosed with pancreatic carcinoma in 1991 were treated with pancreatic resection (97). This percentage of patients resected is even lower for those over the age of 70 years. Although surgical resection is the only potential method of cure, the results remain disappointing. For patients who are able to undergo resection, the mean survival is still only 10.6–24.6 months (99).

The Whipple operation, or pancreaticoduodenectomy, is the operation of choice for the most common lesions, which are located in the head of the pancreas, as well as for periampullary, duodenal, and distal common bile duct neoplasms. In the past, it was associated with an extremely high complication rate and mortality rate as high as 26%. When weighed against the relatively small survival impact seen with successful surgery, many viewed the procedure as an unreasonable option for treatment (100, 101). The role of this operation in elderly patients was fraught with even more concern. However, in more recent years, the morbidity and mortality rates associated with the Whipple operation have decreased significantly (102–104). Mortality rates of between 0 and 5% are more commonly reported (102, 104, 105). Even in the elderly, mortality rates for surgery are acceptable in selected patients (4, 103, 106).

One review of 138 patients over 70 years old who underwent pancreatic resection for malignancy reported an operative mortality rate of 6% and morbidity rate of over 40% (4). Univariate analysis revealed a history of cardiopulmonary disease, an abnormal preoperative electrocardiogram, and an abnormal chest radiograph that were predictors of complications. In multivariate analysis, the only factor found to be a significant predictor of complications was a blood loss of more than 2 L. No significant differences were found in length of hospital stay, rate of intensive care unit admission, and morbidity or mortality rates between patients younger than 70 years old and those older than 70 years. Median survival was 18 months, and a 5-year survival rate of 21% was seen.

In a Veteran's Administration (VA) series of 77 patients with pancreatic cancer between the ages of 70–79 years, the mortality rate was 14%, and for six patients over the age of 80 years, no mortalities were seen (103). Several other smaller series of pancreatic resections have also reported mortality rates in patients over 70 years old to be 5–10% with morbidity rates of 14–48% (107–109). In another small series of selected patients without cardiac, respiratory, or hepatic failure, no difference in morbidity was seen in patients over 70 years old undergoing pancreaticoduodenectomy from those less than 70 years old (8).

One series from Johns Hopkins reported on 145 consecutive pancreaticoduodenectomies without a single mortality (102). The majority of cases were performed for malignancies. Thirty-seven patients in the series were over the age of 70 years. No significant differences were found between the length of stay or rate of complications in patients over 70 years old compared to younger patients. However, the patients were admittedly carefully selected prior to the operation as evidenced by no differences in the preoperative medical risk factors between patients under and over the age of 70 years.

The major causes of morbidity after pancreatic resection are related to complications associated with pancreatic fistula, anastomotic breakdown, and sepsis (8, 105, 110). Other studies have indicated that the routine use of octreotide may help reduce the risk of postoperative morbidity related to pancreatic fistula, pancreatitis, abscess, and sepsis (111, 112).

However, survival rates for resection remain limited (104, 105). Five-year survival rates are not different in the elderly. One series reported a 5-year survival rate for pancreatic cancer of 17% in patients over the age of 70 years and 19% in patients less than 70 years old (106). Periampullary tumor survival rates were better at 38 and 45%, respectively. Despite limited long-term survival, resection remains superior to bypass or laparotomy alone. In a review of over 3000 patients from the 1970s, a mean survival of 12.7 months for resection, 5.7 months for bypass, and 2.6 months for laparotomy alone were reported (99). In the same review of over 2000 patients from the 1980s, mean survival increased significantly in resected patients to 17 months, whereas bypass (6.6 months) and laparotomy alone (3.1) were no different.

Since the survival rate for resectable disease is still poor, adjuvant chemoradiation therapy has been given. An improvement in survival has been demonstrated in small series (113–115). More recently, preoperative chemoradiation therapy has been used in an attempt to increase resectability rates and survival in patients with pancreatic cancer (116). Preliminary results reveal preoperative therapy is safe and well tolerated (116). No specific information on how the elderly tolerate such treatment is available.

Still, the majority of patients with pancreatic cancer are not able to be resected. Surgery is needed in nearly 50% of patients for palliation of the two common complications that occur in the natural course of the disease, biliary and gastric obstruction (99). Pain often also requires palliation. The mean survival of patients after bypass is considerably lower than for resection at 4.0–11.3 months (99). The elderly may not tolerate bypass procedures as well as younger patients. A VA study did indicate a higher 30-day morbidity and mortality rate and a lower median survival rate after bypass procedures which was statistically significant for patients over 70 years old (110). However, VA patients may have unique characteristics which put them at higher risk. Each patient must be judged on an individual basis taking into consideration the overall status of the patient and expected benefit.

The operative mortality rate for biliary bypass ranges from 4 to 33% (mean 19%) and survival from 1.5 to 12 months (mean 5.4 months) (117). However, biliary obstruction can be as effectively managed with stents placed either endoscopically or percutaneously transhepatically as shown in several randomized series (118–121). Mortality rates are lower for stent placement than for surgical bypass and hospital stays are shorter. Although early complication rates are lower, long-term complication rates such as recurrent jaundice and cholangitis are more common than with surgical bypass.

Gastric outlet obstruction, although far less common as a presenting symptom, still requires operative bypass for relief, although the overall value is questioned. Survival after bypass is often limited and, furthermore, does not always result in palliation (122).

In patients explored for pancreatic resection, up to 55% are found to be unresectable (123). In these patients, a decision must be made about whether to perform prophylactic bypass procedures. In the presence of biliary obstruction, an operative biliary bypass may not be needed if a stent is already in place. Some would argue that biliary bypass via choledochoduodenostomy or jejunostomy can often be accomplished with minimal morbidity and avoids future requirements for stent changes and potential infections and episodes of sepsis associated with the presence of stents.

There continues to be controversy regarding the routine performance of prophylactic gastrojejunostomy at the time of exploration. The argument for doing the procedure are that 13–17% of patients will go on to develop gastric outlet obstruction in the future (99, 117). It is estimated that another 10–20% of patients die with duodenal obstruction without undergoing bypass, which may have been prevented if it had been done initially. Doing the bypass adds no morbidity to the procedure (99, 117). But if it is done at a second operation, a mortality rate of 22% and a mean survival of only 3 months have been reported (99). In a more recent series from Johns Hopkins, palliative operations for patients with unresectable pancreatic cancer carried a mortality rate of 3.3%, although the morbidity rate was 37% (123). Forty-one of 118 patients in that series were over 70 years old. These were selected patients who were felt to be able to tolerate a Whipple resection, who are generally in a better overall condition than those patients who are known to have unresectable or advanced disease who subsequently develop indications for palliative bypass. The decision requires clinical judgement. If duodenal impingement is obvious at surgery, a bypass should be done. If gastrojejunostomy is done later when the patient is more debilitated, the risk of complications and mortality increases.

The fact that the majority of patients never go on to develop gastric outlet problems and some patients will develop clinical gastric outlet obstruction or delayed gastric emptying despite having had a bypass argue against the performance of routine gastrojejunostomy (99). Recently, the introduction of laparoscopic techniques has provided a new method of performing the bypass with potentially lower morbidity and mortality in debilitated patients.

VII. GASTRIC CANCER

Nearly 50% of males diagnosed with gastric cancer in the United States and 60% of females are over the age of 70 years (124). Most cases of gastric cancer require surgery for attempted cure or for palliation of symptoms such as bleeding or obstruction. No other curative method of treatment is available.

Several Japanese series have looked at the characteristics of gastric cancer in the elderly. Symptoms at presentation and location of disease in the stomach are similar in younger and older patients (125, 126). One series reports no difference in histological type, whereas another reports a higher incidence of intestinal-type histology in the elderly (125, 126). The macroscopic pattern according to the Borrman criteria appears to be more localized in the elderly, but the occurrence of synchronous multiple primaries is greater and ranges from 7.7 to 13.2% (125–127). The incidence of vascular and lymphatic invasion has been reported to be higher in the elderly, whereas there is no difference in the incidence of lymph node metastases and stage at diagnosis (125, 126).

Curative surgery for gastric cancer requires either partial or total gastrectomy; surgery that is associated with significant operative morbidity and mortality. The exact extent of surgery remains a controversial subject not only in regard to the extent of gastric resection but also in the extent of lymphadenectomy required. Removal of perigastric nodes is termed a D1 resection, whereas removal of more extensive regional lymph nodes outside the perigastric region is termed a D2 resection. It is not clear whether more extensive resections impact on recurrence or survival. It is clear, however, that complication rates are known to be higher after proximal and total gastrectomies and after D2 regional node dissections (128, 129). In one large Western prospective randomized trial, the rate of surgical complications was doubled after D2 resections (128). The rate of nonsurgical complications (with the exception of pulmonary complications, which were also doubled in the D2 group) such as cardiac, urinary tract, and thromboembolic were similar.

The morbidity and mortality rates of performing gastric resections in the elderly appear to be increased over younger patients (Table 7). Although preoperative risk factors are increased in the elderly with gastric cancer, particularly of a cardiac and pulmonary nature, the majority of complications and deaths are caused by infections, anastomotic leaks, and pulmonary problems as in younger patients (3, 128, 129, 132). One small series reported no difference in major surgical complications between older and younger patients, but there was a statistically significant increase in overall septic complications and respiratory infections in older patients (132). The occurrence of multiorgan impairment and malnutrition was statistically related to the incidence of postoperative complications, but it was the degree of organ impairment rather than age that was predictive of postoperative complications.

An important element in deciding about surgical treatment in the elderly is

Table 7   Gastric Resections in the Elderly

Reference (year)	Country	Age	No. of patients	Morbidity (%)	Mortality (%)
130 (1997)[a]	USA-MSKCC[b]	>70	310	47.1	7.1
131 (1996)	Japan	70–79	341	22	5.3
		≥80[c]	43	26	5
128 (1995)	Netherlands	>70	231		
		D1	128	30	7
		D2	103	45	18
129 (1988)	Norway	≥80	106	34	15

[a] 85% > D1 resections.
[b] Memorial Sloan Kettering Cancer Center.
[c] Limited surgical procedures only.

Table 8 Gastric Cancer Survival after Curative Resection

Reference	No. of patients	Age	5-year survival (%)		10-year survival (%)
131			*Cumulative*	*Age corrected*	
	480	50–59	66.3[a]	68.9[b]	59[a]
	578	60–69	58.3	63.2	46
	341	70–79	48.6	62.1	27.4
	43	≥80	28	53	4
126	232	<70	49.4[c]		33.6
		>70	48.6		23.2
3	57	<70	14.5		
	24	≥70	19.4		

[a]Cumulative survival rates significantly different between age groups.
[b]Age-corrected survival not significantly different between age groups.
[c]Survival not significantly different between age groups.

the impact on the quality of life. One series from Japan assessed the quality of life after gastrectomy for gastric cancer in patients over 70 years old compared to those younger than 70 years (133). No significant difference was found in the amount of food intake or weight change after surgery in the elderly compared to younger patients. However, a significant decrease in performance status (PS) was found. Although PS decreased after surgery in both groups, it improved as time passed after the operation in the younger patients. In the older patients, the initial decrease after surgery remained relatively constant and did not improve with time. Performance status was 0–79% of elderly patients before surgery and 56% of patients postoperatively at the time of the questionaire (0 = patient can go out and do full-scale work; 1 = patient's ability is reduced but can look after himself or herself; 2 = patient is in bed more than 50% of daytime and requires others' help in home life; 3 = patient is totally bedridden and always requires others' help). However, most patients were still able to look after themselves. The ''health rate'' and employment rate were lower after surgery for the elderly, but over half of those who did not return to work felt it was not necessary for them to return rather than not possible for physical reasons. The overall conclusion was that the elderly should not be excluded from surgery based on quality of life concerns. In another smaller series of patients over the age of 70 years undergoing total gastrectomy, 70% of patients returned to ''normal life'' after 1 year, although regaining of body weight was slower than in younger patients (134).

The 5-year survival for curatively resected patients with gastric cancer is similar for younger and older patients (Table 8).

VIII. MELANOMA

The overall incidence of melanoma in the United States is increasing. The percentage of cases occurring in the older population also appears to be increasing. In 1985, 21.2% of cases occurred in patients over 70 years of age (135). This number increased to 27.2% of cases in 1990. The cummulative lifetime risk of developing melanoma in the United States by age 85 years is now 1 in 90 (1.1%) (136).

The characteristics of melanoma appear to be slightly different in the elderly. Although the extremities are the most common location for melanomas in females, head and neck melanomas become more frequent with advancing age (137, 138). In men, truncal melanomas are most common, but again head and neck melanomas become more frequent and surpass truncal melanomas after the age of 70 years (137, 138). Older patients have also been reported to have thicker melanomas with deeper levels of invasion and an increase in the incidence of ulceration (139, 140). It is not clear whether this may reflect a delay in the diagnosis of these lesions in the elderly population.

There is no evidence to suggest that the treatment for the elderly should be any different than that for younger individuals. The surgical decisions for melanoma treatment include the width of the margins of resection around the primary lesion and the need for regional lymph node dissection.

The margins of resection are determined by the thickness of the primary melanoma. For lesions less than 1 mm thick, a 1 cm margin is adequate (141, 142). For lesions 1–4 mm thick, a margin of 2 cm is advised based on the results of the Intergroup Melanoma Surgery Trial (143, 144). Age was not used as a criterion for exclusion in this study.

Although age has not been used as a criterion for determining the margins of resection, one large retrospective series did report age to be a significant independent factor in the risk for local recurrence (145). Patients over 60 years old were found to have a local recurrence rate of 7.8%, patients between the ages of 30–59 had a local recurrence rate of 2.5%, and patients less than 30 years old had a local recurrence rate of 1.2% at a median follow-up of 8 years. Other independently significant risk factors for recurrence included tumor thickness, ulceration, and sex. Another series reported a 12.1% local recurrence rate for patients with thin melanomas (<0.76 mm) over the age of 70 years (146). Although an analysis was not performed for potential factors affecting this high recurrence rate, it might be explained by the higher incidence of head and neck melanomas in the elderly with its attendant higher rate of local recurrence. This also raises a concern about adequacy of margins in elderly patients with melanoma. In the prospective randomized trial evaluating margins, no difference was found in the rate of local recurrence for age over 50 years old versus less than 50 years old (44). However, a higher rate of local recurrence was demonstrated for head and neck lesions.

The dissection of regional lymph nodes for melanoma treatment is routine for patients with clinically positive nodes; however, the value of elective node dissection (ELND) for patients with clinically negative lymph nodes has long been debated. Regional node dissections have significant long-term complications, and a clear benefit has not been established. Thin melanomas (<0.76 mm) have a low risk of metastatic spread and ELND is not warranted. For intermediate-thickness melanomas (0.75 or 1.0–4.0 mm), two prospective randomized trials failed to show an improvement in survival from ELND (147, 148). The most recent prospective randomized trial performed by the Intergroup Melanoma Surgical Program for patients with lesions 1–4 mm thick showed no significant difference in the 5-year survival for ELND with a follow-up of 7.4 years (149). Subgroup analysis, however, did reveal a significantly improved survival for patients who underwent ELND with tumors 1–2 mm thick, patients without tumor ulceration, and patients 60 years old or younger with tumors either 1–2 mm thick or without ulceration. It appears that ELND is, therefore, not indicated in the elderly for intermediate-thickness melanomas.

For thick melanomas (>4 mm), the risk of regional nodal metastases is high, as is the risk for distant disease. The ELND can be done with the intention of staging or as palliation prior to the nodes becoming clinically evident, but it may not have an impact on survival (150).

The recent introduction of the sentinel node biopsy technique provides a new approach. In this technique, a blue dye is injected intradermally at the site of the primary melanoma. The dye is then followed into the regional node basin where the first lymph node or nodes to turn blue are identified and removed. These are termed the sentinel lymph nodes. If these nodes are positive for tumor, a full node dissection is performed. If negative, then no dissection is done. Initial experience with this technique showed the blue dye method was able to identify the sentinel lymph node in 82% of patients (151). With more experience, the sentinel node could be identified in 96% of cases (151). The false-negative rate of the technique in identifying the presence of metastatic disease was 1% (151). Because of technical difficulties with the blue dye, radiolymphoscintigraphy using technitium-labeled sulfur colloid has been utilized to locate the sentinel node (152). Now both the dye and the radiolabeling are used conjointly. A prospective trial comparing sentinel node biopsy with observation is being done.

As long as there was no proven benefit to adjuvant therapy for melanoma, the role for lymph node dissection was entirely therapeutic. However, a recent prospective randomized trial demonstrated an improvement in relapse-free and overall survival with the use of adjuvant interferon-α-2b for patients with T4 and N1 lesions (153). The therapy, given for 1 year, had significant toxicity but did prolong survival by approximately 1 year. With the existence of an effective adjuvant, it will become more important to determine nodal status for staging purposes. The toxicity of adjuvant therapy in the elderly was not specifically addressed in this study.

Survival from melanoma is reported to decrease with advancing age (138, 140, 154, 155). From a prognostic standpoint, several factors are known to be associated with survival in malignant melanoma. These include tumor thickness, ulceration, tumor site, gender, and lymph node status (and number of lymph nodes involved) (137, 140, 154, 156–158). Age as a prognostic variable is inconsistent. Some series demonstrate age to be important, whereas others have found no relationship (138, 139, 154, 157). Factors which might account for the difference in survival seen in the elderly include a greater incidence of thicker and ulcerated lesions in the elderly, a more advanced stage at diagnosis with increased age, and a higher incidence of head and neck primaries (137, 139, 140). However, in one study with over 12,000 patients, multivariate analysis showed age to be independently important in the prognosis, especially in women (138). A survival disadvantage was seen in patients over 55 years old. Women, however, had a better outcome, and the influence of hormones on prognosis in women was questioned. Only a slight survival advantage was observed in older women over older men, whereas a much larger survival advantage was observed in younger women as compared to younger men.

IX. LAPAROSCOPY

The role of laparoscopy in cancer surgery and in the elderly is not yet defined. The benefits of laparoscopy over conventional surgical techniques shown for nononcological surgical procedures include the limited incisions with an attendant decrease in postoperative pain and a decreased hospital stay and recuperation period. An additional factor which must be considered for cancer operations is that these benefits must be achieved without a detrimental effect on the ability to cure the cancer. The principles of cancer surgery must be adhered to so as not to compromise the chance for cure. Bowel handling, tumor manipulation, anastomosis formation, attention to margins, and lymph node clearance must be performed with the same delicacy as with open procedures.

Of great concern are reports of trocar site recurrences after laparoscopic resection of cancers. Thirty-five port site recurrences after laparoscopic coloectomy were reported in one literature review (82). In that same review, 23 recurrences were reported after thoracoscopic resection of pulmonary malignancies and another 31 cases of port site recurrence were reported after other laparoscopic procedures, including procedures for ovarian cancer and unsuspected gallbladder cancer. Incisional recurrences are almost unheard of after standard open operative procedures for cancers.

For some cancers in which there is a high rate of unresectability such as hepatobiliary, pancreatic, and gastric cancers, preliminary laparocopic examination may avoid unnecessary laparotomy (159, 160). Laparoscopic splenectomy has been reported in hematological malignancies (161).

There are some limitations to laparoscopic procedures, specifically the limited ability to palpate organs and the inaccessibility of several areas of the abdomen such as the posterior surface of the liver, posterior wall of the stomach, and areas of the retroperitoneum. Until prospective studies are performed, laparoscopy should be used selectively and with caution.

X. CONCLUSIONS

The incidence of most cancers increases with age. Although the risk for surgery increases in the elderly with comorbidities, there are ways to evaluate risk to allow interventions that might potentially decrease morbidity and mortality. Appropriate treatments should be offered to the elderly until studies are performed that demonstrate the elderly can safely be managed in a different manner than younger patients. The elderly should not be denied adequate treatment simply on the basis of age alone.

APPENDIX

Child's Criteria

	Child's Group		
	A (Minimal)	B (Moderate)	C (Advanced)
Serum bilirubin mg%	<2.0	2.0–3.0	>3.0
Serum albumin gm%	>3.5	3.0–3.5	<3.5
Ascites	Absent	Easily controlled	Poorly controlled
Neurologic disorder	None	Minimal	Advanced coma
Nutrition	Excellent	Good	Poor, wasting

Source: Ref. 163.

REFERENCES

1. Record high life expectancy. Statistical Bulletin, Metropolitan Insurance Companies. Jul–Sep 1993, pp 28–35.
2. Goodwin JS, Samet JM, Hunt WC. Determinants of survival in older cancer patients. J Natl Cancer Inst 1996; 88:1031–1038.
3. Bittner R, Schirrow H, Butters M, Roscher R, Krautzberger W, Oettinger W, Beger HG. Total gastrectomy, a 15-year experience with particular reference to the patient over 70 years of age. Arch Surg 1985; 120:1120–1125.
4. Fong Y, Blumgart LH, Fortner JG, Brennan MF. Pancreatic or liver resection for malignancy is safe and effective for the elderly. Ann Surg 1995; 222:426–437.
5. Fong Y, Cohen AM, Fortner JG, Enker WE, Turnbull AD, Coit DG, Marrero AM,

Prasad M, Blumgart LH, Brennan MF. Liver resection for colorectal metastases. J Clin Oncol 1997; 15:938–946.

6. Greenburg AG, Saik RP, Pridham D. Influence of age on mortality of colon surgery. Am J Surg 1985; 150:65–70.

7. Hesterberg R, Schmidt WU, Ohmann C, Roher HD, Sattler J. Risk of elective surgery of colorectal carcinoma in the elderly. Dig Surg 1991; 8:22–27.

8. Kojima Y, Yasukawa H, Katayama K, Note M, Shimada H, Nakagawara G. Postoperative complications and survival after pancreatoduodenectomy in patients aged over 70 years. Surg Today Jpn J Surg 1992; 22:401–404.

9. Morel P, Egeli RA, Wachtl S, Rohner A. Results of operative treatment of gastrointestinal tract tumors in patients over 80 years of age. Arch Surg 1989; 124:662–664.

10. Nagasue N, Chang Y-C, Takemoto Y, Taniura H, Kohno H, Nakamura T. Liver resection in the aged (seventy years or older) with hepatocellular carcinoma. Surgery 1993; 113:148–154.

11. Palmberg S, Hirsjarvi E. Mortality in geriatric surgery, with special reference to the type of surgery, anaesthesia, complicating diseases, and prophylaxis of thrombosis. Gerontology 1979; 25:103–112.

12. Reiss R, Deutsch AA, Nudelman I. Abdominal surgery in elderly patients: statistical analysis of clinical factors prognostic of mortality in 1,000 cases. Mt Sinai J Med 1987; 54:135–140.

13. Evers BM, Townsend CM, Thompson JC. Organ physiology of aging. Surg Clin North Am 1994; 74:23–39.

14. Wynne HA, Cope LH, Mutch E, Rawlins MD, Woodhouse KW, James OF. The effect of age upon liver volume and apparent liver blood flow in healthy man. Hepatology 1989; 9:297–301.

15. Mooney H, Roberts R, Cooksley WGE, Halliday JW, Powell LW. Alterations in the liver with ageing. Clin Gastroenterol 1985; 14:757–771.

16. Rocca R. Psychosocial aspects of surgical care in the elderly patient. Surg Clinics No Amer 1994; 74:223–243.

17. Buxbaum JL, Schwartz AJ. Perianesthetic considerations for the elderly patient. Surg Clin North Am 1994; 74:41–58.

18. Dripps RD, Lamont A, Eckenhoff. The role of anesthesia in surgical mortality. JAMA 1961; 178:261–266.

19. Goldman L. Cardiac risks and complications of noncardiac surgery. Ann Intern Med 1983; 98:504–513.

20. Goldman L, Caldera DL, Nussbaum SR, Southwick FS, Krogstad D, Murray B, Burke DS, O'Malley TA, Goroll AH, Caplan CH, Nolan J, Carabello B, Slater EE. Multifactorial index of cardiac risk in noncardiac surgical procedures. N Engl J Med 1977; 297:845–850.

21. DelGuercio LR, Cohn JD. Monitoring operative risk in the elderly. JAMA 1980; 243:1350–1355.

22. Pulmonary Artery Consensus Conference Participants. Pulmonary artery catheter consensus conference: Consensus statement. New Horizons 1997; 5:175–193.

23. Gagner M, Franco D, Vons C, Smadja C, Rossi RL, Braasch JW. Analysis of morbidity and mortality rates in right hepatectomy with the preoperative APACHE II score. Surgery 1991; 110:487–492.

24. Gagner M. Value of preoperative physiologic assessment in outcome of patients undergoing major surgical procedures. Surg Clin North Am 1991; 71:1141–1150.

25. Hosking MP, Warner MA, Lobdell CM, Offord KP, Melton LJ. Outcomes of surgery in patients 90 years of age and older. JAMA 1989; 261:1909–1915.

26. Osteen RT, Karnell LH. Breast cancer. In: GD Steele, DP Winchester, HR Menck, GP Murphy, eds. National Cancer Data Base: Annual Review of Patient Care 1993. Atlanta: American Cancer Society, 1993; pp. 10–19.

27. Yancik R, Ries LA. Cancer in older persons. Magnitude of the problem-how do we apply what we know? Cancer 1994; 74:1995–2003.

28. Weinberger M, Saunders AF, Samsa GP, Bearon LB, Gold DT, Brown JT, Booher P, Loehrer PJ. Breast cancer screening in older women: Practices and barriers reported by primary care physicians. J Am Geriatrics Society 1991; 39:22–29.

29. Vincent AL, Bradham D, Hoercherl S, McTague D. Survey of clinical breast examinations and use of screening mammography in Florida. South Med J 1995; 88:731–736.

30. Leather DS, Roberts MM. Older women's attitudes towards breast disease, self examination, and screening facilities: implications for communication. Br Med J 1985; 290:668–670.

31. The NCI Breast Cancer Screening Consortium. Screening mammography: a missed clinical opportunity? JAMA 1990; 264:54–58.

32. Habbema JDF, van Oortmarssen GJ, van Putten DJ, Lubbe JT, van der Mass PJ. Age-specific reduction in breast cancer mortality by screening: an analysis of the results of the Health Insurance Plan of Greater New York Study. J Natl Cancer Inst 1986; 77:317–320.

33. Tabar L, Gad A, Holmberg LH, Ljunquist U, Fagerberg CJG, Baldetorp L, Grontoft O, Lundstrom B, Manson JC, Eklund G, Day NE, Pettersson F. Reduction in mortality from breast cancer after mass screening with mammography. Lancet 1985; 13:829–832.

34. Van Dijck JAAM, Verbeek ALM, Beex LVAM, Hendriks JHCL, Holland R, Mravunac M, Straatman H, Werre JM. Mammographic screening after the age of 65 years: evidence for a reduction in breast cancer mortality. Int J Cancer 1996; 66:727–731.

35. Tabar L, Fagerberg G, Chen H-H, Duffy SW, Smart CR, Gad A, Smith RA. Efficacy of breast cancer screening by age. Cancer 1995; 75:2507–2517.

36. Faulk RM, Sickles EA, Sollitto RA, Ominsky SH, Galvin HB, Frankel SD. Clinical efficacy of mammographic screening in the elderly. Radiology 1995; 194:193–197.

37. Mandelblatt JS, Wheat ME, Monane M, Moshief RD, Hollenberg JP, Tang J. Breast cancer screening for elderly women with and without comorbid conditions: a decision analysis model. Ann Intern Med 1992; 116:722–730.

38. Busch E, Kemeny M, Fremgen A, Osteen RT, Winchester DP, Clive RE. Patterns of breast care in the elderly. Cancer 1996; 78:101–111.

39. Allen C, Cox EB, Manton KG, Cohen HJ. Breast cancer in the elderly: Current patterns of care. J Am Geriatrics Society 1986; 34:637–642.

40. Winchester DP, Menck HR, Osteen RT, Kraybill W. Treatment trends for ductal carcinoma in situ of the breast. Ann Surg Oncol 1995; 2:207–213.

41. Ernster VL, Barclay J, Kerlikowske K, Grady D, Henderson IC. Incidence and treatment for ductal carcinoma in situ of the breast. JAMA 1996; 275:913–918.

42. Yancik R, Ries LG, Yates JW. Breast cancer in aging women: a population-based study of contrasts in stage, surgery, and survival. Cancer 1989; 63:976–981.

43. Singletary SE, Shallenberger R, Guinee VF. Breast cancer in the elderly. Ann Surg 1993; 218:667–671.

44. Pujol P, Hilsenbeck SG, Chamness GC, Elledge RM. Rising levels of estrogen receptor in breast cancer over 2 decades. Cancer 1994; 74:1601–1606.

45. McCarty K, Silva JS, Cox EB, Leight GS, Wells SA, McCarty K Sr. Relationship of age and menopausal status to estrogen receptor content in primary carcinoma of the breast. Ann Surg 1983; 197:123–127.

46. Fisher B, Anderson S, Redmond CK, Wolmark N, Wickerham DL, Cronin WM. Re-analysis and results after 12 years of follow-up in a randomized clinical trial comparing total mastectomy with lumpectomy with or without irradiation in the treatment of breast cancer. N Engl J Med 1995; 333:1456–1461.

47. Veronisi U, Saccozzi R, Del Vecchio M, Banfi A, Clemente C, De Lena M, Gallus G, Greco M, Luini A, Marubini E, Muscolino G, Rilke F, Salvadori B, Zecchini A, Zucali R. Comparing radical mastectomy with quadrantectomy, axillary dissection, and radiotherapy in patients with small cancers of the breast. N Engl J Med 1981; 305:6–11.

48. Sarrazin D, Le M, Rousees J, Contesso G, Petit J-Y, Lacour J, Viguier J, Hill C. Conservative treatment versus mastectomy in breast cancer tumors with macroscopic diameter of 20 millimeters or less. Cancer 1984; 53:1209–1213.

49. Liljegren G, Holmberg L, Adami HO, Westman G, Graffman S, Bergh J. Sector resection with or without postoperative radiotherapy for stage I breast cancer: five year results of randomized trial. J Natl Cancer Inst 1994; 86:717–722.

50. NIH Consensus Conference. Treatment of early-stage breast cancer. JAMA 1991; 265:391–395.

51. Wanebo HJ, Cole B, Chung M, Vezeridis M, Schepps B, Fulton J, Bland K. Is surgical management comprimised in elderly patients with breast cancer? Ann Surg 1997; 225:579–589.

52. Nattinger AB, Gottlieb MS, Veum J, Yahnke D, Goodwin JS. Geographic variation in the use of breast-conserving treatment for breast cancer. N Engl J Med 1992; 326:1102–1107.

53. Farrow DC, Hunt WC, Samet JM. Geographic variation in the treatment of localized breast cancer. N Engl J Med 1992; 326:1097–1101.

54. Davis SJ, Karrer FW, Moor BJ, Rose SG, Eakins G. Characteristics of breast cancer in women over 80 years of age. Am J Surg 1985; 150:655–658.

55. Chu J, Diehr P, Feigl P, Glaefke G, Begg C, Glicksman A, Ford L. The effect of age on the care of women with breast cancer in community hospitals. J Gerontol 1987; 42:185–190.

56. Fisher B, Redmond C, Fisher ER, Bauer M, Wolmark N, Wickerham L, Deutsch M, Montague E, Margolese R, Foster R. Ten-year results of a randomized clinical trial comparing radical mastectomy and total mastectomy with or without radiation. N Engl J Med 1985; 312:674–681.

57. Martelli G, DePalo G, Rossi N, Cordini D, Boracchi P, Galante E, Vetrella G. Long-term follow-up of elderly patients with operable breast cancer treated with surgery without axillary dissection plus adjuvant tamoxifen. Br J Cancer 1995; 72:1251–1255.

58. Wazur DE, Erban JK, Robert NJ, Smith TJ, Marchant DJ, Schmid C, DiPetrillo T, Schmidt-Ullrich R. Breast conservation in elderly women for clinically negative axillary lymph nodes without axillary dissection. Cancer 1994; 74:878–883.

59. Swanson RS, Sawicka J, Wood WC. Treatment of carcinoma of the breast in the older geriatric patient. Surg Gynecol Obstet 1991; 173:465–469.
60. Peschel RE, Wilson L, Haffty B, Papadopoulos D, Rosenzweig K, Feltes M. The effect of advanced age on the efficacy of radiation therapy for early breast cancer, local prostate cancer and grade III-IV gliomas. Int J Rad Oncol Biol Phys 1993; 26:539–544.
61. Robertson JFR, Ellis IO, Elston CW, Blamey RW. Mastectomy or tamoxifen as initial therapy for operable breast cancer in elderly patients: 5-year follow-up. Eur J Cancer 1992; 28A:908–910.
62. Veronisi U, Luini A, Del Vecchio M, Greco M, Galimberti V, Merson M, Rilke F, Sacchini V, Saccozzi R, Savio T, Zucali R, Zurrida S, Salvadori B. Radiotherapy after breast-preserving surgery in women with localized cancer of the breast. N Engl J Med 1993; 328:1587–1591.
63. Bates T, Riley DL, Houghton J, Fallowfield L, Baum M. Breast cancer in elderly women: a Cancer Research Campaign trial comparing treatment and optimal surgery with tamoxifen alone. Br J Surg 1991; 78:591–594.
64. Adami H-O, Malker B, Holmberg L, Persson I, Stone B. The relation between survival and age at diagnosis in breast cancer. N Engl J Med 1986; 315:559–563.
65. Mueller CB, Ames F, Anderson GD. Breast cancer in 3558 women: age as a significant determinant in the rate of dying and causes of death. Surgery 1978; 83:123–132.
66. Silliman RA, Troyan SL, Guadagnoli E, Kaplan SH, Greenfield S. The impact of age, marital status, and physician-patient interactions on the care of older women with breast carcinoma. Cancer 1997; 80:1326–1334.
67. Steele GP, Colorectal cancer in Steele GD, Winchester DP, Menck HR, Murphy GP. National Cancer Data Base: Annual Review of Patient Care 1993. Washington, DC: American Cancer Society, 1993, pp 20–36.
68. Kemppainen M, Raiha I, Sourander L. Delay in diagnosis of colorectal cancer in elderly patients. Age Ageing 1993; 22:260–264.
69. Irvin TT, Prognosis of colorectal cancer in the elderly. Br J Surg 1988; 75:419–421.
70. Kemppainen M, Raiha I, Rajala T, Sourander L. Characteristics of colorectal cancer in elderly patients. Gerontology 1993; 39:222–227.
71. Mulcahy HE, Patchett SE, Daly L, O'Donoghue DP. Prognosis of elderly patients with large bowel cancer. Br J Surg 1994; 81:736–738.
72. Kingston RD, Jeacock J, Walsh S, Keeling F. The outcome of surgery for colorectal cancer in the elderly: a 12-year review from the Trafford Database. Eur J Surg Oncol 1995; 21:514–516.
73. Boyd JB, Bradford B, Watne AL. Operative risk factors of colon resection in the elderly. Ann Surg 1980; 192:743–746.
74. Waldron RP, Donovan IA, Drumm J, Mottram SN, Tedman S. Emergency presentation and mortality from colorectal cancer in the elderly. Br J Surg 1986; 73:214–216.
75. Arnaud JP, Schoegel M, Ollier JC, Adloff M. Colorectal cancer in patients over 80 years of age. Dis Colon Rectum 1991; 34:896–898.
76. Vivi AA, Lopes A, Cavalcanti SDF, Rossi BM, Marques LA. Surgical treatment of colon and rectum adenocarcinoma in elderly patients. J Surg Oncol 1992; 51:203–206.
77. Spivak H, Maele DV, Friedman I, Nussbaum M. Colorectal surgery in octogenarians. J Am Cancer Soc 1996; 183:46–50.

78. Fitzgerald SD, Longo WE, Daniel GL, Vernava AM. Advanced colorectal neoplasia in the high-risk elderly patient: Is surgical resection justified? Dis Colon Rectum 1993; 36:161–166.

79. Huscher C, Silecchia G, Croce E, Farello A, Lezoche E, Morina M, Azzola M, Feliciotti, Rosato P, Tarantini M, Basso N. Laparoscopic colorectal resection. Surg Endosc 1996; 10:875–879.

80. Peters WR, Fleshman JW. Minimally invasive colectomy in elderly patients. Surg Laparosc Endosc 1995; 5:477–479.

81. Vara-Thorbeck C, Garcia-Caballero M, Salvi M, Gutstein D, Toscano R, Gomez A, Vara-Thorbeck R. Indications and advantages of laparoscopy-assisted colon resection for carcinoma in elderly patients. Surg Laparosc Endosc 1994; 4:110–118.

82. Johnstone PAS, Rohde DC, Swartz SE, Fetter JE, Wexner SD. Port site recurrences after laparoscopic and thoracoscopic procedures in malignancy. J Clin Oncol 1996; 14:1950–1956.

83. Dohmoto M, Hunerbein M, Schlag PM. Palliative endoscopic therapy of rectal cancer. Eur J Cancer 1996; 32A:25–29.

84. Gardner B, Dotan J, Shaikh, Feldman J, Herbsman H, Alfonso A, Iyer SK. The influence of age upon the survival of adult patients with carcinoma of the colon. Surg Gynecol Obstet 1981; 153:366–368.

85. Hobler KE. Colon surgery for cancer in the very elderly, cost and 3-year survival. Ann Surg 1986; 203:129–131.

86. Hughes K, Simon R, Songhorabobi S, Adson MA, Ilstrup DM, Fortner JG. Resection of the liver for colorectal carcinoma metastases: A multi-institutional study of indications for resection. Surgery 1988; 103:278–288.

87. Sugihara K, Hojo K, Moriya Y, Yamasaki S, Kosuge T, Takayama T. Pattern of recurrence after hepatic resection for colorectal metastases. Br J Surg 1993; 80:1032–1035.

88. Rosen CB, Nagorney DM, Taswell HF, Helgeson SL, Ilstrup DM, van Heerden JA, Adson MA. Perioperative blood transfusion and determinants of survival after liver resection for metastatic colorectal carcinoma. Ann Surg 1992; 216:493–505.

89. van Ooijen B, Wiggers T, Meijer S, van der Heijde MN, Sloff MJH, van de Velde CJH, Obertop H, Gouma DJ, Bruggink EDM, Lange JF, Munting JDK, Rutten APM, Rutten HJT, de Vries JE, Groot G, Zoetmulder FAN, van Putten WLJ. Hepatic resections for colorectal metastases in The Netherlands, a multiinstitutional 10-year study. Cancer 1992; 70:28–34.

90. Scheele J, Stangl R, Altendorf-Hofmann A, Gall FP. Indicators of prognosis after hepatic resection for colorectal secondaries. Surgery 1991; 110:13–29.

91. Nordlinger B, Guiguet M, Vaillant J-C, Balladur P, Boudjema K, Bachellier P, Jaeck D. Surgical resection of colorectal carcinoma metastases to the liver. Cancer 1996; 77:1254–1264.

92. Fortner JG, Lincer RM. Hepatic resection in the elderly. Ann Surg 1990; 211:141–145.

93. Scheele J, Stangl R, Altendorf-Hofmann A, Paul M. Resection of colorectal liver metastases. World J Surg 1995; 19:59–71.

94. Takenaka K, Shimada M, Higashi H, Adachi E, Nishizaki T, Yanaga K, Matsumata T, Sugimachi K. Liver resection for hepatocellular carcinoma in the elderly. Arch Surg 1994; 129:846–850.

95. Yanaga K, Kanematsu T, Takenaka K, Matsumata T, Yoshida Y, Sugimachi K. He-

patic resection for hepatocellular carcinoma in elderly patients. Am J Surg 1988; 155: 238–241.

96. Ezaki T, Yukaya H, Ogawa Y. Evaluation of hepatic resection for hepatocellular carcinoma in the elderly. Br J Surg 1987; 74:471–473.

97. Niederhuber JE, Brennan MF, Menck HR. The national cancer data base report on pancreatic cancer. Cancer 1995; 76:1671–1677.

98. Parker SL, Tong T, Bolden S, Wingo PA. Cancer statistics 1997. CA 1997; 47:5–27.

99. Watanapa P, Williamson RCN. Surgical palliation for pancreatic cancer: developments during the past two decades. Br J Surg 1992; 79:8–20.

100. Connolly MM, Dawson PJ, Michelassi F, Moossa AR, Lowenstein F. Survival in 1001 patients with carcinoma of the pancreas. Ann Surg 1987; 206:366–373.

101. Edis AJ, Kiernan PD, Taylor WF. Attempted curative resection of ductal carcinoma of the pancreas, review of Mayo Clinic experience, 1951–1975. Mayo Clin Proc 1980; 55:531–536.

102. Cameron JL, Pitt HA, Yeo CJ, Lilemoe KD, Kaufman HS, Coleman J. One hundred and forty-five consective pancreaticoduodenectomies without mortality. Ann Surg 1993; 217:430–438.

103. Wade TP, El-Ghazzawy AG, Virgo KS, Johnson FE. The Whipple resection for cancer in US Department of Veterans Affairs Hospitals. Ann Surg 1995; 221:241–248.

104. Michelassi F, Erroi F, Dawson PJ, Pietrabissa A, Noda S, Handcock M, Block GE. Experience with 647 consecutive tumors of the duodenum, ampulla, head of the pancreas, and distal common bile duct. Ann Surg 1989; 210:544–556.

105. Trede M, Schwall G, Saeger H-D. Survival after pancreaticoduodenectomy, 118 consecutive resections without an operative mortality. Ann Surg 1990; 211:447–458.

106. Hannoun L, Christophe M, Ribeiro J, Nordlinger B, Elriwini M, Tiret E, Parc R. A report of forty-four instances of pancreaticoduodenal resection in patients more than seventy years of age. Surg Gynecol Obstet 1993; 177:556–560.

107. Delcore R, Thomas JH, Hermreck AS. Pancreaticoduodenectomy for malignant pancreatic and periampullary neoplasms in elderly patients. Am J Surg 1991; 162:532–536.

108. Spencer MP, Sarr MG, Nagorney DM. Radical pancreatectomy for pancreatic cancer in the elderly. Ann Surg 1990; 212:140–143.

109. Kairaluoma MI, Kiviniemi H, Stahlberg M. Pancreatic resection for carcinoma of the pancreas and the periampullary region in patients over 70 years of age. Br J Surg 1987; 74:116–118.

110. Wade TP, Radford DM, Virgo KS, Johnson FE. Complications and outcomes in the treatment of pancreatic adenocarcinoma in the United States veteran. J Am Coll Surg 1994; 179:38–48.

111. Bassi C, Falconi M, Lombardi D, Briani G, Vesentini S, Camboni MG, Pederzoli P. Prophylaxis of complications after pancreatic surgery: Results of a multicenter trial in Italy. Digestion 1994; 55:41–47.

112. Buchler M, Friess H, Klempa I, Hermanek P, Sulkowski U, Becker H, Schafmayer A, Baca I, Lorenz D, Meister R, Kremer B, Wagner P, Witte J, Zurmayer EL, Saeger H-D, Rieck B, Dollinger P, Glaser K, Teichmann R, Konradt J, Gaus W, Dennler H-J, Welzel D, Beger HG. Role of octreotide in the prevention of postoperative complications following pancreatic resection. Am J Surg 1992; 163:125–131.

113. Whittington R, Bryer MP, Haller DG, Solin LJ, Rosato EF. Adjuvant therapy of re-

sected adenocarcinoma of the pancreas. Int J Rad Oncol Biol Phys 1991; 21:1137–1143.

114. Kalser MH, Ellenberg SS. Pancreatic cancer, adjuvant combined radiation and chemotherapy following curative resection. Arch Surg 1985; 120:899–903.

115. Gastrointestinal Tumor Study Group. Further evidence of effective adjuvant combined radiation and chemotherapy following curative resection of pancreatic cancer. Cancer 1987; 59:2006–2010.

116. Hoffman JP, Weese JL, Solin LJ, Engstrom P, Agarwal P, Barber LW, Guttmann MC, Litwin S, Salazar H, Eisenberg BL. A pilot study of preoperative chemoradiation for patients with localized adenocarcinoma of the pancreas. Am J Surg 1995; 169:71–78.

117. Sarr MG, Cameron JL. Surgical management of unresectable carcinoma of the pancreas. Surgery 1982; 91:123–133.

118. Bornman PC, Tobias R, Harries-Jones EP, Van Stiegmann G, Terblanche J. Prospective controlled trial of transhepatic biliary endoprosthesis versus bypass surgery for incurable carcinoma of head of pancreas. Lancet J 1986; 11:69–71.

119. Shepherd HA, Royle G, Ross APR, Diba A, Arthur M, Colin-Jones D. Endoscopic biliary endoprosthesis in the palliation of malignant obstruction of the distil common bile duct: a randomized trial. Br J Surg 1988; 75:1166–1168.

120. Andersen JR, Sorensen SM, Kruse A, Rokkjer M, Matzen P. Randomised trial of endoscopic endoprosthesis versus operative bypass in malignant obstructive jaundice. Gut 1989; 30:1132–1135.

121. Dowsett JF, Russell RCG, Hatfield ARW, Cotton PB, Williams SJ, Speer AG, Houghton J, Lennon T, Macrae K. Malignant obstructive jaundice: A prospective randomized trial of by-pass surgery versus endoscopic stenting. Gastroenterology 1989; 96:A128.

122. Weaver DW, Wienck RG, Bouwman DL, Walt AJ. Gastrojejunostomy: is it helpful for patients with pancreatic cancer? Surgery 1987; 102:608–613.

123. Lillimoe KD, Sauter PK, Pitt HA, Yeo CJ, Cameron JL. Current status of surgical palliation of periampullary carcinoma. Surg Gynecol Obstet 1993; 176:1–10.

124. Wanebo HJ, Kennedy BJ, Chmiel J, Steele G, Winchester D, Osteen R. Cancer of the stomach, a patient care study by the American College of Surgeons. Ann Surg 1993; 218:583–592.

125. Kitamura K, Yamaguchi T, Taniguchi H, Hagiwara A, Yamane T, Sawai K, Takahashi T. Clinicopathological characteristics of gastric cancer in the elderly. Br J Cancer 1996; 73:798–802.

126. Bandoh T, Isoyama T, Toyoshima H. Total gastrectomy for gastric cancer in the elderly. Surgery 1991; 109:136–142.

127. Maehara Y, Emi Y, Tomisaki S, Oshiro T, Kakeji Y, Ichiyoshi Y, Sugimachi K. Age-related characteristics of gastric carcinoma in young and elderly patients. Cancer 1996; 77:1174–1180.

128. Bonenkamp JJ, Songun I, Hermans J, Sasako M, Plukker JTM, van Elk P, Obertop H, Gouma DJ, Taat CW, van Lanschot J, Meyer S, de Graaf PW, von Meyenfeldt MF, Tilanus H, van de Velde CJH. Randomised comparison of morbidity after D1 and D2 dissection for gastric cancer in 996 Dutch patients. Lancet 1995; 345:745–748.

129. Viste A, Haugstvedt T, Eide GE, Soreide O, The Norwegian Stomach Cancer Trial Members. Postoperative complications and mortality after surgery for gastric cancer. Ann Surg 1988; 207:7–13.

130. Schwartz RE, Karpeh MS, Brennan MF. Factors predicting hospitalization after operative treatment for gastric carcinoma in patients older than 70 years. J Am Coll Surg 1997; 184:9–15.

131. Tsujitani S, Katano K, Oka A, Ikeguchi M, Maeta M, Kaibara N. Limited operation for gastric cancer in the elderly. Br J Surg 1996; 83:836–839.

132. Pacelli F, Bellantone R, Doglietto GB, Perri V, Genovese V, Tommasini O, Crucitti F. Risk factors in relation to postoperative complications and mortality after total gastrectomy in aged patients. Am Surg 1991; 57:341–345.

133. Habu H, Saito N, Sato Y, Takeshita K, Sunagawa M, Endo M. Quality of postoperative life in gastric cancer patients seventy years of age and over. Int Surg 1988; 73:82–86.

134. Koga S, Oda M, Kaibara N, Hisaki T. Total gastrectomy in the aged with special reference to postoperative convalescence and return to normal life. Dig Surg 1985; 2: 31–35.

135. Urist MM, Karnell LH. Melanoma in Steele GD, Winchester DP, Menck HR, Murphy GP. National Cancer Data Base: Annual Review of Patient Care 1993. Washington, DC: American Cancer Society, 1993, pp 52–66.

136. Liu T, Soong S-J. Epidemiology of malignant melanoma. Surg Clin North Am 1996; 76:1205–1222.

137. Thorn M, Adami H-O, Ringborg U, Bergstrom R, Krusemo U. The association between anatomic site and survival in malignant melanoma. An analysis of 12,353 cases from the Swedish cancer registry. Eur J Cancer Clin Oncol 1989; 25:483–491.

138. Kemeny MM, Busch E, Stewart AK, Menck HH. Superior survival of young women with malignant melanoma. Am J Surg 1998; 175:437–445.

139. Masback A, Westerdahl J, Ingvar C, Olsson H, Jonsson N. Cutaneous malignant melanoma in southern Sweden 1965, 1975, and 1985, Prognostic factors and histologic correlations. Cancer 1997; 79:275–283.

140. Austin PF, Cruse W, Lyman G, Schroer K, Glass F, Reintgen DS. Age as a prognostic factor in the malignant melanoma population. Ann Surg Oncol 1994; 1:487–494.

141. Veronisi U, Cascinelli N, Adamus J, Balch C, Bandiera D, Barchuk A, Bufalino R, Craig P, DeMarsillac J, Durand JC, van Geel AN, Holmstrom H, Hunter JA, Jorgensen OG, Kiss B, Kroon B, Lacour J, Lejune F, Mackie R, Mechl Z, Mitrov G, Morabito A, Nosek H, Panizzon R, Prade M, Santi P, Van Slooten E, Tomin R, Trapeznikov N, Tsanov T, Urist M, Wozniak KD. Thin stage I primary cutaneous malignant melanoma, comparison of excision with margins 1 or 3 cm. N Engl J Med 1988; 318:1159–1162.

142. Veronisi U, Cascinelli N. Narrow excision (1-cm margin), a safe procedure for thin cutaneous melanoma. Arch Surg 1991; 126:438–441.

143. Balch CM, Urist MM, Karakousis CP, Smith TJ, Temple WJ, Drzewiecki K, Jewell WR, Bartolucci AA, Mihm MC, Barnhill R, Wanebo HJ. Efficacy of 2-cm surgical margins for intermediate-thickness melanomas (1 to 4 mm), results of a multi-institutional randomized surgical trial. Ann Surg 1993; 218:262–269.

144. Karakousis CP, Balch CM, Urist MM, Ross MM, Smith TJ, Bartolucci AA. Local recurrence in malignant melanoma: Long-term results of the multiinstitutional randomized surgical trial. Ann Surg Oncol 1996; 3:446–452.

145. Urist MM, Balch CM, Soong S-J, Shaw HM, Milton GW, Maddox WA. The influence of surgical margins and prognostic factors predicting the risk of local recurrence in 3445 patients with primary cutaneous melanoma. Cancer 1985; 55:1398–1402.

146. Slingluff CL, Vollmer RT, Reintgen DS, Seigler HF. Lethal "thin" malignant melanoma, identifying patients at risk. Ann Surg 1988; 208:150–161.

147. Veronisi U, Adamus J, Bandiera C, Brennhovd IO, Caceres E, Casinelli N, Claudio F, Ikonopisov VV, Kirov S, Kulakowski A, Lacour J, Lejune F, Mechl Z, Morabito A, Rode I, Sergeev S, van Slooten E, Szczygiel K, Trapeznikov NN, Wagner RI. Inefficacy of immediate node dissection in stage I melanoma of the limbs. N Engl J Med 1977; 297:627–630.

148. Sim FH, Taylor WF, Ivins JC, Pritchard DJ, Soule EH. A prospective randomized study of the efficacy of routine elective lymphadenectomy in management of malignant melanoma. Cancer 1978; 41:948–956.

149. Balch CM, Soong S-J, Bartolucci AA, Urist MM, Karakousis CP, Smith TJ, Temple WJ, Ross MI, Jewell WR, Mihm MC, Barnhill RL, Wanebo HJ. Efficacy of an elective regional lymph node dissection of 1 to 4 mm thick melanomas for patients 60 years of age and younger. Ann Surg 1996; 224:255–266.

150. Crowley NJ, Seigler HF. The role of elective lymph node dissection in the management of patients with thick cutaneous melanoma. Cancer 1990; 66:2522–2527.

151. Morton DL, Wen D-R, Wong JH, Economou JS, Cagle LA, Storm FK, Foshag LJ, Cochran AJ. Technical details of intraoperative lymphatic mapping for early stage melanoma. Arch Surg 1992; 127:392–399.

152. Krag DN, Meijer SJ, Weaver DL, Loggie BW, Harlow SP, Tanabe KK, Laughlin EH, Alex JC. Minimal-access surgery for staging of malignant melanoma. Arch Surg 1995; 130:654–658.

153. Kirkwood JM, Strwderman MH, Ernstoff MS, Smith TJ, Borden EC, Blum RH. Interferon alfa-2b adjuvant therapy of high-risk resected cutaneous melanoma: The Eastern Cooperative Oncology Group Trial EST 1684. J Clin Oncol 1996; 14:7–17.

154. Magnus K, Phil D. Prognosis in malignant melanoma of the skin, significance of stage of disease, anatomical site, sex, age, and period of diagnosis. Cancer 1977; 40:389–397.

155. Stidham KR, Johnson JL, Seigler HF. Survival superiority of females with melanoma, a multivariate analysis of 6383 patients exploring the significance of gender in prognostic outcome. Arch Surg 1994; 129:316–324.

156. Garbe C, Buttner P, Bertz J, Burg G, d'Hoedt B, Drepper H, Guggenmoos-Holzmann I, Lechner W, Lippold A. Orfanos CE, Peters A, Rassner G, Stadler R, Stroebel W. Primary cutaneous melanoma, prognostic classification of anatomic location. Cancer 1995; 75:2492–2498.

157. Garbe C, Buttner P, Bertz J, Burg G, d'Hoedt B, Drepper H, Guggenmoos-Holzmann I, Lechner W, Lippold A. Orfanos CE, Peters A, Rassner G, Stadler R, Stroebel W. Primary cutaneous melanoma, Identification of prognostic groups and estimation of individual prognosis for 5093 patients. Cancer 1995; 75:2484–2491.

158. Balch CM, Soong S-J, Murad TM, Ingalls AL, Maddox WA. A multifactorial analysis of melanoma, III. Prognostic factors in melanoma patients with lymph node metastases (stage II). Ann Surg 1981; 193:377–388.

159. Callery MP, Strasberg SM, Doherty GM, Soper NJ, Norton JA. Staging laparoscopy with laparoscopic ultrasonography: optimizing resectability in hepatobiliary and pancreatic malignancy. J Am Coll Surg 1997; 185:33–39.

160. Burke EC, Karpeh MS, Conlon KC, Brennan MF. Laparoscopy in the management of gastric adenocarcinoma. Ann Surg 1997; 225:262–267.

161. Flowers JL, Lefor AT, Steers J. Heyman M, Graham SM, Imbembo AL. Laparoscopic splenectomy in patients with hematologic diseases. Ann Surg 1996; 224:19–28.

162. Landis SH, Murray T, Bolden S, Wing PA. Cancer Statistics 1999. CA–A Cancer Journal for Clinicians 1999; 49:8–31.

163. Child CG, III. The liver and portal hypertension. In: Dumphy JE (ed), Major Problems in Clinical Surgery, Vol 1, Philadelphia, WB Saunders, 1964.

9
Radiation Therapy and the Elderly

Arno James Mundt
University of Chicago Hospitals
Chicago, Illinois

I. INTRODUCTION

Radiation therapy (RT) occupies an important position in the treatment of cancer. It was not long after the discovery of x-rays that the potential benefits of radiation in the treatment of patients with cancer began to be realized (1). Currently, RT is used as either definitive therapy or as an adjunct to surgery and/or chemotherapy in the treatment of tumors arising in almost every organ system. In addition, RT offers cancer patients an effective means of palliation when cure is not possible.

It has been estimated that over one half of all cancer patients receive RT sometime during the course of their disease (2). Although many are elderly, surprisingly little information exists regarding the use of RT in these patients. Moreover, most of the available data highlight solely the prognostic significance of age, ignoring other important issues including toxicity.

The focus of this chapter is on RT in the elderly. Particular attention is devoted to the issue of toxicity and methods for its reduction. Special uses of RT and its role in palliation in the elderly patient are reviewed. In addition, RT in the treatment of benign conditions arising in the elderly is discussed. A general overview of the biological and physical basis of RT is beyond the scope of this chapter. Interested readers are referred elsewhere (3).

II. BARRIERS TO RT IN THE ELDERLY

Although RT is commonly used in the treatment of many benign and malignant tumors, the elderly have been shown to be less likely to undergo RT in a wide variety of tumors (4–9). The reasons for this difference, however, are not entirely clear. One important reason is that elderly cancer patients are less likely than younger patients to undergo definitive treatment regardless of the extent of their disease (10). In addition, a number of potential barriers to RT have been identified in the elderly. Recognition of these and other factors is important if disparities in treatment and outcome based on age are to be overcome.

A. Toxicity Concerns

Concerns regarding the potential toxicity of RT are a major reason it is less used in the elderly. However, these concerns are often more based on prejudice and anecdote rather than objective data. As will be seen in Sec. III, the preponderance of the available laboratory and clinical data do not support the view that acute and chronic toxicity are more frequent or pronounced in the elderly. Attention should instead be focused on the general health and performance status of the patient. Elderly patients also often have concerns about potential toxicity that may result in their declining therapy. These concerns must be identified and addressed.

B. Myths and Biases About the Elderly and Cancer

Numerous myths and biases about the elderly and cancer held by patients and physicians have been identified as major barriers to RT in the elderly. The elderly often believe that when cancer is diagnosed in their age group, "it's too late" even found early (11). Radiation therapy is also commonly felt to be the treatment of last resort (11). Physicians frequently view the elderly as being less compliant (7). In fact, the elderly are *more* compliant than younger patients (12). Many physicians also feel that the elderly tolerate or do not feel pain in contrast to younger patients (11). Finally, tumors arising in the elderly are often felt to be biologically less aggressive than those arising in younger patients. In fact, tumors arising in the elderly are often more poorly differentiated than those in younger patients (13,14).

C. Social Factors

Several social factors represent potential barriers to RT in the elderly patients. The most important is access to transportation. Goodwin et al. noted that elderly patients who drive or have access to a driver are four times more likely to receive RT (15). Access to transportation is of paramount importance, since most RT courses range from 4 to 5 weeks of daily therapy. Although one third of patients age more than 65 years of age are dependent on others for transportation (16), this figure rises to two thirds in patients older than 85 years old (16). Patients living alone without assistance are also less likely to undergo RT. Unfortunately, 26% of elderly cancer patients live alone, and 38% have either no children or no children in the vicinity (16).

D. Other Factors

Other potential barriers to RT in the elderly include impairments in functional and cognitive status. In a review of newly diagnosed breast, prostatic, and colorectal cancer patients, Goodwin and coworkers reported that poor functional status and poor cognitive status were correlated with a decreased use of RT (15). Certainly, when a patient's cognition is markedly impaired, a prolonged course of definitive RT is not appropriate. However, mild to moderate cognitive impairments are not appropriate contraindications to short-course palliative RT.

III. RADIATION TOXICITY IN THE ELDERLY

Radiation toxicity is traditionally divided into acute and chronic reactions. Acute reactions, for example, skin desquamation, mucositis, and diarrhea, occur during or immediately following treatment and are presumed to be due to the interruption of repopulation of rapidly proliferating tissues. Chronic reactions, for example, fibrosis, fistulae, and necrosis, occur months to years later and result, in part, from damage to slowly proliferating tissues. Other factors, including vascular alterations, may also play a role. Laboratory and clinical data evaluating the impact of aging on acute and chronic tissue reactions are summarized below. Laboratory data are divided into two types (total body and specific organ data) based on the extent of radiation exposure. The clinical data are categorized by organ system by the specific tumors included in the reports.

A. Laboratory Data

1. Total Body Irradiation Data

A consistent finding in the total body irradiation (TBI) experiments is that a direct correlation exists between aging and radiosensivity in mature laboratory animals. Crosfill et al. exposed mice (aged 1 day to 90 weeks) to various TBI doses. The dose resulting in 50% mortality (LD_{50}) was found to rise steeply with age in the very young mice, peak at approximately 40 weeks, and then rapidly decrease (17). Hursh and Casarett also noted a higher mortality rate in 16-month-old versus 6-month-old rats exposed to identical TBI doses (18). Similar results have been reported by others (19).

2. Specific Tissue Data

Unlike the TBI series, most series evaluating specific tissues have not found a correlation between increased radiosensitivity and age. Unfortunately, all the available data are based on the response of *rapidly proliferating* tissues, thereby limiting conclusions to only acute radiation reactions.

Hopewell and Young compared the radiosensivity of pig skin in 12- to 14-, 35-, and 52-week-old animals exposed to various radiation doses (18.0–23.4 Gy). Although higher doses were associated with increased rates of necrosis, no difference was seen in the severity of the reactions based on age (20). Hamlet and Hopewell evaluated the response of skin in rats and noted that advanced age was associated with a statistically significant *lower* radiosensitivity. Necrosis was seen in 55% of the 14-week-old versus 15.5% of the 52-week-old animals following exposure to 30 Gy. Moreover, although the older animals all had complete healing by day 26, healing was more prolonged in the younger animals (21). Other investigators have noted similar findings (22). In contrast, Sargent and Burns noted a higher radiosensitivity in the skin of older rats (23).

Other investigators have similarly noted no correlation between aging and radiosensitivity in other rapidly proliferating tissues. Landuyt et al. found a nonsignificant higher radiosensitivity in the lip mucosa of 18-month-old compared to 2-month-old mice. However, no difference was seen in the rate of repopulation based on age (24). Hamilton et al. found no differences in the sensitivity of gastrointestinal mucosa in 4-month-old and 24-month-old mice. Of note, however, regenerating crypt colonies in the older mice were smaller suggesting a lower rate of repopulation (25). Similar results have been reported by others (26).

B. Clinical Data

1. Central Nervous System Tumors

No data are available directly comparing the incidence and severity of acute sequelae in adult central nervous system (CNS) tumor patients undergoing RT as a function of age. Series consisting of primarily elderly patients have reported few acute sequelae suggesting that advanced age is not associated with untoward acute sequelae in patients undergoing cranial irradiation (27,28). In fact, elderly patients have been shown to tolerate even aggressive chemoradiotherapic regimens (29). Fatigue is common in all patients undergoing cranial irradiation, but it may be particularly difficult in the elderly with baseline functional deficits.

Controversy exists whether the elderly are at higher risk for chronic sequelae including radiation necrosis, optic nerve and chiasmal injuries, neuropsychological deficits, and pituitary-hypothalamic dysfunction. Although series of primarily elderly patients have noted low rates of chronic sequelae (27,28), hypertension, which is more common in the elderly, may increase the risk of radionecrosis (30). Elderly patients may also be at higher risk for chronic neuropsychological sequelae. Maire et al. noted a decline in full-scale intelligence quotients (IQ) in most patients undergoing cranial irradiation. Although improvements were seen at subsequent testing, these improvements were limited to patients below the age of 50 years (31).

2. Head and Neck Cancer

The impact of aging on the risk of radiation sequelae in head and neck cancer (HNC) patients has been the subject of several reports. Chin et al. analyzed acute toxicity in 104 oropharyngeal cancer patients treated with either definitive or adjuvant RT. No correlation was found between the frequency or severity of acute sequelae and advanced age. Moreover, no differences were seen in the number of treatment interruptions nor ability to complete treatment. Although longer hospital stays were noted in older patients, this difference was felt to be due to social factors not toxicity (32). Huegnin et al. similarly noted no differences in the frequency or severity of acute toxicity between elderly (aged ≥75 years) and nonelderly HNC patients treated in a prospective study at the University Hospital in Zurich (33). Pignon and coworkers recently reported the tolerance of HNC patients treated on five consecutive European Organization for Research and Treatment of Cancer (EORTC) trials. All patients received definitive RT with or without concomitant cisplatin. Four hundred and eight patients were older than 65 years (185 aged ≥75 years). Mucositis was noted in 98.5% of patients and was not more pronounced in the patients aged ≥65 years. However, subjective assessment of pain and ability to eat was more pronounced in the older patients. Patients older than 70 years were more likely to report an inability to eat (31.2 vs 7.7%) (P <.001) than patients less than 50 years old. A nonsignificant trend to more weight loss >10% of baseline weight was noted in patients age more than 60 years old (34).

Less data are available regarding the chronic RT toxicity in elderly HNC patients. Unlike acute toxicity, most chronic sequelae, including dental problems, soft-tissue necrosis, and cartilage and bone necrosis, are rare. The notable exception, however, is xerostomia. In the only study evaluating the risk of late toxicity based on age, Pignon et al. noted no difference in the frequency of severity of late sequelae in HNC patients less than 65 years old versus those older than 65 years (34).

3. Lung Cancer

Although RT is commonly used in the treatment of elderly lung cancer (LC) patients, limited data are available evaluating the impact of age on radiation toxicity. In a prospective analysis of 26 elderly LC patients (median age 69.8 years), Larson and coworkers noted that definitive RT was well tolerated apart from fatigue and skin irritation. Patients were able to complete therapy without major disruptions in functional status. An improved functional status was noted at 3 months compared to prior to therapy (35).

Potential chronic sequelae following thoracic RT include pneumonitis, esophageal stricture, carditis, and myelitis. Controversy exists whether elderly LC patients are at higher risk for chronic sequelae. Koga and coworkers compared the risk and severity of radiation pneumonitis in a small study of 33 patients aged less than 70 years old versus 29 patients age more than 70 years old. Severe pneumonitis was more common in the elderly patients regardless of treatment volume (36). In contrast, Segawa et al. evaluated risk factors for pneumonitis in 89 patients (25 aged ≥70 years) undergoing RT with and without chemotherapy. No difference was seen in the incidence and severity of pneumonitis based on age between patients less than 70 versus more than 70 years old (37).

4. Breast Cancer

Two series have evaluated the acute tolerance of RT in elderly breast cancer (BC) patients. Wyckoff et al. compared the acute toxicity in 100 BC patients younger than age 65 years with 63 patients older than age 65 years. No differences were noted in cutaneous or hematological toxicity nor in the frequency of treatment breaks secondary to acute reactions (38). Turesson and coworkers evaluated the acute toxicity in 402 BC patients undergoing breast irradiation. Although age was correlated with worse acute skin toxicity on univariate analysis, age did not remain statistically significant on multivariate analysis after controlling for confounding patient and treatment factors (39).

The risk of late toxicity following breast irradiation (breast and arm edema, fibrosis, mastitis, pneumonitis, brachial plexopathy, rib fracture, and poor cosmesis) is low. Conflicting data exist regarding the impact of age on the risk of late sequelae following breast irradiation. Turesson et al. noted no correlation-significant late skin reactions and advanced age (39). Other investigators have noted no differences in the development of telangiectasias and breast fibrosis between elderly and nonelderly patients (40). Of note, Olsen and coworkers noted a *lower* incidence of brachial plexopathy in elderly patients undergoing breast or chest wall irradiation (41). In contrast, one series noted a higher incidence of impaired shoulder range of motion in elderly patients (42). Advanced age is correlated with arm edema in some (43) but not in all studies (44,45). In addition, although several series have found similar cosmetic outcomes between elderly and nonelderly (46,47) patients, others have reported poorer cosmesis in older patients (48,49).

5. Gastrointestinal Tumors

The relationship between aging and acute radiation toxicity in gastrointestinal (GI) tumor patients has been studied in rectal and anal cancer patients. Leo and coworkers analyzed the tolerance of postoperative RT in 38 patients (18 aged more than 65 years) with low rectal tumors. No differences were seen in the frequency or severity of RT sequelae between the two groups (50). De Gara et al. compared the acute toxicity in 38 anal cancer patients age less than 65 years old versus 38 patients more than 65 years old. Although no significant differences were seen in terms of RT doses or fields between the two groups, older patients had a significantly lower percentage of acute toxicity (48 vs 74%) ($P = .03$) than the younger patients. However, older patients were treated with less aggressive chemotherapy (51).

Chronic radiation sequelae in GI tumor patients differ by site. Esophageal patients may develop esophageal stenosis and pneumonitis. The most serious sequela in intrabdominal and pelvic tumors is small bowel injury. Rectal and anal cancer patients may experience chronic proctitis. Overall, the frequency of severe late sequelae is low. Moreover, the available data suggests that age per se does not increase the risk of their development. Leo et al. compared the frequency and severity of late RT sequelae in rectal cancer patients treated with coloanal anastomosis and adjuvant RT. Only two significant late sequelae (one anastomotic stenosis, one rectal perforation) occurred, both in patients under age 65 years. No difference was seen in the long-term functional results, including the frequency of bowel movements (50). Mak and coworkers reported no correlation between age and late sequelae in rectal and rectosigmoid carcinoma patients undergoing surgery and adjuvant RT (52). Two Japanese centers similarly noted no difference in the risk of significant late toxicity in esophageal cancer patients treated with RT alone. Hishikawa et al. found no difference in the frequency of late sequelae in patients treated with external beam and high-dose rate intraluminal boosts. Mucosal ulceration occurred in 58, 49, and 47% of patients aged less than 69, 70–79, and more than 80 years, respectively. Fistulous sequelae occurred in 2, 8, and 6%, respectively (53). In a smaller series of esophageal cancer patients not receiving intraluminal therapy, Yamakawa et al. reported no difference in chronic toxicity between patients more than 80 versus less than 80 years old (54).

6. Genitourinary Tumors

Several studies have evaluated the toxicity of RT in elderly prostate and bladder cancer patients. Liu and coworkers analyzed acute urinary and intestinal toxicity in 156 prostate cancer patients (86 aged >70 years) treated with RT. No differences were seen in the frequency of intestinal and urinary acute toxicity in patients above and below age 70 years except for a higher rate of mild urinary toxicity in the older group. Of note, older patients reached maximal intestinal and urinary toxicity sooner than younger patients (55). Vijaykumar and coworkers at the University of Chicago similarly found no correlation between advanced age and acute intestinal and urinary sequelae in prostate cancer patients undergoing RT (56). Definitive RT is also well tolerated acutely in elderly bladder cancer patients (57–60).

Potential chronic radiation sequelae in prostate cancer patients includes proctitis, cystitis, and impotency. Bladder cancer patients may develop a stenotic, contracted bladder or fistulae. Sandler et al. evaluated the late sequelae in 721 primarily elderly (median age 71.5 years) prostatic cancer patients treated with definitive RT. Advanced age was not found to be a significant factor on either univariate or multivariate analysis (61). Of note, Hanlon et al. noted a *lower* rate of serious intestinal sequelae in patients older than age 60 years (4 vs 13%) compared to younger patients (62). Serious late sequelae are infrequent in elderly bladder cancer patients even following combined chemoradiotherapy. Shipley et al. reported the outcome of 70 muscle invasive bladder cancer patients ranging from age 46 to 87 years (mean age

70 years) treated with concomitant cisplatin and RT. Four patients (5%) developed a small bowel obstruction. In addition, the incidence of significant hematuria, hip necrosis, and soft-tissue injury were 5, 1, and 6%, respectively (63). Low rates of long-term sequelae were reported by other investigators using concomitant chemoradiotherapy in elderly patient populations (57–60).

7. Reticuloendothelial Malignancies

Two series have addressed the impact of age on the acute RT toxicity in Hodgkin's disease (HD) patients. Zietman et al. reviewed the treatment of 29 stage I–II HD patients age 60 years old or older undergoing RT alone. Although six (21%) required a treatment break secondary to acute toxicity, this was similar to that seen in younger patients (64). Austin-Seymour and coworkers performed a similar analysis on 52 stage I–IV HD patients aged 60–75 years. Stage I–IIA patients received subtotal nodal RT, whereas more advanced patients underwent either total lymphatic irradiation or chemotherapy with or without involved field RT. Acute sequelae were common with 21 patients (40%) experiencing weight loss of more than 10% of baseline body weight or cytopenia requiring treatment breaks (65). No comparative studies have been performed in non–Hodgkin's lymphoma (NHL) patients undergoing RT. However, the available data suggests that RT is well tolerated alone or with chemotherapy in elderly NHL patients (66). Adult patients with acute and chronic leukemia rarely receive RT. One important exception is a patient undergoing high-dose chemotherapy (HDCT) and stem cell rescue. These patients may receive TBI. Such an approach is also occasionally used in relapsed and refractory HD and NHL. Acute sequelae include nausea, emesis, and diarrhea. In part due to the fact that few elderly patients undergo HDCT, no data are available comparing the acute toxicity of TBI as a function of age.

Possible chronic RT sequelae following limited field RT in HD and NHL include pneumonitis, hypothyroidism, carditis, xerostomia, Lhermitte's syndrome, and second malignancies. In the series of Austin-Seymour et al., two patients (4%) developed pneumonitis, one (2%) duodenitis, and one (2%) small bowel obstruction. Second malignancies occurred in six patients (11%) (one NHL, one leukemia, one lung cancer, one melanoma, one unknown primary) (65). Zietman et al. reported small bowel obstruction in one patient (3%) and second malignancy in five (17%). Of note, three of the five patients with a second malignancy had a tumor within the prior RT field (64). Several investigators have also found that increased age is correlated with a higher rate of chronic toxicity, including myeodysplasic syndrome in patients undergoing TBI prior to HDCT (67,68).

8. Gynecological Malignancies

Several investigators have evaluated radiation gynecological malignancies patients as a function of age. Pignon et al. reported the acute toxicity of RT in elderly cervical cancer (CC) patients and noted a higher rate of acute bladder sequelae in the elderly. However, after adjusting for radiation dose, no differences remained (69). Grant and coworkers noted a higher frequency of acute sequelae in CC patients 75 years old or older with 32% unable to complete therapy. However, most received large daily fraction (>200 cGy), which most likely contributed to the high sequelae rate (70). Sablanska et al. reported a higher rate of treatment cessation secondary to acute sequelae in elderly CC patients (41 vs 19%) compared to younger patients. However, no mention was made regarding technique, including daily fraction size, beam energies, and total dose (71). In contrast, Mitsuhashi et al. compared the acute sequelae in 126 CC patients aged 70 years or older versus 160 aged less than 70 years treated with conventional RT techniques. No differences were seen in the frequency of acute intestinal and bladder sequelae (72).

Uterine, cervical, and vaginal cancer patients often receive intracavitary or interstitial brachytherapy in addition to pelvic RT. Although numerous potential acute sequelae exist ranging from uterine perforation to pulmonary emboli, the likelihood of such sequelae is low. It is controversial whether elderly patients are at a higher risk for acute problems during brachytherapy. In a recent review at the University of Chicago, Wollschlaeger et al. noted no difference in the type, frequency, of severity of in-hospital problems in 170 brachytherapic treatments. No differences were seen in the incidence or severity of infectious, gastrointestinal, pulmonary, cardiac, or thromboembolic events between CC patients younger than 65 years of age versus older than 65 years of age. The most factors most significantly correlated with significant sequelae were diabetes and a prior history of abdominal or pelvic surgery (73). Similarly, Chao and coworkers evaluated 150 brachytherapic insertions in 96 medically inoperable stage I endometrial cancer patients (40 age more than 75 years old) and noted only four (3%) significant sequelae, although most had multiple and often significant comorbidities (74). In contrast, Lanciano et al. analyzed 95 brachytherapic treatments and found that an age of more than 50 years was the most significant factor correlated with acute sequelae. In fact, a patient age of more than 50 years remained the only significant factor on multivariate analysis (75).

Potential sequelae in gynecologic patients undergoing RT include proctitis, rectal ulceration, stricture, fistulae, small bowel obstruction, cystitis, vaginal stenosis and necrosis, and leg edema. Several investigators have failed to note a higher frequency of chronic sequelae in elderly patients treated with whole pelvic RT with and without brachytherapy (69,72) Mitsuhashi et al. noted similar rates of severe rectal (9.5 vs 6%), bladder (0.8 vs 1.8%), and small bowel (0 vs 0.6%) in CC patients aged 70 years and older and those aged less than 70 years. Rates of leg edema and bone necrosis were also similar in the two groups (72). Perez and coworkers noted no difference in the incidence of late sequelae in elderly CC patients. However, patients aged more than 65 years were routinely treated with 5–10% lower doses (76). In contrast, Kennedy et al. treated 63 patients more than 75 years old with various gynecological malignancies with definitive or adjuvant RT and noted late complications in 12 (19%) of which 4 (6%) were life threatening. Three patients (5%) developed fistulae (77). However, no details of treatment were given. It thus remains unclear whether poor technique contributed to these sequelae. We recently performed an analysis of rectal sequelae in our CC patients who underwent RT alone. The most significant factors associated with late rectal injury were diabetes mellitus and pelvic doses >50 Gy. An age of more than 65 years was not found to be a significant factor on either univariate or multivariate analysis (78). In contrast, Corn and coworkers, at the Fox Chase Cancer Center in Philadelphia, noted that an age of more than 65 years was significantly correlated on both univariate and multivariate analysis with severe late sequelae in 235 endometrial cancer patients treated with postoperative RT (79).

9. Skin Cancer

Although RT is commonly used in elderly patients with skin cancer, no data exist comparing the toxicity of RT in elderly and nonelderly patients. However, series of predominantly elderly patients report low rates of untoward toxicity. Lovett et al. reviewed the outcome of 339 primarily elderly (majority in their 70s and 80s) skin cancer patients treated with RT at the Mallinckrodt Institute, Washington University, St. Louis, Missouri. Treatment was well tolerated acutely. Moreover, severe late sequelae were seen in only 5.5% of patients. Cosmesis was excellent or good in 92% (80).

10. Soft-Tissue and Bone Tumors

No comparative studies have been published comparing the RT toxicity in elderly and nonelderly patients with soft-tissue and bone tumors. In our two recent series of soft-tissue sarcoma patients undergoing surgery and RT, no correlation was seen between advanced age and radiation toxicity (81,82).

IV. STRATEGIES FOR REDUCING RADIATION TOXICITY IN THE ELDERLY

The radiation oncologist treating the elderly must strive not only to maximize the potential for cure but also minimize the potential for serious treatment sequelae. Unfortunately, these goals may be in conflict. Various strategies available for reducing the potential for acute and chronic RT sequelae in the elderly are outlined below.

A. Radiation Technique

Attention to optimal technique is the most important means of reducing toxicity in the elderly cancer patient. Optimal technique begins with proper positioning and immobilization at simulation. Although most patients are treated in the supine position, several special positions are often useful. The "chin tuck" position is used in pituitary tumors and sphenoid wing meningiomas allowing for the addition of a vertex field that decreases the dose delivered to the temporal lobes (83). The neck is hyperflexed and positioning is assured with a thermoplastic caste. Vaginal and vulvar patients are placed in a "frog leg" position that reduced skin folds in the groin and thus the severity of desquamation. Careful positioning in extremity tumors helps avoid irradiation of the entire limb circumference reducing the risk of edema (84). Although positioning may be difficult in the elderly, particularly in those with impaired joint range of motion, optimal positioning is usually achieved with patience and experience.

Other technical factors impacting on toxicity include field number, beam energy, radiation type, fraction size, and total dose. Multiple fields are almost always preferable to one or two, particularly in the abdomen and pelvis. Several centers now routinely use six field techniques in the treatment of prostatic cancer in an effort to reduce bowel and bladder toxicity (85). High-energy photon beams should be used in the treatment of all deep-seated tumors to reduce hot spots within superficial structures. In selective tumors, electrons or low-energy photons are preferable owing to the sparing of underlying or surrounding critical structures (86). Particle beams (neutrons, protons) are useful in certain sites; for example, the base of skull (87). Conventional daily fractions (1.8–2.0 Gy) are recommended, particularly when surrounding critical structures are included. Large daily fractions are associated with an increased risk of late effects and should be avoided in most definitively treated patients. Modifications of daily and total doses may be necessary in the setting of concomitant chemotherapy and in patients with connective-tissue diseases.

B. New Technology

Various new approaches may help reduce the risk of toxicity in the elderly. Computed tomography (CT)–based treatment planning allows better localization of tumor and areas at risk. Recently, three-dimensional conformal RT (3DCRT) is becoming increasingly popular and allows the high-dose region to be *conformed* to the target volume with increased sparing of neighboring critical structures. One promising use of 3DCRT is the exclusion of the contralateral parotid gland in head and neck cancer patients, thereby reducing the risk of xerostomia (88,89). In addition, the benefits of 3DCRT in prostatic cancer have also been reported (90). The technique is further enhanced by intensity modulation and inverse treatment planning (91).

Another innovative technique that may help reduce toxicity is functional treatment planning. In CNS patients, functional magnetic resonance imaging (fMRI) allows mapping of critical cortical regions aiding in the selection of treatment plans (92). A 3D lung perfusion map can be generated by a means of single-photon emission CT (SPECT). Treatment plans minimizing the irradiation area of maximum perfusion are thus possible reducing the risk of late sequelae (93).

C. Reduction of Treatment Volume

Volume of treatment is a major determinant of late RT toxicity. Treatment volumes can be reduced with the aid of CT-based treatment planning. In addition, many *traditional* volumes can be reduced. For example, early-stage breast cancer patients often receive prophylactic internal mammary nodal irradiation in addition to breast, axillary, and supraclavular nodal irradiation. Many centers now routinely omit internal mammary nodal treatment, thereby greatly reducing the volume of treatment, including treatment of the heart. Additional examples include omission of bilateral neck irradiation in *selective* head and neck cancers (94) and subdiaphragmatic irradiation in favorable early-stage Hodgkin's disease (95). More controversial examples include omission of pelvic irradiation in early-stage testicular tumors (96) and mediastinal irradiation in medically inoperable stage I lung cancer (97). The ultimate means of reducing the volume of treatment is by eliminating treatment altogether. Although traditionally given, adjuvant RT may not be necessary in *selective* unknown head and neck primaries (98), intraductal carcinoma of the breast (99), and subcutaneous soft-tissue sarcoma (100).

D. Drug Therapy

Acute radiation reactions experienced by elderly patients can be ameliorated by a variety of drugs. Head and neck patients with odonyphagia and mucositis benefit from viscous xylocaine (Lidocaine) either alone or with Mylanta and diphenhydramine hydrochloride (Benadryl). Oral candidiasis may exacerbate these symptoms and should be treated promptly with antifungal medications. Lung cancer patients with early signs of pneumonitis benefit from bronchodilators, expectorants, and occasionally oxygen. Corticosteroids are infrequently necessary. When administered, corticosteroids should be tapered slowly to prevent reactivation of symptoms. Corticosteroids are also occasionally needed following cranial RT. However, their use in the elderly needs to be weighed against potential side effects, including alterations in mood, insomnia, and exacerbation of underlying diabetes. Nausea and emesis respond to Prochloperazine (Compazine) and Zofran odansetron (Zofran). Dyspepsia and gastritis are treated with antacids and H_2 blockers. Diarrhea and cramping respond to diphenoxylate hydrochloride with atropine sulfate (Lomotil) or loperamide (Imodium). Steroid suppositories with hydrocortisone (Proctofoam) are helpful in treating proctitis. Antispasmodics such as phenzopyridine hydrochloride (Pyridium) are helpful in patients with dysuria and cystitis.

An alternative approach is the *prophylactic* drug therapy. Two promising agents are pilocarpine and sulcralfate. Pilocarpine prior to and during head and neck irradiation may reduce the incidence of xerostomia (101). Sulcralfate may decrease the severity of esophagitis due to thoracic irradiation (102).

E. Physical Therapy

Physical interventions are another strategy used to reduce chronic toxicity in elderly patients. Vaginal dilators are recommended in cervical and endometrial cancer patients to decrease vaginal stenosis, particularly in patients who are not sexually active. Range of motion exercises are used in breast cancer patients and those with extremity tumors. Although commonly prescribed, no objective data are available evaluating the efficacy of these approaches.

F. Treatment Protraction and Dose Reduction

In the past, treatment protraction, for example, split-course therapy, and reduced total doses were routinely used as a means of reducing acute and chronic toxicity in elderly patients. It is now known, however, that such approaches may adversely impact on outcome. Treatment protraction has been correlated with poorer tumor control and survival in a number of tumor sites, including esophageal (103) and cervical cancer (104). Acute reactions should instead be managed medically. Nonetheless, treatment breaks are inevitable in certain disease sites; for example, vulvar cancer. Dose reductions due to age alone is a practice that should no longer be tolerated and simply results in lower tumor control and survival.

V.   SPECIAL USES OF RT IN THE ELDERLY

A. Radiosurgery

Radiosurgery (RS) is a specialized technique that involves the use of large, single doses of radiation focused on a small intracranial volume with high precision. Initially proposed by Leksell in the 1950s (105), RS has only become popular and widely available in recent years. Treatment is administered with either a dedicated cobalt 60 unit ("gamma knife") or via a modified linear accelerator. Multiple noncoplanar arcs are used to conform the high-dose region to the tumor volume. Immobilization is assured with the aid of surgical pins in the skull. Several centers are now exploring the use of relocatable frames that do not require placement of pins. An example RS treatment plan is shown in Fig. 1.

Radiosurgery provides the elderly patient with a variety of benign and malignant CNS tumors an effective alternative to surgery. Promising results with minimal toxicity have been reported in many primary CNS tumors arising in the elderly, including astrocytomas (106) and acoustic neuromas (107). Radiosurgery has also been used to treat pituitary tumors (108) and meningiomas (109). In addition, RS is a highly efficacious treatment of arteriovenous malformations (AVMs). Published

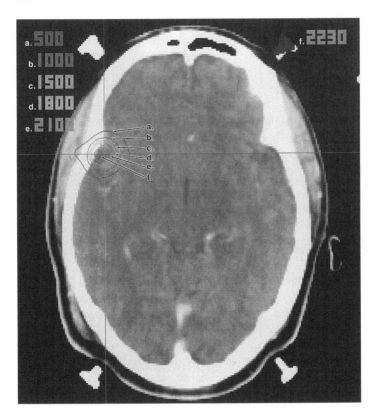

Figure 1   An axial computed tomographic slice of a patient with a solitary brain metastasis from a lung primary undergoing stereotactic radiosurgery. Isodose lines have been superimposed on the scan demonstrating rapid falloff of the dose in the surrounding normal brain: a) 500 cGy, b) 1000 cGy, c) 1500 cGy, d) 1800 cGy, e) 2100 cGy, and f) 2230 cGy.

series report complete obliteration rates ranging from 75 to 90% (110–112). Many centers have recently adopted RS as a treatment of CNS metastases. Although the traditional approach to a patient with an isolated CNS metastasis has been surgery and whole brain irradiation (113), comparable results have been reported with RS, questioning the need for surgery (114,115).

B.   Interstitial Prostate Brachytherapy

Interstitial prostate brachytherapy (IPB) involves the treatment of localized prostatic cancer by the placement of radioactive sources (seeds) within the prostate gland.

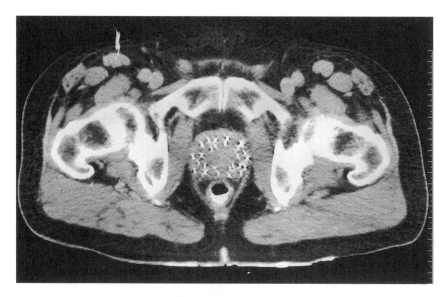

Figure 2 Axial computed tomographic scan of a patient with early stage prostate cancer treated with a permanent implant.

The procedure is performed with either temporary or permanent sources. Fig. 2 illustrates a CT scan of a patient with permanent iodine 125 seeds in place.

In the elderly early-stage prostatic cancer patient, IBP is an appealing approach, because it represents an effective alternative to *both* radical surgery and protracted external beam RT. Promising results in *selective* early-stage patients have been reported, particularly those with low initial prostate-specific antigen (PSA) levels (116,117). Acute and chronic sequelae have been acceptable in these predominantly elderly patients (118). In a review of 321 patients (median age 70 years), Khan et al. noted minor sequelae in 15.9% of patients. However, only 1% required hospitalization or minor surgery (119). Further follow-up is needed before IBP can be considered to be the standard approach in these patients.

C. Endocavitary RT in Rectal Cancer

Endocavitary (contact) therapy is the use of low-energy photon irradiation in patients with early-stage rectal cancer delivered at short distances via a specialized endoscopic applicator. The low-energy beam results in high superficial doses with sparing of underlying tissues. Treatment is delivered on an outpatient basis and requires only local anesthesia. Patients are treated once every 1.5–2.0 weeks for four to five sessions.

Endocavitary therapy is an excellent approach in elderly rectal cancer patients who are poor surgical candidates. Ideal tumors are exophytic, low grade, ≤5 cm in size, and <12 cm from the anal verge. Gerard et al. reported the outcome of 101 early-stage rectal tumors treated with endocavitary RT. Local control in the T1 and T2 tumors were 93 and 60%, respectively. Treatment was well tolerated in these predominantly elderly patients, with only 15% requiring local anesthesia secondary to pain on sphincter dilation. Although mucosal ulceration was noted in approximately one third of patients, none was symptomatic (120). Others have reported similarly favorable results (121). An equivalent alternative approach in these patients is local excision combined with external beam RT. Minsky and coworkers have reported excellent long-term results with this approach (122).

D. Prophylactic Lymph Node RT

Prophylactic lymph node RT (PLNRT) is a means of sterilizing microscopic disease involvement in clinically negative lymph nodes. Moderate doses (45–50 Gy) are delivered over 5–6 weeks to regions at risk. It is an appealing alternative to prophylactic lymph node dissection (PLND) in elderly patients, particularly poor surgical candidates. In early-stage breast cancer, PLNRT results in excellent axillary control with a low risk of chronic arm edema (123). Although the pathological status of the axilla remains unknown, in many patients, the only appropriate adjuvant therapy is tamoxifen. In head and neck cancer, PLNRT is capable of equivalent control rates as PLND (124). Interestingly enough, controversy exists regarding the efficacy of PLNRT in early-stage vulvar cancer. In an influential Gynecology Oncology Group (GOG) study, patients were randomized to either PLND or PLNRT following surgical resection of the primary lesion. Nodal recurrence rates were significantly higher in the PLNRT group (18 vs 0%) (125). However, the RT technique was suboptimal with marked underdosing of the regional lymph nodes. Numerous other studies using superior RT techniques have confirmed the efficacy and low toxicity of PLNRT in these patients (126,127). In all elderly vulvar cancer patients, PLNRT should be considered in place of PLND, particularly those at high risk for poor healing and other long-term sequelae.

E. Reduction or Elimination of Chemotherapy

An interesting role for RT in the elderly is to reduce the dose intensity of chemotherapy. This approach is routinely used in early-stage, intermediate-grade non–Hodgkin's lymphoma (NHL). These patients traditionally received four to six cycles of cyclophosphamide (Cytoxan), hydroxydaunomycin (doxorubicin, Adriamycin), Oncovin (vincristine), and prednisone (CHOP). However, Connors et al. reported a 5-year recurrence free survival of 85% with only three cycles of CHOP and involved field RT (66). The merit of this approach was confirmed in a recent prospective randomized trial (128). Localized RT combined with systemic chemotherapy may potentially allow chemotherapic dose reductions in other disease sites.

A more controversial approach is the use of RT in place of chemotherapy. This is an appealing approach in elderly patients with early-stage "high-risk" ovarian cancer. These patients typically receive four to six cycles of adjuvant chemotherapy. However, RT, in the form of the radiocolloid phosphorus 32 (^{32}P), is associated with equivalent long-term survival (129,130). Moreover, ^{32}P is a one-time treatment with less toxicity. A recent randomized European trial suggested an improved recurrence-free survival with cisplatin. However, approximately one fourth of the radiocolloid group did not receive ^{32}P, questioning the results of this trial (131).

F. High-Dose Rate Brachytherapy

Brachytherapy (intracavitary and interstitial) is traditionally administered with low-dose rate (LDR) techniques. Treatment times range from 1 to 4 days with dose rates of 40–80 cGy/h. An alternative approach that is becoming increasingly popular is high-dose rate (HDR) brachytherapy. High-activity iridium 192 (^{192}Ir) sources are used with dose rates exceeding 200 cGy/min. High-dose rate brachytherapy is currently used in tumors of the head and neck cancer, cervix, uterus, and prostate.

High-dose rate brachytherapy is an excellent approach in elderly patients, particularly those with multiple medical problems. Unlike LDR brachytherapy, HDR brachytherapy is an outpatient procedure requiring only minimal anesthesia. Moreover, prolonged bedrest is not necessary. Although preliminary data suggest that HDR brachytherapy is associated with equivalent outcomes (132,133), considerable controversy exists regarding the potential for late toxicity (134,135). Additional follow-up and randomized studies are clearly needed to resolve this debate.

G. Intraoral Cone Therapy

Definitive RT in certain head and neck cancers (oral tongue, floor of mouth) requires both external beam and interstitial brachytherapy. However, interstitial brachytherapy is not feasible in all elderly patients. An alternative approach is intraoral cone therapy (IOCT). Low-energy photons (250 kV) are delivered via a specialized applicator. Daily fractions of 275–300 cGy are used to a total dose of 15–24 Gy. High doses of radiation are deposited in the tumor with relative sparing of the underlying structures. Unfortunately, IOCT is not feasible in all elderly head and neck patients. Ideal candidates are edentulous, with exophytic tumors that are encompassable by the treatment cone. Wang and coworkers at the Massachusetts General Hospital have reported excellent control rates with IOCT in patients with oral cavity and oropharyngeal tumors suggesting that IOCT is a reasonable alternative to interstitial brachytherapy in these patients (136).

H. Benign Conditions

In addition to its use in malignant disease, RT is also used in the treatment of a number of benign tumors and conditions arising in the elderly.

One important use of RT in the elderly patient without cancer is as prophylaxis against heterotopic ossification (HO) following joint arthroplasty. Approximately

20–30% of arthroplasty patients develop HO, particularly those with severe osteoarthritis, ankylosing spondylitis, and myositis ossificans (137). Several investigators have reported low rates of HO (<5%) without significant treatment sequelae following adjuvant RT (138,139).

Radiation therapy is also capable of inhibiting vessel restenosis following percutaneous transluminal angioplasty in patients with atherosclerotic vascular disease. Restenosis occurs in approximately 30–40% of coronary vessels following coronary angioplasty, typically with 6 months (140). Promising results have been published with endovascular RT following angioplasty (141,142). In a randomized trial, Tierstein et al. reported a statistically lower rate of restenosis in patients receiving RT (17 vs 50%) (*P* = .01) compared to patients treated with coronary stenting and angioplasty alone (143). Numerous centers are now exploring endovascular and external RT in patients at high risk of restenosis following angioplasty of the coronary and peripheral vessels.

Promising results have been reported in other benign conditions arising in the elderly following RT, including macular degeneration (144), pterygium (145), Graves' opthalmoplegia (146), bursitis (147), and Peyronie's disease (148).

I. Palliative RT

Cure is not possible in all elderly cancer patients. In these patients, palliation of symptoms in an effort to improve the quality of life is of paramount importance. Of all the major cancer treatment modalities, RT is the most important means of providing rapid and durable palliation. The role of RT in the palliative treatment of elderly patients with metastatic or locally advanced disease is outlined below.

1. Bone Metastases

Symptomatic bone metastases occur in a wide variety of malignancies arising in the elderly, including breast and prostatic cancer. Treatment is typically administered with limited fields encompassing the symptomatic site(s). Radiation therapy is the single most effective means of treatment in these patients, with pain relief being achieved in approximately 70% of patients (149). Short-course regimens with high daily fractions are typically used (30 Gy in 10 treatments). Toxicity is typically mild and self-limited regardless of patient age (150). The optimal treatment schedule remains unclear. Tong et al. reviewed two Radiation Therapy Oncology Group (RTOG) randomized trials evaluating various schedules ranging from 15.0 to 40.5 Gy over 3 weeks. No differences were seen in the efficacy between the various regimens. Treatment was well tolerated in these primarily elderly patients (151). Some investigators feel that the protracted regimens (30 Gy in 10 or 40 Gy in 15 fractions) are more effective (152). An alternative strategy is hemibody irradiation (153). However, a more appealing approach in the elderly is the radiocolloid strontium 89 (^{89}Sr). Promising results have been reported with ^{89}Sr alone or in conjunction with external beam RT. Strontium 89 is particularly appealing in the elderly, since it is a one-time treatment with few acute side effects (154).

2. Brain Metastases

Brain metastases occur in a number of malignancies in the elderly. Radiation therapy is the single most effective treatment of these patients. Treatment is typically delivered over 10 days to a total dose of 30 Gy to the whole brain. Few acute sequelae are expected even in the elderly (150). However, as in the treatment of bone metastases, the optimal fractionation schedule in patients with CNS metastases remains unclear. Borgelt et al. reviewed the outcome of various treatment schedules ranging from 20 Gy in 5 fractions to 40 Gy in 20 fractions on two consecutive RTOG trials. No differences were seen in terms of frequency nor duration of response. Overall, 50% of patients had significant improvement in neurological symptoms. Responses in terms of headache, motor dysfunction, cranial nerve palsies, and sensory dysfunction were 82, 74, 75, and 77%, respectively. Complete responses were seen in 52, 32, 40, and 41%, respectively. Of note, the less protracted regimens were noted to result in a more rapid overall response (155).

Controversy exists regarding the optimal treatment of patients with solitary CNS metastases. Elderly patients with locally controlled primary lesions and a good performance status should be offered definitive treatment. As seen above, radiosurgery is quickly becoming the standard approach in these patients. Surgery is nonetheless indicated in patients who may benefit from decompression or in whom the diagnosis is in doubt.

3. Spinal Cord Compression

Metastatic vertebral lesions resulting in impingement or compression of the spinal cord (or cauda equina) are infrequent but devastating events in elderly cancer patients. Symptoms may range from pain or sensory loss alone to profound motor and sensory impairments. Radiation therapy is commonly used in the treatment of these patients. Treatment is initiated emergently with concomitant corticosteroids. Most radiation oncologists treat the involved site with a margin of two normal vertrebral bodies. Controversy exists over whether RT alone is sufficient or should be combined with decompressive laminectomy (156). At the University of Chicago, all elderly patients with a good performance status and without widespread metastatic disease undergo laminectomy prior to RT. In most patients, 30 Gy is given in 10 treatments. Selective highly radiosensitive tumors (leukemia, lymphoma) do not require surgery owing to their rapidity of response. Treatment is well tolerated in most patients regardless of age. Patients with cervical or thoracic spine disease typically note transient odonyphagia. The treatment of lumbosacral spine disease is associated with diarrhea and occasionally nausea and emesis. These sequelae are easily controlled with medication.

4. Other Sites

Other indications for palliative RT in the elderly include symptomatic liver metastases (157), orbital metastases (158), and carcinomatous meningitis (159). Palliative RT is also beneficial in elderly patients with symptomatic locally advanced disease, including lung cancer (160) and ovarian cancer (161). An appealing approach in the elderly is the use of intraluminal brachytherapy. This approach is a highly effective means of palliation in patients with bronchial (162), biliary (163), and esophageal (164) obstruction due to locally advanced or metastatic disease.

VI. CONCLUSIONS

Radiation therapy plays an important role in the treatment of the elderly oncologic patient. Although it is commonly believed that the elderly are at high risk for the development of acute and chronic RT sequelae, the majority of the available laboratory and clinical data do not support this view. In fact, age per se should not be used as a reason to withhold definitive or palliative RT. Treatment decisions should instead be based on the general health and performance status of the patient. Novel RT approaches and techniques are appealing in the elderly, particularly those unfit for extensive surgery and/or chemotherapy. Radiation therapy also offers the elderly patient effective palliation when cure is not possible. Further research is needed to define clearly the role of RT in this important and growing group of patients.

REFERENCES

1. Freund L. Ein mit roentgen-strahlen behandelter fall von naevus pigmentosus piliferus. Wien Med Wochensch 1897; 47:428–433.
2. Tobias JS. Clinical practice of radiotherapy. Lancet 1992; 339:159–163.
3. Weichselbaum RR, Hallahan D, Chen G. Biological and physical basis to radiation oncology. In: J Holland, E Frei, R Bast, D Kufe, D Morton, RR Weichselbaum, eds. Cancer Medicine. Malvern, PA: Lea & Febriger, 1993; pp 539–566.
4. Coburn MC, Pricolo VE, Soderberg CH. Factors affecting prognosis and management of carcinoma of the colon and rectum in patients more than eighty years of age. J Am Coll Surg 1994; 179:65–69.
5. Newschaffer CJ, Penberthy L, Desch CE, Retchin SM, Whittemore M. The effect of age and comorbidity in the treatment of elderly women with non-metastatic breast cancer. Arch Intern Med 1996; 156:85–90.
6. Newcomb P, Carbone PP. Cancer treatment and age: patients perspectives. J Natl Cancer Inst 1993; 85:1580–1584.
7. McKenna RJ. Clinical aspects of cancer in the elderly: treatment decisions, treatment choices and follow-up. Cancer 1994; 74:2107–2117.
8. Mor V, Masterson-Allen S, Goldberg RJ, Cummings FJ, Glicksman AS, Fretwell MD.

Relationship between age at diagnosis and treatments received by cancer patients. J Am Geriatr Soc 1985; 33:585–589.

9. Kennedy BJ, Loeb V, Peterson V, Donegan W, Natarajan N, Mettlin C. Survival in Hodgkin's disease by stage and age. Med Pediatr Oncol 1992; 20:100–104.

10. Goodwin JS, Samet JM. Factors affecting the diagnosis and treatment of older patients with cancer. In: L Balducci, GH Lyman, WB Ershler, eds. Geriatric Oncology. Philadelphia: Lippincott, 1992, pp 42–52.

11. Berkman B, Rohan B, Sampson S. Myths and biases related to cancer in the elderly. Cancer 1994; 74:2004–2008.

12. Holland JC, Massie MJ. Psychosocial aspects of cancer in the elderly. Clin Geriatr Med 1987; 3:2766–2770.

13. Holmes FF. Clinical evidence for change in tumor aggressiveness with age. In: L Balducci, GH Lyman, WB Ershler, eds. Geriatric Oncology. Philadelphia: Lippincott, Co., Philadelphia, 1992, pp 86–91.

14. Hakama M, Penttinen J. Epidemiologic evidence for two components of cervical cancer. Br J Obstet Gynaecol 1981; 88:209–214.

15. Goodwin JS, Hunt WC, Samet JM. Determinants of cancer therapy in elderly patients. Cancer 1993; 72:594–601.

16. Goodwin JS, Hunt WC, Key CR, Samet J. Cancer treatment programs: who gets chosen? Arch Intern Med 1988; 148:2258–2260.

17. Crosfill ML, Lindop PJ, Rotblat J. Variations of sensitivity to ionizing radiation with age. Nature 1959; 183:1729–1730.

18. Hursh JB, Casarett GW. The lethal effect of acute X irradiation on rats as a function of age. Br J Radiol 1956; 29:169–171.

19. Sacher GA. Dependence of acute radiosensitivity on age in adult female mouse. Science 1957; 125:1039–1040.

20. Hopewell JW, Young CMA. The effect of field size on the reaction of pig skin to single doses of X rays. Br J Radiol 1982; 55:356–361.

21. Hamlet R. Hopewell JW. The radiation response of skin in young and old rats. Int J Radiat Biol 1982; 42:573–576.

22. Denekamp J. Residual radiation damage in mouse skin 5 to 8 months after irradiation. Radiology 1975; 115:191–195.

23. Sargent EV, Burns FJ. Radioautographic measurement of electron induced epidermal kinetic effects in different aged rats. J Invest Dermatol 1987; 88:320–323.

24. Landuyt W, van der Schueren E. Effect of age on the radiation-induced repopulation in mouse lip mucosa. Strahlen Onkol 1991; 167:41–45.

25. Hamilton E. Cell proliferation and aging in mouse colon. I. Repopulation after repeated X-ray injury in young and old mice. Cell Tissue Kinet 1978; 11:423–431.

26. Olofsen-van Acht MJJ, Hooije CMC, Aardweg GJMJ, Velthuijsen MLF, Levendag PC. Tolerance of rat rectum for radiation as a function of age. Int J Radiat Oncol Biol Phys 1997; 39(Suppl):255.

27. Mirimanoff RO, Dosoretz DE, Linggood RM, Ojemann RG, Martuza RL. Meningioma: analysis of recurrence and progression following neurosurgical resection. J Neurosurg 1985; 62:18–24.

28. Glaholm J. Bloom HJG, Crow JH. The role of radiotherapy in the management of intracranial meningiomas: the royal marsden hospital experience with 186 patients. Int J Radiat Oncol Biol Phys 1990; 18:755–761.

29. Cooper JS, Borok TL, Ransohoff J, Carella RJ. Malignant glioma: results of combined modality therapy. JAMA 1982; 248:62–65.

30. Asscher AW. Arterial hypertension and irradiation damage to the nervous system. Lancet 1962; 2:1343–1344.

31. Maire JP, Coudin B, Guerin J, Caudry M. Neuropyschological impairment in adults with brain tumors. Am J Clin Oncol 1987; 10:156–162.

32. Chin R, Fisher RJ, Smee RI, Barton MB. Oropharyngeal cancer in the elderly. Int J Radiat Oncol Biol Phys 1995; 32:1007–1016.

33. Huguenin P, Glanzman C, Lutolf UM. Acute toxicity of curative radiotherapy. Strahlen Onkol 172:658–663.

34. Pignon T, Horiot JC, Van den Bogaert W, Van Glabbeke M, Scalliet P. No age limit for radical radiotherapy in head and neck tumors. Eur J Cancer 1996; 32A:2075–2081.

35. Larson PJ, Lindsey AM, Dodd MJ, Brecht ML, Packer A. Influence of age on problems experienced by patients with lung cancer undergoing radiation therapy. Oncol Nurs Forum 1993; 20:473–480.

36. Koga K, Kusumoto S, Watanabe K, Nishikawa K, Harada K, Ebihara H. Age factor relevant to the development of radiation pneumonitis in radiotherapy of lung cancer. Int J Radiat Oncol Biol Phys 1988; 14:367–371.

37. Segawa Y, Takigawa N, Kataoka M, Takata I, Fujimoto N, Ueoka H. Risk factors for development of radiation pneumonitis following radiation therapy with or without chemotherapy. Int J Radiat Oncol Biol Phys 1997; 39:91–98.

38. Wyckoff J, Greenberg H, Sanderson R, Wallach P, Balducci L. Breast irradiation in the older woman: a toxicity study. J Am Geriatr Soc 1994; 42:150–152.

39. Turesson I, Nyman J, Holmberg E, Oden A. Prognostic factors for acute and late skin reactions in radiotherapy patients. Int J Radiat Oncol Biol Phys 1996; 36:1065–1075.

40. Bentzen SM, Overgaard J. Patient-to-patient variability in the expression of radiation-induced normal tissue injury. Semin Radiat Oncol 1994; 4:68–80.

41. Olsen NK, Pfeiffer P, Johannsen L, Schroder H, Rose C. Radiation-induced brachial plexopathy: neurological follow-up in 161 recurrence-free breast cancer patients. Int J Radiat Oncol Biol Phys 1993; 26:43–49.

42. Bentzen SM, Overgaard M, Thames HD. Fractionation sensitivity of a functional endpoint: impaired shoulder movement after post-mastectomy radiotherapy. Int J Radiat Oncol Biol Phys 1989; 17:531–537.

43. Calvin DP, Powers C, Awan A, Halpern HJ, Heimann R. Arm lymphedema following breast conservation therapy. Presented at the 20th Annual San Antonio Breast Cancer Symposium, San Antonio, December 3–6, 1997.

44. Martin LM, LePechoux C, Calitchi E, Otmezguine Y, Feuilhade F, Brun B, Piedbois P, Mazeron JJ, Julien M, Le Bourgeois JP. Management of breast cancer in the elderly. Eur J Cancer 1994; 30A:590–596.

45. Larson D, Weinstein M, Goldberg I, Silver B, Recht A, Cady B, Silen W, Harris JR. Edema of the arm as a function of the extent of axillary surgery in patients with stage I-II carcinoma of the breast treated with primary radiotherapy. Int J Radiat Oncol Biol Phys 1986; 12:1575–1582.

46. Hallahan DE, Michel AG, Halpern HJ, Awan AM, Desser R, Bitran J, Recant W, Wyman B, Spelbring DR, Weichselbaum RR. Breast conserving surgery and definitive irradiation for early stage breast cancer. Int J Radiat Oncol Biol Phys 1989; 17:1211–1216.

47. Beadle GF, Silver B, Botnick L, Hellman S, Harris JR. Cosmetic results following primary radiation therapy for early stage breast cancer. Cancer 1984; 54:2911–2918.
48. Steeves RA, Phromratanapongse P, Wolberg WH, Tormey DC. Cosmesis and local control after irradiation in women treated conservatively for breast cancer. Arch Surg 1989; 124:1369–1373.
49. Pezner RD, Patterson MP, Lipsett JA, Odom-Maryon T, Vora NL, Wong JYC, Luk KH. Factors affecting cosmetic outcome in breast cancer treatments: objective quantitative measurement. Breast Cancer Res Treat 1991; 20:85–92.
50. Leo E, Audisio RA, Belli F, Vitellaro M, Baldini MT, Mascheroni L, Patuzzo R, Rigillo G, Rebuffoni G, Filiberti G, Navarria P, Andreola S. Total rectal resection and colo-anal anastomosis for low rectal tumors: comparative results in a group of young and old patients. Eur J Cancer 1994; 30A:1092–1095.
51. De Gara CJ, Basrur V, Figueredo A, Goodyear M, Knight P. The influence of age on the management of anal cancer. Hepatogastroenterology 1995; 42:73–76.
52. Mak AC, Rich TA, Schultheiss TE, Kavanagh B, Ota DM, Romsdahl MM. Late complications of postoperative radiation therapy for cancer of the rectum and rectosigmoid. Int J Radiat Oncol Biol Phys 1994; 28:597–603.
53. Hishikawa Y, Kurisu K, Taniguchi ZM, Kamikonya N, Miura T. Radiotherapy for carcinoma of the esophagus in patients aged eighty or older. Int J Radiat Oncol Biol Phys 1991; 20:685–688.
54. Yamakawa M, Shiojima K, Takahashi M, Saito Y, Matsumoto H, Mitsuhashi N, Niibe H. Radical treatment for esophageal cancer in patients over eighty years old. Int J Radiat Oncol Biol Phys 1994; 30:1225–1232.
55. Liu L, Glicksman AS, Coachman N, Kuten A. Low acute gastroinestinal and genitourinary toxicities in whole pelvic irradiation of prostate cancer. Int J Radiat Oncol Biol Phys 1997; 38:65–71.
56. Vijayakumar S, Awan A, Karrison T, Culbert H, Chan S, Kolker J, Low N, Halpern H, Rubin S, Chen GTY, Weichselbaum RR. Acute toxicity during external-beam radiotherapy for localized porstate cancer: comparison of different techniques. Int J Radiat Oncol Biol Phys 1993; 25:359–371.
57. Rotman M, Macchia R, Silverstein M, Aziz H, Choi K, Rosenthal J, Braverman A, Laungani GB. Treatment of advanced bladder carcinoma with irradiation and concomitant 5-fluorouracil infusion. Cancer 1988; 59:710–714.
58. Jakse G, Frommhold H, Nedden DZ. Combined radiation and chemotherapy for locally advanced transitional cell carcinoma of the urinary bladder. Cancer 1985; 55:1659–1664.
59. Russell KJ, Boileau MA, Higano C, Collins C, Russell AH, Koh W, Cole SB, Chapman WH, Griffin TW. Combined 5-fluorouracil and irradiation for transitional cell carcinoma of the urinary bladder. Int J Radiat Oncol Biol Phys 1990; 19:693–699.
60. Sauer R, Schrott KM, Dunst J, Thiel HJ, Hermanek P, Bornhof C. Preliminary results of treatment of invasive bladder carcinoma with radiotherapy and cisplatin. Int J Radiat Oncol Biol Phys 1988; 15:871–875.
61. Sandler HM, McLaughlin PW, Ten Haken RK, Addison H, Forman F, Lichter A. Three dimensional conformal radiotherapy for the treatment of prostate cancer: low risk of chronic rectal morbidity observed in a large series of patients. Int J Radiat Oncol Biol Phys 1995; 33:797–801.
62. Hanlon AL, Schultheiss TE, Hunt MA, Mousas B, Peter RS, Hanks GE. Chronic rectal

bleeding after high-dose conformal treatment of prostate cancer warrants modification of existing morbidity scales. Int J Radiat Oncol Biol Phys 1997; 38:59–63.

63. Shipley WU, Prout GR, Einstein AB, Coombs J, Wausman Z, Soloway MS, Englander L, Barton BA, Haferman MD. Treatment of invasive bladder cancer by cisplatin and radiation in patients unsuited for surgery. JAMA 1976; 258:931–935.

64. Zietman AL, Linggood RM, Brookes PR, Convery K, Piro A. Radiation therapy in the management of early stage Hodgkin's disease presenting in later life. Cancer 1991; 68:1869–1873.

65. Austin-Seymour MM, Hoppe RT, Cox RS, Rosenberg SA, Kaplan HS. Hodgkin's disease in patients over 60 years old. Ann Intern Med 1984; 100:8–13.

66. Connors JM, Klimo P, Fairey RN, Voss N. Brief chemotherapy and involved field radiation therapy for limited stage histologically aggressive lymphoma. Ann Intern Med 1987; 107:25–30.

67. Darrington DL, Vose JM, Anderson JR. Incidence and characterization of secondary myelodysplastic syndrome and acute myelogeneous leukemia following high-dose chemoradiotherapy and autologous stem-cell transplantation for lymphoid malignancies. J Clin Oncol 1994; 12:2527–2534.

68. Stone RM, Neuberg D, Soiffer R. Myeolodysplastic syndrome as a late complication following autologous bone marrow transplantation for non–Hodgkin's lymphoma. J Clin Oncol 1994; 12:2535–2542.

69. Pignon T, Horiot JC, Bolla M, van Poppel H, Bartelink H, Roelofsen F, Pene F, Gerard A, Einhorn N, Nguyen TD, Vanglabbeke M, Scalliet P. Age is not a limiting factor in radical radiotherapy in pelvic malignancies. Radiother Oncol 1997; 42:107–129.

70. Grant PT, Jeffrey JF, Fraser RC, Tompkins MG, Filbee JF, Wong OS. Pelvic radiation therapy for gynecologic malignancy in geriatric patients. Gynecol Oncol 1989; 33:185–188.

71. Sablinska B. Carcinoma of the uterine cervix in women over 70 years of age. Gynecol Oncol 1979; 7:128–135.

72. Mitsuhashi N, Takahashi M, Nozaki M, Yamakawa M, Takanishi T, Sakurai H, Maebayashi K, Hayakawa K, Niibe H. Squamous cell carcinoma of the uterine cervix: radiation therapy for patients aged 70 years and older. Radiology 1995; 194:141–145.

73. Wollschlaeger K, Mundt A, Powers C, Rotmensch J, Herbst A, Waggoner S. Morbidity associated with low-dose rate intracavitary radiotherapy for carcinoma of the uterine cervix. Gynecol Oncol 1997; 64:315.

74. Chao CKS, Grigsby PW, Perez CA, Mutch DG, Herzog T, Camel HM. Medically inoperable stage I endometrial carcinoma: a few dilemmas in radiotherapeutic management. Int J Radiat Oncol Biol Phys 1996; 34:27–31.

75. Lanciano R, Corn B, Martin E, Schultheiss T, Hogan WM, Rosenblum N. Perioperative morbidity of intracavitary gynecologic brachytherapy. Int J Radiat Oncol Biol Phys 1994; 29:969–974.

76. Perez CA, Camel HM, Walz BJ. Radiation therapy alone in the treatment of carcinoma of the uterine cervix: a 20 year experience. Gynecol Oncol 1986; 23:127–140.

77. Kennedy AW, Flagg JS, Webster KD. Gynecologic cancer in the very elderly. Gynecol Oncol 1989; 32:49–54.

78. Roeske J, Mundt A, Halpern H, Swenney P, Sutton H, Powers C, Rotmensch J,

Waggoner S, Fleming G, Weichselbaum RR. Late rectal sequelae following definitive radiation therapy for carcinoma of the uterine cervix: a dosimetric analysis. Int J Radiat Oncol Biol Phys 1997; 37:351–358.

79. Corn BW, Lanciano RM, Greven KM, Naumoff J, Schultz D, Hanks GE, Fowble BL. Impact of improved irradiation technique, age and lymph node sampling on the severe complication rate of surgically staged endometrial cancer patients: a multivariate analysis. J Clin Oncol 1994; 12:510–515.

80. Lovett RM, Perez CA, Shapiro SJ, Garcia DM. External irradiation of epithelial skin cancer. Int J Radiat Oncol Biol Phys 1990; 19:235–242.

81. Mundt AJ, Awan A, Sibley G, Simon M, Rubin S, Samuels B, Wong W, Beckett M, Vijayakumar S, Weichselbaum RR. Conservative surgery and adjuvant radiation therapy in the management of adult soft tissue sarcoma of the extremities: clinical and radiobiologic results. Int J Radiat Oncol Biol Phys 1995; 32:977–985.

82. Mundt AJ, Gibbs P, Peabody T, Simon M, Awan A, Weichselbaum R. Localized subcutaneous soft tissue sarcoma: implications for the use of adjuvant radiation therapy. Int J Radiat Oncol Biol Phys 1995; 32:166.

83. Medenhall WM, Marcus RB. Verification of vertex fields for radiotherapy of brain tumors. Int J Radiat Oncol Biol Phys 1994; 28:556–557.

84. Lawrence TS, Lichter AS. Soft tissue sarcomas (excluding retroperitoneum). In: CA Perez, LW Brady, eds. Principles and Practice of Radiation Oncology. Philadelphia: Lippincott, 1992, pp 2201–2275.

85. Roach M, Pickett B, Rosenthal SA, Verhey L, Phillips TL. Defining treatment margins for six field conformal irradiation of localized prostate cancer. Int J Radiat Oncol Biol Phys 1994; 28:267–275.

86. Amdur RJ, Kalbaugh KJ, Ewald LM, Parsons JT, Mendenhall WM, Bova FJ, Million RR. Radiation therapy for skin cancer near the eye: kilovoltage x-rays versus electrons. Int J Radiat Oncol Biol Phys 1992; 23:769–779.

87. Berson AM, Castro JR, Petti P. Charged particle irradiation of chordomas and chondrosarcoma of the base of skull and cervical spine: the Lawrence Berkeley Laboratory experience. Int J Radiat Oncol Biol Phys 1988; 15:559–563.

88. Hazuka MB, Martel MK, Marsh L, Lichter AS, Wolf GT. Preservation of parotid function after external beam irradiation in head and neck cancer patients: a feasibility study using 3-dimensional treatment planning. Int J Radiat Oncol Biol Phys 1993; 27:731–737.

89. Nishioka T, Shirato H, Arimoto T, Kaneko M, Kitahara T, Oomori K, Yasuda M, Fukuda S, Inuyama Y, Miyasaka K. Reduction of radiation-induced xerostomia in nasopharyngeal carcinoma using CT simulation with laser patients marking and three-field irradiation technique. Int J Radiat Oncol Biol Phys 1997; 38:705–712.

90. Hanks GE, Schultheiss TE, Hunt MA, Epstein B. Factors influencing incidence of acute grade 2 morbidity in conformal and standard radiation treatment of prostate cancer. Int J Radiat Oncol Biol Phys 1995; 31:25–29.

91. Mohan R, Leibel SA. Intensity modulation of the radiation beam. In: VT Devita, S Hellman, SA Rosenberg, eds.: Cancer: Principles and Practice of Oncology. Philadelphia: Lippincott-Raven, 1997, pp 3107–3175.

92. Hamilton RJ, Sweeney PJ, Pelizzari CA, Yetkin FZ, Holman BL, Garada B, Weichselbaum RR, Chen GTY. Functional imaging in treatment planning of brain lesions. Int J Radiat Oncol Biol Phys 1997; 37:181–187.

93. Marks LB, Spencer JP, Bentel GC, Ray SK, Sherouse GW, Sontag MR, Coleman RE, Jaszczak RJ, Turkington TG, Tapson V. The utility of SPECT lung perfusion scans in minimizing and assessing the physiologic consequences of thoracic irradiation. Int J Radiat Oncol Biol Phys 1993; 26:659–668.

94. Murthy AK, Hendrickson FR. Is contralateral neck treatment necessary in early carcinoma of the tonsil? Int J Radiat Oncol Biol Phys 1980; 6:91–95.

95. Sutcliffe SB, Gospodarowicz MK, Bersagel DE. Prognostic groups for management of localized Hodgkin's disease. J Clin Oncol 1985; 3:393–397.

96. Kircuta IC, Sauer J, Bohndorf W. Omission of the pelvic irradiation in stage I testicular seminoma: a study of postorchiectomy paraortic radiotherapy. Int J Radiat Oncol Biol Phys 1996; 35:293–298.

97. Kupelian PA, Komaki R, Allen P. Prognostic factors in the treatment of node-negative nonsmall cell lung carcinoma with radiotherapy alone. Int J Radiat Oncol Biol Phys 1996; 36:607–613.

98. Coster JR, Foote RL, Olden KD, Jack SM, Schaid DJ, DeSanto LW. Cervical nodal metastasis of squamous cell carcinoma of unknown origin: indications for withholding radiation therapy. Int J Radiat Oncol Biol Phys 1992; 23:743–749.

99. Lagios M, Margolin F, Westdahl P. Mammographically detected duct carcinoma in situ: frequency of local recurrence following tylectomy and prognostic effect of nuclear grade on local recurrence. Cancer 1989; 63:618–623.

100. Gibbs P, Peabody T, Mundt AJ, Montag A, Simon M. Oncologic outcomes of subcutaenous sarcomas of the extremities. J Bone J Surg 1997; 79A:888–897.

101. LeVeque FG, Montgomery M, Potter D, Zimmer MB, Rieke JW, Steiger BW, Gallagher SC, Muscoplat CC. A multicenter, randomized, double-bling, placebo-controlled, dose-titration study of oral pilocarpine for treatment of radiation-induced xerostomia in head and neck cancer patients. J Clin Oncol 1993; 11:1124–1131.

102. Meredith R, Salter M, Kim R, Spencer S, Wepelmann B, Rodu B, Smith J, Lee J. Sulcralfate for radiation mucositis: results of a double-blind randomized trial. Int J Radiat Oncol Biol Phys 1997; 37:275–279.

103. Kajanti M, Kaleta R, Kankooranata L, Muhonen T, Holsti L. Effect of overall treatment time on local control in radical radiotherapy for squamous cell carcinoma of the esophagus. Int J Radiat Oncol Biol Phys 1995; 32:1017–1023.

104. Girinsky T, Rey A, Roche B, Haie C, Gerboulet A, Randrianavivello H, Chassagne D. Overall treatment time in advanced cervical carcinoma: a critical parameter in treatment outcome. Int J Radiat Oncol Biol Phys 1993; 27:1051–1056.

105. Leksell L. The stereotaxic method and radiosurgery of the brain. Acta Chir Scand 1951; 102:316–320.

106. Pozza F, Colombo F, Chierego G. Low grade astrocytomas: treatment with unconventionally fractionated external beam stereotactic radiation therapy. Radiology 1989; 171:565–569.

107. Linskey ME, Lunsford LD, Flickinger JC. Tumor control after stereotactic radiosurgery in neurofibromatosis patients with bilateral acoustic tumors. Neurosurgery 1992; 31:829–838.

108. Flickinger JC, Nelson BP, Martinez AJ, Deutsch M, Taylor F. Radiosurgery of nonfunctioning adenomas of the pituitary gland: results with and long term followup. Cancer 1989; 63:2409–2414.

109. Engenhart R, Kimmig B, Hover KH, Wowra B, Sturm V, van Kaick G, Wannenmacher

M. Stereotactic single high dose radiation therapy of benign intracranial meningiomas. Int J Radiat Oncol Biol Phys 1990; 19:1021–1026.

110. Colombo F, Benedetti A, Fozza F, Marchetti C, Chierego G. Linear accelerator radiosurgery of cerebral arteriovenous malformations. Neurosurgery 1989; 24:833–840.

111. Steiner L, Lundquist C, Adler JR, Torner JC, Alves W, Steiner M. Clinical outcome of radiosurgery for cerebral arteriovenous malformations. J Neurosurg 1992; 77:1–8.

112. Steinberg GK, Fabrikant JI, Marks MP, Levy RP, Frankel KA, Phillips MH, Shuer LM, Silverberg GD. Stereotactic heavy-charged-particle bragg-peak radiation for intracranial arteriovenous malformations. N Engl J Med 1990; 323:96–101.

113. Patchell RA, Tibbs PA, Walsh JW, Dempsey RJ, Maruyama Y, Kryscio RJ, Markesbery WR, Masdonald JS, Young B. A randomized trial of surgery in the treatment of single metastases to the brain. N Engl J Med 1990; 322:494–500.

114. Adler JR, Cox RS, Kaplan I, Martin DP. Stereotactic radiosurgery treatment of brain metastases. J Neurosurg 1992; 76:444–449.

115. Mehta MP, Rozenthal JM, Levin AB, Mackie TR, Kubsad SS, Gehring MA, Kinsella TJ. Defining the role of radiosurgery in the management of brain metastases. Int J Radiat Oncol Biol Phys 1992; 24:619–625.

116. Wallner K, Roy J, Zelefsky M, Fuks Z, Harrison L. Short-term freedom from disease progression after I-125 postate implantation. Int J Radiat Oncol Biol Phys 1994; 30: 405–409.

117. Grimm PD, Blasko JC, Ragde H, Sylvester J, Clarke D. Does brachytherapy have a role in the treatment of prostate cancer? Hematol Oncol Clin North Am 1996; 10:653–673.

118. Blasko JC, Ragde H, Cuse RW, Sylvester JE, Cavanagh W, Grimm PD. Should brachytherapy be considered a therapeutic option in localized prostate cancer. Urol Clin North Am 1996; 23:633–650.

119. Khan K, Thompson FC, Bush S, Stidley C. Transperineal percutaneous iridium-192 interstitial template implant of the prostate: results and complications in 321 patients. Int J Radiat Oncol Biol Phys 1992; 22:935–939.

120. Gerard JP, Ayzac L, Coquard R, Romestaing P, Ardiet JM, Rocher FP, Barbet N, Cenni JL, Souquet JC. Endocavitary irradiation for early rectal carcinomas T1 (T2). A series of 101 patients treated with the Papillon's technique. Int J Radiat Oncol Biol Phys 1996; 34:775–783.

121. Sischy B, Hinson EJ, Wilkinson DR. Definitive radiation therapy for selected cancers of the rectum. Br J Surg 1988; 75:901–903.

122. Minsky BD, Enker WE, Cohen AM, Lauwers G. Local excision and postoperative radiation therapy for rectal cancer. Am J Clin Oncol 1994; 17:411–416.

123. Wazer DE, Erban JK, Robert NJ, Smith TJ, Marchant DJ, Schmid C, DiPetrillo T, Schmidt-Ullrich BA. Breast conservation in elderly women for clinically negative axillary lymph nodes without axillary dissection. Cancer 1994; 74:878–883.

124. Mendenhall WM, Million RR, Cassissi NJ. Elective neck irradiation in squamous cell carcinoma of the head and neck. Head Neck Surg 1980; 3:15–20.

125. Keys H. Gynecology Oncology Group trials of combined technique therapy for vulvar cancer. Cancer 1993; 71:1691–1696.

126. Petereit DG, Mehta MP, Buchler DA, Kinsella TJ. Is inguinal-femoral irradiation as effective as lymphadenectomy for N0, N1 vulvar disease? Int J Radiat Oncol Biol Phys 1992; 24(Suppl):210.

127. Henderson RH, Parsons JT, Morgan L, Million RR. Elective ilioinguinal lympy node irradiation. Int J Radiat Oncol Biol Phys 1984; 10:811–819.
128. Glick J, Kim K, Earle J, O'Connell M. An ECOG ranomized phase III trial of CHOP vs CHOP + radiotherapy for intermediate grade early stage non–Hodgkin's lymphoma. Proc Am Soc Clin Oncol 1995; 14:391.
129. Vergote IB, Vergote-De Vos LN, Abeler VM, Aas M, Lindegaard MW, Kjorstad KE, Trope CG. Randomized trial comparing cisplatin with radioactive phosphorus or whole-abdomen irradiation as adjuvant treatment of ovarian cancer. Cancer 1992; 69: 741–749.
130. Young RC, Walton LA, Ellenberg SS. Adjuvant therapy in stage I and stage II epithelial ovarian cancer: results of two prospective randomized trials. N Engl J Med 1990; 322:1021–1027.
131. Bolis G, Colombo N, Pecorelli S, Torri V, Marsoni S, Bonazzi C, Chiari S, Favalli G, Mangili G, Presti M. Adjuvant treatment for early epithelial ovarian cancer: results of two randomised clinical trials comparing cisplatin to no further treatment or chromic phosphate (^{32}P). Ann Oncol 1995; 6:887–893.
132. Stitt JA, Fowler JF, Thomadsen BR, Buchler DA, Paliwal BP, Kinsella TJ. High dose rate intracavitary brachytherapy for carcinoma of the cervix: the Madison system: I. Clinical and radiobiological considerations. Int J Radiat Oncol Biol Phys 1992; 24: 335–348.
133. Inoue T, Teshima T, Muraya S, Shimizutani K, Fuchihata H, Furukawa S. Phase III trial of high and low dose rate interstitial radiotherapy for early oral tongue cancer. Int J Radiat Oncol Biol Phys 1996; 36:1201–1204.
134. Eifel PJ. High-dose-rate brachytherapy for carcinoma of the cervix: high tech or high risk? Int J Radiat Oncol Biol Phys 1992; 24:383–386.
135. Orton CG, Seyedsadr M, Somnay A. Comparison of high and low dose rate remote afterloading for cervix cancer and the importance of fractionation. Int J Radiat Oncol Biol Phys 1992; 21:1425–1434.
136. Wang CC. Cancer of the head and neck. In: CC Wang, ed. Clinical Radiation Oncology: Indications, Techniques and Results. Littleton, MA: PSG, 1988, pp 201–275.
137. Ritter MA, Vaughn RB. Ectopic ossification after total hip arthroplasty: predisposing factors, frequency and effect on results. J Bone J Surg 1977; 59A:345–348.
138. Anthony P, Keys H, McCollister E. Prevention of heterotopic bone formation with early postoperative irradiation in high risk patients undergoing total hip arthroplasty: comparison of 10.0 Gy vs 20.0 Gy schedules. Int J Radiat Oncol Biol Phys 1987; 3: 365–369.
139. Lo TCM, Healy WL, Covall DJ. Heterotopic bone formation after hip surgery: prevention with single dose post-operative hip irradiation. Radiology 1988; 168:851–855.
140. Popma JJ, Califf RM, Topol EJ. Clinical trials of restenosis after coronary angioplasty. Circulation 1991; 84:1426–1436.
141. Popowski Y, Verin V, Urban P. Endovascular beta-irradiation after percutaneous transluminal coronary balloon angioplasty. Int J Radiat Oncol Biol Phys 1996; 36:841–845.
142. Schopohl B, Liermann D, Pohlit LJ, Heyd R, Strassman G, Bauersachs R, Schulte-Huermann D, Rahl CG, Manegold K-H, Kollath J, Bottcher HD. Iridium-192 endovascular brachytherapy for avoidance of initimal hyperplasia after percutaneous translumi-

nal angioplasty and stent implantation in peripheral vessels: 6 years of experience. Int J Radiat Oncol Biol Phys 1996; 36:829–833.

143. Tierstein PS, Massullo V, Jani S, Popma JJ, Mintz GS, Russo RJ, Schatz RA, Guaneri EM, Steuterman S, Morris NB, Leon MB, Tripuranemi P. Catheter-based radiotherapy to inhibit restenosis after coronary stenting. N Engl J Med 1997; 336:1697–1703.

144. Berson AM, Finger PT, Sherr DL, Emery R, Alfieri AA, Bosworth JL. Radiotherapy for age-related macular degeneration: technique and preliminary subjective response. Int J Radiat Oncol Biol Phys 1996; 36:861–866.

145. Van den Brenck HAA. Results of prophylactic postoperative irradiation in 1300 cases of pterygium. Am J Roentgenol 1968; 103:723–727.

146. Donaldson SS, Bagshaw MS, Kriss JP. Supervoltage orbital radiotherapy for Graves' opthalmopathy. J Clin Endocrinol Metab 1973; 37:276–279.

147. Milone FP, Copeland MM. Calcific tendonitis of the shoulder joint. Am J Roentgenol 1986; 159:793–796.

148. Mira JG, Chahbazian CM, del Regato JA. The value of radiotherapy for Peyronie's disease: presentation of 56 new case studies and review of the literature. Int J Radiat Oncol Biol Phys 1980; 6:161–165.

149. Price P, Hoskin PJ, Easton D. Low dose single fraction radiotherapy in the treatment of metastatic bone pain: a pilot study. Radiother Oncol 1988; 12:297–301.

150. Crocker I, Prosnitz L. Radiation therapy of the elderly. Clin Geriatr Med 1987; 3:473–481.

151. Tong C, Gillick L, Hendrickson FR. The palliation of symptomatic osseous metastases: final results of the study by the Radiation Therapy Oncology Group. Cancer 1982; 50:893–896.

152. Blitzer PH. Reanalysis of the RTOG study of the palliation of symptomatic osseous metastasis. Cancer 1985; 55:1468–1473.

153. Salazar OM, Rubin P, Hendrickson FR, Poulter C, Zagars G, Feldman MI, Asbell S, Doss L. Single-dose half-body irradiation for the palliation of multiple bone metastases from solid tumors: a preliminary report. Int J Radiat Oncol Biol Phys 1981; 7:773–781.

154. Scher HI, Chung LWK. Bone metastases: improving the therapeutic index. Semin Oncol 1994; 21:630–635.

155. Borgelt BB, Gelber R, Brady LW, Griffin T, Hendrickson FR. The palliation of hepatic metastases: results of the radiation therapy oncology group pilot study. Int J Radiat Oncol Biol Phys 1981; 7:587–591.

156. Findlay GFG. Adverse effects of the management of malignant spinal cord compression. J Neurol Neurosurg Psychiatry 1984; 47:761–765.

157. Liebel SA, Pajak TF, Massullo V, Order SE, Komaki RU, Chang CH, Wasserman TH, Phillips TL, Lipshutz J, Durbin LM. A comparison of misonidazole sensitized radiation therapy to radiation therapy alone for the palliation of hepastic metastases: results of a Radiation Therapy Oncology Group randomized prospective trial. Int J Radiat Oncol Biol Phys 1987; 13:1057–1062.

158. Dobrowsky W. Treatment of choroid metastases. Br J Radiol 1988; 61:140–144.

159. Zachariah B, Zachariah SB, Vorghese R, Balducci L. Carcinomatous meningitis: clinical manifestations and management. Int J Clin Pharmacol Ther 1985; 33:7–12.

160. Rees GJ, Tevrell CE, Barley VC, Newman HF. Palliative raiotherapy for lung cancer: two versus five fractions. Clin Oncol 1997; 9:90–95.

161. Adelson MD, Wharton JT, Delclos L, Copeland L, Gershenson D. Palliative radiotherapy for ovarian cancer. Int J Radiat Oncol Biol Phys 1987; 13:17–21.

162. Cotter GW, Larscy C, Ellingwood KE, Herbert D. Inoperable endobronchial obstructing lung cancer treated with combined endobronchial and external beam irradiation: a dosimetric analysis. Int J Radiat Oncol Biol Phys 1993; 27:531–535.

163. Montemaggi P, Costamagna, G, Dobelbower RR, Cellini N, Morganti AG, Mutignani M, Perri V, Brizi G, Marano P. Intraluminal brachytherapy in the treatment of pancreas and bile duct carcinomas. Int J Radiat Oncol Biol Phys 1995; 32:437–441.

164. Taal BG, Aleman BM, Koning CC, Boot H. High dose rate brachytherapy before external beam radiotherapy in inoperable oesophageal cancer. Br J Cancer 1996; 74: 1452–1457.

10

Chemotherapeutic Treatment Issues in the Elderly

Marc Gautier
Dartmouth Hitchcock Medical Center
Lebanon, New Hampshire

Harvey Jay Cohen
Veterans Administration Medical Center and
Duke University Medical Center
Durham, North Carolina

I. INTRODUCTION

Approximately 50% of all tumors occur in people over the age of 65 years. Chemotherapy has demonstrated beneficial effects in the treatment of cancer, but it has principally been studied in patients under the age of 65 years. The question remains, how does chemotherapy effect elderly patients, who are frequently afflicted with cancer? In this chapter, we discuss the changes in pharmacokinetics and pharmacodynamics associated with aging that alter the outcome of chemotherapy.

Much of what we know about the use of chemotherapic drugs in cancer patients is derived from clinical trials. When new chemotherapeutic drugs are initially brought to clinical trials, they are studied in phase I studies. The goal of these studies is to determine the maximum tolerated dose of the chemotherapeutic agent. Once the appropriate dose of the chemotherapeutic drug is established, phase II studies attempt to determine if there is any activity against specific disease types. Frequently, elderly patients are excluded from these early studies, and thus there is limited knowledge about how many of these drugs are altered with the normal process of aging (1). Phase I and II studies initially describe how a drug is handled in the human system. These studies usually show a high degree of variability between patients in how a given drug is handled.

This variability in drug handling is sometimes due to measurable differences in organ function, but more frequently, it is due to unknown processes. This extensive variability is manifested by variable responses and toxicity of the same dose of chemotherapy in different patients. The standard practice is to dose chemotherapy in uniform fashion by calculating that dose on the basis of the body surface area. The origin of this practice stems not so much from reducing intrapatient variability as attempting to control the dose when moving from animal studies to humans. This chapter examines some of the sources of the variability between patients receiving chemotherapy. We also suggest how chemotherapeutic doses should be adjusted in the face of known determinants of this variability. A clear message from the data is that age alone is a poor predictor of the variability between patients. In fact, in older age groups, the intrapatient variability is even higher than in younger age groups.

One other issue needs to be explored in understanding the use of chemotherapy in elderly patients. The narrow therapeutic index of most chemotherapic drugs is well known to patients and physicians alike. Frequently, the question is, "Is the benefit worth the toxicity?" To approach that issue one needs to know the goal of the chemotherapy. In modern oncology, there are several accepted roles for the use of chemotherapy. Chemotherapy is frequently used after surgery or radiation in the adjuvant setting. Chemotherapy also can be used alone with curative intent. Frequently, palliation is the only goal for chemotherapy. One important perception among oncologists is that chemotherapy is less effective and more toxic in elderly patients. With the impression of this altered ratio of toxicity to benefit, there is some tendency to avoid doses of chemotherapy that would be more likely to provide cure and a subtle shift toward the use of chemotherapy as palliation, or not all. This tendency for less use of intense chemotherapy with advancing age has been noted by several investigators (2, 3). Although the dose of chemotherapy can be associated with both toxicity and response rates, modification of the dose of chemotherapy is almost always contingent on toxicity considerations. Because toxicity can be life threatening, many oncologists avoid doses of chemotherapy that they believe will be associated with significant toxicity. There are clear examples where aggressive chemotherapy is tolerated less well in older patients than younger patients (acute myclogenous leukemia [AML] induction therapy) (4). However, multiple studies have demonstrated that older patients can tolerate standard-dose chemotherapy with similar toxicity as younger patients (5). Moreover, some studies suggest that older patients have less emotional distress associated with taking chemotherapy (6). Despite these data many older patients continue to have "adjusted" regimens owing to concerns about how age alone will place them at risk for toxicity from chemotherapy.

II. PHARMACOKINETICS

The term *pharmacokinetics* describes the principles that apply to the handling of many drugs in the body. These principles can be summarized in the following fashion: (a) an optimal outcome is likely if the drug concentration in the serum reaches a target level; (b) there are several definable interactions that account for the differences among patients in achieving a target drug level; and (c) thus, a wide range of drug doses may be required to achieve the optimal clinical response in different patients. These principles do not expressly consider the factors involved in obtaining the clinical response. *Pharmacodynamics* is the study of the interactions between these serum levels of drugs and outcomes (see see. III).

There are four major factors controlling most pharmacokinetic alterations: categories are absorption, distribution, metabolism, and excretion. We will examine each of these in turn and assess how aging affects each process. Although these four principles define most of the pharmacokinetic variability among patients, there are other processes that can add to intrapatient variabiltiy.

A. Absorption

Most cancer chemotherapy is delivered intravenously; however, there are many drugs that are delivered orally, either alone or in combinations. Melphalan, cyclophosphamide, and methotrexate are commonly used for a variety of neoplasms that occur in the elderly. More recently, other drugs that have been available intravenously may be more advantageously used in an oral regimen. Etoposide is an example of a drug that may be more active in a variety of diseases if given in low doses orally over 3 weeks. Research to find oral formulations of the commonly used drug flourouracil is proceeding. For many reasons, it may be preferable to use the oral route of administration of chemotherapy.

Aging affects gastrointestinal physiology in a variety of ways (7). It is clear that gastric acidity decreases with age. The amount of secretions from the intestinal tract also decreases with age. Absorptive surface area, splanchnic blood flow, and bowel motility have less clear alterations with aging. In younger patients, there is a wide variation in the absorption of these oral medicines. In elderly patients, one can expect the same wide variability without any clinically relevant change due to aging (8). Most investigators recommend following the effects of the oral medicine to confirm adequate absorption. Practically, for example, in the use of melphalan for multiple myeloma one should check a white blood cell count (WBC) 2–3 weeks after the dose is administered orally to confirm a 50% decrease in the WBC. If the WBC has not fallen this much, then the oral dose needs to be increased to account for the observed lack of absorption. For many drugs serum levels can be checked to assure adequate absorption (9).

B. Distribution

Once the chemotherapeutic drug has reached the systemic circulation, either by parental administration or oral dosing with absorption, there will be some changes in the distribution of the drug that are predictable with aging. There are well-described changes in body composition that occur with aging (8). There is an increased percentage of body weight due to fat, with decreases in body weight due to muscle and water. The fat content is estimated to increase from 15% of body weight to 30%, whereas intracellular water decreases from 42 to 33% from the ages of 25–75 years. This will alter distribution volumes for both fat- and water-soluble compounds.

Another factor affecting distribution is related to binding by plasma proteins to certain drugs. Albumin decreases with age by about 15%. Chronic illness, such as cancer, and poor nutrional status also can significantly lower the level of serum albumin. For drugs that are tightly protein bound, the amount of free drug available to interact with target receptors will be affected by this change in albumin. Drugs such as etoposide are clearly affected by this mechanism. Although this is not isolated to elderly patients, it does point out the need to individualize therapy and to consider elderly patients as a subset (10). The frequency of other drug use in the elderly population raises the likelihood of drug-drug interactions via competition for binding sites on albumin. This is more likely to occur in elderly patients then younger patients because of the frequency of the use of polypharmacy in elderly patients (11).

Despite these clear-cut and predicatable changes that occur in the factors controlling distribution in elderly patients, there is little actual data to aid in adjusting the dose of chemotherapy. Nonetheless, these principles should be taken into account by the physician caring for elderly patients.

C. Metabolism

Once the drug has achieved serum levels and been distributed into the compartments of the body, the terminal phase of the presence of the drug in the body is primarily related to metabolism and excretion. Activation of drug is a large component of the metabolism of many drugs. Any alteration in activation or metabolism of a drug will affect the exposure of the patient to the drug. Hepatic metabolism is a critical element in the pharmacokinetics of many drugs.

Hepatic metabolism is dependent on three critical elements: (a) hepatic blood flow, (b) liver size, and (c) activity of drug-metabolizing enzymes. Each of these elements can be affected by the normal process of aging (12). There is an abundance of data confirming that hepatic blood flow decreases with age. There are also data showing that liver size decreases with age. The amount of decrease in the size of the liver approaches 20–40% and may account for the majority of the alterations in the hepatic metabolism of drugs in elderly patients.

Changes associated with aging in the drug-metabolizing enzymes within the liver have been controversial (13). Animal models have given mixed results. Some liver enzyme functions appear to decrease with age in some animals but not in others. Specific information regarding chemotherapeutic drug processing by the hepatic enzyme systems in older patients is not available.

Given that there is an agreed change in some hepatic functions associated with advancing age, one would expect that there have been evaluations of specific chemotherapeutic drugs in patients of advanced age. Unfortunately, there is a lack of clinical data regarding age-related changes in pharmacokinetics of chemotherapeutic drugs. There is current interest in these issues, and groups such as the Cancer and Leukemia Group B (CALGB) are currently evaluating these issues in pharmacokinetic phase II studies in elderly patients with relapsed malignancies.

To this point, we have examined just age-related changes in liver function. In the setting of known liver dysfunction, there is additional information. However, there is much disagreement regarding the measurement of the alterations in hepatic function to best reflect drug metabolism. Liver function tests, as commonly obtained, do not accurately reflect the ability of the liver to metabolize drugs. Furthermore, other drugs, such as barbituates, will significantly affect metabolism without altering liver function tests. Nonetheless, recommendations regarding dose adjustments of chemotherapy based on liver abnormalities and concomitant medications can be made. Table 1 outlines some of the recommendations that can be made for dose adjustments in the face of known hepatic dysfunction for some common chemotherapeutic drugs.

D. Excretion

The clearest example of age-related decline in organ function relates to the excretion phase of drug handling. There is a clear age-related decrease in renal function as demonstrated by a decrease in the glomerular filtration rate (GFR). The importance of altered renal function on the kinetics of chemotherapeutic drugs is most clear for carboplatin and methotrexate. The key feature though is related to altered renal function and not to age. Thus, a younger patient with a reduced GFR should have a dose adjustment greater than an older person with an intact GFR. This continues to confirm the impression that age alone is a poor indicator for adjustment of chemotherapy, and that the alterations in underlying organ function are the critical elements to optimize individual therapy.

Other drugs are thought to be affected by renal excretion as well. Dose adjustment recommedations have been made despite a lack of rigorous clinical data relating these dose adjustments to optimal clinical outcomes. Nonetheless, Table 1 includes frequently recommended dose adjustments in the setting of renal dysfunction.

Some drugs undergo both hepatic metabolism and hepatic excretion via bile. The anthracyclines are most closely associated with biliary excretion. Once again,

Table 1 Recommended Dose Adjustments for Selected Agents

Drug	Clearance mechanism	Dose modification
Alkylating agents		
Cyclophosphamide	Renal	Decrease 50% if Cr Cx <25 mL/min/m2
Cisplatin	Renal	Decrease proportional to Cr Cx
Chlorambucil	Metabolic	No recommendations
Antimetabolites		
Methotrexate	Renal	Decrease if Cr Cx <60 mL/min/m2
Fluorouracil	Metabolic	No recommendations
Fludarabine	Renal/metabolic	Decrease proportional to Cr Cx
Hydroxyurea	Renal/metabolic	Decrease proportional to Cr Cx
Plant derivatives		
Vincristine	Metabolic	Decrease 50% if bilirubin >1.5 ULN
Etoposide	Renal/metabolic	Decrease proportional to Cr Cx and consider dose adjustment with impaired liver funtion
Paclitaxel	Metabolic	Consider dose adjustment with impaired liver function
Antitumor antibiotics		
Doxorubicin	Metabolic	Decrease 50% if bilirubin 1.2–3.0 decrease 75% if bilirubin 3.1–5.1
Bleomycin	Renal	Decrease 50–75% if Cr Cx <25 mL/min/m^2

Cr Cx, creatinine clearance; ULN, upper limits of normal.

the relationship of biliary excretion to age is questionable. Animal studies do not support decreases in biliary excretion with aging. Thus, no specific age adjustments for drugs that have a significant biliary excretion are required. However, in the setting of significant hepatic dysfunction (as demonstrated by an elevated bilirubin), drugs that undergo significant excretion in the bile should be dose adjusted. Table 1 has common recommendations.

III. PHARMACODYNAMICS

Now that we have evaluated some of the common changes in pharmacokinetics, it is time to evaluate what is known about the pharmacodynamic changes that occur with aging. Recall that pharmacokinetics describes the behavior of the drug in the body, whereas pharmacodynamics more accurately describes what the drug does to the body. The field of pharmacodynamics is quite complex and there are limited amounts of data specific to elderly patients and chemotherapy.

One reason it is difficult to study pharmacodynamics is that frequently only serum levels are measured, and this may not reflect the level of drug exposure at the target site. Age-related changes in a variety of cellular processes may account for some pharmacodynamic alterations. We know, for example, that the changes in autonomic nervous system function with age render elderly patients more sensitive to the toxicity of beta-blockers. Unfortunately, there is little mechanistic data exploring these issues for cancer chemotherapy.

Several suggestions have been made to account for the pharmacodynamic alterations with aging (13). Changes in p-glycoprotein drug expulsion, abnormal protein synthesis, membrane transport, abnormal DNA repair, altered drug receptors, or target enzymes have all been implicated to account for some pharmacodynamic variability. As noted, however, there are no direct clinical data to prove these claims.

IV. AGE AND TOXICITY OF CHEMOTHERAPY

In this section, we will initially evaluate the clinical data suggesting that there is a difference in end organ susceptibility to chemotherapy with advancing age. Subsequently, we will evaluate specific agents and classes of chemotherapies (e.g., anthracycline cardiotoxicity). The observed age-related changes in chemotherapeutic sensitivity may have many sources. We will evaluate some of the organ sensitivity that has been noted. The most common age-related chemotherapeutic sensitivity appears to be myelosupression (14).

Attempting to separate out the process of aging verses comorbid illnesses can be quite difficult. Myelosupression, which does appear to be more common in the elderly after chemotherapy, has not clearly been associated with age alone. When one examines the bone marrow function of healthy elderly people, there is little discernible decline with age. There have been a variety of studies examining the effects of aging on numbers of stem cells, hematopoietic stroma, and growth factors in normal volunteers. These studies have not clearly shown a decrease in function with advancing age. This implies that any changes may be related to other comorbid illnesses and not to the aging process itself. Clinically, excessive hematological toxicity has been noted in elderly patients. In a series of studies reviewing large numbers of patients and a variety of treatment regimens, there was an increased incidence of hematological toxicity in the elderly noted (15). In a study of over 16,000 patients, excessive hematological side effects in older patients were associated with certain chemotherapeutic drugs (actinomycin, doxorubicin, methotrexate, methyl-N-[2-chloroethyl]-N′-cyclonitrosourea [CCNU], vinblastine, and etoposide). Most of these drugs are characterized by biliary excretion, and this may account for their excess toxicity. Other studies have demonstrated comparable hematological toxicity for younger and older patients with a variety of chemotherapeutic regimens, such as the combination of cyclophosphamide, methotrexate, and fluorouracil (CMF) for breast cancer, provided the dose is adjusted for the GFR (16). There are some specific regimens that are frequently associated with excessive hematological toxicity in the elderly.

Induction chemotherapy for AML has been associated with higher early death rates in older patients, principally due to the complications of myelosupression. An Eastern Cooperative Oncology Group (ECOG) study evaluated elderly patients with AML comparing induction chemotherapy to low-dose treatment (17). Although there was no difference in the complete response rate (28%), early deaths were more common in the induction arm (60%) compared to the low-dose arm (25%). This study is typical of studies demonstrating excessive toxicity to chemotherapy in the hematopoietic organ for elderly patients.

Support for hematological toxicity is now available. Hematopoietic growth factors work equally well in older patients as in younger patients (18). No longer is the only option for hematological toxicity dose reduction. Hopefully, this will translate into improved outcomes for patients who might benefit from full-dose chemotherapy, although this has not been demonstrated to date. This is most important in diseases where full doses of chemotherapy are associated with higher cure rates and improved survival. Hodgkin's disease, non–Hodgkin's lymphoma, and breast cancer are all diseases in which dose intensity is associated with improved survival.

Gastrointestinal complaints are frequent in patients taking chemotherapy. Nausea and vomiting are common complaints. Mucositis, usually manifested by a sore mouth, may be more common in the elderly. At least one study suggests that patients older than the age of 65 years treated with 5-fluorouracil (5-FU) had increased rates of mucositis (19). Regardless of the frequency of mucositis, elderly patients are less tolerant to the complications of mucositis, including dehydration, that can accompany lack of oral intake.

Cardiac toxicity is a serious problem, especially in association with anthracycline therapy. Low-output congestive heart failure occurring with high total doses of doxorubicin is the typical clinical scenario. It appears that age may predispose to this toxicity even at lower total doses of doxorubicin for patients over the age of 70 years (20). Whether this represents subclinical cardiac disease or reflects the normal physiological aging process resulting in a lack of homeostatic reserve is unclear. Nonetheless, current recommendations advise that elderly patients have a less total dose of doxorubicin than younger patients. The mechanism of doxorubicin cardiotoxicity is related to the generation of oxygen free radicals. Recently, the free radical scavenger dexrazoxane has been shown to be protective of doxorubicin cardiotoxicity (21).

Few chemotherapies are toxic to the pulmonary system. Bleomycin is the most common drug associated with pulmonary toxicity. At least one study has suggested an increased rate of pulmonary toxicity in patients over the age of 70 years receiving bleomycin (22). Age-related declines in elasticity of lung tissue makes this toxicity more morbid when it does occur. The pulmonary toxicity associated with bleomycin, like doxorubicin, is associated with high cumulative total doses. No formal recommendations are available for dose adjustments for elderly patients.

Although we know there is an age-related decline in renal function as manifested by a decrease in the GFR, there is little evidence to suggest that there is an age-associated increased risk of renal dysfunction from chemotherapy. Cisplatinum-induced renal toxicity is clearly associated with poor renal function rather than advancing age.

Neurological toxicity, principally neuropathy, is a major concern. Although many chemotherapic agents are known to be associated with a neuropathy (vincas and taxanes), there is scant evidence relating this risk to advancing age. Some studies have shown a higher rate of peripheral neuropathy in older patients, but clearly comorbid illnesses, such as diabetes, increase the disposition toward the development of peripheral neuropathy, which can sometimes produce profound functional impairment. Conclusive data associating age and central nervous system toxicity are limited to cerebellar toxicity associated with high doses of cytarabine used in induction chemotherapy for AML (23). Dose reduction is routine for elderly patients receiving cytarabine in high doses for AML.

V. DRUGS

Chemotherapeutic agents are frequently classified into general categories. Although there is no standard system for categorizing chemotherapeutic agents, most are classified according to mechanisms of action. Even though we have limited knowledge about all the mechanisms of action of most chemotherapeutic agents, this is a useful system. Common categories include the alkylating agents (e.g., cyclophosphamide) and antimetabolites (e.g., methotrexate). Some antineoplastic agents are classified according to their derivation. Plant derivatives (e.g., paclitaxel [Taxol]) and antibiotics (e.g., doxorubicin) are also useful chemotherapeutic agents. We will examine the most commonly used agents by category. We will also briefly review characteristic mechanisms of action and general toxicity associated with each class of drug. These issues have been well reviewed in detail by a variety of investigations and the interested reader is referred to these sources for more information (24, 25).

A. Alkylating Agents

Alkylating agents have been classic chemotherapeutic agents since their development as part of chemical warfare. These chemicals produce highly reactive compounds that form a covalent bond, usually with DNA. This leads to cross linking between the two strands of DNA, and other alterations to the DNA structure. Although they seem to be more active against actively dividing cells, possibly because these cells have less time to repair any alkylator damage to the DNA before the next division, alkylating agents are thought to be cell cycle phase nonspecific (will kill both actively dividing and resting cells). This makes these compounds effective against tumors with small growth fractions. The most commonly used alkylating agents include cyclophosphamide, chlorambucil, and melphalan.

Alkylating agents come in a variety of preparations, including intravenous and oral formulations. There is a wide dose range, and both cyclophosphamide and melphalan are used in low oral doses as well as very high-dose therapy, as in bone marrow transplant regimens. Toxicity is dose related and includes moderate nausea and myelotoxicity. Cyclophosphamide causes a serious cystitis via its metabolite, acrolein. Secondary malignancy, especially leukemia, is a well-recognized complication of exposure to these agents and is likely due to the intercalation of these alkylating agents into the DNA of normal host cells causing genetic changes leading to this malignant process.

Although alkylating agents share a common mechanism of action, they have a variety of other characteristics that are quite divergent because of different chemical structures. Thus, pharmacokinetic differences exist from agent to agent with regard to renal clearance (carboplatin) and the requirement for hepatic metabolism to be active (cyclophosphamide). Because of these differences, there is less cross resistance within the class of alkylating agents than other classes of chemotherapeutic agents.

B. Antimetabolites

The antimetabolites represent the most rational and well-studied class of cancer therapeutic agents. Methotrexate is widely used in clinical situations with activity against a variety of neoplasms (e.g., leukemia, lymphoma, breast cancer, osteogenic sarcoma) as well as nonmalignant disorders (e.g., psoriasis, rheumatoid arthritis, graft-vs-host disease). Methotrexate exerts its wide therapeutic activity via its ability to act as a folate antagonist. Although there are several possible ways to act as a folate antagonist, the major mechanism is via inhibition of the dihydrofolate reductase enzyme (DHFR) in the target cell. This depletes the cell of available reduced folates and inhibits de novo synthesis of purines and pyrimidines.

High doses of methotrexate can be safely given with an increased therapeutic window by providing a rescue dose of leucovorin several hours after the methotrexate. Toxicity from methotrexate includes myelotoxicity and gastrointestinal mucosal irritation. Chronic oral methotrexate can cause a severe hepatotoxicity.

Other critical intracellular pathways have been successfully targeted. The development of analogues to both purine and pyrimidine, the essential building blocks of DNA, have resulted in active chemotherapeutic agents. The pyrimidine analogue fluorouracil is widely used in colorectal carcinoma. Cytosine arabinoside (araC) is a nucleoside analogue of deoxycytidine and is active against a variety of hematological malignancies. Purine analogues include mercaptopurine, thioguanine, and hydroxyurea. The relatively newly discovered purine analogues 2-fluoroadenosine-5-phosphate (fludarabine), 2-chlorodeoxyadenosine (2-CDA), and deoxycoformycin (pentostatin) have further expanded this class of drugs. We will briefly discuss the mechanism of action of two representatives of this group.

Fluorouracil is a commonly used analogue of pyrimidine. There are many potential sites of action of fluorouracil. Fluorouracil requires intracellular activation to exert its antitumor effect. The major target appears to be thymidylate synthase, and the setting of reduced folate availability can further augment antitumor activity. Other mechanisms exist to explain fluorouracil's antitumor activity. Unfortunately, resistance is common, and each of the mechanisms of action can be evaded by tumor cells. The major toxicity from the fluorouracil is dose related and specifically affects the gastrointestinal mucosa and myeloid elements. Toxicity is related to the schedule of administration of the drug. Diarrhea can be severe and life threatening, especially when a regimen of continuous infusion is used. When leucovorin is used to augment the activity of fluorouracil, gastrointestinal symptoms are increased.

Fludarabine, one of the new nucleoside analogues, has become important in the treatment of cancer because of its activity in hematological malignancies like chronic lymphocytic leukemia. This is especially important to elderly patients because of the frequency of chronic lymphocytic leukemia in this population. Fludarabine is active against DNA polymerase-α and acts to stop DNA chain growth. Fludarabine also decreases concentrations of critical nucleotides. Fludarabine causes significant myelosupression and in high doses causes a severe neurotoxicity. The drug is cleared by the kidney, and emerging evidence suggests that the dose should be decreased as creatine clearance decreases.

C. Plant Derivatives

Many chemotherapeutic agents are natural products that originated from plants. There are three commonly used classes of drugs in this category. The vinca alkaloids (e.g., vincristine), the epipodophyllotoxins (e.g., etoposide), and taxanes (e.g., taxol) will be discussed.

The vincas are active in a wide range of cancers. The mechanism of action involves a disruption of microtubular assembly. Vincristine is one member of this family. The drug binds to tubulin and prevents mitoses, which is dependent on the microtubular assembly process for productive cell division. Vincristine is primarily metabolized in the liver. There is a high degree of protein binding and binding to cellular elements (platelets) in the blood stream. Toxicity is principally peripheral neuropathy, which is age related and occurs more frequently in older patients. Navelbine, a relatively newer vinca alkaloid, is less toxic to the peripheral nerves but has more hematological toxicity. Its activity profile has made it an attractive drug for use in elderly patients with breast cancer and lung cancer. The drugs in this family are vesicants and can cause significant local damage if they escape the venous system.

Etoposide represents the family of drugs from the mandrake plant, the epipodophyllotoxins. Like the vincas, etoposide exerts its antineoplastic activity via disruption of the microtubular assembly process, although the site of action is different than the vincas. Etoposide also has an additional mechanism of action. By binding to and disrupting topoisomerase II, etoposide induces direct strand breakage in DNA. This is probably the more clinically relevant action as an antineoplastic agent.

Etoposide appears to be cleared by a combination of renal and metabolic processes. Because of significant protein binding, the dose should be adjusted for patients with both renal and hepatic insufficiency. The major dose-limiting toxicity has been myelosupression. Because of the DNA strand breakage, etoposide has been associated with secondary malignancies, including leukemia.

The bark of the yew tree yielded a new compound known as Taxol. This family of drugs also includes taxotere. There is wide antitumor activity, initially noted in ovarian cancer. Taxol also acts via microtubule assembly. Taxol appears to stabilize the microtubules and prevent their normal disassembly. Taxol is hepatically metabolized and excreted in the bile and thus needs dose adjustments in the setting of hepatic insufficiency.

A high percentage of hypersensitivity reactions initially limited the wide use of Taxol, but with adequate premedications, these can be controlled. Toxicity is dose dependent and is reflected in neutropenia. Neurological toxicity can also occur. Initially, the drug was infused over 24 h, but now 3-h infusions are standard.

D. Antitumor Antibiotics

Several chemotherapeutic drugs have been derived from antibiotics. The anthracyclines have been extensively studied. These agents are widely active and used in a variety of tumors. They were originally isolated from the *Streptomyces* species of bacteria. Doxorubicin and daunorubicin were the first two drugs in this family, but there are now many representative anthracyclines. Other antitumor antibiotics include bleomycin and mitomycin C, but we will focus on anthracyclines in this section.

The anthracyclines are active in a wide range of tumors, including breast cancer, lung cancer, and sarcomas, as well as leukemias and lymphomas. The mechanism of action continues to be studied. Toposiomerase II inhibition with resultant DNA strand breakage appears to be an important mechanism. Additionally, he formation of oxygen radicals also enhances cytotoxicity. The anthracyclines appear to be metabolized significantly in the liver with minimal renal clearance. Dose adjustments on the basis of serum bilirubin are common.

The major toxicity from the anthracyclines includes myelosuppression and mucositis. The drugs are vesicants and local reactions can be severe. Cardiac toxicity is related to the cumulative dose over time and appears to be directly related to oxygen radical development. Preexisting cardiac dysfunction increases the risk of cardiac toxicity secondary to the drug. The antitumor antibiotics are also subject to the multidrug resistance (MDR) pump (see Sec. V. E). As such, resistance to these agents is frequently shared with other naturally occurring compounds.

E. Drug Resistance and Supportive Care

Many of the naturally occurring anticancer drugs share a mechanism of resistance. The MDR pump has the ability actively to pump chemotherapy drugs out of target cells. Many cancer cells become resistant to the chemotherapeutic drugs through this mechanism. Elderly patients may be particularly prone to this problem. In AML, for example, older patients have greater expression of the MDR gene product then younger ones. Methods to reverse resistance have focused on poisoning the MDR pump and represent an active area of research.

Chemotherapeutic treatments for cancer patients have long been associated with significant toxicity. Elderly patients have frequently suffered from many of the toxicities as previously noted. It is hoped that advances in supportive care will provide improvements in the toxicity to the therapeutic ratio of chemotherapeutic drugs.

One of the major advances in supportive care for chemotherapy has been the discovery of recombinant growth factors for hematopoietic cells. Currently, treatments to improve the neutrophil count are approved by the U.S., Food and Drug Administration (FDA). There has been extensive commentary on the appropriateness of the use of these growth factors. In acute leukemia, these growth factors can speed the recovery of neutrophil counts for patients going through high doses of chemotherapy but they do not appear to impart improved survival (26). Importantly, the use of these myeloid growth factors appears to be safe without clinically significant stimulation of the leukemic process.

Clinically important endpoints such as a decrease in the number of hospital days, fewer antibiotic days, and cost savings are important and can be improved with the use of these growth factors. Nonetheless, until there are clear survival benefits, there will be continued debate regarding the appropriateness of these expensive factors. The American Society of Clinical Oncology (ASCO) has formulated guidelines for the use of these growth factors (27). The interested reader is referred to that publication. Although there are no specific recommendations based on age alone (outside the situation in acute leukemia), the general recommendations in those guidelines are appropriate in elderly patients with cancer. Erythropoietin has been useful in the treatment of elderly patients with severe anemia, and it can be effective in the setting of transfusion dependency. Through experience, it can be a valuable adjunct in improving and maintaining the functional status of such patients.

Chemotherapy is an important part of the armamentarium for cancer treatment. With appropriate administration and monitoring, it can be used effectively for elderly cancer patients in adjuvant and curative as well as palliative settings.

REFERENCES

1. Borkowski JM, Duerr M, Donehower RC, Rowinsky EK, Chen TL, Ettinger DS, Grochow LB. Relation between age and clearance rate of nine investigational anticancer drugs from phase I pharmacokinetic data. Cancer Chemother Pharmacol 1994; 33:493–496.
2. Samet J, Hunt WC, Key C, Humble CG, Goodwin JS. Choice of cancer therapy varies with age of patient. JAMA 1986; 255:3385–3390.

3. Mor V, Masterson-Allen S, Goldberg RJ, Cummings FJ, Glicksman AS, Fretwell MD. Relationship between age at diagnosis and treatment received by cancer patients. J Am Geriatr Soc 1985; 33:585–589.
4. Champlin RE, Gajewski JL, Gdde DW. Treatment of acute myelogenous leukemia in the elderly. Semin Oncol 1989; 16:51–56.
5. Leslie WT. Chemotherapy in older cancer patients. Oncology 1992; 6(2):74–80.
6. Nerenz DR, Lov RR, Leventhal H, Easterling DV. Phychosocial consequences of cancer chemotherapy for elderly patients. Health Serv Res 1986; 6(2):961–76.
7. Vestal RE, Montamat SC, Nielson CP. Drugs in special patient groups: the elderly. In: Clinical Pharmacology—Basic Principles in Therapeutics, 3rd ed. KL Melmon, HF Morrelli, BB Hoffman, DW Nierenberg, eds. New York: McGraw-Hill, 1992, pp 851–874.
8. Vestal RE. Aging and pharmacology. Cancer 1997; 80(7):1302–1310.
9. Gautier M, Cohen HJ. Multiple Myeloma in the Elderly. Geriatr Soc 1994; 42:46.
10. Verbeeck RK, Cardinal J-A, Wallace SM. Effect of age and sex on the plasma binding of acidic and basic drugs. Eur J Clin Pharmacol 1984; 27:91–97.
11. Chrischilles EA, Foley DJ, Wallace RB, Lemke JH, Semla TP, Hanlon JT, et al. Use of medications by persons 65 and over: data from the established populations for epidemiologic studies of the elderly. J Gerontol 1992; 47:M137–44.
12. Woodhouse K, Wynne HA. Age-related changes in hepatic function. Implications for drug therapy. Drugs-Aging 1992; 2:243–255.
13. Ratain MJ, Schilsky RL, Conley BA, Egorin MJ. Pharmacodynamics in cancer therapy. J Clin Onc 1990; 8(10):1739–1753.
14. Walsh SJ, Begg CB, Carbone PP. Cancer chemotherapy in the elderly. Semin in Onc 1989; 16(1):66–75.
15. Begg CB, Elson PJ, Carbone PP. A study of excess hematologic toxicity in elderly patients treated on cancer chemotherapy protocols. In: Yancik R, ed. Cancer in the Elderly: Approaches to Early Detection and Treatment. New York: Springer-Verlag, 1989, pp 149–163.
16. Gelman RS, Taylor SC. Cychlophosphamide, methotrexate, and 5-flourouracil chemotherapy in women more than 65 years old with advanced breast cancer: The elimination of age trends in toxicity by using doses based on creatinine clearance. J Clin Oncol 1984; 2:1404–1413.
17. Kahn SB, Begg C, et al: Full dose versus attenuated dose daunorubicin, cytosine arabinoside, and 6-thioguanine in the treatment of acute nonlymphocytic leukemia in the elderly. J Clin Oncol 1984; 2:865–870.
18. Vose JM. Cytokine use in the older patient. Semin Oncol. 1995; 22(1),6–8.
19. Brower M, Asbury R, Kramer Z et al. Adjuvant chemotherapy of colorectal cancer in the elderly. Population-based experience. Proc Am Soc Clin Oncol 1993; 12:195.
20. Van Hoff DD, Layard MW, Basa P, et al. Risk factors for doxorubicin-induced congestive heart failure. Ann Intern Med 1979; 91:710–717.
21. Swain SM, Whaley FS, Gerber MC et al. Cardioprotection with dexrazoxane for doxorubicin-containing therapy in advanced breast cancer. J Clin Oncol 1997; 15(4):1318–1332.
22. Ginsberg SL, Comis RL. The pulmonary toxicity of antineoplastic agents. Semin Oncol 1982; 9:34–51.

23. Damon LE, Mass R, Linher CA: The association between high-dose cytarabine neurotoxicity and renal insufficiency. J Clin Oncol 1989; 7:1563.

24. Balducci L, Extermann M. Cancer chemotherapy in the older patient. Cancer 1997; 80(7):1317–1322.

25. Conti JA, Christman K. Cancer chemotherapy in the elderly. J Clin Gastroenterol 1995; 21(1):65–71.

26. Dombret H, Chastang C, Fenaux P et al. A controlled study of recombinant human granulocyte colony-stimulating factor in elderly patients after treatment for acute myelogenous leukemia. N Eng J Med 1993; 332:1678–1683.

27. Ozer H, Anderson JR, Anderson PN et al. American Society of Clinical Oncology Recommendations for the use of hematopoietic colony-stimulating factors: evidence-based, clinical practice guidelines. J Clin Oncol 1994; 12(11):2471–2508.

11

Breast Cancer

Gretchen Kimmick
Wake Forest University School of Medicine
Winston–Salem, North Carolina

I. INTRODUCTION

The foremost cancer diagnosis and the second leading cause of cancer-related death in American women, breast cancer, is becoming a "common disease" and is greatly feared. In 1997, the American Cancer Society estimated that there would be 181,600 new cases and 44,190 deaths due to breast cancer (1). Despite the great research effort to decrease the impact of this disease, few major advances have been made. The thrust of efforts must now be directed at prevention and early detection. In the geriatric population, this is no less of an issue. An estimated 48% of women diagnosed with metastatic breast cancer and 52% of all breast cancer deaths are in women greater than 65 years of age (2). In fact, breast cancer incidence and mortality rates increase with age (3, 4). In the SEER (Surveillance, Epidemiology, and End Results) Program database, breast cancer occurs in 60 per 100,000 women age less than 65 years old; 322 per 100,000 women aged over 65 years; and 375 per 100,000 women over 85 years old (2). Breast cancer–related mortality rates reach 172 women per 100,000 women over the age of 85 years as compared to 18 per 100,000 and 80 per 100,000 women aged 35–44 and 55–64 years, respectively (Fig. 1) (2). The size of the geriatric population is also growing. Since 1900, the population over the age of 65 years has increased 10-fold. Today, approximately 30 million Americans, or 1 in 9, are over 65 years old compared to only 1 in 15 persons in 1940. It is projected that in 2020, one in five Americans will be over 65 years old. Presently, almost half of all newly diagnosed breast cancers in the United States occur in women over age 65 years (2, 5), and it is estimated that, by 2030, two thirds of patients with breast cancer will be 65 years old or older (6).

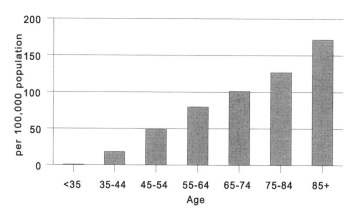

Figure 1   Age-adjusted breast cancer mortality rates

In general, the guiding principles of breast cancer therapy are early detection, aggressive local therapy to prevent recurrence of breast cancer at the primary tumor site, and systemic therapy to prolong survival by preventing the development or slowing the progression of metastatic disease. Treatment of the geriatric population should follow these principles—weighing risks and benefits of treatment and keeping in mind the remaining life span and presence of comorbid conditions. Historically, less aggressive management of breast cancer in older women has been reported. They are less likely to be screened (7, 8), more frequently diagnosed at advanced stage (2, 9, 10), more likely to have inadequate initial therapy, and less likely to participate in clinical trials (2, 11–14). Current research is directed at increasing the number of older women who have screening mammography; increasing breast cancer awareness; specifically defining the utility of surgical, medical, and radiation approaches to breast cancer in older women; and determining why older women do not participate in clinical trials.

Although not unique to older individuals, chronic disease is more common with advancing age. Almost 80% of people over the age of 65 years will have at least one chronic disease and approximately one third will have three or more chronic diseases (15). This is critically important for two distinct reasons: (a) the choice of therapy is influenced by the presence of coexisting diseases that may increase therapeutic complications, and (b) in clinical trials, the best measure of success of cancer treatment is survival, which may be limited by coexisting illness. Since older women with breast cancer are likely to suffer from more than one illness, and the risk of death increases as the number of major comorbid conditions increases, it is important to identify the specific cause of death in assessing the impact of breast cancer treatment on survival in a trial. Attempts have been made to develop a ''comorbidity index'' to assess the risk of dying from specific concurrent conditions among women diagnosed with breast cancer (16). Interestingly, Satariano and

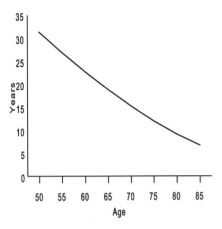

Figure 2 Average life expectancy by age for women.

coworkers found that even after adjusting for other confounding factors, women with two or more comorbidities are two times more likely than those without comorbid conditions to die from breast cancer (17). A second study by Satariano and Ragland examined the effect of comorbidity and breast cancer stage on 3-year survival in women with primary breast cancer (15). This longitudinal, observational study of 936 women aged 40–84 years found that women with three or more comorbid conditions had a 20-fold higher rate of mortality from causes other than breast cancer. The effects of comorbidity were independent of age, disease stage, tumor size, histological type, type of treatment, race, and social and behavioral factors. Comorbidity, therefore, increases the risk of death, in general, and increases breast cancer-related death.

The main goal of breast cancer therapy is to prolong survival. The life expectancy of older women is frequently viewed as limited. In actuality, the average life expectancy at various ages is longer than expected (Fig. 2) (3). An otherwise healthy woman who lives to be 65 years old is expected to live another 18.8 years and an 85-year old woman, 6.6 years.

II. STAGING AND PROGNOSTIC INDICATORS

Breast cancer stage is directly related to risk of recurrence and to survival (Fig. 3). Staging, as described by the American Joint Committee for Cancer (AJCC) guidelines (18), is useful in all patients for determination of prognosis and for making treatment-related decisions. The AJCC breast cancer staging criteria categorize the extent of malignancy according to the size of the primary lesion (T), the extent of

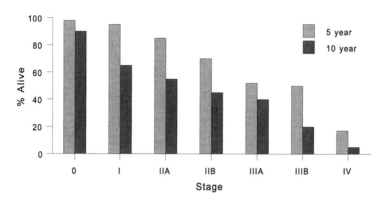

Figure 3   Breast cancer survival by stage. *Source*: Data from Ref. 176.

nodal involvement (N), and the occurrence of metastases (M) (Table 1). Tumor size
(the largest diameter of the infiltrating component) and the extent of nodal involvement (number of axillary nodes removed and number positive) are determined from
specimen pathology. For the extent of nodal involvement to reflect the prognosis
accurately, at least six nodes should be examined. The pathology report should also
include histological type and tumor grade; assessment of tumor necrosis, vascular
invasion, lymphatic invasion, and skin involvement; percentages of ductal carcinoma in situ and invasive carcinoma in the primary lesion; and analysis of estrogen
(ER) and progesterone (PR) receptors in the primary lesion. In the past, ER and PR
determinations were done using biochemical methods that required $0.5-1.0$ cm^3 of
tumor tissue; current immunohistochemical methods allow accurate receptor assays
on even the smallest tissue samples and can be done on paraffin-embedded material.
Other markers such as tumor DNA content and S-phase activity by flow cytometry,
Mib-1, oncogene expression such as c-*erbB*-2 (HER-2/neu), epidermal growth factor receptors, and protease activity such as cathepsin-D can also be determined from
paraffin sections and may be useful prognostically.

Preoperative evaluation includes complete history and physical examination,
mammography, chest radiograph, complete blood count, and serum chemistries
(with liver function tests and calcium). These studies are helpful in determining the
presence of comorbid illness in addition to finding metastases. Bilateral mammography should be performed on all patients to evaluate both the ipsilateral and contralateral breast for other nonpalpable lesions. Asymptomatic patients with an unremark-
able preliminary evaluation require no further staging procedures. Skeletal surveys,
radionuclide bone scanning, and computerized tomographic (CT) scanning of the
brain, chest, abdomen, and pelvis are unnecessary in asymptomatic patients with
normal physical findings and initial blood work. The use of tumor markers, such

Table 1 Staging System for Cancer of the Breast—AJCC Criteria

Symbol TNM system	Meaning
TX	Primary tumor cannot be assessed
T0	No evidence of primary tumor
Tis	Carcinoma in situ: intraductal carcinoma, lobular carcinoma in situ, or Paget's disease of the nipple with no tumor
T1	Tumor ≤ 2 cm in greatest dimension
	T1a ≤ 0.5 cm in greatest dimension
	T1b > 0.5 cm but not >1 cm in greatest dimension
	T1c > 1 cm but not >2 cm in greatest dimension
T2	Tumor >2 cm but not >5 cm in greatest dimension
T3	Tumor >5 cm in greatest dimension
T4	Tumor of any size with direct extension to chest wall[a] or skin (includes inflammatory carcinoma)
NX	Regional lymph nodes cannot be assessed (e.g., previously removed)
N0	No regional lymph-node metastases
N1	Metastasis to movable ipsilateral axillary nodes
N2	Metastases to ipsilateral axillary nodes fixed to one another or to other structures
N3	Metastases to ipsilateral internal mammary lymph nodes
MX	Presence of distant metastasis cannot be assessed
M0	No evidence of distant metastasis
MI	Distant metastases (including metastases to ipsilateral supraclavicular lymph nodes)
Clinical Stage	
0	Tis, N0, M0
1	T1, N0, M0
IIA	T0, N1, M0
	T1, N1, M0
	T2, N0, M0
IIB	T2, N1, M0
	T3, N0, M0
IIIA	T0 or T1, N2, M0
	T2, N2, M0
	T3, N1 or N2, M0
IIIB	T4, any N, M0
	Any T, N3, M0
IV	Any T, any N, MI

[a] The chest wall includes the ribs, intercostal muscles, and serratus anterior muscle, but not the pectoral muscle.
Source: Ref. 14.

as the carcinoembryonic antigen (CEA) and mucin antigen (CA 15-3) in patient management is controversial and not recommended on a routine basis.

Infiltrating ductal carcinoma is the most common histological breast tumor type in older women, and it accounts for 75–80% of cases (2, 19). Reports claim that aggressive tumor types, medullary carcinoma and inflammatory cancer, are seen less frequently and that indolent histologies, colloid and papillary carcinoma, are more common in older than in younger women (19, 20). These are rare histologies, however, representing less than 10% of mammary carcinomas in women aged 85 years and older. Prognostic markers vary with age and indicate that breast tumors in the older population may be slower growing, more differentiated, and more hormone responsive. The thymidine-labeling index is lower (21), a greater proportion of cells are estrogen receptor positive (22), and tumors are more frequently moderately to well-differentiated (20, 23). Despite this, survival is similar in older and younger women with localized and regional stages of breast cancer, and, paradoxically, older women seem to fare worse with metastatic disease (2, 24).

III. PREVENTION AND DIAGNOSIS

A. Prevention

Risk factors for breast cancer include older age, white race, family history of breast cancer, early menarche, late age at birth of first child, late menopause, history of benign breast disease (hyperplasia/atypical hyperplasia), radiation exposure, obesity, taller stature, oral contraceptive use, postmenopausal estrogen-replacement therapy, and alcohol use (25). Still other factors which remain controversial include high dietary fat intake; low consumption of micronutrients such as vitamins A, E, and C and selenium; and high coffee consumption (25). Primary prevention of breast cancer would require modification of known predisposing factors. Unfortunately, there are no easily modifiable risk factors for breast cancer, and no method of primary prevention has yet proven effective. The National Surgical Adjuvant Breast and Bowel Project Prevention Trial (NSABP P1) is examining the potential protective effect of tamoxifen in women at high risk for breast cancer, including all women over the age of 60 years (26). Results are not yet available.

A family history of breast cancer, implying a genetic defect, may be important in 6–19% of all cases of breast cancer (27, 28). Genetic predisposition is particularly important in early-onset breast cancer, diagnosed before age 50 years, but is probably not a major factor in the geriatric population. BRCA1, the first gene found to be related to breast cancer, has been located on chromosome 17q, and accounts for approximately 2–3% of breast cancers and 16–45% of familial breast cancers; it portends an increased risk for both breast and ovarian cancers (29–31). Women who are carriers for BRCA1 and have a strong family history of breast cancer are estimated to have an 85% lifetime risk for developing breast cancer; 51% will develop breast cancer by the time they are 50 years old and 87% by the age of 70 years (32,

33). Women with BRCA1 who live to the age of 70 years have a cumulative risk of 65% for bilateral breast cancers.

Another gene, BRCA2, has been located on chromosome 13q (34). Linkage studies suggest that 35% of high-risk families may have BRCA2 gene mutations (33). BRCA2 may be more important in postmenopausal cases of breast cancer. The lifetime breast cancer risk for BRCA2 mutation carriers in families where breast cancer is common is estimated to be 85%. In women who have a BRCA1 or BRCA2 mutation but not necessarily a strong family history of breast cancer, the estimated risk of breast cancer is lower—only 56% by the age of 70 years (31). There are probably many modifying factors, including genetic, hormonal, and environmental, that determine whether a genetic mutation will lead to cancer.

B. Screening

Secondary prevention of breast cancer involves screening mammography and breast physical examination. Promotion of these two measures of early detection has reduced breast cancer–related mortality. Current guidelines for screening mammography recommend its use in women between the ages of 40 and 75 years (35, 36). In women aged 50–59 years, the use of mammography and physical examination biennially reduces mortality by 60% over 3–7 years; the use of mammography alone reduces mortality by 40% (37). Swedish trials have included women up to 74 years old and found a significant reduction in mortality for women up to the age of 70 years (RR 0.71, CI 0.56–0.91 for screened versus nonscreened women aged 60–69 years), and a trend toward reduced mortality, although not significant, for women aged 70–74 years (RR 0.94, CI 0.60–1.46) (38).

No large randomized trials have been done to evaluate the use of screening mamography in women over 65 years old. With age, however, the breast changes from a dense glandular organ to a less dense, smaller organ containing more fat; this change in architecture increases the contrast between normal and abnormal breast tissue making it easier to find malignancies by mamography in older women. Theoretically, mammography should be beneficial. There is evidence from retrospective data and decision analyses supporting its use.

Faulk and colleagues compared age-specific screening results in 10,915 women old than age 65 years (old) and 21,226 women aged 50–64 years (young) who were referred by a physician for mammography (39). The overall rate of abnormal interpretations was 5% in both young and old age groups. Older women were twice as likely to have abnormal screening findings judged to be suspicious for malignancy (10 vs 5%, P = NS) and were also more likely to have abnormalities judged to be characteristic of malignancy (4 vs 1%, P = NS). The number of breast cancer cases among abnormal screening interpretations (positive predictive value, PPV), the number of malignancies among biopsies prompted by screening (biopsy yield), and the number of women with cancer per 1000 examinations (cancer detection rate) were all higher in the older subgroup (Table 2). The cancers diagnosed

Table 2 PPV, Biopsy Yield, and Cancer Detection Rate Among Younger and Older Women

Age (years)	PPV (%)	Biopsy yield (%)	Cancer detection rate[a]
50–64	12	40	5.7
65+	20	56	9.2

PPV, positive predictive value.
[a] Number of women with cancer per 1000 examinations.

in the older group were also smaller and more frequently node negative. In this study, the differences observed were too small to reach statistical significance. A consistent trend toward improved prognosis for older women, however, was noted and further study is warranted. In fact, screening older women may find tumors at a smaller size. Wilson and colleagues retrospectively reviewed clinical records and radiological examinations of 52 women over the age of 75 years with breast cancer, comparing cancers found at screening with those identified by symptoms (40). Breast cancers were significantly smaller and of earlier stage in the screened women (Table 3). Although this was a small study, the results were statistically significant; that is, mammographically detected breast cancers are of earlier stage than those manifested as palpable masses. Because the prognosis of breast cancer is directly proportional to tumor size, screened women over 75 years old have a better prognosis than those diagnosed based on symptoms.

The decision to screen older women is complicated by considerations of increased comorbidity and reduced life expectancy (41–43). The life expectancy of healthy women who live to 65, 75, and 85 years old is 18.8 years, 11.9 years, and 6.6 years, respectively (3). To evaluate the cost–benefit ratio of breast cancer screening (clinical examination and mammography) in women older than 65 years with and

Table 3 Breast Cancers in Screened and Unscreened Women Over Age 75 years

	Screened	Unscreened	P value[a]
n	16	36	
Tumor size (cm)	1.1	2.1	<.0005
In situ (%)	6	11	<.0005
Minimal stage[b] (%)	82	33	<.0005
Lymph Nodes +(%)	0	47	.009

[a] P values for mean size determined by t-test; all others were by χ^2 test.
[b] Minimal stage defined as nonpalpable and/or <2 cm in size.
Source: Data from Ref. 40.

without comorbid conditions, Mandelblatt et al. used a decision analysis model (44). In this report, early detection of breast cancer by screening yielded increases in life expectancy for all older women despite age and coexisting medical conditions, although the magnitude of benefit decreased with increasing age. In this model, screening increased life expectancy by 617 days and 178 days in average-health women aged 65–69 and ≥85 years, respectively, who were found to have breast cancer. With congestive heart failure, screening increased life expectancy by 311 and 126 days for women found to have breast cancer, aged 65–69 and ≥85 years, respectively. The cost-effectiveness ratio of screening mammography and breast examination during a routine office visit compared favorably to other commonly used screening tests such as cervical cancer screening and fecal occult blood testing in older persons. There is no inherent reason, therefore, to impose an upper age limit for breast cancer screening.

In summary, recent guidelines do not recommend the use of screening mammograms in women older than 75 years, because there is no evidence that it decreases breast cancer–related mortality. Only a large randomized trial, focused on women 75 years old and older, will define the value of mammography in this population. Since randomized controlled trials have already proven the benefit of screening mammography in women aged 50–64 years, and the average life expectancy of women age up to 85 years is greater than 10 years (3), it can be inferred that screening will benefit women aged 65–85 years. It is of questionable benefit to use screening mammography in women more than 85 years old because of the limited life expectancy, anxiety, and discomfort.

Older women are less likely to be screened (7, 8). In 1991, only 35–59% of women aged 65–74 years used mammography (45), and according to a retrospective review of 1990 Medicare bills, mammography use decreases with increasing age (46). On January 1, 1991, Medicare began offering reimbursement for screening mammography every 2 years. Despite this, mammography use in women over 65 years old remains low. Only 36.9% of a representative sample of 4110 women 65 years and older had mammography during the years 1991 and 1992; 14.4% of those lacking supplemental insurance versus 44.7% of those with employer-sponsored supplemental insurance, 40.1% of those with self-purchased supplemental insurance, and 23.9% of those with Medicaid supplemental insurance (47). Barriers that prevent optimum screening in these women include negative physician and patient attitudes, lack of accessibility, lack of information, and competing concurrent acute medical conditions (48).

With respect to patient compliance, it appears that the physician's enthusiastic recommendation is key. In a telephone survey of 972 women, 724 of whom were older than 65 years, the factors that influenced utilization of mammography included age, race, health status, and physician-patient communication (49). Only physician-patient communication significantly predicted a recent mammogram or clinical breast examination. In an analysis by Leather and Roberts, older patients who were alerted to the importance of mammography by a physician were more likely to have the procedure done (50). The use of nonphysician personnel to enhance breast cancer screening in older women has also proven to be successful in improving screening rates (51–53).

Primary care physicians recommend fewer screening mammograms for older than for younger women (48). Reasons that physicians do not recommend screening mammograms in older women include cost to older patients and lack of insurance, older patient refusal, physician forgetfulness, confusion regarding guidelines, discomfort or pain, coexisting medical illnesses that limit life expectancy, patient's living situation, and age alone (48, 54, 55). In a cross-sectional survey utilizing clinical case vignettes, and questions about breast cancer screening practices and attitudes toward ACS guidelines, Marwill and colleagues analyzed the impact of patients' age, comorbidity, functional status, and quality of life on the physicians' decisions to recommend screening mammograms for older women (55). Surveys were mailed to a random sample of Massachusetts internists, obstetrician/gynecologists, family/general practice physicians, and geriatricians. Sixty-five percent responded. Respondents recommended periodic clinical breast examinations and mammograms in 94% of women aged 65 to 74 years; 89% reported performing periodic clinical breast examinations and 79% recommended mammography for women aged 75–84 years. Only 48% strongly agreed with ACS guidelines for annual mammography for women over the age of 65 years. Age, dementia, and nursing home residence were patient factors associated with decreased mammogram use. Limited mobility and chronic medical problems were not.

C. Diagnosis

In a postmenopausal woman, any palpable breast mass requires biopsy. Mammography may be helpful in characterizing the mass and/or finding other suspicious areas; however, mammography may not image palpable lesions in as many as 20% of patients (56). The majority of palpable masses in older women are malignant. Fine-needle aspiration (FNA) biopsy is a highly reliable method of tissue diagnosis. If the FNA is negative or inconclusive, unless the mass proves to be a cyst and resolves after aspiration, further biopsy, either repeat FNA or excision, is necessary. For patients who have a mass that is characteristic of malignancy on either physical examination or mammography, initial excision of the lesion or mastectomy and axillary dissection may be preferable to a two-stage procedure involving an FNA or excisional biopsy followed by definitive surgery.

Mammographically detected breast lesions, palpable or not, also require biopsy. If these are nonpalpable, either stereotactic or needle-localized biopsy is necessary. Stereotactic large-core needle biopsy is now widely accepted as a reliable method of providing a histological diagnosis for mammographically detected suspicious and indeterminate breast lesions (57–59). This technique is relatively noninvasive and allows pathological evaluation of a mammographic abnormality. Needle-localization biopsy allows for removal of the abnormal lesion for tissue diagnosis.

For some patients, after careful discussion, follow-up with physical examination and repeat mammography in several months is appropriate. For most patients, the fear of breast cancer and the possibility that even a low-risk lesion may prove to be malignant is a compelling motive for lesion biopsy or excision.

IV. BREAST CARCINOMA IN SITU

Widespread use of screening mammography has led to a major increase in the diagnosis of ductal carcinoma in situ (DCIS) (60–62). These tumors are suggested by microcalcifications found on screening mammography and are usually nonpalpable. Before the use of mammography, DCIS lesions were uncommon and usually detected as a large breast mass. Mastectomy cures almost all patients, but lesser procedures such as lumpectomy and breast irradiation probably are as effective for patients with lesions less than 2.5 cm (63, 64). Axillary dissection finds metastases in less than 1% of patients and is generally not recommended. Excision alone, without local radiation therapy, may be appropriate for patients with lesions <2.0–2.5 cm in diameter with generous ($\geq$ 1 cm) margins of normal tissue surrounding the in situ component (65).

Lobular carcinoma in situ (LCIS) is more common in premenopausal patients, lacks clinical and mammographic signs, is bilateral in 25–35% of patients. It is not a palpable lesion and is usually an incidental finding after breast biopsy. Treatment options range from observation to bilateral mastectomy (66). Of note, 20–40% of patients with LCIS subsequently develop invasive ductal cancer, with both the ipsilateral and contralateral breast at similar risk. The diagnosis of LCIS, therefore, serves as marker of subsequent risk of breast cancer. Most experts recommend close follow-up of these patients without aggressive surgery.

V. MANAGEMENT OF NONMETASTATIC BREAST CANCER

A. Local Therapy of Breast Cancer

For the older woman with stage I–II breast cancer, the major options for local treatment include modified radical mastectomy and lumectomy followed by radiation. The choice of therapy must be individualized and based on overall health status (whether or not general anesthesia will be tolerated), preference for breast preservation, and ability and willingness to attend daily radiation sessions for 4–6 weeks.

1. Mastectomy

Modified radical mastectomy with axillary dissection and lumpectomy with axillary dissection followed by local radiation are the accepted local treatments for early breast cancer (67–69). Long-term follow-up and an overview of randomized trials claim equivalent survival for the two modalities (67, 70, 71) and local recurrence rates are generally less than 5% (72). There are now a number of studies confirming that healthy older people tolerate surgery, such as mastectomy, well (73–75) and that survival following surgery is similar in older and younger groups (73, 76, 77). Operative mortality is generally in the range of 1–3%. The most common causes of postoperative morbidity noted are cardiovascular and neurological problems (78). Herbsman and coworkers analyzed survival based on age in a retrospective analysis of 1780 patients with breast cancer, 138 of whom were over the age of 70 years (76). These women all underwent some form of mastectomy: simple mastectomy, modified radical mastectomy, or radical mastectomy. Survival was similar in all age groups, irrespective of race, type of surgery, histology, tumor size, or stage (Table 4).

Mastectomy, although not as cosmetically pleasing as conservative local surgery in most cases, is an excellent method of obtaining local control of breast cancer with a minimum number of hospital visits. In older women, with serious comorbid conditions and/or limited mobility or transportation, limiting the required number of hospital trips may be a major consideration. It is important, however, to include the patient in the treatment decision, research shows that the quality of life and the adjustment to the diagnosis of breast cancer is better in women who participate in treatment planning and decisions (79–82).

Sandison and colleagues reported the definitive treatment decisions of 50 women over 70 years old (83). All had a new diagnosis of breast cancer and were offered four treatment options (a) tamoxifen alone, (b) complete local excision and tamoxifen, (c) modified radical mastectomy and tamoxifen, and (d) complete local excision, radiotherapy, and tamoxifen. Thirty-eight of the 50 women in the study chose their treatment and the remainder elected to let the surgeon decide. One patient chose tamoxifen alone, 2 chose complete local excision and tamoxifen, 4 chose mastectomy, and 31 chose conservative surgery, radiotherapy, and tamoxifen. All

Table 4 Survival of Women with Early Breast Cancer by Age and Stage

	Age (years)			
	<50	50–59	60–69	>70
Overall survival (%)				
5-year	54.7	65.4	59.9	53.5
10-year	39.5	53.5	42.6	41.1
5-year survival (%)				
local disease	70	81	74	65
regional disease	39	48	50	47

Source: Data from Ref. 76.

patients who underwent breast-conserving therapy were either very happy or happy with the cosmetic result at 6 and 12 months. All but two of the women who chose their treatment considered that they had made the right choice. At 12 months of follow-up, only two women were unhappy with their choice of treatment.

Postmastectomy radiation therapy may decrease the incidence of systemic metastases and prolong survival (84). In premenopausal women with axillary lymph node involvement, the data are quite convincing (85, 86). In healthy older women with large tumors or axillary node involvement, local adjuvant radiotherapy, even if mastectomy is the chosen surgery, should be considered.

2. Breast-Conserving Surgery

Historically, older women are less likely than younger women to have breast-conserving surgery (BCS). Lazovich and colleagues noted that the likelihood of BCS decreases with increasing age ($P < .01$), in their study of 8095 women with stages I and II breast cancer, 42.4% of women under the age of 50 years underwent BCS compared to 31.5, 26.7, and 25.4% of women aged 60–69, 70–79, and $\geq$80 years, respectively (87). Crivellari and coworkers found only 7.5% of 115 women with a mean age of 75 years underwent BCS followed by RT (88). The reasons for this trend have not been fully defined but probably include both patient and physician preferences. In the absence of contraindications to surgery, however, we recommend that the option of breast-conserving surgery followed by RT be discussed with older patients.

Women over 70 years old were not generally included in the trials comparing mastectomy to lumpectomy and radiation therapy. The biological rationale for breast preservation, however, can be extrapolated to older women. In fact, nonrandomized data suggest that older women may have a particularly low rate of breast recurrence after lumpectomy and radiotherapy compared to younger women (78). A study of 518 women treated at the Institut Curie in Paris observed 10-year local control rates of 97, 85, and 71% in women over 55, 33–45, and 32 years of age or younger, respectively (72). Other reports support that the frequency of breast recurrences decreases with increasing age (89, 90). The local recurrence rates for patients treated with quadrantectomy alone in the report of Veronesi et al. were 3.8 and 8.7% for women age more than 55 years old and 46–55 years old, respectively (89). The long-term results of a randomized trial comparing mastectomy versus conservative therapy followed by local radiotherapy also support this contention (91). In node-negative patients, the relative risk of local recurrence is 1.9 (95% CI 1.1–3.4, $P = .02$) for women younger than 50 years old versus 50 years old or older.

Local breast recurrence after lumpectomy adversely effects the quality of life and can be substantially diminished using RT. In a randomized study at 12 years of follow-up, Fisher and coworkers demonstrated that the rate of local failure after lumpectomy to histologically negative margins was decreased from 35 to 10% by the addition of postoperative irradiation ($P < 0.001$) (67). In this study, the majority of local recurrences were observed in the first 5 postoperative years.

Breast radiation is well tolerated in older women. Wyckoff and coworkers found a comparable number of treatment interruptions, overall length of treatment, and frequency of cutaneous and hematological toxicity in women who underwent conservative surgery and radiation, aged 65 years or older versus younger than 65 years old (92). Kantorowitz and coworkers retrospectively reviewed the outcome in patients treated with segmental mastectomy with or without RT and confirmed the benefit and tolerability of RT in women older than 60 years of age (74). One third to one half of women who underwent segmental mastectomy alone versus only 2 of 77 women treated with segmental mastectomy and RT had local failure. Complications of segmental mastectomy and RT (such as breast and arm edema, pneumonitis, pulmonary fibrosis, and myositis) were modest, cosmesis was acceptable, and there was no significant increase in morbidity. With a follow-up of 4 years, disease-free and overall survival were longer in the RT-treated patients; they were also more likely to retain their breast compared to women who had a segmental mastectomy alone.

3. Axillary Dissection

The role of axillary dissection in women, especially older women, with very small breast tumors is under scrutiny. This procedure is regarded primarily as a staging procedure and secondarily as a form of locoregional control. Currently, some form of systemic therapy is recommended for any woman with a tumor ≥ 1 cm in size regardless of lymph node status (93). The value of axillary dissection as a staging procedure, therefore, must be carefully weighed against the possible complications.

Major complications of axillary dissection are infrequent and include injury or thrombosis of the axillary vein and injury to the motor nerves of the axilla. However, there is significant morbidity, both short- and long-term, associated with axillary dissection. In women undergoing breast-conserving surgery, axillary dissection makes both general anesthesia and hospitalization necessary, whereas lumpectomy alone is an outpatient procedure that can be done using local anesthetic. Other potential problems associated with axillary dissection include seroma formation, shoulder dysfunction, anesthesia in intercostobrachial nerve distribution, lymphedema of the arm, increased breast edema after lumpectomy and radiotherapy, and unsatisfactory cosmesis.

Lymphedema is particularly troubling. Its incidence is reported to range from 1.5 to 62.5% (78). This wide range is probably a reflection of the fact that lymphedema is not life threatening, usually mild, rarely limits function, and is underreported. In older women with comorbid conditions such as arthritis and neurological deficits, in whom mobility and use of the upper extremities may already be a concern, lymphedema and the pain associated with axillary dissection may severely restrict motion and functional capacity.

It has been suggested that axillary dissection be foregone in certain subgroups of women with small primary breast cancers. In women with very small tumors (defined as <1 cm), axillary node involvement has been found in 12–37% (94, 95). Physical examination may assist in predicting nodal involvement, but its false-negative and false-positive rates of 27–32 and 25–31% are high (96). Barth et al. examined the influence on axillary lymph node metastases of 11 clinical and pathological factors: tumor size, lymphovascular invasion, nuclear grade, S-phase, ploidy, palpability, age, estrogen and progesterone receptor status, HER2/neu, and histology (94). Twenty-three percent of the 918 patients reviewed had axillary lymph node metastases. In multivariate analysis, lymphovascular invasion, tumor palpability, nuclear grade, and tumor size were the only independent predictors of axillary lymph node metastases. Among 117 patients with nonpalpable, non–high-grade, ≤1 cm tumors without lymphovascular invasion, the incidence of axillary lymph node involvement was only 3%. In the 43 patients with palpable Tlc tumors of high grade and with lymphovascular invasion, 43% had axillary lymph node metastases. Fein and colleagues also performed a large (1598 patients with T1 and 2 breast tumors who had level I/II axillary dissection) retrospective study to define a subset of women who were at low risk for axillary lymph node metastases (95). Axillary lymph node metastases were present in 27.8% of this patient population. By multivariate analysis, the presence of lymphovascular invasion, clinically as opposed to mammographically detected tumors, and larger tumors predicted axillary lymph node involvement. Women with mammographically detected, nonpalpable tumors measuring ≤5 mm had no axillary lymph node metastases. Parameters of tumor size, whether or not the primary lesion is palpable, and lymphovascular invasion are key to predicting lymph node metastases; women with small (<0.5 cm), nonpalpable tumors that are not invading lymphovascular spaces have a very low probability of lymph node metastases and may be appropriate candidates to forego axillary dissection.

Some investigators suggest that older women do not require axillary lymph node dissection, because the knowledge gained does not influence adjuvant treatment choice. Feigelson and coworkers reviewed 10 years of tumor registry data for women 70 years old and older with T1 breast cancers; 78 cases were identified (97). When women were divided into groups by the approach taken toward the axilla, no difference in adjuvant treatment, axillary recurrence rates, or survival was found. Naslund et al. retrospectively reviewed case notes of 166 women aged 75 years or more who underwent primary surgery for breast cancer at Danderyd Hospital in Stockholm, Sweden, to see if the information gained from axillary dissection influenced postoperative adjuvant treatment. Axillary dissection was performed in 83% of cases. According to the treatment guidelines for breast cancer, the information gained from the procedure influenced postoperative treatment in only 36% of patients at their institution. In a retrospective study of Haffty and colleagues, systemic therapy practice patterns and long-term outcome were examined with respect to axillary dissection (98). Current practice patterns of 292 patients with invasive breast cancer who underwent conservative surgery and were treated within a 3-year time period were reviewed with respect to patient age, primary tumor size, clinical nodal status, and presenting symptoms. Of the 292 patients, 17.8% had axillary lymph node involvement yet the vast majority (91.8%) received some form of systemic adjuvant therapy, 38% chemotherapy and 53.8% tamoxifen. When broken down by age, in patients older than 50 years who presented with nonpalpable disease axillary dissection appeared to have a minimal impact on subsequent management. Of patients older than 50 years who presented with nonpalpable disease, 94.9% had node-negative disease and, of these, 82% received adjuvant tamoxifen. Long-term outcome measures of distant metastasis, disease-free survival, and overall survival were also examined in 565 patients who underwent axillary dissection as part of their initial surgery and were compared to 390 patients who had not undergone axillary dissection. Interestingly, there was no statistically significant difference in these.

In order to decrease the complication rate of axillary dissection, less invasive procedures are under investigation. The most promising of these is lymphatic mapping and sentinel node biopsy (99). This procedure allows identification and sampling of the first node in the lymphatic basin to receive lymphatic flow; that is, presumptive removal of the initial site of metastatic disease. Promising results using this technique have been achieved. Clinical trials are now being developed to compare sentinel lymph node biopsy and axillary dissection. In healthy older women who are candidates for clinical trials where lymph node status is a basis for patient selection, we do recommend that axillary dissection be performed.

B. Hormone Therapy as an Alternative to Definitive Surgery

For many older patients, especially those with advanced but localized tumors (T3 or T4 tumors) and those with serious comorbid conditions or frailty, the antiestrogen tamoxifen may be a reasonable initial treatment. Retrospective series and prospective trials, however, have demonstrated tamoxifen alone to be the least effective single modality for local control in patients with operable breast cancer. Response rates range from 28 to 67% with one third to two thirds of patients developing progressive local disease necessitating salvage therapy with radiotherapy or surgery (100–113) (Table 5). Local failure is the major concern in patients treated with tamoxifen only (114). Since the morbidity associated with local recurrence adversely affects the quality of life, treatment with mastectomy or lumpectomy and radiation therapy are preferred.

The combination of tamoxifen and hypofractionated once-weekly radiation (6.5 Gy per fraction for a total of five fractions to the breast and seven to the tumor bed) has recently been studied in older women (115). Local control was achieved in 81% for T1 and 96% for T2 tumors at 3 years. Overall and disease-free survival at 3 years were comparable to other treatment approaches. This strategy may be useful in older women who are unable to undergo surgery. Giving weekly, as opposed to daily, radiation treatments is more convenient for frail older people and has been proven to be effective in early-stage breast cancer in other studies.

Table 5 Local Treatment of Early Breast Cancer in Older Women[a]

	Overall survival	Disease-free survival	Breast recurrence	References
Modified radical mastectomy	82–85% at 5 yrs	83–95% at 5 yrs	0–30[b]	67,169,170
Lumpectomy and radiation	65–90% at 5 yrs 50–77% at 10 yrs	85% at 5 yrs 70–90% at 10 yrs	0–13%	171,172
Radiation and tamoxifen	87% at 3 yrs	72% at 3 yrs	14%	173
Wide excision and tamoxifen	67–75% at 5 yrs	75–92% at 5 yrs	3–32%	174,175 111,169 170
Wide excision alone	69% at 5 yrs 30–41% at 9 yrs	85% at 5 yrs	3–19%	74,89,90
Tamoxifen alone	47–80% at 2 yrs 47–50% at 5 yrs 42% at 10 yrs	NA	30–60%	103,106,107, 111,112,113

NA, not applicable.
[a] Data for overall and disease-free survivals were pooled from the references given.
[b] Breast, chest wall, and regional lymph node recurrences.

C. Systemic Adjuvant Therapy

Current management guidelines recommend the use of adjuvant systemic treatment for any woman with an invasive breast cancer measuring >1 cm in size (93). Tamoxifen has a well established role in adjuvant therapy for postmenopausal women with estrogen receptor–positive, node-positive or node-negative, breast cancer.

After initial management with mastectomy or lumpectomy followed by RT, women with stages I and II breast cancer have a 10-year risk of recurrence of 25–30 and 50–90%, respectively (116). Breast cancer recurrence is, therefore, a major concern. In older women with breast cancer metastatic to axillary lymph nodes, breast cancer–related deaths are more common than deaths due to other nonmalignant disease (15). In two large adjuvant trials of tamoxifen therapy in older patients with node-positive breast cancer, only 10–20% of patients died of causes unrelated to breast cancer (117, 118).

1. Adjuvant Hormonal Therapy

Adjuvant therapy for stage II breast cancer in women over the age of 70 years typically consists of hormonal manipulation, usually with the antiestrogen tamoxifen, regardless of hormone receptor status. The recent comprehensive meta-analysis by the Early Breast Cancer Trial Collaborative Group (EBCTCG) of adjuvant therapy trials showed that postmenopausal patients treated with tamoxifen, including those more than 70 years old, had a significantly lower risk of tumor recurrence (29% lower) and death (20% lower) when compared to those randomized to observation alone (119). This benefit was noted in women with hormone receptor–negative (reduced tumor recurrence by 16% and death by 16%) as well as hormone receptor–positive (reduced tumor recurrence by 36% and death by 23%) tumors.

Other trials have confirmed tamoxifen's value in older women with hormone receptor–positive tumors (118, 120, 121). Castiglione and coworkers studied 320 women aged 66 to 80 years treated for 1 year with tamoxifen and low-dose prednisone or placebo (117). The 8-year disease-free survival was 36 versus 22% in the treatment and placebo groups, respectively. Cummings and coworkers compared tamoxifen to placebo as adjuvant therapy in a group of 168 women 65–84 years old with stage II breast cancer, the tamoxifen-treated patients had longer median times to relapse (7.4 years vs 4.4 years), less contralateral breast cancers, and less distant and bone-only first recurrences (118).

Five years of adjuvant tamoxifen therapy is currently recommended (122). Early trials proved the benefit of tamoxifen administered for 1 or 2 years (123). More recent studies using longer durations of treatment have produced superior results (119, 124), but 10 years has not been shown to be superior to 5 years (122).

2. Adjuvant Chemotherapy

Combination chemotherapy in stage II premenopausal and postmenopausal (<70 years old) patients, with or without lymph node involvement, unequivocally improves relapse-free and overall survival (119). Chemotherapy has not yielded as impressive results in postmenopausal women, however, as it has in premenopausal women. In the 1992 meta-analysis (119), adjuvant chemotherapy, compared to no chemotherapy, reduced mortality by 10% in women aged 60–69 years compared to 25% in women younger than 50 years old. Many of the breast cancer adjuvant trials included in the meta-analysis excluded women over the age of 70 years (125–129). Of the 75,000 patients in the meta-analysis, only 300 women over the age of 70 years received chemotherapy (119).

Arbitrarily lower doses of chemotherapy are sometimes used in older women and may partially explain the lower effectiveness of chemotherapy in postmenopausal women (130, 131). However, healthy older women with metastatic breast cancer tolerate standard chemotherapy regimens as well as younger women (132, 133). One study of doxorubicin-containing adjuvant regimens showed similar tolerability in patients 65 years old and older compared to those 50–69 years old (134).

The value of chemotherapy when added to tamoxifen in stage II, ER-positive postmenopausal women remains controversial; several trials have suggested no benefit compared to tamoxifen alone (128, 135–138), whereas other reports suggest a role for chemotherapy in addition to tamoxifen (5, 125, 126, 139). Although prospective trials have addressed the use of adjuvant chemotherapy when added to tamoxifen in postmenopausal women, no such trial has addressed the issue specifically in women over the age of 70 years. Since the value of adjuvant chemotherapy decreases with increasing age (119), trials are needed to determine the effect of adjuvant chemotherapy, when added to tamoxifen, on relapse-free survival, overall survival, and quality of life.

D. Follow-up for Women with Early Breast Cancer

After completion of primary management for early breast cancer, follow-up is required to monitor for tumor recurrence and toxicities of treatment. Although there is no evidence that close follow-up results in improved overall survival, the detection of early skin or lymph node (soft tissue) recurrence may result in more effective palliation. Moreover, follow-up visits provide an opportunity for patients to express concerns and for physicians to give reassurance. Extensive laboratory and radiological procedures are now available for detection of metastatic disease, but trials have indicated that a brief, focused history, and a limited physical examination (skin, chest, breast, and abdominal examination) detects more than 75% of metastases (140, 141). Mammography is an exception and should be performed yearly to detect new primary lesions, since a history of breast cancer is a risk factor for another breast cancer.

Recently, because of the growing concern over health care costs, many organizations are formulating guidelines for follow-up. The American Society of Clinical Oncology guidelines are presented in Table 6 (35). In addition to mammograms and follow-up visits with the oncologist and the gynecologist, patients should be edu-

Table 6 Follow-up of Women with Early Breast Cancer After Diagnosis and Initial Treatment

	Frequency of examination		
	0–3 years	3–5 years	5+ years
History/physical exam	Every 3–6 months	Every 6–12 months	Yearly
Breast self-exam	Monthly	Monthly	Monthly
Mammogram	Yearly	Yearly	Yearly
Gyn exams	Yearly	Yearly	Yearly
Other	PRN	PRN	PRN

PRN, as required.
Source: Adapted from Recommended Breast Cancer Surveilance Guidelines, American Society of Clinical Oncology, 1997.

cated about the symptoms of breast cancer recurrence so that these are reported and evaluated promptly.

VI. METASTATIC BREAST CANCER

Currently available treatment modalities for metastatic breast cancer are not curative and most likely do not significantly extend life expectancy. Palliation of symptoms and optimization of the quality of life are the major goals of therapy. Tamoxifen, because of its low toxicity, is the treatment of choice for first-line therapy in metastatic breast cancer unless the patient has rapid progression of metastases or major visceral organ dysfunction (142, 143). As initial therapy, tamoxifen elicits complete and partial responses in 30–40% of unselected patients with response durations averaging about 1 year. Half of those with ER-positive breast tumors respond, which is important in postmenopausal women, since ER positivity is higher (144). In fact, older postmenopausal women (>65 years) appear to have a slightly better prognosis with regard to response, time to progression of disease, and overall survival when treated with tamoxifen (145). When disease becomes refractory to tamoxifen, second-line hormonal agents such as progestins, aromatase inhibitors, estrogens, and corticosteroids or chemotherapeutic regimens are considered.

Initial response rates are generally higher with chemotherapy than with endocrine therapy. Eventual survival, however, is not significantly influenced by the initial treatment choice (146). In one randomized comparison of tamoxifen versus chemotherapy (cyclophosphamide, methotrexate, and fluoromacil) in women older than 65 years old, survival was similar and women whose tumors initially failed to respond to tamoxifen subsequently responded to chemotherapy (147). In patients with ER-negative tumors, 43% responded to CMF and 21% to tamoxifen.

In another trial comparing chemotherapy, chemotherapy plus tamoxifen, and tamoxifen alone, response rates were 45, 51, and 22%, respectively (148). Both trials found higher initial response rates to the chemotherapy but similar survival for all groups.

Patients who respond initially to endocrine therapy are likely to respond to further endocrine manipulation (142). The majority of older patients, because they have ER-positive tumors, fall into this group. Other hormonal therapies, including progestins, aromatase inhibitors, and estrogen, have similar response rates but more side effects than tamoxifen and are reserved for second-line therapy. Megace, a progestin, or anastrozole, a selective aromatase inhibitor, are typical choices for second-line hormonal therapy (142, 149, 150). Other newer hormonal agents such as the pure antiestrogens, newer aromatase inhibitors, such as formestane (151), and combinations of hormonal agents and biologics are currently under investigation and may be more effective with comparable or less toxicity.

Chemotherapy is generally offered to those patients with progressive metastatic breast cancer whose tumors have demonstrated resistance to endocrine therapy. Healthy older women with metastatic breast cancer treated with standard chemotherapy have response rates and toxicity profiles similar to those of younger women (132, 133). Chemotherapy-related myelosuppression is more common in older patients, although its duration and severity have not resulted in major differences in bleeding or in mortality related to neutropenia and infection (132, 133, 152). In patients with solid tumors treated with palliative doses of chemotherapy, severe nonhematological toxicity is similar for both young and old (132). Gelman and colleagues treated 92 patients from 65 to 90 years old with a CMF regimen, modifying the methotrexate dosage based on creatinine clearance (153). Response rates were substantially lower for these patients compared to a younger cohort treated with CMF, but duration of response, time to failure, and survival were all longer in the older women. In a retrospective analysis of women treated with chemotherapy on state of the art research protocols, Christman and colleagues showed no difference in response, time to failure, or survival for older when compared to younger patients (133).

The anthracyclines are considered to be the most effective agents against breast cancer (154, 155). Cardiac toxicity related to anthracycline compounds is more common in older people (156). ICRF-187, a cardioprotective agent, may be useful in ameliorating anthracycline-induced cardiotoxicity (157). Mitoxantrone is less cardiotoxic and has similar efficacy compared to doxorubicin; it is a reasonable alternative in older women (158, 159). Overall tolerability of doxorubicin-based chemotherapy has been retrospectively studied in older women ($\geq$65 years) versus younger women (<65 years) (160). Records of 1011 women (252 aged 50–54, 254 aged 55–59, 261 aged 60–64, 158 aged 65–69, 64 aged 70–74, 21 aged 75–79, and 1 over age 80), were reviewed. Comparing women less than 65 years old with those 65 years old or older, response rates were higher in younger women ($P =$ .001), but overall survival times were similar ($P =$ .06). Dose intensity was comparable between the two groups ($P = .49$). Neutropenic fevers occurred with equal frequency (16%), but fever was more common in women 65 years old or older (12 vs 17%, $P = .05$).

Paclitaxel (161, 162) and docetaxel (163, 164) are also very effective in metastatic breast cancer. Paclitaxel can be used at similar dose intensities in older and younger women (165).

Another potentially useful chemotherapeutic agent is vinorelbine, which requires weekly administration but has a low toxicity (166, 167). Sorio and coworkers examined the pharmacokinetics and tolerance of vinorelbine (30 mg/m^2 iv on days 1 and 8 every 3 weeks) in 25 women older than 65 years with metastatic breast cancer (168). The systemic clearance rate was large (mean 23.4 L/kg), the terminal half-life was long (mean 26.2 h), and the systemic clearance rate large (mean 1.2 L/kg); these were all similar to parameters previously noted in younger women. Tolerance was also acceptable with only 37% experiencing severe neutropenia. Of 20 evaluable patients, there were 6 partial responses.

In metastatic disease, radiation therapy (RT) can be very useful to relieve bone pain, treat isolated metastatic lesions in other sites, and treat intracranial metastases or spinal cord compression. There is very little information about the use of RT for metastatic breast cancer in older women. Extrapolation of data in the adjuvant setting implies that it is useful with minimal excess toxicity. Clearly, if RT is indicated because of intracranial metastases or bone pain, the benefits of therapy outweigh the possible risks.

VII. CONCLUSIONS AND RECOMMENDATIONS

Breast cancer in older women is a major national health concern. Over 50% of breast cancers are diagnosed in women older than 65 years, a quickly growing segment of our population. Healthy older women should be offered state of the art screening and treatment for breast cancer. This includes mamography, surgery, radiation therapy, and adjuvant therapy for early-stage tumors. Clinical trials focusing on the role of adjuvant treatment in older women with breast cancer are of paramount imporatnce. In older women with comorbid conditions or frailty that may limit survival or jeopardize surgical or other treatment outcomes, primary treatment with tamoxifen or adjuvant therapy with tamoxifen alone after surgery may be warranted. Outside of the clinical trials setting, metastatic disease should be treated similarly in all age groups.

REFERENCES

1. Parker SL, Tong T, Bolden S, Wingo PA. Cancer statistics, 1997. CA Cancer J Clin 1997; 47:5–27.

2. Yancik R, Ries LG, Yates JW. Breast cancer in aging women. A population-based study of contrasts in stage, surgery, and survival. Cancer 1989; 63:976–981.

3. National Center for Health Statistics. Vital Statistics of the United States, 1989, Vol II–Mortality Part A. 1993; Washington, DC. Public Health Service DHHS Publication No. (PHS) 93–1101, US Government Printing Office.

4. Kessler LG. The relationship between age and incidence of breast cancer. Population and screening program data. Cancer 1992; 69:1896–1903.

5. Balducci L, Schapira DV, Cox CE, Greenberg HM, Lyman GH. Breast cancer of the older woman: an annotated review. J Am Geriatr Soc 1991; 39:1113–1123.

6. Stewart JA, Foster RS, Jr. Breast cancer and aging (review). Semin Oncol 1989; 16: 41–50.

7. Brown JT, Hulka BS. Screening mammography in the elderly: a case-control study. J Gen Intern Med 1988; 3:126–131.

8. Robie PW. Cancer screening in the elderly. J Am Geriatr Soc 1989; 37:888–893.

9. Allen C, Cox EB, Manton KG, Cohen HJ. Breast cancer in the elderly. Current patterns of care. J Am Geriatr Soc 1986; 34:637–642.

10. Rosen PP, Lesser ML, Kinne DW. Breast carcinoma at the extremes of age: a comparison of patients younger than 35 years and older than 75 years. J Surg Oncol 1985; 28:90–96.

11. Bergman L, Dekker G, van Leeuwen FE, Huisman SJ, Van Dam FS, van Dongen JA. The effect of age on treatment choice and survival in elderly breast cancer patients. Cancer 1991; 67:2227–2234.

12. Greenfield S, Blanco DM, Elashoff RM, Ganz PA. Patterns of care related to age of breast cancer patients. JAMA 1987; 257:2766–2770.

13. Mor V, Masterson-Allen S, Goldberg RJ, Cummings FJ, Glicksman AS, Fretwell MD. Relationship between age at diagnosis and treatments received by cancer patients. J Am Geriatr Soc 1985;33:585–589.

14. Silliman RA, Guadagnoli E, Weitberg AB, Mor V. Age as a predictor fo diagnostic and initial treatment intensity in newly diagnosed breast cancer patients. J Gernontol 1989; 44:M46–M50.

15. Satariano WA, Ragland DR. The effect of comorbidity on 3-year survival of women with primary breast cancer. Ann Intern Med 1994; 120:104–110.

16. Satariano WA. Aging, comorbidity, and breast cancer survival: an epidemiologic view (review). Adv Exp Med Biol 1993; 330:1–11.

17. Satariano WA, Ragheb NE, Dupuis MA. Comorbidity in older women with breast cancer: an epidemiologic approach. In: Yancik R, Yates J, eds. Cancer in the Elderly: Approaches to Early Detection and Treatment. 71th ed. New York: Springer, 1989, pp 71–107.

18. American Joint Committee on Cancer. Manual for Staging of Cancer. 4th ed. Philadelphia: Lippincott, 1992.

19. Schottenfeld D, Robbins GF. Breast cancer in elderly women. Geriatrics 1971; 26: 121–131.

20. Schaefer G, Rosen P, Lesser M, et al. Breast carcinoma in elderly women: Pathology, prognosis, survival. Pathol Ann 1984;19:195–219.

21. Meyer JS, Hixon B. Advanced stage and early relapse of breast carcinomas associated with high thymidine labeling indices. Cancer Res 1979; 39:4042–4047.

22. McCarty KS, Silva JS, Cox EB, Leight GS, Wells SA. Relationship of age and meno-

pausal status to estrogen receptor content in primary carcinoma of the breast. Ann Surg 1983; 197:123–127.

23. Henderson IC. Biologic variations of tumors. Cancer 1992; 69(Suppl):1888–1895.

24. Adami HO, Malker B, Holmberg L, Persson I, Stone B. The relation between survival and age at diagnosis in breast cancer. N Engl J Med 1986;315:559–563.

25. Harris JR, Lippman ME, Veronesi U, Willett W. Breast cancer. N Engl J Med 1992; 327:319–328, 390–398, 473–480.

26. Ganz PA, Day R, Ware JE, Jr., Redmond C, Fisher B. Base-line quality-of-life assessment in the National Surgical Adjuvant Breast and Bowel Project Breast Cancer Prevention Trial. J Natl Cancer Inst 1995; 87:1372–1382.

27. Colditz GA, Willett WC, Hunter DJ, Stampfer MJ, Manson JE, Hennekens CH, et al. Family history, age, and risk of breast cancer: prospective data from the Nurses' Health Study. JAMA 1993; 270:338–343.

28. Slattery ML, Kerber RA. A comprehensive evaluation of family history and breast cancer risk. The Utah Population Database. JAMA 1993;270:1563–1568.

29. Miki Y, Swensen J, Shattuck-Eidens D, Futreal PA, Harshman K, Tavtigian S, et al. A strong candidate for the breast and ovarian cancer susceptibility gene BRCA 1. Science 1994; 266:66–71.

30. Couch FJ, Deshano ML, Blackwood MA, Calzone K, Stopfer J, Campeau L, et al. BRCA1 mutations in women attending clinics that evaluate the risk of breast cancer. N Engl J Med 1997;336:1409–1415.

31. Struewing JP, Hartge P, Wacholder S, Baker SM, Berlin M, McAdams M, et al. The risk of cancer associated with specific mutations of BRCA1 and BRCA2 among Ashkenazi Jews. N Engl J Med 1997; 336:1401–1408.

32. Easton DF, Bishop DT, Ford D, Crockford GP, Breast Cancer Linkage Consortium. Genetic linkage analysis in familial breast and ovarian cancer: results from 214 familes. Am Hum Genet 1993; 52:678–701.

33. Weber BL, Garber JE. Harris JR, Lippman ME, eds. Familial Breast Cancer: Recent Advances. 1. 1997; Cedar Knolls, NJ: Lippman-Raven Healthcare. Diseases of the Breast Updates.

34. Wooster R, Neuhausen SL, Mangion J, Quirk Y, Ford D, Collins N, et al. Localization of a breast cancer susceptibility gene, BRCA2, to chromosome 13q12-13. Science 1994; 265:2088–2090.

35. Anonymous. Recommended breast cancer surveillance guidelines. Amercian Society of Clinical Oncology. J Clin Oncol 1997; 15:2149–2156.

36. Anonymous. National Institutes of Health Consensus Development Conference Statement: Breast Cancer Screening for Women Ages 40–49, January 21–23, 1997. National Institutes of Health Consensus Development Panel (review). J Natl Cancer Inst 1997; 89:1015–1026.

37. Rimer BK. Breast cancer screening. In: Harris JR, Lippman ME, Morrow M, Hellman S, eds. Diseases of the Breast. 3rd ed. Philadelphia: Lippincott, 1996, pp 307–322.

38. Costanza ME. Issues in breast cancer screening in older women (review). Cancer 1994; 74:2009–2015.

39. Faulk RM, Sickles EA, Sollitto RA, Ominsky SH, Galvin HB, Frankel SD. Clinical efficacy of mammographic screening in the elderly. Radiology 1995; 194:193–197.

40. Wilson TE, Helvie MA, August DA. Breast cancer in the elderly patient: early detection with mammography. Radiology 1994; 190:203–207.

41. Satariano WA. Comorbidity and functional status in older women with breast cancer: implications for screening, treatment, and prognosis. J Gerontol 1992; 47(Spec No.): 24–31.

42. Mor V, Pacala JT, Rakowski W. Mammography for older women: who uses, who benefits? J Gerontol 1992; 47(Spec No.):43–49.

43. Kopans DB. Screening mammography in women over age 65. J Gerontol 1992; 47(Spec No.):59–62.

44. Mandelblatt JS, Wheat ME, Monane M, Moshief RD, Hollenberg JP, Tang J. Breast cancer screening for elderly women with and without comorbid conditions. A decision analysis model. Ann Intern Med 1992; 116:722–730.

45. Coleman EA, Feuer EJ. Breast cancer screening among women from 65 to 74 years of age in 1987–88 and 1991. NCI Breast Cancer Screening Consortium. Ann Intern Med 1992; 117:961–966.

46. Burns RB, McCarthy EP, Freund KM, Marwill SL, Shwartz M, Ash A, et al. Variability in mammography use among older women. J Am Geriatr Soc 1996; 44:922–926.

47. Blustein J. Medicare coverage, supplemental insurance, and the use of mammography by older women. N Engl J Med 1995;332:1138–1143.

48. Weinberger M, Saunders AF, Samsa GP, Bearon LB, Gold DT, Brown JT, et al. Breast cancer screening in older women: practices and barriers reported by primary care physicians. J Am Geriatr Soc 1991; 39:22–29.

49. Fox SA, Siu AL, Stein JA. The importance of physician communication on breast cancer screening of older women. Arch Intern Med 1994; 154:2058–2068.

50. Leather DS, Roberts MM. Older women's attitudes towards breast disease, self examination, and screening facilities: implications for communication. Br Med J 1985; 290: 668–670.

51. Herman CJ, Speroff T, Cebul RD. Improving compliance with breast cancer screening in older women. Results of a randomized controlled trial. Arch Intern Med 1995; 155: 717–722.

52. Smith MK. Implementing annual cancer screenigns for elderly women. J Gerontolo Nurs 1995; 21:12–17.

53. Sitzes CR. A community-based breast cancer education and screening program for elderly women. Geriatr Nurs 1995; 16:151–154.

54. McCool WF. Barriers to breast cancer screening in older women. A review (review). J Nurse-Midwifery 1994; 39:283–299.

55. Marwill SL, Freund KM, Barry PP. Patient factors associated with breast cancer screening among older women. J Am Geriatr Soc 1996; 44:1210–1214.

56. Donegan WL. Evaluation of a palpable breast mass. N Engl J Med 1992; 327:937–942.

57. Bassett L, Winchester DP, Caplan RB, Dershaw DD, Dowlatshahi K, Evans, et al. Stereotactic core-needle biopsy of the breast: a report of the Joint Task Force of the American College of Radiology, American College of Surgeons, and College of American Pathologists (review). CA Cancer J Clin 1997; 47:171–190.

58. Parker SH, Lovin JD, Jobe WE, Burke BJ, Hopper KD, Yakes WF. Nonpalpable breast lesions: stereotactic automated large-core biopsies. Radiology 1991; 180:403–407.

59. Parker SH, Burbank F, Jackman RJ, Aucreman CJ, Cardenosa G, Cink TM, et al. Percutaneous large-core breast biopsy: a multi-institutional study. Radiology 1994; 193:359–364.

60. Ernster VL, Barclay J, Kerlikowske K, Grady D, Henderson C. Incidence of and treatment for ductal carcinoma in situ of the breast. JAMA 1996; 275:913–918.

61. Zheng T, Holford TR, Chen Y, Jones BA, Flannery J, Boyle P. Time trend of female breast carcinoma in situ by race and histology in Connecticut, U.S.A. Eur J Cancer 1997; 33:96–100.

62. Schnitt SJ, Silen W, Sadowsky NL, Connolly JL, Harris JR. Ductal carcinoma in situ (intraductal carcinoma) of the breast N Engl J Med 1988; 318:898–903.

63. Solin LJ, Kurtz J, Fourquet A, Amalric R, Recht A, Bornstein BA, et al. Fifteen-year results of breast-conserving surgery and definitive breast irradiation for the treatment of ductal carcinoma in situ of the breast. J Clin Oncol 1996; 14:754–763.

64. Fisher B, Costantino J, Redmond C, Fisher E, Margolese R, Dimitrov N, et al. Lumpectomy compared with lumpectomy and radiation therapy for the treatment of intraductal breast cancer. N Engl J Med 1993; 328:1581–1586.

65. Schwartz GF. The role of excision and surveillance alone in subclinical DCIS of the breast. Oncology 1994; 8:21–26.

66. Osborne MP, Hoda SA. Current management of lobular carcinoma in situ of the breast. Oncology 1994; 8:45–49.

67. Fisher B, Anderson S, Redmond CK, Wolmark N, Wickerham DL, Cronin WM. Reanalysis and results after 12 years of follow-up in a randomized clinical trial comparing total mastectomy with lumpectomy with or without irradiation in the treatment of breast cancer. N Engl J Med 1995; 333:1456–1461.

68. Fowble BL, Solin LJ, Schultz DJ, Goodman RL. Ten year results of conservative surgery and irradiation for stage I and II breast cancer. Int J Radiat Oncol Biol Phys 1991; 21:269–277.

69. Jacobson JA, Danforth DN, Cowan KH, d'Angelo T, Steinberg SM, Pierce L, et al. Ten-year results of a comparison of conservation with mastectomy in treatment of stage I and II breast cancer. N Engl J Med 1995; 332:907–911.

70. Anonymous. Effects of radiotherapy and surgery in early breast cancer. An overview of the randomized trials. Early Breast Cancer Trialists' Collaborative Group. N Engl J Med 1995; 333:1444–1455.

71. Morris AD, Morris RD, Wilson JF, White J, Steinberg S, Okunieff P, et al. Breast-conserving therapy vs mastectomy in early-stage breast cancer: a meta-analysis of 10-year survival. Cancer J Sci Am 1997; 3:6–12.

72. Fourquet A, Campana F, Zafrani B, Mosseri V, Vielh P, Durand J-C, et al. Prognostic factors of breast recurrence in the conservative management of early breast cancer: a 25-year follow-up. Int J Radiat Oncol Biol Phys 1989; 17:719–725.

73. Hunt KE, Fry DE, Bland KI. Breast carcinoma in the elderly patient: an assessment of operative risk, morbidity and mortality. Am J Surg 1980; 140:339–342.

74. Kantorowitz DA, Poulter CA, Sischy B, Paterson E, Sobel SH, Rubin P, et al. Treatment of breast cancer among elderly women with segmental mastectomy or segmental mastectomy plus postoperative radiotherapy. Int J Radiat Oncol Biol Phys 1988; 15:263–270.

75. Svastics E, Sulyok Z, Besznyak I. Treatment of breast cancer in women older than 70 years. J Surg Oncol 1989; 41:19–21.

76. Herbsman H, Feldman J, Seldera J, Gardner B, Alfonso AE. Survival following breast cancer surgery in the elderly. Cancer 1981; 47:2358–2363.

77. Masetti R, Antinori A, Terribile D, Marra A, Granone P, Magistrelli P, et al. Breast cancer in women 70 years of age or older. J Clin Oncol 1996; 13:2722–2730.

78. Morrow M. Breast disease in elderly women. [Review]. Surgical Clinics of North America 1994; 74:145–161.

79. Fallowfield LJ, Hall A, Maguire P, Baum M, A'Hern RP. Psychological effects of being offered choice of surgery for breast cancer. BMJ 1994; 309:448

80. Leinster SJ, Ashcroft JJ, Slade PD, Dewey ME. Mastectomy versus conservative surgery: psychosocial effects of the patient's choice of treatment. J Psychosoc Oncol 1989; 7:179–192.

81. Morris J, Royle GT. Offering patients a choice of surgery for early breast cancer: a reduction in anxiety and depression in patients and their husbands. Soc Sci Med 1988; 26:583–585.

82. Morris J, Ingham R. Choice of surgery for early breast cancer: psychosocial considerations. Soc Sci Med 1988; 27:1257–1262.

83. Sandison AJ, Gold DM, Wright P, Jones PA. Breast conservation or mastectomy: treatment choice of women aged 70 years and older. Br J Surg 1996; 83:994–996.

84. Arriagada R, Rutqvist LE, Mattsson A, Kramar A, Rotstein S. Adequate locoregional treatment for early breast cancer may prevent secondary dissemination. J Clin Oncol 1995; 13:2869–2878.

85. Ragaz J, Jackson SM, Le N, Plenderleith IH, Spinelli JJ, Basco VE, et al. Adjuvant radiotherapy and chemotherapy in node-positive premenopausal women with breast cancer. N Engl J Med 1997; 337:956–962.

86. Overgaard M, Hansen PS, Overgaard J, Rose C, Andersson M, Bach F, et al. Postoperative radiotherapy in high-risk premenopausal women with breast cancer who receive adjuvant chemotherapy. N Engl J Med 1997; 337:949–955.

87. Lazovich DA, White E, Thomas DB, Moe RE. Underutilization of breast-conserving surgery and radiation therapy among women with stage I or II breast cancer. JAMA 1991; 266:3433–3438.

88. Crivellari D, Galligioni E, Foladore S, Errante D, Conte G, Nascimben O, et al. Treatment patterns in elderly patients (greater than or equal to 70 years) with breast carcinoma. A retrospective study of the Gruppo Oncologico Clinico Cooperativo del nord-Est (GOCCNE). Tumori 1991; 77:136–140.

89. Veronesi U, Luini A, Del Vecchio M, Greco M, Galimberti V, Merson M, et al. Radiotherapy after breast-preserving surgery in women with localized cancer of the breast. N Engl J Med 1993; 328:1587–1591.

90. Clark RM, McCulloch PB, Levine MN, Lipa M, Wilkinson RH, Mahoney LJ, et al. Randomized clinical trial to assess the effectiveness of breast irradiation following lumpectomy and axillary dissection for node-negative breast cancer. J Natl Cancer Inst 1992; 84:683–689.

91. Veronesi U, Banfi A, Salvadori B, Luini A, Saccozzi R, Zucali R, et al. Breast conservation is the treatment of choice in small breast cancer: long-term results of a randomized trial. Eur J Cancer 1990; 26:668–670.

92. Wyckoff J, Greenberg H, Sanderson R, Wallach P, Balducci L. Breast irradiation in the older woman: a toxicity study. J Am Geriatr Soc 1994; 42:150–152.

93. Carlson RW, Goldstein LJ, Gradishar WJ, Lichter AS, McCormick B, Moe RE, et al. NCCN Breast cancer practice guidelines. Oncology 1996; 10(11 Suppl):47–75.

94. Barth A, Craig PH, Silverstein MJ. Predictors of axillary lymph node metastases in patients with T1 breast carcinoma. Cancer 1997; 79:1918–1922.

95. Fein DA, Fowble BL, Hanlon AL, Hooks MA, Hoffman JP, Sigurdson ER, et al. Identification of women with T1–T2 breast cancer at low risk of positive axillary nodes. J Surg Oncol 1997; 65:34–39.

96. Harris JR, Hellman S. Natural history of breast cancer. In: Harris JR, Lippman ME, Morrow M, Hellman S, eds. Diseases of the Breast. Philadelphia: Lippincott-Raven, 1996, pp 375–391.

97. Feigelson BJ, Acosta JA, Feigelson HS, Findley A, Saunders EL. T1 breast carcinoma in women 70 years of age and older may not require axillary lymph node dissection. Am Surg 1996; 172:487–490.

98. Haffty BG, Ward B, Pathare P, Salem R, McKhann C, Beinfield M, et al. Reappraisal of the role of axillary lymph node dissection in the conservative treatment of breast cancer. J Clin Oncol 1997; 15:691–700.

99. Veronesi U, Paganelli G, Galimberti V, Viale G, Zurrida S, Bedoni M, et al. Sentinel-node biopsy to avoid axillary dissection in breast cancer with clinically negative lymph-nodes. Lancet 1997; 349:1864–1867.

100. Allan SG, Rodger A, Smyth JF, Leonard RC, Chetty U, Forrest AP. Tamoxifen as primary treatment of breast cancer in elderly or frail patients: a practical management. Br Med J Clin Res 1985; 290:358.

101. Preece PE, Wood RA, Mackie CR, Cuschieri A. Tamoxifen as initial sole treatment of localised breast cancer in elderly women: a pilot study. Br Med Clin Res 1982; 284:869–870.

102. Robertson JF, Todd JH, Ellis IO, Elston CW, Blamey RW. Comparison of mastectomy with tamoxifen for treating elderly patients with operable breast cancer. Br Med J 1988; 297:511–514.

103. Akhtar SS, Allan SG, Rodger A, Chetty UD, Smyth JF, Leonard RC. A 10-year experience of tamoxifen as primary treatment of breast cancer in 100 elderly and frail patients. Eur J Surg Oncol 1991; 17:30–35.

104. Bergman L, van Dongen JA, van Ooijen B, van Leeuwen FE. Should tamoxifen be a primary treatment choice for elderly breast cancer patients with locoregional disease? Breast Cancer Res Treat 1995; 34:77–83.

105. Ciatto S, Bartoli D, Iossa A, Grazzini G, Cirillo A. Response of primary breast cancer to tamoxifen alone in elderly women. Tumori 1991; 77:328–330.

106. Gazet JC, Markopoulos C, Ford HT, Coombes RC, Bland JM, Dixon RC. Prospective randomised trial of tamoxifen versus surgery in elderly patients with breast cancer. Lancet 1988; 1:679–681.

107. Gazet JC, Ford HT, Coombes RC, Bland JM, Sutcliffe R, Quilliam J, et al. Prospective randomized trial of tamoxifen vs surgery in elderly patients with breast cancer. Eur J Surg Oncol 1994; 20:207–214.

108. Mustacchi G, Milani S, Pluchinotta A, De Matteis A, Rubagotti A, Perrota A. Tamoxifen or surgery plus tamoxifen as primary treatment for elderly patients with operable breast cancer: The G.R.E.T.A. Trial. Group for Research on Endocrine Therapy in the Elderly. Anticancer Res 1994; 14:2197–2200.

109. Ciatto S, Cirillo A, Confortini M, Cardillo C, de L. Tamoxifen as primary treatment of breast cancer in elderly patients. Neoplasma 1996; 43:43–45.

110. van Dalsen AD, de Vries JE. Treatment of breast cancer in elderly patients. J Surg Oncol 1995; 60:80–82.

111. Bates T, Riley DL, Houghton J, Fallowfield L, Baum M. Breast cancer in elderly women: a Cancer Research Campaign trial comparing treatment with tamoxifen and optimal surgery with tamoxifen alone. The Elderly Breast Cancer Working Party. Br J Surg 1991; 78:591–594.

112. Horobin JM, Preece PE, Dewar JA, Wood RA, Cuschieri A. Long-term follow-up of elderly patients with locoregional breast cancer treated with tamoxifen only. Br J Surg 1991; 78:213–217.

113. Robertson JF, Ellis IO, Elston CW, Blamey RW. Mastectomy or tamoxifen as initial therapy for operable breast cancer in elderly patients: 5-year follow-up. Eur J Cancer 1992; 28A:908–910.

114. Fowble B. An assessment of treatment options for breast conservation in the elderly woman with early stage breast cancer. Int J Radiat Oncol Biol Phys 1995; 31:1015–1017.

115. Rostom AY, Pradhan DG, White WF. Once weekly irradiation in breast cancer. Int J Radiat Oncol Biol Phys 1987; 13:551–555.

116. Henderson IC. Adjuvant systemic therapy for early breast cancer. Curr Probl Cancer 1987; 11:127–207.

117. Castiglione M, Gelber RD, Goldhirsch A. Adjuvant systemic therapy for breast cancer in the elderly: competing causes of mortality. International Breast Cancer Study Group. J Clin Oncol 1990; 8:519–526.

118. Cummings FJ, Gray R, Tormey DC, Davis TE, Volk H, Harris J, et al. Adjuvant tamoxifen versus placebo in elderly women with node-positive breast cancer: long-term follow-up and causes of death. J Clin Oncol 1993; 11:29–35.

119. Anonymous. Systemic treatment of early breast cancer by hormonal, cytotoxic, or immune therapy. 133 randomised trials involving 31,000 recurrences and 24,000 deaths among 75,000 women. Early Breast Cancer Trialists' Collaborative Group. Lancet 1992; 339:1–15, 71–85.

120. Cummings FJ, Gray R, Davis TE, Tormey DC, Harris JE, Falkson G, et al. Adjuvant tamoxifen treatment of elderly women with stage II breast cancer. A double-blind comparison with placebo. Ann Intern Med 1985; 103:324–329.

121. Wander HE, Nagel GA, Luig H, Emrich D. Intensive short-term chemotherapy in patients with advanced breast cancer. Klini Wochenschr 1987; 65:317–323.

122. Fisher B, Digman J, Wieand S, Wolmark N, Wickerham DL. Duration of tamoxifen therapy for primary breast cancer: 5 versus 10 years (NSABP B-14). Proceedings of ASCO 1996; 15:113 (abstr).

123. Anonymous. Controlled trial of tamoxifen as a single adjuvant agent in the management of early breast cancer. 'Nolvadex' Adjuvant Trial Organisation. Br J Cancer 1988; 57:608–611.

124. Fisher B, Brown A, Wolmark N, Redmond C, Wickerham DL, Wittliff J, et al. Prolonging tamoxifen therapy for primary breast cancer. Findings from the National Surgical Adjuvant Breast and Bowel Project clinical trial. Ann Intern Med 1987; 106:649–654.

125. Fisher B, Redmond C, Legault-Poisson S, Dimitrov NV, Brown AM, Wickerham DL, et al. Postoperative chemotherapy and tamoxifen compared with tamoxifen alone in

the treatment of positive-node breast cancer patients aged 50 years and older with tumors responsive to tamoxifen: results from the National Surgical Adjuvant Breast and Bowel Project B-16. J Clin Oncol 1990; 8:1005–1018.

126. Fisher B, Redmond C, Fisher ER, Wolmark N. Systemic adjuvant therapy in treatment of primary operable breast cancer: National Surgical Adjuvant Breast and Bowel Project experience. NCI Monographs 1986; pp 35–43.

127. Taylor SG, Knuiman MW, Sleeper LA, Olson JE, Tormey DC, Gilchrist KW, et al. Six-year results of the Eastern Cooperative Oncology Group trial of observation versus CMFP versus CMFPT in postmenopausal patients with node-positive breast cancer. J Clin Oncol 1989; 7:879–889.

128. Boccardo F, Rubagotti A, Bruzzi P, Cappellini M, Isola G, Nenci I, et al. Chemotherapy versus tamoxifen versus chemotherapy plus tamoxifen in node-positive, estrogen receptor-positive breast cancer patients: results of a multicentric Italian study. Breast Cancer Adjuvant Chemo-Hormone Therapy Cooperative Group. J Clin Oncol 1990; 8:1310–1320.

129. Bonadonna G, Valagussa P, Tancini G, Rossi A, Brambilla C, Zambetti M, et al. Current status of Milan adjuvant chemotherapy trials for node-positive and node-negative breast cancer. NCI Monographs 1986, pp 45–50.

130. Henderson IC, Hayes DF, Gelman R. Dose-response in the treatment of breast cancer: a critical review. J Clin Oncol 1988; 6:1501–1515.

131. Hryniuk WM, Levine MN, Levin L. Analysis of dose intensity for chemotherapy in early (stage II) and advanced breast cancer. NCI Monographs 1986, pp 87–94.

132. Begg CB, Cohen JL, Ellerton J. Are the elderly predisposed to toxicity from cancer chemotherapy? An investigation using data from the Eastern Cooperative Oncology Group. Cancer Clin Trials 1980; 3:369–374.

133. Christman K, Muss HB, Case LD, Stanley V. Chemotherapy of metastatic breast cancer in the elderly. The Piedmont Oncology Association experience. JAMA 1992; 268: 57–62.

134. Muss H, Cooper MR, Hoen H, Cruz J, Powell B, Richards F, Spurr C, White D. Adjuvant chemotherapy in older women with node positive breast cancer: The Piedmont Oncology Association experience. Proc Am Soc Clin Oncol 1992; 11:12x (abstr).

135. Anonymous. Consensus conference. Adjuvant chemotherapy for breast cancer. JAMA 1985; 254:3461–3463.

136. Anonymous. Effects of adjuvant tamoxifen and of cytotoxic therapy on mortality in early breast cancer. An overview of 61 randomized trials among 28,896 women. Early Breast Cancer Trialists' Collaborative Group. N Engl J Med 1988; 319:1681–1692.

137. Fisher B, Redmond C, Brown A, Fisher ER, Wolmark N, Bowman D, et al. Adjuvant chemotherapy with and without tamoxifen in the treatment of primary breast cancer: 5-year results from the National Surgical Adjuvant Breast and Bowel Project Trial. J Clin Oncol 1986; 4:459–471.

138. Pritchard KI, Paterson AH, Fine S, Paul NA, Zee B, Shepherd LE, et al. Randomized trial of cyclophosphamide, methotrexate, and fluorouracil chemotherapy added to tamoxifen as adjuvant therapy in postmenopausal women with node-positive estrogen and/or progesterone receptor-positive breast cancer: a report of the National Cancer Institute of Canada Clinical Trials Group. Breast Cancer Site Group. J Clin Oncol 1997; 15:2302–2311.

139. Anonymous. Effectiveness of adjuvant chemotherapy in combination with tamoxifen for node-positive postmenopausal breast cancer patients. International Breast Cancer Study Group. J Clin Oncol 1997; 15:1385–1394.

140. Rosselli Del Turco M, Palli D, Cariddi A, Ciatto S, Pacini P, Distante V. Intensive diagnostic follow-up after treatment of primary breast cancer. A randomized trial. National Research Council Project on Breast Cancer follow-up. JAMA 1994; 271:1593–1597.

141. Anonymous. Impact of follow-up testing on survival and health-related quality of life in breast cancer patients. A multicenter randomized controlled trial. The GIVIO Investigators [see comments]. JAMA 1994; 271:1587–1592.

142. Kimmick G, Muss HB. Current status of endocrine therapy for metastatic breast cancer (review). Oncology 1995; 9:877–886.

143. Robinson E, Kimmick GG, Muss HB. Tamoxifen in postmenopausal women a safety perspective (review). Drugs Aging 1996; 8:329–337.

144. Henderson IC. Endocrine therapy of metastatic breast cancer. In: Harris JR, Hellman S, Henderson IC, Kinne DW, editors. Breast Diseases. 2nd ed. Philadelphia: Lippincott, 1991, pp 559–603.

145. Dhodapkar MV, Ingle JN, Cha SS, Mailliard JA, Wieand HS. Prognostic factors in elderly women with metastatic breast cancer treated with tamoxifen: an analysis of patients entered on four prospective clinical trials. Cancer 1996; 77:683–690.

146. Kiang DT, Gay J, Goldman A, Kennedy BJ. A randomized trial of chemotherapy and hormonal therapy in advanced breast cancer. N Engl J Med 1985; 313:1241–1246.

147. Taylor SG, Gelman RS, Falkson G, Cummings FJ. Combination chemotherapy compared to tamoxifen as initial therapy for stage IV breast cancer in elderly women. Ann Intern Med 1986; 104:455–461.

148. Anonymous. A randomized trial in postmemopausal patients with advanced breast cancer comparing endocrine and cytotoxic therapy given sequentially or in combination. The Australian and New Zealand Breast Cancer Trials Group, Clinical Oncological Society of Australia. J Clin Oncol 1986; 4:186–193.

149. Jonat W, Howell A, Blomqvist C, Eiermann W, Winblad G, Tyrrell C, et al. A randomised trial comparing two doses of the new selective aromatase inhibitor anastrozole (Arimidex) with megestrol acetate in postmenopausal patients with advanced breast cancer. Eur J Cancer 1996; 32A:404–412.

150. Buzdar A, Jonat W, Howell A, Jones SE, Blomqvist C, Vogel CL, et al. Anastrozole, a potent and selective aromatase inhibitor, versus megestrol acetate in postmenopausal women with advanced breast cancer: results of overview analysis of two phase III trials. Arimidex Study Group. Journal of Clinical Oncology 1996; 14:2000–2011.

151. Zilembo N, Buzzoni R, Celio L, Noberasco C, Ferrari L, Laffranchi A, et al. Formestane as treatment of advanced breast cancer in elderly women. Tumori 1994; 80:433–437.

152. Begg CB, Elson PJ, Carbone PP. A study of excess hematologic toxicity in elderly patients treated on chemotherapy protocols. In: Yancik R, ed. Cancer in the Elderly: Approaches to Early Detection and Management. New York: Springer-Verlag, 1989, pp 149–161.

153. Gelman RS, Taylor SG. Cyclophosphamide, methotrexate, and 5-fluorouracil chemotherapy in women more than 65 years old with advanced breast cancer: the elimination of age trends in toxicity by using doses based on creatinine clearance. J Clin Oncol 1984; 2:1404–1413.

154. Overmoyer BA. Chemotherapy in the management of breast cancer (review). Cleve Clin J Med 1995; 62:36–50.

155. Norton L. Salvage chemotherapy of breast cancer (review). Semin Oncol 1994; 21: 19–24.

156. Von Hoff DD, Layard MW, Basa P, Davis HL, Jr., Von Hoff AL, Rozencweig M, et al. Risk factors for doxorubicin-induced congestive heart failure. Ann Intern Med 1979; 91:710–717.

157. Speyer JL, Green MD, Zeleniuch-Jacquotte A, Wernz JC, Rey M, Sanger J, et al. ICRF-187 permits longer treatment with doxorubicin in women with breast cancer. J Clin Oncol 1992; 10:117–127.

158. Hainsworth JD. The use of mitoxantrone in the tratment of breast cancer (review). Semin Oncol 1995; 22:17–20.

159. Benjamin RS. Rationale for the use of mitoxantrone in the older patient: cardiac toxicity (review). Semin Oncol 1995; 22:11–13.

160. Ibrahim NK, Frye DK, Buzdar AU, Walters RS, Hortobagyi GN. Doxorubicin-based chemotherapy in elderly patients with metastatic breast cancer. Arch Intern Med 1996; 156:882–888.

161. Gianni L, Capri G, Munzone E, Straneo M. Paclitaxel (Taxol) efficacy in patients with advanced breast cancer resistant to anthracyclines. Semin Oncol 1994; 21(Suppl 8): 29–33.

162. Holmes FA, Walters RS, Theriault RL, Forman AD, Newton LK, Raber MN, et al. Phase II trial of taxol, an active drug in the treatment of metastatic breast cancer. J Natl Cancer Inst 1991; 83:1797–1805.

163. Valero V, Holmes FA, Walters RS, Theriault RL, Esparza L, Fraschini G, et al. Phase II trial of docetaxel: a new, highly effective antineoplastic agent in the management of patients with anthracycline-resistant metastatic breast cancer. J Clin Oncol 1995; 13:2886–2894.

164. Ravdin PM, Burris HA, Cook G, Eisenberg P, Kane M, Bierman WA, et al. Phase II trial of docetaxel in advanced anthracycline-resistant or anthracenedione-resistant breast cancer. J Clin Oncol 1995; 13:2879–2885.

165. Bicher A, Sarosy G, Kohn E, Adamo DO, Davis P, Jacob J, et al. Age does not influence taxol dose intensity in recurrent carcinoma of the ovary. Cancer 1993; 71:594–600.

166. Weber BL, Vogel C, Jones S, Harvey H, Hutchins L, Bigley J, et al. Intravenous vinorelbine as first-line and second-line therapy in advanced breast cancer. J Clin Oncol 1995; 13:2722–2730.

167. Marty M, Extra JM, Dieras V, Giacchetti S, Ohana S, Espie M. A review of the antitumour activity of vinorelbine in breast cancer. Drugs 1992; 44(Suppl 4):29–35.

168. Sorio R, Robieux I, Galligioni E, Freschi A, Colussi AM, Crivellari D, et al. Pharmacokinetics and tolerance of vinorelbine in elderly patients with metastatic breast cancer. Eur J Cancer 1997; 33:301–303.

169. von Rueden DG, Sessions SC. Alternative therapy for elderly patients with breast cancer. Am Surg 1994; 60:72–78.

170. van Zyl JA, Muller AG. Tumour excision plus continuous tamoxifen compared with modified radical mastectomy in patients over 70 years of age with operable breast cancer. J Surg Oncol 1995; 59:151–154.

171. Solin LJ, Schultz DJ, Fowble BL. Ten-year results of the treatment of early-stage

breast carcinoma in elderly women using breast-conserving surgery and definitive breast irradiation. Int J Radiat Oncol Biol Phys 1995; 33:45–51.

172. Wazer DE, Erban JK, Robert NJ, Smith TJ, Marchant DJ, Schmid C, et al. Breast conservation in elderly women for clinically negative axillary lymph nodes without axillary lymph nodes without axillary dissection. Cancer 1994; 74:878–883.

173. Maher M, Campana F, Mosseri V, Dreyfus H, Vilcoq JR, Gautier C, et al. Breast cancer in elderly women: a retrospective analysis of combined treatment with tamoxifen and once-weekly irradiation. Int J Radiat Oncol Biol Phys 1995; 31:783–789.

174. Dunser M, Haussler B, Fuchs H, Margreiter R. Tumorectomy plus tamoxifen for the treatment of breast cancer in the elderly. Eur J Surg Oncol 1993; 19:529–531.

175. Martelli G, Moglia D, Boracchi P, Del Prato I, Galante E, De Palo G. Surgical resection plus tamoxifen as treatment of breast cancer in elderly patients: a retrospective study. Eur J Cancer 1993; 29A:2080–2082.

176. Haskell CM, Barsky SH, Bassett LW, Love SM. Natural history and pretreatment assessment of breast cancer. In: Haskel CM, Berek JS, eds. Cancer Treatment, 4th ed. Philadelphia, PA: W.B. Saunders Company, 1995, pp 324–337.

12
Gynecological Cancers

David H. Moore
Indiana University School of Medicine
Indianapolis, Indiana

I. INTRODUCTION

During the 20th century, the number of persons under 65 years of age living in the United States has tripled; however, the number of persons over 65 years of age has multiplied by a factor of 11 (1). The older population is expected to double by the year 2030 (Fig. 1). The percentage of women 65 years of age and older has also continued to increase from 13.1% in 1980 to 14.6% in 1990 (2). Among this age group, an estimated 157,800 women died of cancer in 1990, which is second only to cardiovascular disease as the leading cause of mortality (3). Cancer is the leading cause of mortality in women between the ages of 35–75 years. The incidence of most cancers increases with age. Approximately 50% of all cancers, and 60% of cancer deaths, occur in people over 65 years of age (4). As the population continues to age and the number of elderly cancer patients continues to increase, it is essential that the medical community not only learn and understand cancer biology pertinent to the aged but also appreciate the unique concerns and quality of life expectations of the elderly. For these patients, it is unfortunate that most of what we know about the diagnosis, treatment, and prognosis of specific cancers comes from studies conducted in younger patient populations (5).

Cancers arising in the female genital tract are some of the more common malignancies in women. Gynecological cancers comprise approximately 13.7% of all new cancer diagnoses and 9.9% of all cancer deaths among women in the United States (6). It is the purpose of this chapter to describe current staging, diagnosis, and treatment strategies for cancers of the female genital tract: vulva, cervix, uterus, and ovary. Because of the extreme rarity of vaginal and fallopian tube cancers, the interested reader is encouraged to consult other sources. Whenever possible, this

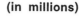

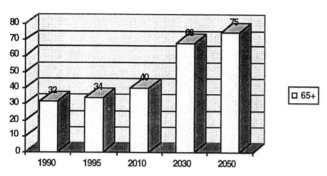

Figure 1   Population of the United States by age, 1990–2050 (From Ref. 1.)

chapter will also discuss gyncological cancer epidemiology, diagnosis, treatment, and prognosis pertaining to the elderly patient.

II. VULVAR CANCER

Invasive cancers of the vulva constitute approximately 5% of all gynecological cancers. It is the fourth most common gynecological cancer in the United States, with approximately 3300 new cases and 800 deaths (6). Although Bartholin's gland adenocarcinomas, various sarcomas, malignant melanomas, and a number of other cutaneous tumors may arise on the vulva, squamous cell carcinomas account for over 90% of invasive vulvar cancers. Unless specified otherwise, 'vulvar cancer' implies a squamous cell carcinoma. Most of what is known about vulvar cancer is derived from studies of squamous cell carcinomas, on which this section will focus.

Traditionally, vulvar cancer has been considered to be a disease the elderly, with most cases occurring during the sixth decade of life, although 15% of vulvar cancers develop in women less than 40 years of age (7, 8). It has been reported in very young women (9) and in pregnancy (10). The epidemiology of vulvar cancer is not well understood. The lower genital tract neoplasias—vulva, vagina, cervix— have several risk factors in common. One risk factor for the development of vulvar cancer is neoplasia elsewhere in the lower genital tract. Obesity, hypertension, and diabetes mellitus have been considered to be putative risk factors (11); however, these more likely reflect associations with comorbid conditions encountered in an aging population rather than causation. Chronic vulvar dermatoses such as lichen sclerosis and squamous cell hyperplasia are often found simultaneously with squamous cell carcinoma and have been suggested as precursor lesions of invasive vulvar cancer. A longitudinal study of 350 patients with lichen sclerosis showed that only

3% developed invasive vulvar cancer (12). Earlier studies linking cigarette smoking to the development of vulvar cancer (13) have been confirmed by two important case-control analyses (14, 15). There is a strong correlation between infection with the human papillomavirus (HPV) and vulvar neoplasia. DNA of HPV has been identified in both in situ and invasive vulvar cancers. Although other HPV types have been found, most vulvar cancers are believed to be associated with HPV type 16 (16, 17). In a report by Brinton and colleagues, genital warts (condylomata) were a significant risk factor for the development of vulvar carcinoma; furthermore, patients who both smoked and had a history of genital warts had a 35-fold increase in risk (15).

Recent observations have suggested that squamous cell vulvar cancer may have two different etiologies (18, 19). Younger patients with vulvar cancer tend to have squamous cell carcinomas of basaloid or warty histological subtype, often found adjacent to areas of vulvar intraepithelial neoplasia, and associated with the presence of HPV. Younger women are also more likely to report a history of multiple sexual partners, early initiation of intercourse, and cigarette smoking. Conversely, older women tend to have keratinizing squamous cell carcinomas, often found in association with lichen sclerosis, and HPV is not present. Given the marked increase in human papillomavirus infection among the U.S. population, there may be a subsequent sharp increase in the incidence of HPV-associated vulvar cancers and may explain the increasing incidence of vulvar cancer in younger women. There presently does not seem to be any prognostic difference between HPV-positive versus HPV-negative tumors (20, 21).

There is no effective screening procedure aside from a meticulous inspection of the external genitalia and vestibule at the time of annual gynecological examination. The vast majority of women who present with vulvar carcinoma are not found through routine gynecological examination but present with symptoms of burning or pruritus in the vulvar area, pain, bleeding, or a mass (Fig. 2). The initial step in the management of cancer is to first confirm the diagnosis, which in the case of vulvar cancer may be easily accomplished with an office punch biopsy under local analgesia. Other vulvar lesions such as large condylomata accuminata or verrucous carcinomas may mimic an invasive squamous cancer, and histological confirmation will prevent the misapplication of radical treatment.

Vulvar cancers metastasize by three mechanisms: (a) local growth and extension; (b) embolization to groin lymph nodes; and (c) vascular dissemination to distant sites (infrequent). Treatment planning in all patients should include pelvic examination with careful palpation of groin nodes and a chest radiograph. For patients with large tumors encroaching on the urethra or bladder, a cystourethroscopy may provide useful information, and proctosigmoidoscopy or barium enema may be useful for the evaluation of patients with tumors extending to the anus or infiltrating the rectovaginal septum. In 1988, the International Federation of Gynecology and Obstetrics (FIGO) staging classification for vulvar cancer was changed to a surgical system (Table 1). Reasons for this change included (a) practically all patients with

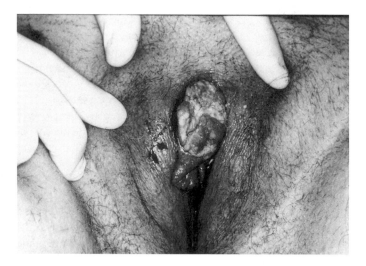

Figure 2 FIGO stage II squamous cell carcinoma of the vulva. The patient presented with complaints of bleeding and pain in the vulvar area of 6–8 weeks' duration. The tumor involved the clitoris but did not extend to the urethra. The cancer was excised via partial radical vulvectomy and bilateral groin node dissection. All lymph nodes were negative for metastatic cancer. She remains without evidence for recurrent cancer 3 years after primary surgery.

vulvar cancer undergo operative treatment to include biopsy or excision of the inguinal–femoral lymph nodes; (b) the presence of cancer metastatic to the groin lymph nodes is the singlemost important prognostic factor for recurrence and survival; and (c) the accuracy of clinical evaluation of the groin lymph nodes is poor.

Since the turn of the century radical deep resection of the entire vulva and dissection of the groin lymph nodes has been used for invasive carcinoma of the vulva, and this became standard therapy with the surgical refinements reported by Taussig (22) and Way (23). In an effort to reduce physical and psychosexual morbid-

Table 1 FIGO Staging Classification for Vulvar Cancer

Stage 0:   Carcinoma in situ, intraepithelial carcinoma
Stage I: Tumor confined to the vulva and/or perineum, ≤2 cm in greatest diameter
Stage II: Tumor confined to the vulva and/or perineum, >2 cm in greatest diameter
Stage III: Tumor of any size with adjacent spread to the lower urethra and/or the vagina, or the anus, and/or unilateral regional lymph node metastasis
Stage IVA: Tumor invades the upper urethra, bladder mucosa, rectal mucosa, or pelvic bone, and/or bilateral regional lymph node metastasis
Stage IVB: Any distant metastasis including pelvic lymph nodes

ity with such a radical operation, without compromising survival, DiSaia and colleagues were the first to report a successful and more conservative resection in patients with stage I vulvar cancer (24). Subsequent reports have applied this same operation to patients with larger primary tumors (25, 26). Various terms have been used to describe this operation, including *radical wide excision, radical hemivulvectomy,* or *partial radical vulvectomy.* Combined with the removal of groin lymph nodes through separate incisions instead of through an en bloc excision of intervening vulva and perineum (27), the morbidity of vulvar surgery has been greatly reduced without compromising efficacy. For tumors that do not involve midline structures, removal of the groin lymph nodes is sufficient; when the ipsilateral nodes are negative, the risk for recurrence in the contralateral groin is exceedingly small (25, 28, 29). Radiation therapy has an established role in the treatment of vulvar cancer. A randomized controlled trial conducted by the Gynecologic Oncology Group established the superiority of postoperative pelvic and groin irradiation over pelvic lymphadenectomy in patients with vulvar cancer metastatic to the inguinal–femoral lymph nodes (30). Attempts to replace groin node dissection with elective groin irradiation have been more controversial (31). Primary radiation therapy has been used as an alternative to ultraradical surgery (e.g., pelvic exenteration) for patients with locally advanced vulvar carcinoma, and it has also been investigated as an alternative to surgery for patients with smaller tumors (32, 33).

Predictors of survival in vulvar cancer include the presence and number of involved groin nodes, FIGO stage, and age. Five-year survival ranges from stage I, 80%; stage II, 70%; stage III, 65%; to stage IV, 24% (34). Elderly women with vulvar cancer do appear to have a worse prognosis (34, 35). Five-year survival declines from 87% for women less than 40 years of age to 65.8% for women over the age of 70 years (34). Whether these age-based differences in survival reflect differences in tumor biology, clinical presentation (FIGO stage), or treatment is unknown; nonetheless, multivariate analysis has confirmed that age is an independent prognostic factor.

Elderly women with vulvar cancer are often faced with problems of long-term disability from vulvectomy and/or radiation therapy. Although surgical treatment over the past 20 years has become more conservative, vulvar surgery is still disfiguring and affects sexuality and psychosocial well-being. Unfortunately, very few studies have addressed these problems. It will become increasingly important that we not only develop new approaches to the treatment of vulvar cancer but also understand what impact those treatments have on the quantity and quality of life of elderly patients.

III. CERVICAL CANCER

Worldwide cervical cancer is second only to breast cancer in incidence and mortality. In the United States, cervical cancer is less common because of the development and implementation of screening programs based on the Papanicolaou (Pap) smear. It is the third most common gynecological cancer, with approximately 14,500 cases each year (2% of all cancers in women) and 4800 deaths (6). Approximately 85–90% of invasive cervical cancers are squamous cell carcinomas and 10–15% are adenocarcinomas.

Although the epidemiology of squamous cell carcinoma of the cervix continues to evolve, the influence of sexual behaviors has long been recognized. Young age at first intercourse, multiple sexual partners, and high parity are all important risk factors (36, 37). Sexual behaviors by male partners also contribute to a woman's risk of developing cervical neoplasia (38). These factors suggest that a sexually transmitted agent may be responsible, and the agent that is most likely responsible is the HPV family of DNA tumor viruses (39, 40). Over 70 HPV types have been identified, each with a predilection to infect specific tissue sites. The types most prevalent in cervical cancer are HPV 16, and HPV 18, and these are rarely isolated in women who have not experienced sexual intercourse (41–43). Approximately 50–60% of male sexual partners of women with cervical neoplasia or condylomata will have evidence of HPV infection (44, 45). The oncogenic potential of HPV is believed to result from integration of viral DNA into the host cell and expression of a viral transforming protein (E6) which binds to and enhances the degradation of the p53 gene product important in cell cycle regulation. It is interesting that p53 mutations are present in the very few patients with cervical carcinoma without associated HPV (46). Not all women who harbor HPV develop cervical neoplasia. Other factors which may contribute to cervical carcinogenesis include nutrition, immunological status, and cigarette smoking. Carcinogens present in cigarette smoke are concentrated in cervical mucus (47) and may interfere with host immunity (48). Several studies have clearly linked exposure to cigarette smoke to an increased risk for cervical cancer (49, 50).

With the advent of cytological screening, many women are diagnosed and treated with preinvasive cervical disease (cervical intraepithelial neoplasia, or CIN). Pap smear screening is thus a means of primary prevention. Women may develop cervical cancers undetected by conventional screening, but the vast majority of patients who develop this disease do not attend screening clinics. Patients with cervical cancer may present with complaints of pain, vaginal bleeding or discharge, or postcoital spotting. The diagnosis is established through biopsy and histopathological study of cervical tissue.

Cervical cancer spreads primary by means of local infiltration into surrounding tissues. Extension laterally may result in renal failure from ureteral obstruction. Invasion into the bladder or rectum may also occur. Cervical cancers may also metastasize via lymphatic dissemination to regional lymph nodes and uncommonly by vascular dissemination to distant organs (51). The FIGO staging classification for cervical cancer is based on clinical findings (Table 2). Although a number of studies may be performed for staging and treatment planning, none provides more useful information than the pelvic examination.

Table 2 FIGO Staging Classification for Cervical Cancer

Stage 0:	Carcinoma in situ, intraepithelial carcinoma
Stage IA1:	Tumor confined to the cervix, identified only microscopically, measured invasion of stroma ≤3 mm in depth and ≤7 mm in width
Stage IA2:	Tumor confined to the cervix, identified only microscopically, measured invasion of stroma >3 and ≤5 mm in depth and ≤7 mm in width
Stage IB1:	Tumor confined to the cervix, preclinical lesions greater than IA or clinical lesions ≤4 cm in diameter
Stage IB2:	Tumor confined to the cervix, clinical lesions >4 cm in diameter
Stage IIA:	Tumor extends beyond the cervix, involves the vagina but not the lower 1/3, no obvious parametrial involvement
Stage IIB:	Tumor extends beyond the cervix, obvious parametrial involvement but does not extend to the pelvic wall
Stage IIIA:	Tumor extends beyond the cervix, involves the lower 1/3 of the vagina
Stage IIIB:	Tumor extends beyond the cervix with extension to the pelvic wall and/or hydronephrosis or nonfunctioning kidney
Stage IVA:	Spread of the tumor to adjacent organs (rectum, bladder)
Stage IVB:	Spread of the tumor to organs beyond the true pelvis

Approximately 50% of women with cervical cancer present with a tumor clinically confined to the cervix (6). These patients may be treated either with radical hysterectomy (with or without removal of the fallopian tubes and ovaries) or pelvic radiation therapy with essentially equivalent results (52–55). Proponents of surgical treatment claim ovarian preservation and better sexual function as advantages of radical hysterectomy. Proponents of radiation therapy claim less short-term morbidity—advantageous for elderly patients with comorbid conditions or those who wish to approximate normal daily functions during an outpatient treatment—and the fact that, pending operative selection criteria, many of the patients who undergo radical hysterectomy will require postoperative radiation therapy. Unfortunately, no prospective studies exist to address patient preferences or outcome measures such as treatment convenience, morbidity, and long-term effects on physical and sexual functions. In general, women who undergo surgical treatment tend to be younger and otherwise healthier than those patients who receive radiation therapy—likely reflecting a strong selection bias on the part of the treating physicians. It does appear that the use of hysterectomy for the treatment of early-stage cervical cancer is increasing (56).

Patients with "bulky" tumors confined to the cervix (stage IB2) may also undergo primary treatment with radical hysterectomy or radiation therapy. An alternative therapeutic approach for this group of women is the use of preoperative pelvic radiation therapy followed by extrafascial (nonradical) hysterectomy. Although the superiority of this combined treatment approach has been reported in retrospective series, it has yet to be validated in prospective controlled trials (57, 58).

Patients who undergo radical hysterectomy receive postoperative pelvic radiation therapy if there is microscopic tumor extension to the parametrical tissues or surgical margins or positive pelvic lymph nodes (59, 60). For patients who present with locally advanced (stage IIB-IVA) cervical cancer, primary radiation therapy with a combination of external beam radiation and brachytherapy is the appropriate treatment. Patterns of care studies have demonstrated a steady improvement in cervical cancer cure rates from 1973 to 1983 attributed to the use of higher radiation therapy doses to the pelvis and increased use of brachytherapy (61). Further improvements may be possible by avoiding unnecessary prolongation of overall treatment time (62).

Chemotherapy for the treatment of cervical cancer has been used in three contexts: (a) concomitant to radiation therapy (''radiosensitizer''); (b) prior to definitive radiation therapy or surgery (''neoadjuvant''); and (c) palliative. Few prospective trials of concomitant chemotherapy and radiation therapy have been conducted, although the Gynecologic Oncology Group has reported results from two randomized controlled trials demonstrating superiority of hydroxyurea plus pelvic radiation over radiation therapy alone (63) and superiority of hydroxyurea over misonidazole as a radiation sensitizer (64, 65). Neoadjuvant chemotherapy prior to radiation therapy has been disappointing (66). Neoadjuvant chemotherapy prior to surgery has improved rates of tumor resectability and may improve overall survival (67, 68). The use of neoadjuvant chemotherapy prior to radical hysterectomy is being studied in an ongoing Gynecologic Oncology Group protocol. When cervical cancer is no longer amenable to curative intent with surgery or radiation therapy, then chemotherapy is the only treatment option. Despite the identification of a number of active drugs and regimens, it is uncertain whether chemotherapy has any impact on either symptoms (palliation) or survival. Objective responses occur in fewer than 40% of patients with very few complete responses. One observor has stated that standard chemotherapy for advanced cervical cancer should therefore be participation in a clinical trial (69).

In general, elderly women with cervical carcinoma have a worse prognosis. In her review of 17,119 cases of cervical cancer in the SEER (Surveillance, Epidemiology, and End Results) database, Kosary (34) reported 5-year relative survival steadily decreased as age increased: under 30 years old (87.5%); 30–39 years (80.9%); 40–49 years (71.3%); 50–59 years (63.1%); 60–69 years (57.6%); 70 years and older (46.0%). The poor prognosis associated with advancing age was independent of disease extent at diagnosis. At all FIGO stages (except stage IA), elderly women did worse (34). In a review of Gynecologic Oncology Group data it was noted that increasing age was associated with a poorer performance status and more advanced stage (70).

It is unknown whether these age-based differences in survival reflect differences in cervical cancer biology, clinical presentation (FIGO stage), or treatment efficacy. More information is needed regarding the epidemiology of cervical cancer in the older versus younger patient. Given the worse prognosis associated with aging, it is important that elderly women be given the opportunity to participate in cervical cancer screening programs. Several reports suggest that Pap smear screening of the elderly is cost effective (71, 72). Finally, eligibility criteria for participation in clinical treatment protocols should not inappropriately exclude elderly women.

IV. UTERINE CANCER

Cancer of the uterus is the fourth most common cancer in women (6% of all female cancers) and the most common gynecological malignancy. There are an estimated 34,900 new cases and 6000 deaths from uterine cancer each year (6). Sarcomas account for 3–5% and adenocarcinomas arising from the uterine endometrium account for 95–97% of uterine cancers (Fig. 3). The focus of this section will be endometrial cancer.

Classic risk factors for the development of endometrial adenocarcinoma are obesity, hypertension, and diabetes mellitus (73). Obesity as a risk factor is believed to be mediated by endogenous estrogens, a common denominator for endometrial cancer. Hence, prolonged use of unopposed estrogens, history of nulliparity/infertility, chronic anovulation, and early age at menarche or late age at menopause are established risk factors. Conversely, the use of combination oral contraceptives decreases the risk for endometrial cancer (74). Inheritable genetic factors contribute to a small percentage of cases. Endometrial cancer is the most common extracolonic cancer to arise in women with Lynch II (hereditary nonpolyposis colorectal) syndrome and occurs in 4–11% of these women (75, 76). Endometrial cancer is a disease associated with aging. Three fourths of endometrial cancers occur in postmenopausal women, and the incidence increases from approximately 12 cases per 100,000 women at age 40 years to 84 cases per 100,000 women at age 60 years (77).

There is no screening test for endometrial cancer. Pap smears are abnormal in only 30–50% of women known to have endometrial cancer. Various cytological and histological endometrial sampling methods have been developed and eventually discarded because of low sensitivity or high cost. Ultrasonography is emerging as an important means to evaluate the endometrium, but, at present, it cannot be recommended as a screening test in asymptomatic women. Consideration for endometrial cancer screening is rational for the woman taking tamoxifen for breast cancer (prophylaxis or treatment). These women are being seen on a regular basis by the medical community and are at increased risk for developing endometrial cancer. The estimated annual risk of endometrial cancer in tamoxifen-treated patients is approximately 2/1000 women (78). However, these women do not have a worse prognosis than other patients with uterine adenocarcinoma, and, in the absence of symptoms, there are insufficient data to recommend routine screening with endometrial biopsy or ultrasonograph (79, 80).

The patient with endometrial cancer in almost all cases presents with abnormal bleeding. The diagnosis may be suspected with ultrasonography but is confirmed

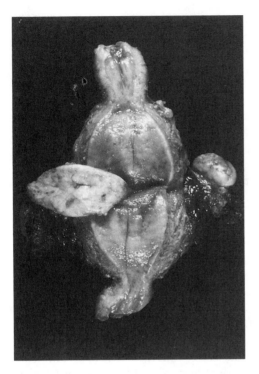

Figure 3 FIGO stage IB adenocarcinoma of the endometrium. The patient presented with postmenopausal bleeding and an office endometrial biopsy showed well-differentiated (grade 1) adenocarcinoma. The hysterectomy specimen has been opened to reveal a polypoid tumor arising from the endometrium and histopathological study demonstrated limited myometrial invasion. No postoperative therapy was administered, and the patient remains without evidence for recurrent cancer 5 years after primary surgery.

with an office endometrial biopsy or dilatation and curettage (D&C) in the operating room. Hysteroscopy may be useful to assist with tissue collection and can be performed as an office procedure. Despite the absence of a suitable screening modality, approximately 90% of women present with tumor clinically confined to the uterus. Endometrial cancer spreads by local infiltration, lymphatic dissemination, and transperitoneal seeding. Rarely, hematogenous spread may also occur. Because over 95% of women with endometrial cancer undergo primary surgical therapy, and clinical staging is highly inaccurate, the FIGO staging classification for endometrial cancer is based on surgical–pathologic findings Table 3.

For the 90% of women with cancer clinically confined to the uterus, optimal treatment consists of total abdominal hysterectomy, bilateral salpingo-oophorectomy, pelvic washings for cytological evaluation, pelvic and aortic lymph node biop-

Table 3 FIGO Staging Classification for Uterine Cancer

Stage IA:	Tumor limited to the endometrium
Stage IB:	Invasion to less than one half the myometrium
Stage IC:	Invasion to more than one half the myometrium
Stage IIA:	Endocervical glandular involvement only
Stage IIB:	Cervical stromal invasion
Stage IIIA:	Tumor invades the serosa and/or adnexae, and/or positive peritoneal cytology
Stage IIIB:	Vaginal metastasis
Stage IIIC:	Metastasis to the pelvic and/or aortic lymph nodes
Stage IVA:	Tumor invasion of the bladder or rectum
Stage IVB:	Distant metastasis including intraabdominal and/or inguinal lymph nodes

Note: Cases of carcinoma of the corpus should be graded according to the degree of histological differentiation as follows:
Grade 1 = 5% or less of a nonsquamous or nonmorular solid-growth pattern.
Grade 2 = 6–50% of a nonsquamous or nonmorular solid-growth pattern.
Grade 3 = more than 50% of a nonsquamous or nonmorular solid-growth pattern.

sies, and abdominal exploration (81). This operation permits removal of the primary tumor in and the assessment for metastatic disease important to postoperative treatment planning. Most gynecological surgeons are not trained in lymph node dissection procedures. In experienced hands, pelvic and aortic lymphadenectomy does not significantly contribute to increased postoperative morbidity (82–84). A prospective study reported by the Gynecologic Oncology Group provides important information on the relationship between tumor grade, depth of myometrial invasion, and lymph node metastasis for stage I endometrial cancer (85). Given the low risk (<3%) of lymph node metastasis in grade 1 endometrial adenocarcinoma, it is questionable whether routine lymph node sampling is necessary for these patients. Furthermore, the risk of aortic lymph node metastasis was negligible if pelvic lymph nodes were negative. In this series, almost 50% of positive lymph nodes were not detected by intraoperative inspection or palpation, and thus these cursory procedures are insufficient for patients at significant risk for nodal disease (85).

For the morbidly obese patient with endometrial cancer, abdominal surgery can be a difficult exercise for the surgeon, and the risk for postoperative complications such as wound infection or separation are high. Many of these women have well-differentiated cancers, a low risk for lymph node metastasis, and a good prognosis, and for them vaginal hysterectomy may be preferable (86, 87). Laparoscopic-assisted vaginal hysterectomy is being developed as another surgical approach to endometrial cancer. It allows for removal of the adnexae and completion of surgical staging, including retroperitoneal lymph node dissection (88). Laparoscopic lymph node sampling has also been performed to complete surgical staging in women with incompletely staged endometrial cancer (89). For selected patients, these promising approaches may reduce morbidity without compromising surgical adequacy.

A number of high-risk factors for endometrial cancer have been identified, including high tumor grade, papillary serous or clear cell histology, deep myometrial invasion, tumor extension to the cervix, adnexal metastasis, positive peritoneal cytology, or metastasis to the pelvic/aortic lymph nodes. Postoperative pelvic radiation therapy is commonly recommended for patients with one or more high-risk factors and disease confined to the uterus or pelvis. Vaginal brachytherapy is often administered if the tumor involves the cervix. Pelvic radiation therapy is quite effective in diminishing the likelihood for recurrent cancer within the pelvis, but its effect on improving overall survival is questionable (90, 91). A significant proportion of patients who develop recurrent endometrial cancer confined to the pelvis can be treated with radiation therapy and achieve long-term remission (91, 92). This would minimize the benefit of, and questions the need for, postoperative pelvic radiation in selected patients with high-risk factors. When endometrial cancer has metastasized to the aortic lymph nodes, a combination of pelvic plus para-aortic ("extended-field") radiotherapy is effective (93, 94). Patients with small-volume residual stage IVB endometrial cancer confined to the abdominal cavity may be treated with whole abdominal radiotherapy (95, 96). The Gynecologic Oncology Group has completed a prospective trial of whole abdominal radiotherapy for patients with stages III–IV adenocarcinoma and stages I–IV papillary serous or clear cell adenocarcinoma; the results of this study have not been published. Adjuvant chemotherapy may also be useful for the treatment of high-risk endometrial cancer, although this has yet to be confirmed by prospective studies (97).

There are considerable data suggesting that elderly women with endometrial cancer have worse outcomes. Morrow and colleagues from the Gynecologic Oncology Group (COG) reviewed the relationship between surgical–pathological risk factors and outcomes for patients with stages I–II endometrial cancer who underwent hysterectomy with/without postoperative radiation therapy (GOG protocol #33). The relative risk for recurrence was 1.8 times greater for patients more than 75 years of age and 1.4 times greater for patients 65–75 years of age (98). In an analysis of 41,120 cases from the SEER database, Kosary (34) noted a steady decrease in the 5-year survival with increasing age: less than 40 years (93.1%); 40–49 years (91.8%); 50–59 years (91.3%); 60–69 years (84.8%); and over 70 years (70.6%). Within each FIGO stage, the 5-year survival declines with increasing age (34). There is emerging evidence that elderly women with endometrial cancer do worse, because they have worse cancers. Two types of endometrial cancers have been postulated. Type I endometrial cancers usually occur in women who are obese, nulliparous, infertile, or have taken estrogens. Type I cancers are better differentiated (grade 1 or 2), rarely have deep myometrial invasion or nodal metastasis, and have an excellent prognosis. Type II endometrial cancers typically do not have estrogen-related features, are usually poorly differentiated (grade 3), are often of high risk (papillary serous or clear cell) histology, frequently have deep myometrial invasion or node metastasis, and are associated with a poorer prognosis (99). The proportion of type II cancers among elderly women with endometrial cancer is greater. Aside from tumor biology considerations, another reason that elderly women with endometrial cancer may do worse is because of the presence of coexisting medical conditions precluding operative treatment. For these medically inoperable patients, radiation therapy alone can be curative (100, 101). However, in a study by Chao et al., primary radiation therapy for endometrial cancer was less effective in elderly women, because they tended to die of their underlying medical illness (102).

V. OVARIAN CANCER

Ovarian cancer is the second most common gynecological cancer and the most common cause of gynecological cancer death. Each year there are approximately 26,800 new cases and 14,200 deaths from ovarian cancer (6). Ovarian cancer is the fifth leading cause of cancer mortality in women after tumors of the lung, breast, colon, and pancreas (6). Primary ovarian neoplasia is subdivided into three broad categories: epithelial tumors, germ cell neoplasms, and stromal tumors. Over 90% of malignant ovarian tumors are of the epithelial type and include serous, mucinous, endometrioid, and clear cell adenocarcinomas. Unless otherwise specified, *ovarian cancer* is synonymous with an epithelial ovarian malignancy.

The cause of ovarian cancer is unknown. A number of high-risk factors have been identified, including nulliparity or infertility, history of endometrial/colon/ breast cancer, family history, and age. Epithelial ovarian cancer may be viewed as a disease of the elderly. The incidence increases with age and peaks in the seventh and eighth decades of life (103). An ''incessant ovulation'' theory of ovarian cancer is supported by the marked reduction in risk which occurs by interrupting ovulation naturally (through pregnancy) or artificially (oral contraceptive use) (104). Furthermore, Schildkraut and colleagues showed that a women with ovarian cancers overexpressing p53 had a higher number of lifetime ovulatory cycles. They theorized that a higher number of ovulatory cycles may be associated with increased amounts of proliferation-associated DNA damage (105).

Approximately 3–5% of epithelial ovarian cancers occur as part of a familial syndrome. In most families affected by the breast–ovary or the site-specific ovarian cancer syndrome, genetic linkage has been found to the BRCA1 locus on chromosome 17q21 (106, 107). However, (spontaneous) germline *BRCA1* gene mutations are uncommon in nonfamilial ovarian cancer (108). The age of onset of ovarian cancer in hereditary syndromes is considerably younger than the general population mean of ovarian cancer patients (59 years) (109, 110). Furthermore, cancers associated with *BRCA1* mutations appear to have a more favorable clinical course (111).

There is no effective screening test for ovarian cancer and 75% of patients present with advanced disease, accounting for the high mortality from ovarian cancer. The CA-125 antigen is elevated in 85–90% of nonmucinous epithelial ovarian cancers and has been investigated as a possible screening test (112, 113). Transvaginal sonography is excellent for adnexal imaging, and it has also been investigated as a possible screening test (114, 115). Unfortunately, neither of these two modalities is sufficiently sensitive, specific, or cost effective for mass screening. Patients with ovarian cancer present with symptoms. Complaints may at first be vague or nonspecific (abdominal cramping or bloating, pain, changes in bowel or bladder habits, nausea, decreased appetite), but the diagnosis is not suspected until a mass or ascites is detected by examination, ultrasonography, or radiographic imaging (Fig. 4).

A detailed review of ovarian cancer treatment is beyond the scope of this chapter. Briefly, the FIGO staging classification (Table 4) is based on surgical findings, because almost all patients with ovarian cancer initially undergo surgical therapy: (a) to establish the diagnosis; (b) to determine the extent of the disease; and (c) to remove tumor. The comprehensive staging operation for ovarian cancer includes total abdominal hysterectomy and bilateral salpingo-oophorectomy (TAH& BSO), peritoneal washings or collection of ascitic fluid for cytological evaluation, omentectomy, appendectomy, pelvic and aortic lymph node biopsies, inspection of all abdominal viscera and peritoneal surfaces, and aggressive resection of metastatic disease (116).

All patients with ovarian cancer require postoperative chemotherapy except (a) patients with stage IA or IB ovarian cancer, grades 1–2; and (b) patients with low malignant potential ovarian cancer (117–120). Cisplatin-based chemotherapy

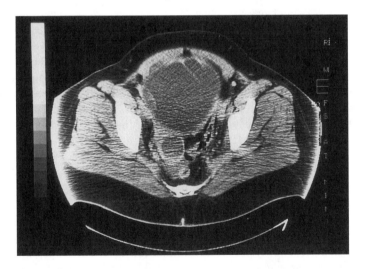

Figure 4 Computed tomogram revealing a large, cystic neoplasm in the pelvis and lower abdomen without ascites or obvious metastatic cancer. The patient underwent total abdominal hysterectomy, bilateral salpingo-oophorectomy, and surgical staging for what proved to be FIGO stage IA papillary serous adenocarcinoma (low malignant potential) of the ovary. No additional therapy was administered, and the patient remains without evidence for recurrent cancer 4 years after primary surgery.

Table 4 FIGO Staging Classification for Ovarian Cancer

Stage IA:	Growth limited to one ovary, no tumor on the external surface, capsule intact, no malignant ascites
Stage IB:	Growth limited to both ovaries, no tumor on the external surface, capsule intact, no malignant ascites
Stage IC:	Tumor classified as stage IA or IB but with tumor on the surface of one or both ovaries, ruptured capsule(s), or malignant ascites or positive peritoneal washings
Stage IIA:	Metastasis to the uterus or fallopian tubes
Stage IIB:	Extension or metastasis to other pelvic organs
Stage IIC:	Tumor classified as stage IIA or IIB but with tumor on the surface of one or both ovaries, ruptured capsule(s), or malignant ascites or positive peritoneal washings
Stage IIIA:	Tumor grossly limited to the pelvis but with histologically confirmed microscopic seeding of the abdominal peritoneal surface
Stage IIIB:	Tumor of one or both ovaries with histologically confirmed implants of the abdominal peritoneal surface ≤2 cm in diameter, negative nodes
Stage IIIC:	Implants >2 cm in diameter and/or positive pelvic or aortic or inguinal lymph nodes
Stage IV:	Tumor of one or both ovaries with distant metastasis such as pleural effusion (cytological confirmation) or parenchymal liver involvement

has become the standard treatment for epithelial ovarian cancer (121). Prospective controlled trials have confirmed the superiority of cisplatin-containing regimens over drug combinations which do not contain cisplatin (122, 123). Paclitaxel was identified as a drug with significant activity against epithelial ovarian cancer approximately 10 years ago (124). Clinical development of paclitaxel was initially hampered by its scarcity. After supply problems were alleviated, the National Cancer Institute initiated a trial of paclitaxel salvage treatment for patients with cisplatin-refractory ovarian cancer. Among the over 1000 patients who participated in this important study, objective responses were reported in 22% (125). Subsequently, the Gynecologic Oncology Group completed a randomized controlled trial of cisplatin plus paclitaxel versus cisplatin plus cyclophosphamide in patients with advanced, suboptimal ovarian cancer. The paclitaxel-containing regimen yielded superior objective response rates and survival (126). Paclitaxel has subsequently been combined with both cisplatin and carboplatin at various doses and infusion rates ranging anywhere from 1 h to 4 days. Ongoing and future investigations are attempting to identify the ideal platinum–paclitaxel drug combination, dose, and schedule.

Despite aggressive surgery and chemotherapy, mortality from epithelial ovarian cancer over the past 30 years has not changed substantially (6). The prognosis for advanced disease is poor at any age, but it appears to be dismal in the elderly. Between 1973 and 1988, ovarian cancer mortality decreased by 25% in younger women but increased by 16% in elderly patients (127). In a review of 21,240 cases of ovarian cancer from the SEER database multivariate analysis showed that age is an independent predictor for survival. Within FIGO staging, the 5-year survival decreases with increasing age. Comparing women less than 40 years of age versus more than 70 years of age, survival for stages III and IV ovarian cancer decreases from 63.2 to 17.6% and from 50.0 to 7.7%, respectively (34). Only in recent years has information regarding the poor survival for elderly women with ovarian cancer become available. Yancik and associates reviewed the clinical outcomes of 11,062 women treated for epithelial ovarian cancer between 1973 and 1982. Compared to younger patients, women 65 years of age and older were more likely to have advanced disease at initial diagnosis and were more likely to receive single-modality treatment. More than 10% of elderly women with stage III/IV ovarian cancer received no treatment, and 60% of the patients who did not undergo surgery were elderly (128). In their analysis of the American College of Surgeons database, Hightower and colleagues reported that elderly women with ovarian cancer had a worse prognosis. Successful tumor cytoreduction decreased from 43.7 to 21.7%, respectively, for patients less than 60 years of age versus more than 80 years of age. Only 15% of elderly patients had tumors that were completely resected. There was also a significant difference in the use of postoperative chemotherapy for younger (72%) versus older (42%) patients (129).

Although these reports suggest that elderly women with ovarian cancer do worse, statistical databases cannot control for all variables which could influence outcome, including the completeness and accuracy of data reporting, and differences in treatment. Nonetheless, analyses from two cooperative cancer study groups of patients participating in prospective clinical trials suggest that age is an independent prognostic variable. Multivariate analysis of 2123 evaluable patients treated by the Gynecologic Oncology Group in six randomized controlled studies identified three factors associated with age: volume of residual disease, tumor grade, and performance status. The survival analysis suggested that age was a significant prognostic factor (130). Multivariate analysis of 291 patients treated in a single Southwest Oncology Group trial revealed that age, race, stage, and performance status were significant prognostic factors for survival. Elderly patients with a poor performance status and all African-American patients regardless of age, stage, or performance status, were particularly likely to do poorly (131).

VI. CONCLUSIONS

The risk for developing gynecological cancer increases with age. Elderly patients with gynecological cancers of the vulva, cervix, endometrium, or ovary appear to have a poorer prognosis. Accepting for the present that age is an important factor influencing outcome, it is important to ask whether age is an independent prognostic variable or whether patient age reflects other known prognostic factors. Do elderly patients do worse because they are elderly, because they receive different treatments, or because they have more biologically aggressive cancers? If elderly patients receive different treatments, is it because of complicating medical conditions, physician or family biases, or unique patient expectations and needs? Are there genetic and biological differences between gynecological cancers arising in younger versus older women and, if so, how can these differences be exploited with treatment? The answers to these and many other questions pertaining to gynecological cancers in the elderly are unknown.

REFERENCES

1. U.S Census Bureau, Office of Statistics: Statistical brief: sixty-five plus in the United States. Washington, DC: U.S. Census Bureau, Office of Statistics, 1997.
2. U.S. Bureau of the Census, Current Population Reports, series P-25, No. 1045.
3. U.S. National Center for Health Statistics, Vital Statistics of the United States, annual.
4. Yancik R. Frame of reference: old age as the context for the prevention and treatment of cancer. In: Yancik R, ed. Perspectives on Prevention and Treatment of Cancer in the Elderly. New York: Raven Press, 1983:5–17.
5. Silliman RA, Balducci L, Goodwin JS, et al. Breast cancer care in old age: what we know, don't know, and do. J Natl Cancer Inst 1993; 85:190–199.
6. Parker SL, Tong T, Bolden S, Wingo PA. Cancer statistics, 1997. CA Cancer J Clin 1997; 47:5–27.
7. Zaino RJ. Carcinoma of the vulva, urethra, and Bartholin's glands. In: Wilkinson EJ, ed. Pathology of the Vulva and Vagina. New York: Churchill Livingstone, 1987:119–153.
8. Henson D, Tarone R. An epidemiologic study of cancer of the cervix, vagina, and vulva based on the Third National Cancer Survey in the United States. Am J Obstet Gynecol 1977; 129:525–532.
9. Nilsson T, Malmstrom H, Simonsen E, Trope C. Case report: a 16-year-old girl with invasive carcinoma in the vulva. Acta Obstet Gynecol Scand 1990; 69:551–552.
10. Moore DH, Fowler WC, Currie JL, Walton LA. Case report: Squamous cell carcinoma of the vulva in pregnancy. Gynecol Oncol 1991; 41:74–77.
11. Franklin EW, Rutledge FD. Epidemiology of epidermoid carcinoma of the vulva. Obstet Gynecol 1972; 39:165–172.
12. Thomas RHM, Ridley CM, McGibbon DH, Black MM. Lichen sclerosis et atrophicus and autoimmunity: a study of 350 women. Br J Dermatol 1988; 118:41–46.
13. Sturgeon SR. In situ and invasive vulvar cancer incidence trends (1973–1987). Am J Obstet Gynecol 1992; 166:1482–1485.
14. Mabuchi K, Bross DS, Kessler II. Epidemiology of cancer of the vulva: a case control study. Cancer 1985; 55:1843–1848.
15. Brinton LA, Nasca PC, Mallin K, et al. Case control study of cancer of the vulva. Obstet Gynecol 1990; 75:859–866.
16. Hording U, Daugaard S, Iversen AKN, et al. Human papillomavirus type 16 in vulvar carcinoma, vulvar intraepithelial neoplasia, and associated cervical neoplasia. Gynecol Oncol 1991; 42:22–26.

17. Buscema J, Naghashfar Z, Sawada E, et al. The predominance of human papillomavirus type 16 in vulvar neoplasia. Obstet Gynecol 1988; 71:601–606.

18. Hording U, Junge J, Daugaard S, et al. Vulvar squamous cell carcinoma and papillomaviruses: indications for two different etiologies. Gynecol Oncol 1994; 52:241–246.

19. Trimble CL, Hildesheim A, Brinton LA, et al. Heterogeneous etiology of squamous carcinoma of the vulva. Obstet Gynecol 1996; 87:59–64.

20. Nuovo GJ, Delvenne P, MacConnell P, et al. Correlation of histology and detection of human papillomavirus DNA in vulvar cancers. Gynecol Oncol 1991; 43:275–280.

21. Kurman RJ, Toki T, Schiffman MH. Basaloid and warty carcinoma of the vulva. Am J Surg Pathol 1993; 17:133–145.

22. Taussig FJ. An analysis of 155 cases of vulvar carcinoma. Am J Obstet Gynecol 1949; 40:764–769.

23. Way S. The anatomy of the lymphatic drainage of the vulva and its influence on the radical operation for carcinoma. Ann R Coll Surg Engl 1948; 3:187–209.

24. DiSaia PJ, Creasman WT, Rich WM. An alternative approach to early cancer of the vulva. Am J Obstet Gynecol 1979; 133:825–832.

25. Burke TJ, Levenback C, Coleman RL, et al. Gershenson DM. Surgical therapy of T1 and T2 vulvar carcinoma: further experience with radical wide excision and selective inguinal lymphadenectomy. Gynecol Oncol 1994; 57:515–520.

26. Berman ML, Soper JT, Creasman WT, et al. Conservative surgical management of superficially invasive stage I vulvar carcinoma. Gynecol Oncol 1989; 35:352–357.

27. Hacker NF, Leuchter RS, Berek JS, et al. Radical vulvectomy and bilateral inguinal lymphadenectomy through separate groin incisions. Obstet Gynecol 1981; 58:574–579.

28. Hacker NJ. Current treatment of small vulvar cancers. Oncology 1990; 4:21–25.

29. Stehman FB, Bundy BN, Dvoretsky PM, Creasman WT. Early stage I carcinoma of the vulva treated with ipsilateral superficial inguinal lymphadenectomy and modified radical hemivulvectomy: a prospective study of the Gynecologic Oncology Group. Obstet Gynecol 1992; 79:490–497.

30. Homesley HD, Bundy BN, Sedlis A, Adcock L. Radiation therapy versus pelvic node resection for carcinoma of the vulva with positive groin nodes. Obstet Gynecol 1986; 68:733–740.

31. Stehman FB, Bundy BN, Thomas G, et al. Groin dissection versus groin radiation in carcinoma of the vulva. Int J Radiat Oncol Biol Phys 1992; 24:389–396.

32. Boronow RC. Therapeutic alternative to primary exenteration for advanced vulvovaginal cancer. Gynecol Oncol 1973; 1:233–255.

33. Perez CA, Grigsby PW, Galakatos A, et al. Radiation therapy in management of carcinoma of the vulva with emphasis on conservative therapy. Cancer 1993; 71:3707–3716.

34. Kosary CL. FIGO stage, histology, histologic grade, age and race as prognostic factors in determining survival for cancers of the female gynecological system: an analysis of 1973–87 SEER cases of cancers of the endometrium, cervix, ovary, vulva, and vagina. Semin Surg Oncol 1994; 10:31–46.

35. Rosen C, Malmstrom H. Invasive cancer of the vulva. Gynecol Oncol 1997; 65:213–217.

36. Brinton LA, Hamman RF, Huggins GR, et al. Sexual and reproductive risk factors for invasive squamous cell cervical cancer. J Natl Cancer Inst 1987; 79:23–30.

37. La Vecchia C, Franceschi S, Decarli A, et al. Sexual factors, venereal diseases, and the risk of intraepithelial and invasive cervical neoplasia. Cancer 1986; 58:935–941.

38. Agarwal SS, Sehgal A, Sardana S, et al. Role of male behavior in cervical carcinogenesis among women with one lifetime sexual partner. Cancer 1993; 72:1666–1669.

39. Schiffman MH. Recent progress in defining the epidemiology of human papillomavirus infection and cervical neoplasia. J Natl Cancer Inst 1992; 84:394–398.

40. Hines JF, Jenson AB, Barnes WA. Human papillomaviruses: their clinical significance in the management of cervical carcinoma. Oncol 1995; 9:279–285.

41. Das BC, Gopalkrishna V, Das DK, et al. Human papillomavirus DNA sequences in adenocarcinoma of the uterine cervix in Indian women. Cancer 1993; 72:147–153.

42. Koutsky LA, Holmes KK, Critchlow CW, et al. A cohort study of the risk of cervical intraepithelial neoplasia grade 2 or 3 in relation the papillomavirus infection. N Engl J Med 1992; 327:1272–1278.

43. Rylander E, Ruusuvaara L, Almstromer MW, et al. The absence of vaginal human papillomavirus 16 DNA in women who have not experienced sexual intercourse. Obstet Gynecol 1994; 83:735–737.

44. Bergman A, Nalick R. Prevalence of human papillomavirus infection in men: comparison of the partners of infected and uninfected women. J Reprod Med 1992; 37:710–712.

45. Levine RU, Crum CP, Herman E, et al. Cervical papillomavirus infection and intraepithelial neoplasia: a study of male sexual partners. Obstet Gynecol 1984; 64:16–20.

46. Paquette RL, Lee YY, Wilczynski SP, et al. Mutations of p53 and human papillomavirus infection in cervical carcinoma. Cancer 1993; 72:1272–1280.

47. Hellberg D, Nilsson S, Haley NJ, et al. Smoking and cervical intraepithelial neoplasia: nicotine and cotinine in serum and cervical mucus in smokers and nonsmokers. Am J Obstet Gynecol 1988; 158:910–913.

48. Barton SE, Maddox PH, Jenkins D, et al. Effect of cigarette smoking on cervical epithelial immunity: a mechanism for neoplastic change? Lancet 1988; 2:652–654.

49. Slattery ML, Robison LM, Schuman KL, et al. Cigarette smoking and exposure to passive smoke are risk factors for cervical cancer. JAMA 1989; 261:1593–1598.

50. Sood AK. Cigarette smoking and cervical cancer: meta-analysis and critical review of recent studies. FAX 1991; 6:31–36.

51. Moore DH. Anatomy, natural history, and patterns of spread of invasive cervical cancer. In: Rubin SC, Hoskins WJ, eds. Cervical Cancer and Preinvasive neoplasia. Philadelphia: Lippincott-Raven, 1996:161–170.

52. Landoni F, Maneo A, Colombo A, et al. Randomised study of radical surgery versus radiotherapy for stage Ib-IIa cervical cancer. Lancet 1997; 350:535–540.

53. Newton M. Radical hysterectomy or radiotherapy for stage I cervical cancer: a prospective comparison with 5 and 10 year follow-up. Am J Obstet Gynecol 1975; 123:535–539.

54. Roddick JW, Greenelaw RH. Treatment of cervical cancer: a randomized study of operation and radiation. Am J Obstet Gynecol 1971; 109:754–759.

55. Perez CA. Part 2: Radiation therapy in the management of cancer of the cervix. Oncology 1993; 7:61–69.

56. Shingleton HM, Jones WB, Russell A, et al. Hysterectomy in invasive cervical cancer: a national patterns of care study of the American College of Surgeons. J Am Coll Surg 1996; 183:393–400.

57. Gallion HH, Van Nagell JR, Donaldson ES, et al. Combined radiation therapy and extrafascial hysterectomy in the treatment of stage IB barrel-shaped cervical cancer. Cancer 1985; 56:262–265.

58. Perez CA, Grigsby PW, Camel HM, et al. Irradiation alone or combined with surgery in stage IB, IIA, and IIB carcinoma of uterine cervix: update of a nonrandomized comparison. Int J Radiat Oncol Biol Phys 1995; 31:703–716.

59. Larson DM, Stringer CA, Copeland LJ, et al. Stage IB cervical carcinoma treated with radical hysterectomy and pelvic lymphadenectomy: role of adjuvant radiotherapy. Obstet Gynecol 1987; 69:378–381.

60. Stock RG, Chen ASJ, Flickinger JC, et al. Node-positive cervical cancer: impact of pelvic irradiation and patterns of failure. Int J Radiat Oncol Biol Phys 1995; 31:31–36.

61. Komaki R, Brickner TJ, Hanlon AL, et al. Long-term results of treatment of cervical carcinoma in the United States in 1973, 1978, and 1983: patterns of Care Study (PCS). Int J Radiat Oncol Biol Phys 1995; 31:973–982.

62. Petereit DG, Sarkaria JN, Chappell R, et al. The adverse effect of treatment prolongation in cervical carcinoma. Int J Radiat Oncol Biol Phys 1995; 32:1301–1307.

63. Hreshchyshyn MM, Aron BS, Boronow RC, et al. Hydroxyurea or placebo combined with radiation to treat stages IIIB and IV cervical cancer confined to the pelvis. Int J Radiat Oncol Biol Phys 1979; 5:317–322.

64. Stehman FB, Bundy BN, Keys H, et al. A randomized trial of hydroxyurea versus misonidazole adjunct to radiation therapy in carcinoma of the cervix: a preliminary report of a Gynecologic Oncology Group study. Am J Obstet Gynecol 1988; 159:87–94.

65. Stehman FB, Bundy BN, Thomas G, et al. Hydroxyurea versus misonidazole with radiation in cervical carcinoma: long-term follow-up of a Gynecologic Oncology Group trial. J Clin Oncol 1993; 11:1523–1528.

66. Edelmann DZ, Anteby SO. Neoadjuvant chemotherapy for locally advanced cervical cancer—where does it stand?: a review. Obstet Gynecol Surv 1996; 51:305–313.

67. Panici PB, Scambia G, Baiocchi G, et al. Neoadjuvant chemotherapy and radical surgery in locally advanced cervical cancer: prognostic factors for response and survival. Cancer 1991; 67:372–379.

68. Sardi JE, Giaroli A, Sananes C, et al. Long-term follow-up of the first randomized trial using neoadjuvant chemotherapy in stage Ib squamous carcinoma of the cervix: the final results. Gynecol Oncol 1997; 67:61–69.

69. Omura GA. Current status of chemotherapy for cancer of the cervix. Oncology 1992; 6:27–32.

70. Stehman FB, Bundy BN, DiSaia PJ, et al. Carcinoma of the cervix treated with radiation therapy: a multi-variate analysis of prognostic variables in the Gynecologic Oncology Group. Cancer 1991; 67:2776–2785.

71. Mandelblatt J, Gopaul I, Wistreich M. Gynecological care of elderly women: another look at Papanicolaou smear testing. JAMA 1986; 256:367–371.

72. Mandelblatt J, Fahs MC. The cost-effectiveness of cervical cancer screening for low-income elderly women. JAMA 1988; 259:2409–2413.

73. Wharton JT, Mikuta JJ, Mettlin C, et al. Risk factors and current management in carcinoma of the endometrium. Surg Gynecol Obstet 1986; 162:515–520.

74. The Cancer and Steroid Hormone Study of the Centers for Disease Control and the National Institute of Child Health and Human Development. Combination oral contraceptive use and the risk of endometrial cancer. JAMA 1987; 257:796–800.

75. Watson P, Lynch HT. Extracolonic cancer in hereditary nonpolyposis colorectal cancer. Cancer 1993; 71:677–685.

76. Mecklin JP, Jarvinen HJ. Tumor spectrum in cancer family syndrome (hereditary nonpolyposis colorectal cancer). Cancer 1991; 68:1109–1112.

77. Kosary CL, Reis LAG, Miller BA, et al., eds. SEER cancer statistics review, 1973–1992: tables and graphs. Bethesda, MW: National Cancer Institute (NIH publication #95-2789), 1995:171–181.

78. Barakat RR. The effect of tamoxifen on the endometrium. Oncology 1995; 9:129–139.

79. Cohen I, Tepper R, Rosen DJD, et al. Continuous tamoxifen treatment in asymptomatic, postmenopausal breast cancer patients does not cause aggravation of endometrial pathologies. Gynecol Oncol 1994; 55:138–143.

80. ACOG Committee Opinion #169. Tamoxifen and endometrial cancer. Washington, DC: American College of Obstetricians and Gynecologists, 1996.

81. Moore DH. Surgical staging of endometrial carcinoma. Clin Consult Obstet Gynecol 1993; 5:100–107.

82. Homesley HD, Kadar N, Barrett RJ, Lentz SS. Selective pelvic and periaortic lymphadenectomy does not increase morbidity in surgical staging of endometrial carcinoma. Am J Obstet Gynecol 1992; 167:1225–1230.

83. Larson DM, Johnson K, Olson KA. Pelvic and para-aortic lymphadenectomy for surgical staging of endometrial cancer: morbidity and mortality. Obstet Gynecol 1992; 79:993–1001.

84. Moore DH, Fowler WC, Walton LA, Droegemueller W. Morbidity of lymph node sampling in cancers of the uterine corpus and cervix. Obstet Gynecol 1989; 74:180–184.

85. Boronow RC, Morrow CP, Creasman WT, et al. Surgical staging in endometrial cancer: clinical-pathologic findings of a prospective study. Obstet Gynecol 1984; 63:825–832.

86. Peters WA, Andersen WA, Thornton WN, Morley GW. The selective use of vaginal hysterectomy in the management of adenocarcinoma of the endometrium. Am J Obstet Gynecol 1983; 146:285–289.

87. Lelle RJ, Morley GW, Peters WA. The role of vaginal hysterectomy in the treatment of endometrial carcinoma. Int J Gynecol Cancer 1994; 4:342–347.

88. Childers JM, Brzechffa PR, Hatch KD, Surwit EA. Laparoscopic assisted surgical staging (LASS) of endometrial carcinoma. Gynecol Oncol 1993; 51:33–38.

89. Childers JM, Spirtos NM, Brainard P, Surwit EA. Laparoscopic staging of the patient with incompletely staged early adenocarcinoma of the endometrium. Obstet Gynecol 1994; 83:597–600.

90. Aalders J, Abeler V, Kolstad P, Onsrud M. Postoperative external irradiation and prognostic parameters in stage I endometrial carcinoma: clinical and histopathologic study of 540 patients. Obstet Gynecol 1980; 56:419–426.

91. Roberts JA, Brunetto VL, Keys HM, et al. A phase III randomized study of surgery

versus surgery plus adjunctive radiation therapy in intermediate risk endometrial adenocarcinoma (GOG #99). Gynecol Oncol (in press).

92. Ackerman I, Malone S, Thomas G, et al. Endometrial carcinoma—relative effectiveness of adjuvant irradiation vs therapy reserved for relapse. Gynecol Oncol 1996; 60: 177–183.

93. Potish RA, Twiggs LB, Adcock LL, et al. Paraaortic lymph node radiotherapy in cancer of the uterine corpus. Obstet Gynecol 1985; 65:251–256.

94. Rose PG, Cha SD, Tak WK, et al. Radiation therapy for surgically proven para-aortic node metastasis in endometrial carcinoma. Int J Radiat Oncol Biol Phys 1992; 24: 229–233.

95. Greer BE, Hamberger AD. Treatment of intraperitoneal metastatic adenocarcinoma of the endometrium by the whole-abdomen moving-strip technique and pelvic boost irradiation. Gynecol Oncol 1983; 16:365–373.

96. Loeffler JS, Rosen EM, Niloff JM, et al. Whole abdominal irradiation for tumors of the uterine corpus. Cancer 1988; 61:1332–1335.

97. Smith MR, Peters WA, Drescher CW. Cisplatin, doxorubicin hydrochloride, and cyclophosphamide followed by radiotherapy in high-risk endometrial carcinoma. Am J Obstet Gynecol 1994; 170:1677–1682.

98. Morrow CP, Bundy BN, Kurman RJ, et al. Relationship between surgical-pathological risk factors and outcome in clinical stage I and II carcinoma of the endometrium: a Gynecologic Oncology Group study. Gynecol Oncol 1991; 40:55–65.

99. Bokhman JV. Two pathogenetic types of endometrial carcinoma. Gynecol Oncol 1983; 15:10–17.

100. Kupelian PA, Eifel PJ, Tornos C, et al. Treatment of endometrial carcinoma with radiation therapy alone. Int J Radiat Oncol Biol Phys 1993; 27:817–824.

101. Rose PG, Baker S, Kern M, et al. Primary radiation therapy for endometrial carcinoma: a case controlled study. Int J Radiat Oncol Biol Phys 1993; 27:585–590.

102. Chao CKS, Grigsby PW, Perez CA, et al. Medically inoperable stage I endometrial carcinoma: a few dilemmas in radiotherapeutic management. Int J Radiat Oncol Biol Phys 1996; 34:27–31.

103. Averette HE, Hoskins W, Nguyen HN, et al. National survey of ovarian carcinoma: I. A patient care evaluation of the American College of Surgeons. Cancer 1993; 71: 1629S–1638S.

104. Ramcharan S, Pellegrin FA, Ray R, Hsu J-P. Volume 3: The Walnut Creek contraceptive drug study: a prospective study of the side effects of oral contraceptives. Bethesda, MD; National Institute of Child Health and Human Development, 1981.

105. Schildkraut JM, Bastos E, Berchuck A. Relationship between lifetime ovulatory cycles and overexpression of mutant p53 in epithelial ovarian cancer. J Natl Cancer Inst 1997; 89:932–938.

106. Easton DF, Bishop DT, Ford D, Crockford GP. Genetic linkage analysis in familial breast and ovarian cancer: results from 214 families: The Breast Cancer Linkage Consortium. Am J Hum Genet 1993; 52:678–701.

107. Steichen-Gersdorf E, Gallion HH, Ford D, Girodet C. Familial site-specific ovarian cancer is linked to BRCA1 on 17q12-21. Am J Hum Genet 1994; 55:870–875.

108. Stratton JF, Gayther SA, Russell P, et al. Contribution of BRCA1 mutations to ovarian cancer. N Engl J Med 1997; 336:1125–1130.

109. Amos CI, Shaw GL, Tucker MA, Hartge P. Age at onset for familial epithelial ovarian cancer. JAMA 1992; 268:1896–1899.
110. Lynch HT, Watson P, Bewtra C, et al. Hereditary ovarian cancer: heterogeneity in age at diagnosis. Cancer 1991; 67:1460–1466.
111. Rubin SC, Benjamin I, Behbakht K, et al. Clinical and pathological features of ovarian cancer in women with germ-line mutations of BRCA1. N Engl J Med 1996;335:1413–1416.
112. Jacobs I, Stabile I, Bridges J, et al. Multimodal approach to screening for ovarian cancer. Lancet 1988; 1988;268–271.
113. Einhorn N, Sjovall K, Schoenfeld S. Early detection of ovarian cancer using the CA125 radioimmunoassay (RIA). Proc ASCO 1990; 9:157 (absr #607).
114. Bourne TH, Whitehead MI, Campbell S, et al. Ultrasound screening for familial ovarian cancer. Gynecol Oncol 1991; 43:92–97.
115. DePriest PD, Van Nagell JR, Gallion HH, et al. Ovarian cancer screening in asymptomatic postmenopausal women. Gynecol Oncol 1993; 51:205–209.
116. Moore DH. Primary surgical management of early epithelial ovarian carcinoma. In: Rubin SC, Sutton GP, eds. Ovarian Cancer. New York: McGraw-Hill, 1993:219–239.
117. Young RC, Walton LA, Ellenberg SS, et al. Adjuvant therapy in stage I and stage II epithelial ovarian cancer: results of two prospective randomized trials. N Engl J Med 1990; 322:1021–1027.
118. Schilder RJ, Boente MP, Corn BW, et al. The management of early ovarian cancer. Oncology 1995; 9:171–182.
119. Kennedy AW, Hart WR. Ovarian papillary serous tumors of low malignant potential (serous borderline tumors): a long term follow-up study, including patients with microinvasion, lymph node metastasis, and transformation to invasive serous carcinoma. Cancer 1996; 78:278–286.
120. Sykes PH, Quinn MA, Rome RM. Ovarian tumors of low malignant potential: a retrospective study of 234 patients. Int J Gynecol Cancer 1997; 7:218–226.
121. Ehrlich CE, Einhorn L, Williams SD, Morgan J. Chemotherapy for stage III-IV epithelial ovarian cancer with *cis*-dichlorodiammineplatinum (II), adriamycin, and cyclophosphamide: a preliminary report. Cancer Treat Rep 1979; 63:281–288.
122. Omura GA, Blessing JA, Ehrlich CE, et al. A randomized trial of cyclophosphamide and doxorubicin with or without cisplatin in advanced ovarian carcinoma: a Gynecologic Oncology Group study. Cancer 1986; 57:1725–1730.
123. Neijt JP, ten Bokkel Huinink WW, van der Burg ME, et al. Randomised trial comparing two combination chemotherapy regimens (Hexa-CAF vs CHAP-5) in advanced ovarian carcinoma. Lancet 1984; 2:594–600.
124. Donehower RC, Rowinsky EK, Grochow LB, et al. Phase I trial of taxol in patients with advanced cancer. Cancer Treat Rep 1987; 71:1171–1177.
125. Trimble EL, Adams JD, Vena D, et al. Paclitaxel for platinum-refractory ovarian cancer: results from the first 1000 patients registered to National Cancer Institute Treatment Referral Center 9103. J Clin Oncol 1993; 11:2405–2410.
126. McGuire WP, Hoskins WJ, Brady MF, et al. Cyclophosphamide and cisplatin compared with paclitaxel and cisplatin in patients with stage III and IV ovarian cancer. N Engl J Med 1996; 334:1–6.
127. Ries LAG, Hankey BF, Miller BA, et al. Cancer statistics review 1973–1988. Bethesda, MD: National Institutes of Health, National Cancer Institute, 1991.

128. Yancik R, Ries LG, Yates JW. Ovarian cancer in the elderly: An analysis of Surveillance, Epidemiology, and End Results Program data. Am J Obstet Gynecol 1986; 154: 639–647.

129. Hightower RD, Nguyen HN, Averette HE, et al. National survey of ovarian carcinoma: IV. Patterns of care and related survival for older patients. Cancer 1994; 73:377S–383S.

130. Thigpen JT, Brady MF, Omura GA, et al. Age as a prognostic factor in ovarian carcinoma. Cancer 1993; 71:606S–614S.

131. Alberts DS, Dahlberg S, Green SJ, et al. Analysis of patient age as an independent prognostic factor for survival in a phase III study of cisplatin-cyclophosphamide versus carboplatin-cyclophosphamide in stages III (suboptimal) and IV ovarian cancer. Cancer 1993; 71:618S–627S.

13
Genitourinary Cancer

Christopher W. Ryan and Nicholas J. Vogelzang
University of Chicago Medical Center
Chicago, Illinois

I. INTRODUCTION

Cancers of the genitourinary system include those of the prostate, bladder, adrenal, kidney, and testicle. All but testicular cancer are primarily diseases of the elderly. For example, when a malignant testicular mass is discovered in an elderly man, it is much more likely to be lymphoma than a germ cell testicular cancer. Genitourinary cancers encompass a spectrum from asymptomatic, latent tumors that may never be of clinical consequence to aggressive and painful metastatic processes. Treatment regimens for the elderly patient with genitourinary cancer must be carefully chosen, with the morbidity of therapy weighed against that of the disease. Appropriate treatment for these cancers may range from conservative "watchful waiting" to aggressive, multimodality therapies that include surgery, radiation, and chemotherapy.

In this chapter, the current recommendations for screening, staging, and treatment of prostatic, bladder, and kidney cancer are reviewed. Special consideration is given to the management of elderly patients. As germ cell testicular cancer is essentially nonexistent in this population, this disease will not be discussed.

II. PROSTATIC CANCER

Prostatic cancer is the most common cancer in American men. Although prostatic cancer does affect younger men, it is mostly a disease of the elderly, with a median age at diagnosis of 66 years (1). Although the 1996 estimated number of new cases of prostatic cancer was over 340,000 (2), in 1999, it was estimated that only 179,000 new cases of prostate cancer would be diagnosed in the United States (3). Nonetheless with nearly 37,000 deaths attributable to the disease, prostatic cancer is the second leading cause of cancer death in men. At autopsy, over two thirds of men over 80 years of age have asymptomatic "latent" prostate cancer (4). Older age remains the greatest risk factor for the development of prostatic carcinoma, with a 70-year-old male having an approximately 1 in 8 risk compared to a 50-year-old with a 1 in 100 risk. The cause of prostatic cancer is unknown, although racial, genetic, and dietary factors have been implicated (1). Approximately 9% of prostatic cancers can be attributed to inherited mutations in prostatic cancer–susceptibility genes (5). A major susceptibility locus for prostatic cancer has been mapped to chromosome 1q and has been designated *HPC1* (hereditary prostate cancer 1) (6). No research has yet linked aging to mutations of this gene. Recent evidence suggests that a CAG repeat polymorphism in the androgen receptor gene confers risk for prostatic cancer, with fewer repeats in the germline associated with an increased likelihood of developing the disease (7).

The increasing (and now decreasing) incidence of prostatic cancer can be attributed to widespread screening using prostate-specific antigen (PSA). The increasing use of the assay in the late 1980s, coupled with the ease of transrectal prostatic biopsies using spring-loaded devices and transrectal ultrasonography, caused an "explosion" in prostatic cancer detection probably peaking in 1996, and greater public awareness of the disease has also contributed to this rapid increase in detection. Since the median time to death from prostate cancer is 8–10 years, clinicians face a dilemma in managing patients diagnosed after the age of 65 years: What are the risks and benefits of aggressive therapy in a geriatric population that may not live long enough to succumb to the effects of this slow-growing malignancy?

The American Cancer Society recommends annual digital rectal examination in combination with PSA testing for prostatic cancer screening beginning at age 50 years, or at a younger age for African-Americans or those with a family history of the disease (8). Retrospective analysis has suggested that biannual PSA testing may be an acceptable screening interval when the initial PSA level is less than 2 ng/mL (9). Families with an altered *HPC1* gene exhibit more advanced stage and younger age at diagnosis, thus supporting initiation of annual screening at age 40 years in susceptible families (10).

The use of the PSA assay as a screening tool has been the center of much controversy. The PSA is a serine protease of the kallikrein family (11) that is found only in prostatic tissue. Increases in prostatic volume, prostatic infarctions, ejaculation, and other nonspecific factors leads to an elevation of PSA as men age even in the absence of malignancy. The low specificity of the PSA test has lead to many unnecessary workups for men with false-positive results. Conversely, 20% of prostatic cancers are diagnosed in men with low PSAs (<4 ng/mL). The normal range that is in common use, regardless of age, is 0–4 ng/mL. Some investigators have recommended the institution of age-specific reference ranges, with higher levels of PSA accepted as "normal" for older patients. One such reference range was developed by Oesterling et al., who studied a group of men between the ages of 40 and 79 years and found a longitudinal increase in serum PSA as men age (Table 1) (12). Institution of age-specific reference ranges may decrease the number of biopsies performed on older patients, whereas increasing the sensitivity for detecting prostatic cancer in younger men. The use of PSA "density" (amount of PSA per unit volume of prostate gland, as determined by transrectal ultrasound) and PSA "velocity" (prostatic cancer causes a more rapid increase in PSA over time) have been investigated as methods to increase screening specificity, but neither refinement has proven useful (13, 14). Prostate-specific antigen complexed with α_1-antichymotrypsin, so-called "bound-PSA," is the form preferentially elevated in prostatic carcinoma, and the combined measurements of free (nonbound) PSA with total PSA may increase the positive predictive value of the test (15). Before employing the PSA assay to screen a patient for prostatic cancer, discussion with the patient should be undertaken to explain the nature of the test and the implications and consequences of the potential results. Some investigators have concluded that PSA screening may be highly cost effective, costing less than $5000 per year of life saved, which compares well to the cost of other cancer-screening practices, such as the $50,000 per year of life saved with mammography (16).

Most commonly, PSA is used to measure response to therapy. Values of PSA should drop to undetectable levels after radical prostatectomy for localized disease (17). Detectable PSA after surgery may indicate residual local disease or distant metastases. Increasing PSA levels after treatment of metastatic disease is usually the earliest sign of relapse. Likewise, a decreasing PSA during treatment of metastatic disease can be used as a response marker and may be indicative of improved survival (18). The acid phosphatase level is another serum marker that was formerly most useful for detecting extracapsular disease in untreated patients, and it is helpful in determining which patients may benefit from surgery.

Prostatic cancer usually causes few clinical symptoms in its early stages. As prostatic cancer progresses, symptoms of urinary obstruction may occur, including hesitancy,weakness of stream, postvoid dribbling, incomplete voiding, and nocturia.

Table 1 PSA Age-Specific Reference Ranges

Age (years)	Serum PSA Concentration (ng/mL)
40–49	0–2.5
50–59	0–3.5
60–69	0–4.5
70–79	0–6.5

PSA, prostate-specific antigen.
Source: Adapted from Ref. 12.

Pain from bony metastases occurs in late-stage disease. Anemia or pancytopenia may result from bone marrow replacement in very advanced disease.

Staging of prostatic cancer is described either using the older Whitmore-Jewett classification system or the newer tumor, node, and metastases (TNM) system (Table 2) (19, 20). A typical staging workup includes measurement of PSA and serum acid phosphatase, chest radiograph, and bone scan (if the PSA is >10 ng/mL). Although there is a high rate of inaccurate staging, as extracapsular or lymph node spread is often difficult to assess clinically and may not be detected until the time of surgery, PSA levels are increasingly being used as a surrogate staging tool. Levels of PSA over 20 ng/mL are virtually synonymous with more advanced local disease.

The most common grading system in use is the Gleason system. A score of 2 through 10 is applied based on the primary and secondary growth patterns of the tumor. The higher the grade, the more undifferentiated the tumor and the less discrete

Table 2 Prostate Cancer Staging

	Whitmore–Jewet	TNM
Found at time of TURP		
<5% Ca, ≤3 foci, low-grade	A1	T1a
>5% Ca, >3 foci, high-grade	A2	T1b
Found at time of TRUS[a] biopsy, prompted by elevated PSA		T1c
Organ Confined		
Palpable tumor		
One lobe	B1	T2a
Both lobes	B2	T2b
Locally Invasive		
Extracapsular extension (unilateral or bilateral)	C1	T3a
To base of seminal vesicles	C2	T3b
Beyond base of seminal vesicles	C3	T3b
Invades bladder neck, external sphincter, rectum, levator muscles, or pelvic side wall		T4
Metastatic Disease		
Elevated acid phosphate only	D0	
Pelvic nodes only	D1	T1-4N1-3M0
Bone	D2	T1-4N1-3M1b
Lung, liver, brain		T1-4N1-3M1c
Hormone refractory	D3	

[a] Transrectal ultrasound
Source: Ref. 20.

the glandular architecture. A higher grade is associated with a higher rate of local tumor spread and metastais (21).

A. Localized Prostatic Cancer

Stage A1 (T1a) prostatic cancer is defined as a normal gland on rectal examination with three or less foci, or less than 5% of tissue containing well-differentiated adenocarcinoma (Gleason sum <4). The acid phosphatase level is normal. This stage of disease is usually found at the time of transurethral resection of the prostate (TURP). Stage A1 prostatic cancer is treated with observation alone, as disease progression is found to occur in only 2% of patients (22). Such conservative therapy has been challenged, as longer follow-up has shown disease progression in 16% of men followed for at least 8 years after diagnosis (23). Lowe and Listrom found that the probability of disease progression increases with age, and they recommend further treatment for patients with a life expectancy of at least 5 years and have Gleason ≥4 disease (24). Although stage A1 disease is unlikely to progress to clinical significance in the life span of many elderly men, annual PSA and rectal examinations remain necessary.

Stage A2 (T1b) of prostatic cancer is defined as a normal gland on rectal examination with more than three foci, or greater than 5% of tissue containing moderately or poorly differentiated adenocarcinoma (Gleason sum ≥4). The acid phosphatase level is normal. Again, this stage is found incidently during TURP. Radical prostatectomy or radiation therapy is offered, especially to men under 65 years old, as median time to disease progression is 4–5 years and death from untreated cancer will occur in 50% of untreated patients within 10–15 years (25). Survival can improve to 70–90% at 10–15 years with such treatment (26). Thus, it is important to distinguish this stage from A1 disease, as treatment can be of benefit.

Stage T1c of prostatic cancer was added to the TNM staging system in 1992. It is defined as carcinoma found on needle biopsy performed solely for an elevated PSA with no palpable tumor. These carcinomas have a tendency to be of higher grade and have higher tumor volumes than T1a tumors and clinically behave like T1b tumors. A 93% disease-free survival at 8 years has been reported in T1c patients treated with radical prostatectomy (27). There appears to be stage migration within T1c disease, with progressive declines in PSA values at diagnosis as a function of calendar year. Therefore, deciding which elderly patients may benefit from definitive therapy should be based on pretreatment PSA levels and pathological findings at biopsy (28).

Stage B1 (T2a) prostatic can is defined as a palpable nodule localized to one lobe of the gland with a normal serum acid phosphatase. Radical prostatectomy or radiotherapy have nearly the same efficacy with a 50–60% survival at 10 years, although some evidence indicates a higher recurrence rate with radiotherapy (29). Interestingly, Alexander et al. noted that older patients with clinical stage B1 disease were found to have a higher pathological stage and grade at radical prostatectomy, possibly due to masking of prostatic induration by benign glandular hypertrophy (30). Stage B2 disease is defined as a palpable nodule involving both lobes of the gland, with a normal serum acid phosphatase. The lateral sulcus is not obliterated. There is controversy regarding how pathologically to distinguish B1 from B2 disease, although in practice the best prognostic indicator is probably the PSA level and Gleason score.

The management of clinically localized prostatic cancer in the elderly is challenging. Without PSA substaging, nearly half of patients thought to have organ-confined disease are found to have cancer spread beyond the prostate at the time of radical prostatectomy (31). With PSA-driven substaging, there is an increasing risk of non–organ-confined disease with each incremental increase in the PSA above 4 ng/mL. For example, with PSA levels over 10 ng/mL, about 50% of patients have non–organ-confined disease. The use of PSA testing combined with clinical stage and Gleason score can help predict the likelihood of lymph node spread, and thus stratify those patients who are more likely to achieve cure from radical prostatectomy (32).

The efficacy of radical prostatectomy versus external beam radiotherapy in the management of localized prostate cancer has been a controversial topic for many years. The only randomized trial to date indicated an advantage for radical prostatectomy, but the study was small and not controlled for pretreatment PSA values (29). During the last 5 years, the concept of PSA or "biochemical" failure as a surrogate endpoint for survival has been used to compare radiation with surgery. Biochemical failure is defined as detectable levels of PSA (usually ≥ 0.2 ng/mL) after radical prostatectomy or a rising PSA on two to three consecutive occasions following a radiotherapy-induced nadir (usually <1.0 ng/mL). Pretreatment PSA and Gleason score are used to stratify high-risk patients, and some series suggest that radical prostatectomy offers improved biochemical relapse-free survival compared to radiation therapy (33). That position is controversial, since Lattanzi et al. estimate that a PSA of less than 8 ng/mL is the level at which the majority of patients can obtain long-term biochemical relapse-free control with radiation (34). A study of surgically staged cases of node-negative, localized prostatic cancer revealed that although biochemical "cure" was not achieved with radiation therapy, cause-specific survival at 10 years still exceeded 80% (35). In summary, we believe that radiotherapy or surgery for prostatic cancer, as they are for breast cancer, are equivalent modalities when stratified by pretreatment PSA and Gleason scores.

Elderly men are often given the option of watchful waiting in the case of clinically localized disease, and several studies have shown that this is a reasonable approach. The Veterans Administration Cooperative Urological Research Group (VACURG) was unable to show a survival benefit in patients with localized disease undergoing radical prostatectomy compared to observation alone, but this study lacked statistical power (36). The study did conclude that localized prostatic cancer in patients greater than 70 years of age with a low Gleason score (<7) is unlikely to decrease that patient's life expectancy if no initial treatment is instituted. A non-randomized observational study by Albertsen et al. suggested that observation alone may be appropriate in older men who have low-volume, low-grade disease (37). The study retrospectively examined men aged 65–75 years who were treated with observation or hormonal therapy alone. Men with low-grade (Gleason 2–4) cancer showed no lowering of life expectancy in comparison to the general population, whereas men with moderate-grade (Gleason 5–7) disease showed up to a 4- to 5-year lowering of life expectancy, and those with high-grade (Gleason 8–10) showed up to 6 to 8 years of lowering of life expectancy. In 1993, the Prostate Patient Outcomes Research Team (PORT) published a decision analysis for management of clinically localized prostatic cancer that showed little benefit to curative intent therapy in elderly men (38). The group modeled radiation therapy, radical prostatectomy, and watchful waiting, with the benefit of treatment being a decrease in death or disability from metastatic disease. They determined that there was less than a 6-month improvement in quality-adjusted survival for men between 70–75 years of age who received radiotherapy or radical prostatectomy, and that in men older than 75 years, no benefits from these therapies were seen in comparison to watchful waiting. The methodology of the PORT analysis was criticized by those favoring surgical or radiation treatment, and a repeat decision analysis with updated data suggested benefit for aggressive therapy in men with moderately or poorly differentiated cancers up to age 75 years (39, 40). A prospective trial, the Prostate Cancer Intervention Versus Observation Trial (PIVOT) started in 1994 to compare the effectiveness of radical prostatectomy versus observation in localized prostatic cancer and has accrued over 400 of a planned 2100 men (41). Hopefully, the results of such a study will help better to define appropriate treatment of localized prostatic cancer.

The decision between conservative versus aggressive management of locally invasive prostatic cancer is an important one, as poorer quality of life has been reported in men undergoing radical prostatectomy or radiation therapy, including significantly worse sexual, urinary, and bowel functions (42). An analysis of radical prostatectomies performed on Medicare patients reported a 1.4% mortality rate for men aged 75–79 years and a 4.6% mortality rate in those over aged 79 years (43). Besides the risk of perioperative mortality, other long-term complications from surgery include impotence, incontinence, and urethral stricture. A survey of Medicare patients aged 65 years and older who had undergone radical prostatectomy reported that over 30% of men needed to use pads or clamps for wetness and 60% had absence of partial or full erections (44). The impairment of postoperative sexual function has been shown to be related to the age of the patient, with older patients faring worse (45). Although nerve-sparing radical prostatectomy has greatly decreased the incidence of postoperative impotency in recent years, these techniques have not been as beneficial in the older patient. Although overall potency rates after radical prostatectomy approach 75%, the rate for men over the age of 70 years is only 20% (46). Several types of treatment are available for postoperative or post-radiation sexual dysfunction, including vacuum devices, pharmacological injection therapy, and implantation of penile protheses (47).

The complications of radiotherapy include acute toxicity such as diarrhea, cystitis, and fatigue, and late toxicity, including procotitis, urinary incontinence, impotence, and urethral stricture (48). The incidence of urinary or rectosigmoid sequelae has been reported to be 3% for severe and 7–10% for moderate complications (49). Despite these risks, definitive radiation therapy is generally well tolerated in the elderly if comorbid conditions are absent.

Despite the potential complications, the use of both radical prostatectomy and radiation therapy increased in men over 80 years of age from less than 10% in 1984 to 25% in 1991 as reported by the National Cancer Institute's Surveillance, Epidemiology, and End Results (SEER) Program (50). Data from the Metropolitan Detroit Cancer Surveillance System showed that the rate of hormonal therapy as first-line treatment for men 75 years of age and older remained constant between the early 1970s and 1992, whereas the rate of radiation therapy increased 11-fold and the rate of radical prostatectomy increased 60-fold (51). A review of Medicare patients undergoing radical prostatectomy between 1990 and 1993 revealed a tripling of the procedure rate among men 70 to 74 years of age and a doubling of the rate among those 75 years or older (52). However, elderly men do not receive intensive therapy as frequently as younger men do, and they tend to receive more hormonal therapy (53). There is no evidence to suggest that such a discrepancy in treatment methods leads to a worse outcome in older patients.

Despite the adverse effects associated with curative-intent therapy for prostatic cancer, a study of a veteran population indicated that a majority of older patients were willing to accept both impotence and incontinence if there was a chance of at least a 10% 5-year survival advantage with treatment (54). Frank discussions need to be undertaken between the physician and patient explaining the risks and benefits of the various treatment options. Other investigational therapies for localized prostatic cancer include brachytherapy and cryosurgery (55). These methods have the potential to be reasonable, well-tolerated alternatives for elderly patients, but they need further study and refinement.

B. Locally Invasive Disease

Stage C (T3a/T3b/T4) prostatic cancer is defined as extension of the disease beyond the capsule of the gland or involving the seminal vesicles, pelvic side wall, bladder, or rectum. The serum acid phosphatase level is elevated and PSA (not used in formal staging) is often above 20 ng/mL. Surgery, radiation therapy, and hormone therapy may be used singly, but most patients receive radiation therapy, which helps to control local symptoms, plus hormonal therapy prior to and during radiation to decrease the amount of tissue to be irradiated and increase symptom-free survival

(56, 57). Although previous studies have not shown a survival advantage, a recent study comparing external radiation alone versus radiation plus hormone ablation with goserelin (a gonadotropin-releasing hormone agonist) showed that combination therapy resulted in an improved 5-year overall survival of 79% compared to 62% in patients treated with radiation alone (58). The use of hormonal therapy alone is attractive for some elderly patients and may be a viable choice in men with significant comorbidity. A currently open international trial is attempting to compare hormonal therapy alone to hormonal therapy plus radiotherapy. Based on the Pilepich et al. (57) and Bolla et al. (58) data, we currently recommend radiation therapy plus hormonal therapy for 1–3 years for treatment of stage T3/T4 disease.

C. Metastatic Disease

Stage D1 (M-1) refers to metastatic disease. Historically, Stage D has been divided into three stages: D0, an elevated acid phosphatase level without evidence of metastatic disease probably indicating micrometastatic disease; D1, metastatic disease localized to the pelvic nodes only; and D2 defined as bony metastases. Some clinical trials refer to stage D3 as hormone-refractory metastatic disease, but D3 is not an accepted staging term. Twenty-five to 30% of newly diagnosed prostate cancers in older men are metastatic at the time of diagnosis, but this figure is dropping with the use of PSA screening (59).

The management of node-positive (D1) cancer is controversial. Most patients will eventually die of their disease, whereas a minority survive long periods apparently free of further metastases. Five-year survival rates vary from 61 to 97%, partly as a function of the number and size of positive nodes (60). Some advocate aggressive therapy with radical prostatectomy or radiotherapy to control local, symptomatic spread of the disease. External beam radiation as a single-modality treatment has shown mixed results, with some evidence suggesting a delay in disease progression but no long-term survival benefit (61, 62). There is some evidence that radical prostatectomy may show improved local control in comparison to expectant management (60). There is also evidence that adjuvant hormonal therapy may improve outcome following radical prostatectomy, especially in patients with tumors of diploid DNA ploidy (63). Hormonal ablation as sole therapy is frequently used in stage D1 disease, but whether treatment should be initiated early or late in the course of metastatic prostate cancer has long been debated (64). Recent data from the British Medical Research Council trial has suggested an advantage to early initiation of hormonal therapy. A decrease in metastatic complications and cancer-related deaths was seen in those patients who received hormonal treatment immediately at the time of diagnosis of locally advanced or asymptomatic metastatic prostatic cancer as compared to those who began treatment when clinical progression occurred (65). We currently recommend radiotherapy to the local disease combined with hormonal therapy for 3 years to control distant disease.

Hormone ablation has been the mainstay of treatment for stage D2 disease since Huggins and Hodges documented the palliative effects of castration in 1941 (66). Options for primary androgen withdrawal include orchiectomy or injection of luteinizing hormone–releasing hormone (LHRH) agonists. Orchiectomy remains the standard modality by which all other forms of hormonal therapy are measured. Although effective, this procedure can be psychologically detrimental and, like all forms of hormonal therapy, will cause decreased potency and hot flashes. Orchiectomy has the advantage of immediate hormonal control, relatively low cost, and elimination of issues of patient compliance. Despite these advantages, the majority of men choose a nonsurgical modality when given a choice between orchiectomy and other forms of therapy (67). The LHRH agonists have become the most popular form of hormonal therapy, although these expensive agents have similar side effects and are less convenient than orchiectomy. The two analogues in common use in the United States are leuprolide and goserelin, which are administered via monthly, 3-monthly, and now 4-monthly depot injections. The agents have been shown to be equally efficacious as orchiectomy (68). They rapidly bind to all luteinizing hormone (LH) receptors causing an initial surge in LH production followed by downregulation of LH production. The initial LH release and resultant rise in testosterone will cause a flare of disease activity when treatment is first begun. Because of this, patients with severe vertebral metastases or acute urethral obstruction should not be given LHRH agonists without the coadministration of an antiandrogen during the first few weeks of treatment (69). Diethylstilbesterol, in spite of being a cheap and nonsurgical alternative to surgical castration (66), is associated with excessive cardiovascular complications and has been withdrawn from the market.

Androgen blockade can also be accomplished by administration of antiandrogenic agents which competitively block binding of dihydrotestosterone to the androgen receptor. Examples include flutamide, bicalutamide, and nilutamide. These drugs do not have the progestational side effects of the steroidal antiandrogens cyproterone acetate and megesterol acetate, nor are they as effective as medical or surgical castration (70). The antiandrogens have hepatotoxic effects, and close monitoring of liver function may be a hardship for older patients. Past enthusiasm for so-called "total androgen blockade" using a combination of an antiandrogen with orchiectomy or LHRH agonist has been lessened by mixed results in subsequent studies (69, 71). The extra cost of such oral treatment may be a drawback in older patients. Flutamide costs $200–$300 per month and is not covered by Medicare, but it is covered by the Veterans Administration (72).

Nearly all patients with metastatic disease will eventually progress after initial hormone therapy, with a median time to PSA progression of 15 – 18 months and clinical progression of 24–36 months. These so called "hormone-refractory" cancers (HRPC) are particularly difficult to manage. Withdrawal of antiandrogens should be the initial intervention in the management of HRPC, as 15–25% of patients demonstrate an objective and/or PSA response with this maneuver (73).

Whether antiandrogens should be added after failure of medical or surgical castration is unknown but is widely done (74). Administration of low-dose glucocorticoids is also an accepted practice that improves pain and can induce both pain and PSA responses (75, 76). Recent evidence indicates that mutations in the androgen receptor (AR) gene may be a factor in the development of hormone resistance and that responses to withdrawal of antiandrogen therapy may be related to stimulation of the mutated AR by antiandrogens (77).

Cytotoxic chemotherapy plays a major role in the palliation of HRPC (78). Chemotherapy is surprisingly well tolerated even in elderly patients, although the common occurrence of bone marrow involvement may curtail the use of chemotherapy. A phase III trial of cyclophosphamide versus 5-fluorouracil versus standard treatment demonstrated a survival advantage to chemotherapy (79). Numerous phase II studies have been performed in patients with HRPC, and the following drugs have demonstrated activity: mitoxantrone (80), doxorubicin, oral cyclophosphamide, and estramustine. The combination of estramustine and vinblastine has shown reproducible activity, with approximately one third of patients obtaining a PSA reduction of greater than 50% (81, 82). Estramustine in combination with either etoposide, docetaxel, paclitaxel, or vinorelbine are active regimens (78, 83). Because of its favorable toxicity profile, mitoxantrone has been investigated as a potential agent for elderly patients and has shown beneficial effects on disease-related symptoms (80). Two randomized phase III trials have compared mitoxantrone plus a glucocorticoid to a glucocorticoid alone in HRPC (84, 85). Both trials showed an advantage for mitoxantrone in terms of pain control, improved quality of life, time to tumor progression, and decline in PSA. There was no survival advantage for mitoxantrone; perhaps due to the widespread use of other drugs as second-line therapy. Additional studies with mitoxantrone are ongoing, including dose-intensive regimens (86). More effective and less toxic agents need to be developed, but currently mitoxantrone plus a glucocorticoid should be offered to all patients with HRPC (87).

The management of bony pain in patients with metastatic disease is an important component of care. The use of narcotic analgesics or nonsteroidal anti-inflammatory agents must be carefully administered given their propensity to cause side effects in older patients (88). External beam radiation is an effective modality in controlling individual sites of painful metastasis (89). Suramin, a drug with unique mechanisms of action benefits 20–35% of patients with bone pain from HRPC, although response rates were confounded (in early trials) by simultaneous withdrawal of flutamide and the activity of coadministered corticosteroids (90, 91). Radiopharmaceuticals such as strontium 89 and samarium 153 are also effective in pain control of skeletal disease (92, 93). Some degree of myelosuppression can be expected with both external beam therapy and radiolabeled compounds, which may exacerbate preexisting anemia from marrow infiltration or chronic disease. Administration of bisphsophonates may also be helpful in controlling symptoms from diffuse bony metastases and in treating or preventing osteoporosis, which regularly accompanies androgen-deprivation therapy (94). Spinal cord compression and pathological fractures are two feared complications of bone metastases for which the clinician must retain a high index of suspicion.

III. BLADDER CANCER

It was be an estimated that there would be 54,200 new cases of bladder cancer in the United States in 1999 (3). Bladder cancer is the second most common genitourinary malignancy, and it is the ninth leading cause of cancer death in men, with more than 11,000 deaths per year. The incidence of bladder cancer has increased only slightly during the last two decades, whereas mortality from the disease has declined approximately 20% (95). Bladder cancer is a disease of the elderly, rarely occurring before the age of 40, with a mean age at diagnosis of 65 years (96).

A number of carcinogens have been implicated in the etiology of bladder carcinoma. These carcinogens are thought to be excreted in the urine, where they have a direct effect on the bladder epithelium. Smokers demonstrate a twofold excess risk over nonsmokers, and cigarette smoking (active or passive) accounts for about one half of all transitional carcinoma of the bladder (97). Arylamines are another well-known cause of bladder cancer and include such compounds as 2-naphthyl-amine, aniline, and 4-aminobiphenyl. Arylamines have long been used in the textile dye and rubber tire industries, but regulatory standards have now essentially elimi-nated occupational exposure to these compounds. Other causes of bladder cancer include heavy phenacetin use and cyclophosphamide exposure (98, 99). Schistoso-miasis of the bladder is a risk factor for squamous cell carcinoma, and it is commonly seen in countries where this infection is endemic (96, 97).

Ninety percent of bladder cancers are transitional cell carcinomas. Adenocarci-noma, squamous cell carcinoma, and atypical carcinomas such as small-cell cancer compose the remaining 10% (100). Transitional cell carcinoma is further classified as papillary or nonpapillary, and it is graded from grade I (well differentiated) to grade III (poorly differentiated). ''Flat'' nonpapillary tumors tend to be more aggres-sive than papillary cancers, and they occur in both in situ (CIS) and invasive forms (96).

Bladder cancer is staged either by the Jewett–Strong–Marshall system or by the TNM system (Table 3), and it is divided into superficial, muscle invasive, and metastatic disease (101). Histological grade and clinicopathological stage are the most important predictors of outcome. Superficial cancers are treated with conserva-tive resection and/or intravesical therapy, whereas muscle-invasive tumors require cystectomy with or without additional chemotherapy or radiotherapy.

Bladder cancer has been cited as an ideal disease for which to institute routine screening for the elderly and other at-risk populations. Almost all cancers cause hematuria at some point, which can be detected with inexpensive and noninvasive urinalysis. Early-stage, superficial carcinomas carry an excellent prognosis with

Table 3 Bladder Cancer Staging

	Jewett-Strong-Marshall	TNM
Superficial		
Tumor in situ		Tis
Tumor confined to mucosa	0	Ta
Subepithelial connective tissue invasion	A	T1
Muscle-invasive		
Superficial muscle invasion (inner half)	B1	T2a
Deep muscle invasion (outer half)	B2	T2b
Perivesical Fat Invasion	C	
Microscopic		T3a
Macroscopic		T3b
Other organ invasion		T4
Prostate, uterus or vagina invasion	D1	T4a
Pelvic or abdominal wall invasion		T4b
Regional lymph nodes cannot be assessed		NX
No regional lymph node metastases		N0
Single node metastasis, 2 cm or less in size		N1
Single node metastasis, >2 cm but <5 cm or multiple lymph nodes, none >5 cm in size		N2
Lymph node metastasis >5 cm in size		N3
Distant metastases cannot be assessed		MX
No distant metastases		M0
Metastatic Disease		
Distant metastases	D2	M1

Source: Ref. 101.

treatment, and thus early detection can be of clear benefit. A retrospective study in men 50 years of age and older who were screened at home with hematuria reagent strips on 14 consecutive days showed an earlier detection of high-grade cancers and reduced mortality compared to an unscreened population of bladder cancer patients (102). Furthermore, screening of men more than 50 years of age has been found to be cost effective (103). These results need confirmation in randomized, prospective studies. Urine cytology, flow cytometry, and molecular probes may add refinement to screening techniques in the future (100, 103). Patients with a previous history of bladder cancer have a high rate of recurrence and represent a population that requires diligent, regular surveillance with cystoscopy and bladder wash cytology, usually at 3-month intervals. An immunoassay for urinary nuclear matrix protein, NMP22, has recently been approved U.S. Food and Drug Administration (FDA) for detection of recurrent bladder cancer and is likely to become a routine component of such surveillance (104).

Hematuria is the most common presenting sign of bladder cancer. Evidence of bladder irritability, including dysuria, urgency, and urinary frequency may be presenting symptoms. Although the usefulness of complete urological screening in all patients with microscopic hematuria has been debated, such investigation should be recommended in older individuals, especially those with higher grade hematuria because of the high incidence of urological malignancy in such populations (105). Delay in referring patients with hematuria for cystoscopy remains a common problem. The older patient presenting with hematuria should undergo a thorough history and physical along with urinalysis and urine cytology. Cystoscopy with biopsy is the mainstay of diagnosis and staging, and should include bimanual examination under anesthesia, bladder washings, and mucosal biopsies distant from the primary tumor to detect CIS. Cytology is positive in more than 90% of patients with high-grade transitional cell carcinoma, whereas low-grade carcinomas give positive results in only 34–63% (100). Intravenous pyelography is of limited value in detecting bladder cancer but can screen for collecting system lesions and will define ureteral obstruction. Abdominal/pelvic computed tomographic (CT) scanning is of no value for screening but does aid in staging for tumors invading the muscle.

A. Superficial Bladder Cancer

Superficial bladder cancer (Ta, T1, CIS) generally has an excellent prognosis. The median 5-year survival with treatment was found to be 86% in a 1983 literature review, with approximately 10% of patients developing invasive disease (106). Most superficial tumors are low grade and papillary, although a subset of superficial cancers are carcinoma in situ (CIS), which has a higher rate of progression and can be more difficult to treat because of its diffuse nature. The most important prognostic factor in superficial bladder cancer is histological grade; overexpression of p53 has recently been shown to be another important independent predictor of outcome (107, 108).

The standard management of superficial bladder cancer is transurethral resection of the bladder tumor with electrocautery (TURB). This is a well-tolerated procedure which is performed as an outpatient procedure, although elderly patients may be at higher risk for complications secondary to blood loss or bladder perforation. Superficial bladder cancer has a variable rate of recurrence, those with poor-prognosis features have a 40–85% recurrence rate, usually within 1 year. Intravesical chemotherapy or immunotherapy after resection is often employed to decrease the rate of tumor recurrence and progression, and it may delay the need for cystectomy (109). Intravesical therapy is indicated in cancers which have a high risk for recurrence and progression, including any patient with CIS or T1 disease. Patients with Ta disease that is high grade or multifocal disease regardless of grade or stage probably also benefit from intravesical therapy. Other patients with stage Ta or those with grade 1 tumors have a low rate of progression and recurrence, and therefore do not necessarily require intravesical therapy (106). The first choice of intravesical therapy is bacillus Calmette–Guérin vaccine (BCG), but selection of an intravesical agent may be influenced by patient age, as the potential harm of agents such as BCG or thiotepa may be greater than mitomycin C or doxorubicin (48).

Approximately 50% of CIS lesions, in the absence of intravesical therapy, progress to invasive disease by 4 years (110). With an average complete response (CR) rate of 70%, intravesical BCG immunotherapy has become the first-line treatment for diffuse CIS, and it was approved by the FDA in 1990. In combination with TURB, BCG has been shown to be superior to TURB alone in patients with superficial bladder cancer, improving survival and decreasing disease progression (111). The mechanism of action of BCG in bladder cancer is poorly understood, but it is thought to stimulate a nonspecific immune response against tumor cells. The side effects of BCG therapy are directly related to this immunogenic process. Unfortunately, the toxicity of BCG can be quite severe, and this may limit its use in the elderly. Cystitis develops in the majority of patients, resulting in dysuria, frequency, and sometimes hematuria. Prolonged symptoms can be treated with 300 mg of isoniazid per day. Although fever and flulike symptoms are common, true "BCG sepsis" with hemodynamic compromise is a rare but dangerous occurrence (112).

After initial therapy, maintenance treatments with BCG can reduce long-term disease recurrence and may prolong survival. This is a distinct advantage over intravesical cytotoxic therapy, the benefit of which is only short term. The current maintenance regimen employs 3 weekly installations of BCG every 6 months for 3 years. Such treatments may be somewhat inconvenient but should be considered in elderly patients who can tolerate therapy.

Other intravesical immunotherapy agents under investigation for treatment of superficial disease include interferon-α (113) and bropirimine, an oral interferon inducer that has been successfully used to treat CIS and may be useful in patients who have failed BCG (114). Photodynamic therapy employs the administration of an intravenous photosensitizing dye followed by intravesical activation with laser treatment, and it may play an important role in treatment of refractory CIS (115).

B. Muscle-Invasive Bladder Cancer

The 5-year survival for muscle-invasive bladder cancer ranges from 50 to 88% for T2 disease to 12–40% for T3b disease (96). A large amount of clinical error complicates staging and many patients thought preoperatively to have T2 disease are found to have T3 or node-positive disease at the time of cystectomy. Muscle-invasive tumors with occult metastases generally become clinically apparent within 12 months, but late relapses 3–5 years after diagnosis can occur (116).

Muscle-invasive bladder cancer (T2–T3) is typically treated with radical cystectomy, a procedure that historically has carried substantial morbidity but low mortality (117). Physicians often avoid recommending radical cystectomy in very elderly patients with invasive disease. Despite this prevalent opinion, radical cystectomy is actually tolerated quite well, and early aggressive surgery should not be avoided on the basis of age alone (118). In fact, repeated TURB with the risk of bleeding, urinary obstruction, and anaesthesia toxicity is considerably more morbid than radical cystectomy (119).

In radical cystectomy, the bladder is removed along with the prostate in males (or the uterus, fallopian tubes, and ovaries in females) along with regional lymph nodes en bloc. Two troublesome sequelae are impotence and the need for urinary diversion. The development of techniques for preserving the neurovascular bundles has improved impotence rates. The ileal conduit has been the standard urinary diversion for many years, but it results in an incontinent stoma. Continent urinary diversions such as the Kock pouch or Indiana pouch are now commonly created, employing an ileal or ileal cecal segment as a reservoir that is marsupialized to the skin (120, 121). The patient self-catheterizes several times a day to drain the urine. Within the past 10 years, surgeons have successfully developed techniques to anastomose the isolated ileal neobladder to the urethra, allowing true continence. Such continent neobladders offer a large improvement over the ileal conduit and are frequently a viable option for elderly patients. Patients must be properly selected for adequate functional status, as regular penile or urethral self-catheterization may be necessary if urinary continence is not complete. Since the colon is slightly more susceptible to malignant transformation with the Indiana pouch, these patients may need yearly cystoscopies of the neobladder. Those procedures that remove a large segment of terminal ileum predispose to metabolic acidosis and vitamin B_{12} deficiency.

The use of adjuvant or neoadjuvant chemotherapy in combination with radical cystectomy has been investigated widely during the last decade. The two most common chemotherapy regimens, methotrexate, vinblastine, and cisplatin (CMV) and methotrexate, vinblastine, doxorubicin, and cisplatin (MVAC), have shown efficacy in metastatic bladder cancer, as described below. They have also shown efficacy in the neoadjuvant setting, with overall response rates of up to 70% (122, 123). Whether such therapy improves survival is less clear. In a large-scale randomized trial of over 950 patients, Hall et al. did not find an overall survival advantage with the use of three cycles of CMV prior to either cystectomy or radiotherapy (124).

Bladder-preservation strategies involve combinations of TURB, partial cystectomy, radiation therapy, and chemotherapy. In patients unfit to undego more aggressive regimes, TURB alone can be considered, but favorable survival rates are seen only in patients with limited disease (125). Patrtial cystectomy offers preservation of continence, sexual function, and decreased morbidity, but this again is restricted to selected patients (126).

Radiotherapy can be used as single, definitive treatment or in combination with cystectomy. Single-modality radiotherapy probably has a slightly worse 5-year survival rate compared with preoperative radiotherapy and cystectomy (127). Preoperative radiotherapy does not add any benefit to cystectomy alone (128). Definitive radiotherapy with the option of salvage cystectomy in case of recurrence probably results in only a small loss of survival advantage as compared to radical cystectomy with preoperative radiotherapy and may be preferable in some older patients. Additionally, the survival difference seems to be less pronounced in elderly patients (129). Unfortunately, elderly patients tend to do poorly with radical radiotherapy and may suffer from considerable local toxicity, including bladder contracture and chronic bleeding. Because of this, some have advocated hypofractionated, split-course, or once weekly radiotherapy as an alternative for patients unable to tolerate conventional treatment (130, 131). In phase II trials, the addition of 5-fluorouracil or cisplatin to radiation therapy has apparently increased the complete response rates to radiation alone (132). However, randomized phase III trials have shown no benefit to the addition of cisplatin or CMV to radiation alone (96). Palliative, short-term radiotherapy may have a role in stopping bladder hemorrhage in patients with metastatic disease (133).

Multimodality bladder-salvage regimens have shown encouraging results, but randomized phase III trials have not been completed. Encouraging results of a bladder-sparing protocol have been reported from the Massachusetts General Hospital in Boston: TURB was followed by CMV and this was followed by radiation therapy with concomitant cisplatin. A 52% overall survival rate at 5 years has been realized, with 43% surviving with an intact, functioning bladder (134). Multimodality, bladder-sparing regimens have been investigated by other groups and high response rates have been reported (135). Some have advocated such therapies for elderly patients unable to undergo surgery, although if these patients cannot undergo a cystectomy, they are unlikely to be able to tolerate multiple cycles of cisplatin-based therapy (136).

Aggressive chemotherapy with a regimen such as MVAC or CMV are often not realistic options for elderly patients. Toxicities include myelosuppression and neutropenic sepsis, mucositis, and renal toxicity. An age-related reduction in renal and cardiac function may limit the use of cisplatin or doxorubicin. Sella et al. reported a series of patients aged 76 years and older who received cisplatin-containing regimens such as CMV and MVAC in both the adjuvant setting and as treatment for metastatic disease. Toxicity was significant, but there was no treatment-related mortality and response rates were similar to those seen in younger patients (137). Less toxic multimodality treatment regimens for elderly patients have been investigated but show decreased efficacy. TURB followed by administration of 5-fluorouracil (5-FU), epirubicin, and cisplatin and followed by radiotherapy for residual disease was studied in patients greater than 70 years of age with locally advanced bladder cancer. A response rate of 55% was obtained with an overall median survival of 11.6 months (138). TURB followed by single agent carboplatin or methotrexate has also been suggested as an alternative for elderly patients with muscle-invasive disease, but this cannot be recommended without further testing (139).

C. Metastatic Bladder Cancer

Metastatic bladder cancer is an aggressive disease with median survival of less than 1 year. Systemic chemotherapy has a definite role in management, but comorbid conditions in many elderly patients make them ineligible to receive aggressive regimens. Age alone should not be a contraindication to such treatment (140). Chemotherapy of advanced bladder cancer has largely centered on cisplatin-based regimens, as this drug is thought to be the most active single agent, with response rates around 30% (140). Methotrexate has also demonstrated significant single-agent activity with similar response rates as cisplatin (141). Unfortunately, only short durations of response are seen with these agents, usually 3–5 months. Other drugs with activity as single agents include cyclophosphamide, ifosfamide, doxorubicin, pirarubicin, mitoxantrone, vincristine, etoposide, trimetrexate, and piritrexim (142).

Combination regimens containing cisplatin and methotrexate, such as CMV and MVAC, have been the focus of numerous investigations. MVAC has been one of the most studied combinations. Developed at Memorial–Sloan Kettering, an excellent response rate of 72% was reported with a CR of 36% (143). However, toxicity from MVAC includes severe thrombocytopenia, neutropenia, mucositis, and infection, and the reported median survival is still only 13 months. MVAC has become the standard of therapy in advanced bladder carcinoma, with improved efficacy over both single agent cisplatin and CISCA (cisplatin, cyclophosphamide, doxorubicin), as demonstrated in two phase III trials (144, 145). Several dose-escalated trials of MVAC have been performed which have resulted in increased toxicity with no demonstrable improvement in efficacy (146, 147).

Although regimens such as MVAC have shown benefit, median survival of advanced bladder cancer remains approximately 1 year, and such regimens are associated with toxicities that may be unacceptable for elderly patients with comorbid conditions. Identification and testing of new active agents in advanced bladder carcinoma remains a priority. Paclitaxel and docetaxel have shown encouraging response rates in small studies (148, 149). Paclitaxel's main side effect is myelosuppression, and its lack of significant renal toxicity makes this agent a reasonable choice in older patients. Gemcitabine has shown favorable results in phase II studies, with response rates of up to 38% (150, 151). The addition of cisplatin to gemcitabine leads to increased myelotoxicity, but it has resulted in impressive response rates of up to 75%, and a randomized trial comparing this combination to MVAC has completed accrual and will be analyzed in late 1999 (152, 153). Because of its favorable toxicity profile, gemcitabine alone, or perhaps in combination with carboplatin, could be considered in older patients with severe comorbid conditions. Metastatic bladder cancer has been shown to be a chemotherapy-sensitive disease, and more clinical trials are needed to investigate new therapies.

IV. RENAL CELL CARCINOMA

Renal cell carcinoma (RCC) is a relatively rare tumor that affects mostly elderly patients. It occurs most commonly in the seventh and eight decades of life and affects twice as many men as women. In 1999, it was estimated that there would be 30,000 new cancers of the kidney and renal pelvis in the United States, and 11,900 people would die of these diseases (3). A number of risk factors beyond gender and age have been identified, including cigarette smoking, obesity, hypertension, and occupational exposures (154, 155).

The most common histological form of RCC is clear cell carcinoma, which comprises 85% of kidney cancers. Other forms include granular cell carcinoma and the "sarcomatoid" variant, which carries a particularly poor prognosis. Oncocytoma and papillary RCC are unusual histological subtypes which tend to have less aggressive clinical courses; the former with nearly 100% survival.

Most cases of kidney cancer are random occurrences, but there are several inherited forms. The short arm of chromosome three (3p) is frequently mutated in both sporadic and familial cases of the disease. Familial clear cell kidney cancer is associated with a germline translocation t(3;8)(p14.2;q24.1) and is inherited in an autosominal dominant pattern (156). Von Hippel–Lindau (VHL) syndrome is an autosomal dominant disorder that leads to development of tumors in multiple organs, including the central nervous system, retina, and kidneys. The VHL gene has been mapped to 3p25–26 and is a tumor suppressor gene (157). Hereditary papillary renal carcinoma is another autosomal dominant disorder that does not seem to involve the short arm of chromosome 3 (158). The hereditary forms of RCC tend to occur at younger ages, and new cases of kidney cancer in the elderly patient are much more likely to represent sporadic occurrences.

Classically, RCC has been referred to as the "internist's tumor" owing to its variety of systemic signs and symptoms (159). Although the most frequent manifestations are hematuria, abdominal pain, and palpable mass, these three findings occur together as the "classic triad" in less than 10% of patients (160). Nonspecific symptoms may include weight loss, fever, and night sweats. In men, a varicocele occasionally results from tumor thrombus of the gonadal vein at its junction with the renal vein. Rare but fascinating paraneoplastic syndromes have been associated with RCC, including erythrocytosis, hypercalcemia, amyloidosis, and nonmetastatic hepatic dysfunction (Stauffer's syndrome) (159, 160). Often, renal carcinomas are found incidentally during imaging studies performed for unrelated reasons. Patients with incidental tumors ("incidentalomas") have a better prognosis, as these carcinomas tend to be smaller and more confined than symptomatic cancers (161).

Intravenous pyelography is often the first imaging study ordered by the clinician, prompted by hematuria or physical findings. This procedure may detect renal masses but lacks sensitivity or specificity. Ultrasonography and CT are the main imaging modalities used to detect and define renal masses. Nonmalignant lesions such as cysts and angiomyolipomas have distinguishing characteristics on ultrasound and CT that often eliminate the need for biopsy. Periodic ultrasound evaluation of a benign-appearing lesion is warranted to monitor for change. Suspicious mass lesions may be sampled with impunity via percutaneous cyst puncture or needle aspiration biopsy under ultrasound or CT guidance.

The most accurate method for preoperative staging is CT, but it is limited in its ability to detect minimally enlarged lymph nodes (162). Magnetic resonance imaging (MRI) is superior to CT for evaluating vena caval involvement and is com-

Table 4 Kidney Cancer Staging

	Robson	TNM
Confined to renal capsule		
≤7 cm	I	T1
>7 cm		T2
Perirenal fat invasion but confined to Gerota's fascia	II	T3a
Renal vein invasion	IIIA	T3b
Vena cava invasion above the diaphragm		T3c
Lymph node invasion	IIIB	
Single regional node		N1
More than one regional node		N2
Organ invasion beyond Gerota's fascia	IVA	T4
Distant metastases	IVB	M1

Source: Ref. 168.

parable to inferior venacavography (163, 164). Renal arteriography is sometimes used in operative planning. Evaluation for metastatic disease should include blood chemistries, bone scan, and a chest radiograph. Given the speed and sensitivity of chest CT imaging, many oncologists recommend this in addition to a chest radiograph.

Either the Robson or the TNM systems is used to stage RCC (Table 4) (165, 166). Stage is the most important predictor of survival. Stage I patients have a 75% survival at 5 years, whereas stage II patients have a 60–70% survival. Stage IIIA has a 40–50% 5-year survival rate, whereas survival for stage IIIB drops to less than 20% at 5 years. Those patients with stage IV disease have a median survival of less than 1 year (167).

A. Localized Disease

Surgery is the mainstay of treatment for localized RCC, as this is the only curative therapy available. In the 1960s, Robson et al. established radical nephrectomy as the gold standard with their reported survival of greater than 60% in stages I and II disease (165). Radical nephrectomy involves ligation of the renal vessels and en bloc removal of Gerota's fascia and its contents, including the kidney and adrenal gland. Vena caval resection is required if the tumor extends into this vessel, and extensive thrombi may require cardiopulmonary bypass with deep hypothermic circulatory arrest. Regional lymphadenectomy is advocated by some because of a few reports of improved survival in patients with nodal metastases alone (168). Neoadjuvant or adjuvant radiotherapy offers no clear benefit and may be associated with significant toxicity, but postoperative radiation may be considered in patients with evidence of deep invasion of Gerota's fascia, adjacent organs, or regional lymph nodes (169, 170). There is no evidence that adjuvant immunotherapy is beneficial in the management of localized RCC (169).

Nephron-sparing surgery (partial nephrectomy) is indicated if there is anatomical or functional absence of the ipsilateral kidney or in cases of bilateral RCC, which occurs in less than 2% of patients (171). Relative indications include impaired kidney function from conditions such as calculus disease, renal artery stenosis, hypertension, or diabetes, all common disorders in the elderly patient (172). Nephron-sparing surgery carries an increased risk of local tumor recurrence, but it has been shown to be efficacious in properly selected patients with low-stage RCC. Because of similar overall survival as patients undergoing radical nephrectomy, nephron-sparing surgery is being more commonly performed in patients with small tumors and a normal (or near-normal) contralateral kidney (169).

Surgical resection, especially radical nephrectomy, can be a risky procedure in patients with comorbid conditions. There is a paucity of literature on the management of elderly patients with resectable RCC. Several reports have indicated that elderly patients, even those with localized disease, are less often treated with surgery than their younger counterparts (173, 174). Whether this reluctance to perform surgery is secondary to poor physical condition or to patient and physicain reluctance is unclear.

B. Metastatic Disease

Thirty percent of patients with RCC present with metastatic disease (169). The most common site of metastasis is the lung followed by soft tissues, bone, liver, and central nervous system. Median survival is less than 1–2 years, and patient age does not seem to affect prognosis (175).

Unfortunately, metastatic RCC is one of the most chemoresistant cancers. No single agent has yet emerged as a standard therapy for RCC. Vinblastine, 5-FU, and floxuridine (FUDR) have been studied the most, but only 5-FU and its metabolite FUDR have demonstrated a 10–12% activity rate (176). The RCC tumor lines have been shown to express highly mRNA for the multidrug resistance gene *MDR1* and its product, P-glycoprotein (177). This may partially explain the tumor's high-level resistance to cytotoxic chemotherapy. Hormonal therapy for RCC has been investigated in the past, but success with such therapy has been poor (176).

The introduction of biological response modifier therapy gave new hope to the treatment of disseminated RCC when it was introduced in the 1978–1982 period. Because of cases of prolonged disease stabilization and spontaneous regression, RCC has been implicated as being susceptible to host immune responses. Interferon-α (INF-α) has been widely studied and has shown an overall response rate of 14% (169). Interleukin-2 (IL-2) (T-cell growth factor) was approved by the FDA in 1992 for treatment of metastatic RCC based on reports of complete and durable tumor responses. Initial studies performed at the National Cancer Institute using high-dose IL-2 and infusions of autologous lymphokine-activated killer (LAK) cells showed response rates of greater than 30%, although subsequent studies have yielded overall response rates of 15–20% and with 2–5% long-term survivors (178, 179). Additional studies have indicated that LAK cells are not a necessary component of treatment (180). No clear benefit has been seen with the addition of IFN-α to high-dose intravenous IL-2 therapy (181), although low-dose subcutaneous IFN may be synergistic or additive when added to low-dose subcutaneous IL-2 (182).

High-dose IL-2 is usually administered as a dose of 720,000 IU/kg intravenous bolus every 8 h up to 14 doses per cycle or until toxicity develops (179). Toxicity is mainly related to increased vascular permeability with septic shock–like hemodynamics being frequently encountered (183). Capillary leak often leads to pulmonary edema and dysfunction that can be similar to that of the adult respiratory distress syndrome. Cardiac toxicity can be life threatening, including myocardial ischemia, infarction, and arrhythmias. Oliguria and renal failure can occur and are thought to be prerenal in origin. Mental status changes range from confusion to obtundation and may continue to progress even after IL-2 is discontinued. Thrombocytopenia and anemia are among the hematological effects of therapy. Obviously, because of the large index of toxicity, the use of high-dose IL-2 is very limited in elderly patients (184). Few elderly patients have been included in the studies to date. Normal cardiac, pulmonary, and renal function are prerequisite to treatment, and evaluation of potential candidates should include cardiac stress testing for patients older than 50 years of age.

Low-dose IL-2 has been advocated by some as an alternative treatment for RCC; with its lower index of toxicity, this treatment may be more reasonable for elderly patients. Although side effects are not as severe as with high-dose therapy, fatigue, fluid-retention, azotemia, and anemia are still common. Outpatient-based IL-2 therapy using subcutaneous injections with or without IFN-α has been investigated in a number of phase I and II studies (182). Response rates seem to be comparable to high-dose therapy, but randomized trials are still underway. We recommend low-dose IFN and IL-2 to virtually all patients regardless of age. IL-2 is administered subcutaneously at a dose of 11×10^6 IU for 4 consecutive days per week with IFN-α at 10×10^6 IU for 2 nonconsecutive days per week and 4 weeks per cycle.

The role of surgery in metastatic RCC has been reevaluated with renewed interest since the advent of successful immunotherapy. Evidence suggests that decreasing the tumor burden with surgery may improve immunoreactivity against the malignancy by the host. Up-front nephrectomy results in a high postoperative morbidity and renal dysfunction rate which often prevents administration of subsequent immunotherapy (185). Delayed adjuvant nephrectomy should be pursued in patients who demonstrate excellent response to immunotherapy but with persistence of the primary lesion (186). Surgical excision of recurrent or residual metastatic lesions after an initial response to nephrectomy and immunotherapy has been advocated (187).

Because of lack of well-tolerated, effective therapy, treatment of metastatic

RCC must be carefully chosen for the elderly patient. Withholding treatment until disease progression is evident may be prudent in some cases, as RCC may have a protracted course and spontaneous regression is a rare but well-known occurrence. Unlike other metastatic genitourinary cancers, systemic therapy cannot not be relied on to palliate symptoms. Analgesia, surgery, and radiotherapy should be employed as needed to manage complications. Continued research into the aging immune system and disease progression rates in RCC is warranted (188).

REFERENCES

1. Oesterling J, Fuks Z, Lee CT, Scher HI. Cancer of the prostate. In: DeVita VT Jr, Hellman S, Rosenberg SA, eds. Cancer: Principles and Practice of Oncology. Philadelphia: Lippincott-Raven, 1997: 1322–1386.
2. Parker SL, Tong T, Bolden S, Wingo PA. Cancer Statistics, 1997. CA Cancer J Clin 1997; 47:5–27.
3. Landis SH, Murray T, Bolden S, et al. Cancer Statistics, 1999. CA Cancer J Clin 1999; 49:8–31.
4. Franks LM, Durh MB. Latency and progression in tumors: the natural history of prostate cancer. Lancet 1956; 17:1036–1037.
5. Carter BS, Beaty TH, Steinberg GD, Childs B, Walsh PC. Mendelian inheritance of familial prostate cancer. Proc Natl Acad Sci USA 1992; 89:3367–3371.
6. Smith JR, Freije D, Carpten JD, et al. A genome-wide search reveals a major susceptibility locus for prostate cancer on chromosome 1. Science 1996; 274:1371–1373.
7. Giovannucci E, Stampfer MJ, Krithivas K, et al. The CAG repeat within the androgen receptor gene and its relationship to prostate cancer. Proc Natl Acad Sci USA 1997; 94:3320–3323.
8. Mettlin C, Jones G, Averette H, Gusberg SB, Murphy GP. Defining and updating the American Cancer Society guidelines for the cancer related check up: prostate and endometrial cancer. CA Cancer J Clin 1993; 43:42–46.
9. Carter HB, Epstein JI, Chan DW, Fozard JL, Pearson JD. Recommended prostate-specific antigen testing intervals for the detection of curable prostate cancer. JAMA 1997; 277:1456–1460.
10. Gronberg H, Isaacs SD, Smith JR, Carpten JD, Bova GS, Freije D, Xu J, Meyers DA, Collins FS, Trent JM, Walsh PC, Isaacs WB. Characteristics of prostate cancer in families potentially linked to the hereditary prostate cancer (HPC1) locus. JAMA 1997; 278:1251–1255.
11. Watt KWK, Lee PJ, M'Timkulu T, Chan WP, Loor R. Human prostate-specific antigen: structural and functional similarity with serine protease. Proc Natl Acad Sci USA 1986; 83:3166–3170.
12. Oesterling JE, Jacobsen SJ, Chute CG, Guess HA, Girman CJ, Panser LA, Lieber MM. Serum prostate-specific antigen in a community-based population of healthy men. JAMA 1993; 270:860–864.
13. Hostetler RM, Mandel IG, Marshburn J. Prostate cancer screening. Med Clin North Am 1996; 80:83–98.

14. Carter HB, Pearson JD, Metter EJ, Brant LJ, Chan DW, Andres R, Fozard JL, Walsh PC. Longitudinal evaluation of prostate-specific antigen levels in men with and without prostate disease. JAMA 1992; 267:2215–2220.

15. Woodrum DL, Brawer MK, Partin AW, Catalona WJ, Southwick PC. Interpretation of free prostate specific antigen clinical research for detection of prostate cancer. J Urol 1998; 159:5–12.

16. Benoit RM, Naslund MJ. The economics of prostate cancer screening. Oncology 1997; 11:1533–1543.

17. Stamey TA, Yang N, Hay AR, McNeal JE, Freiha FS, Redwine E. Prostate-specific antigen as a serum marker for adenocarcinoma of the prostate. N Engl J Med 1987; 317:909–916.

18. Kelly WK, Scher HI, Mazumdar M, Vlamis V, Schwartz M, Fossa SD. Prostate-specific antigen as a measure of disease outcome in hormone-refractory prostatic cancer. J Clin Oncol 1993; 11:607–615.

19. Whitmore WF Jr. Natural history and staging of prostate cancer. Urol Clin North Am 1984; 11: 205–220.

20. American Joint Committee on Cancer: Prostate. In: Fleming ID, Cooper JS, Henson DE, et al., eds. Cancer Staging Manual. 5th ed. Philadelphia: Lippincott, 1997: 219–222.

21. Gleason DF. Histologic grading of prostate cancer: a perspective. Hum Pathol 1992; 23:273–279.

22. Cantrell BB, DeKlerk DP, Eggleston JC, Boitnott JK, Walsh PC. Pathological factors that influence prognosis in stage A prostatic cancer: the influence of extent versus grade. J Urol 1981; 125:516–520.

23. Epstein JI, Paull G, Eggleston JC, Walsh PC. Prognosis of untreated stage A1 prostatic carcinoma: a study of 94 cases with extended follow up. J Urol 1986; 136:837–839.

24. Lowe BA, Listrom MB. Incidental carcinoma of the prostate: an analysis of the predictors of progression. J Urol 1988; 140:1340–1344.

25. Brockstein BE, Vogelzang NJ. Chemotherapy of genitourinary cancers. In: The Chemotherapy Source Book. Baltimore: Williams & Wilkins, 1996: 1215–1251.

26. Elder JS, Gibbons RP, Correa RJ Jr, Brannen GE. Efficacy of radical prostatectomy for stage A2 carcinoma of the prostate. Cancer 1985; 56:2151–2154.

27. Epstein JI, Walsh PC, Carmichael M, Brendler CB. Pathologic and clinical findings to predict tumor extent of nonpalpable (stage T1c) prostate cancer. JAMA 1994; 271: 368–374.

28. Carter HB, Sauvageot J, Walsh PC, Epstein JI. Prospective evaluation of men with stage T1c adenocarcinoma of the prostate. J Urol 1997; 157:2206–2209.

29. Paulson DF, Lin GH, Hinshaw W, Stephani S, and the Uro-Oncology Research Group. Radical surgery versus radiotherapy for adenocarcinoma of the prostate. J Urol 1982; 128:502–504.

30. Alexander RB, Maguire MG, Epstein JI, Walsh PC. Pathological stage is higher in older men with clinical stage B1 adenocarcinoma of the prostate. J Urol 1989; 141: 880–882.

31. Garnick MB, Fair WR. Prostate cancer: emerging concepts. Part I. Ann Intern Med 1996; 125:119–125.

32. Partin AW, Kattan MW, Subong ENP, Walsh PC, Wojno KJ, Oesterling JE, Scardino

PT, Pearson JD. Combination of prostate-specific antigen, clinical stage, and Gleason score to predict pathological stage of localized prostate cancer. JAMA 1997; 277: 1445–1451.

33. Kupelian P, Katcher J, Levin H, et al. External beam radiotherapy versus radical prostatectomy for clinical stage T1-2 prostate cancer: therapeutic implications of stratification by pretreatment PSA levels and biopsy Gleason scores. Cancer J Sci Am 1997; 3:78–87.

34. Lattanzi JP, Hanlon AL, Hanks GE. Early stage prostate cancer treated with radiation therapy: stratifying an intermediate risk group. Int J Radiat Oncol Biol Phys 1997; 38: 569–573.

35. Powell CR, Huisman TK, Riffenburgh RH, et al. Outcome for surgically staged localized prostate cancer treated with external beam radiation therapy. J Urol 1997; 157: 1754–1759.

36. Graversen PH, Nielsen KT, Gasser TC, Corle DK, Madsen PO. Radical prostatectomy versus expectant primary treatment in stages I and II prostate cancer: a fifteen year follow-up. Urology 1990; 36:493–498.

37. Albertsen PC, Fryback DG, Storer BE, Kolon TF, Fine J. Long-term survival among men with conservatively treated localized prostate cancer. JAMA 1995; 274:626–631.

38. Fleming C, Wasson JH, Albertsen PC, Barry MJ, Wennberg JE. A decision analysis of alternative treatment strategies for clinically localized prostate cancer. JAMA 1993; 269:2650–2658.

39. Beck JR, Kattan MW, Miles BJ. A critique of the decision analysis for clinically localized prostate cancer. J Urol 1994; 152:1894–1899.

40. Kattan MW, Cowen ME, Miles BJ, et al. Modeling the impact of comorbidity on the decision to treat clinically localized prostate cancer. Med Decis Making 1996; 16:460.

41. Wilt TJ, Brawer MK. The prostate cancer intervention versus observation trial: a randomized trial comparing radical prostatectomy versus expectant management for the treatment of clinically localized prostate cancer. J Urol 1994; 152:1910–1914.

42. Litwin MS, Leake B, Hays RD, Fink A, Ganz PA, Leake B, Leach GE, Brook RH. Quality-of-life outcomes in men treated for localized prostate cancer. JAMA 1995; 273:129–135.

43. Lu-Yao GL, McLerran D, Wasson J, Wennberg JE, for the Prostate Patient Outcomes Research Team. An assessment of radical prostatectomy. JAMA 1993; 269:2633–2636.

44. Fowler FJ, Barry MJ, Lu-Yao G, Roman A, Wasson J, Wennberg JE. Patient-reported complications and follow-up treatment after radical prostatectomy. The national Medicare experience: 1988–1990 (updated June 1993). Urology 1993; 42:622–629.

45. Quinlan DM, Epstein JI, Carter BS, Walsh PC. Sexual function following radical prostatectomy: influence of preservation of neurovascular bundles. J Urol 1993; 145:998–1002.

46. Walsh PC. Retropubic prostatectomy for benign and malignant diseases. In: Marshall FF ed. Operative Urology. Philadelphia: Saunders, 1991: 264–289.

47. NIH Consensus Development Panel on Impotence. JAMA 1993; 270:83–90.

48. Dreicer R, Cooper CS, Williams RD. Management of prostate and bladder cancer in the elderly. Urol Clin North Am 1996; 23:87–97.

49. Perez CA, Hanks GE, Leibel SA, Zietman AL, Fuks Z, Lee WR. Localized carcinoma of the prostate (stages T1B, T1C, T2, and T3): review of management with external beam radiation therapy. Cancer 1993; 72:3156–3173.

50. Harlan L, Brawley O, Pommerenke F, Wali P, Kramer B. Geographic, age and racial variation in the treatment of local/regional carcinoma of the prostate. J Clin Oncol 1995; 13:93.

51. Severson RK, Montie JE, Porter AT, Demers RY. Recent trends in incidence and treatment of prostate cancer among elderly men. J Natl Cancer Inst 1995; 87:532–534.

52. Imperato PJ, Nenner RP, Will TO. Trends in radical prostatectomy in New York state. Am J Med Qual 1996; 11:205–213.

53. Bennett CL, Greenfield S, Aronow H, Ganz P, Vogelzang NJ, Elashoff RM. Patterns of care related to age of men with prostate cancer. Cancer 1991; 67:2633–2641.

54. Mazur DJ, Merz JF. Older patients' willingness to trade off urologic adverse outcomes for a better chance at five-year survival in the clinical setting of prostate cancer. J Am Geriatr Soc 1995; 43:979–984.

55. Garnick MB, Fair WR. Prostate cancer:emerging concepts. Part II. Ann Intern Med 1996; 125:205–212.

56. Forman JD, Kumar R, Haas G, Montie J, Porter AT, Mesina CF. Neoadjuvant hormonal downsizing of localized carcinoma of the prostate: effects on the volume of normal tissue irradiation. Cancer Invest 1995; 13:8–15.

57. Pilepich MV, Krall JM, Al-Sarraf M, John MJ, Doggett RL, Sause WT, Lawton CA, Abrams RA, Rotman M, Rubin P. Androgen deprivation with radiation therapy compared with radiation therapy alone for locally advanced prostate carcinoma: a randomized comparative trial of the Radiation Therapy Oncology Group. Urology 1995; 45: 616–623.

58. Bolla M, Gonzalez D, Warde P, Dubois JB, Mirimanoff RO, Storme G, Bernier J, Kuten A, Sternberg C, Gil T, Collette L, Pierart M. Improved survival in patients with locally advanced prostate cancer treated with radiotherapy and goserelin. N Engl J Med 1997; 337:295–300.

59. Stephenson RA, Smart CR, Mineau GP, James BC, Janerich DT, Dibble RL. The fall in incidence of prostate cancer: on the down side of a prostate specific antigen induced peak in incidence-data from the Utah Cancer Registry. Cancer 1995; 77:1342–1348.

60. Steinberg GD, Epstein JI, Piantadosi S, Walsh PC. Management of stage D1 adenocarcinoma of the prostate: the Johns Hopkins experience 1974 to 1987. J Urol 1990; 144: 1425–1432.

61. Smith JA, Haynes TH, Middleton RG. Impact of external irradiation on local symptoms and survival free of disease in patients with pelvic lymph node metastasis from adenocarcinoma of the prostate. J Urol 1984; 131:705–707.

62. Paulson DF, Cline WA, Koefoot RB, et al. Extended field radiation therapy versus delayed hormonal therapy in node positive prostatic adenocarcinoma. J Urol 1982; 172:935.

63. Myers RP, Larson-Keller JJ, Bergstralh EJ, Zincke H, Oesterling JE, Leiber MM. Hormonal treatment at the time of radical retropublic prostatectomy for stage D1 prostate cancer: results of long-term follow up. J Urol 1992; 147:910–915.

64. Frose GS, Messing EM. Optimal management of stage D1 prostate cancer. In: Dawson NA, Vogelzang NJ, eds. Prostate Cancer. New York: Wiley-Liss, 1994:197–213.

65. The Medical Research Council Prostate Cancer Working Party Investigators Group. Immediate versus deferred treatment for advanced prostatic cancer: initial results of the medical research council trial. Br J Urol 1997; 79:235–246.

66. Huggins C, Hodges CV. Studies on prostatic cancer I: the effect of castration, estrogen and androgen injections on serum phosphatase in metastatic carcinoma of the prostate. Cancer Res 1941; 1:293–297.

67. Cassileth BR, Soloway MS, Vogelzang NJ, Schellhammer PS, Seidmon EJ, Hait HI, Kennealey GT. Patient's choice of treatment in stage D prostate cancer. Urology 1989; 33(Suppl 5):57–62.

68. Vogelzang NJ, Chodak G, Soloway MS, Block NL, Schellhammer PH, Smith JA, Caplan RJ, Kennealey GT of the Zoladex Prostate Study Group. Goserelin versus orchiectomy in the treatment of advanced prostate cancer: Final results of a randomized trial. Urology 1995; 46:220–226.

69. Thrasher B, Crawford ED. Combined androgen blockade. In: Vogelzang NJ, Scardino PT, Shipley WU, Coffey D, eds. Comprehensive Textbook of Genitourinary Oncology. Baltimore: Williams & Wilkins, 1995:875–884.

70. Kolvenbag GJCM, Furr BJA. Bicalutamide ('Casodex') development: from theory to therapy (review). Can J Sci Am 1997; 3:192–203.

71. Prostate Cancer Trialist's Collaborative Group. Maximum androgen blockade in advanced prostate cancer: an overview of 22 randomized trials with 3283 deaths in 5710 patients. Lancet 1995; 346:265–269.

72. Matchar DB, McCrory DC, Bennett. Treatment considerations for persons with metastatic prostate cancer: survival versus out-of-pocket costs. Urology 1997; 49:218–224.

73. Scher HI, Kelly WK. Flutamide withdrawal syndrome: its impact on clinical trials in hormone-refractory prostate cancer. J Clin Oncol 1993; 11:1566–1572.

74. Small EJ, Vogelzang NJ. Second line hormonal therapy for advanced prostate cancer: a shifting paradigm. J Clin Oncol 1997; 15:382–388.

75. Tannock I, Gospodarowicz M, Meakin W, Panzarella T, Stewart L, Rider W. Treatment of metastatic prostate cancer with low-dose prednisone: evaluation of pain and quality of life as pragmatic indices of response. J Clin Oncol 1989; 7:590–597.

76. Storlie JA, Buckner JC, Wiseman GA, Burch PA, Hartmann LC, Richardson RL. Prostate specific antigen levels and clinical response to low dose dexamethasone for hormone-refractory metastatic prostate carcinoma. Cancer 1995; 76:96–100.

77. Taplin ME, Bubley GJ, Shuster TD, Frantz ME, Spooner AE, Ogata GK, Keir HN, Balk, SP. Mutation of the androgen-receptor gene in metastatic androgen-independent prostate cancer. N Engl J Med 1995; 332:1393–1398.

78. Vogelzang NJ, Crawford ED, Zietman A. Current clinical trial design issues in hormone-refractory prostate cancer: report of a consensus panel. Cancer 1998; 82:2093–2101.

79. Scott WW, Gibbons RP, Johnson PE, Prout GR, Schmidt JD, Saroff J, Murphy GD. The continued evaluation of the effects of chemotherapy in patients with advanced carcinoma of the prostate. J Urol 1976; 116:211–213.

80. Moore MJ, Osoba D, Murphy K, Tannock IF, Armitage A, Findlay B, Coppin C, Neville A, Venner P, Wilson J. Use of palliative end points to evaluate the effects of mitoxantrone and low-dose prednisone in patients with hormonally resistant prostate cancer. J Clin Oncol 1994; 12:689–694.

81. Seidman AD, Scher HI, Petrylak D, Dershaw DD, Curley T. Estramustine and vinblas-

tine: use of prostate specific antigen as a clinical trial end point in hormone refractory prostatic cancer. J Urol 1992; 147:931–934.

82. Hudes GR, Greenberg R, Krigel RL, Seidman AD, Scher HI, Petrylak D, Dershaw D, Curley T. Estramustine and vinblastine: use of prostate specific antigen as a clinical trial endpoint for hormone refractory prostate cancer. J Urol 1992; 147:931–934.

83. Pienta KJ, Redman BG, Bandekar RG, Bandekar R, Strawderman M, Cease K, Esper PS, Naik H, Smith DC. A phase II trial of oral estramustine and oral etoposide in hormone refractory prostate cancer. Urology 1997; 50:401–407.

84. Tannock IF, Osoba D, Stockler MR, Ernst DS, Neville AJ, Moore MJ, Armitage GR, Wilson JJ, Venner PM, Coppin CM, Murphy KC. Chemotherapy with mitoxantrone plus prednisone or prednisone alone for symptomatic hormone-resistant prostate cancer: a Canadian randomized trial with palliative endpoints. J Clin Oncol 1996; 14:1756–1764.

85. Kantoff PW, Conaway M, Winer E, Picus J, Vogelzang NJ. Hydrocortisone (HC) with or without mitoxantrone (M) in patients (pts) with hormone refractory prostate cancer (HRPC): preliminary results from a prospective randomized Cancer and Leukemia Group B Study (9182) comparing chemotherapy to best supportive care (abstr). J Clin Oncol 1996; 14:1748.

86. Levine EG, Halabi S, Hars V, Rago R, Vogelzang NJ. Preliminary results of CALGB 9680: a phase II trial of high dose mitoxantrone/GM-CSF and low dose steroids in hormone-refractory prostate cancer (HRPC). Proc Am Soc Clin Oncol, 1998; 17(Suppl):1297.

87. Kantoff PW. New agents in the therapy of hormone-refractory patients with prostate cancer. Semin Oncol 1995; 22(Suppl 1):32–34.

88. Smith DC, Trump DL. Prostate cancer. In: Cassel CK, Cohen HJ, Larson EB, Meier DE, Resnick NM, Rubenstein LZ, Sorensen LB, eds. Geriatric Medicine. 3rd ed. New York: Springer, 1997:305–315.

89. Benson RC, Hasan JM, Jones AG, Schlise S. External beam radiotherapy for palliation of pain from metastatic carcinoma of the prostate. J Urol 1981; 127:69–71.

90. Kobayaski K, Vokes EE, Vogelzang NJ, Janisch L, Soliven B, Ratain MJ. A phase I study of suramin (NSC 34936) given by intermittent infusion without adaptive control in patients with advanced cancer. J Clin Oncol 1995; 13:2196–2207.

91. Rosen PJ, Mendoza EF, Landaw EM, Mondino B, Graves MC, McBride JH, Turcillo P, deKernion J, Belldegrun A. Suramin in hormone-refractory metastatic prostate cancer: a drug with limited efficacy. J Clin Oncol 1996; 14:1626–1636.

92. Porter AT, McEwan AJB, Powe JE, Reid R, McGowan DG, Lukka H, Sathyanarayana JR, Takemchuk VN, Thomas GM, Erlich LE. Results of a randomized phase III trial to evaluate the efficacy of strontium-89 adjuvant to local field external beam irradiation in the management of endocrine resistant prostate cancer. Int J Radiat Oncol Biol Phys 1993; 25:805–813.

93. Quick D, Reid R, Hoskin P, Duschene G, Sartor O, and the [153]Sm-EDTMP Phase 3 Study Group. Efficacy and safety of [153]Sm-EDTMP in alleviating the pain of bone metastases in patients with prostate carcinoma (abstr). Proc Am Soc Clin Oncol 1996; 15(Suppl):514.

94. Purohit OP, Anthony C, Radstone CR, Owen J, Coleman RE. High dose intravenous pamidronate for metastatic bone pain. Br J Cancer 1994; 70:554–558.

95. Pevesa SS, Blot WJ, Stone BJ, Miller BA, Tavone RE, Fraumenti JF. Recent cancer trends in the United States. J Natl Cancer Inst 1995; 87:175–182.

96. Scher HI, Shipley WU, Herr HW. Cancer of the bladder. In: DeVita VT Jr, Hellman S, Rosenberg SA. Cancer: Principles and Practice of Oncology. Philadelphia: Lippincott-Raven, 1997:1300–1322.

97. Fradet Y. Epidemiology of bladder cancer In: Vogelzang NJ, Scardino PT, Shipley WU, Coffey D, eds. Comprehensive Textbook of Genitourinary Oncology. Baltimore: Williams & Wilkins, 1996:298–304.

98. McCredie M, Stewart JH, Ford JM, MacLennan RA. Phenacetin-containing analgesics and cancer of the bladder or renal pelvis in women. Br J Urol 1983; 55:220–224.

99. Levine LA, Richie JP. Urological complications of cyclophosphamide. J Urol 1989; 141:1063–1069.

100. Young RH. Pathology of bladder cancer. In: Vogelzang NJ, Scardino PT, Shipley WU, Coffey D, eds. Comprehensive Textbook of Genitourinary Oncology. Baltimore: Williams & Wilkins, 1996:326–337.

101. American Joint Committee on Cancer: Urinary bladder. In: Fleming ID, Cooper JS, Henson DE, et al., eds. Cancer Staging Manual. 5th ed. Philadelphia: Lippincott, 1997: 241–243.

102. Messing EM, Young TB, Hunt VB, Gilchrist KW, Newton MA, Brown LL, Hisgu WJ, Greenberg EB, Kuglitsch ME, Wegenke JD. Comparison of bladder cancer outcome in men undergoing hematuria home screening versus those with standard clinical presentations. Urology 1995; 45:387–397.

103. Kryger JV, Messing E. Bladder cancer screening. Semin Oncol 1996; 23:585–597.

104. Soloway MS, Briggman JV, Carpinito GA, Chodak GW, Church PA, Lamm DL, Lange P, Messing E, Pasciak RM, Reservitz GB, Rukstalis DB, Sarosdy MF, Stadler WM, Thiel RP, Hayden CL. Use of a new tumor marker, urinary NMP22, in the detection of occult or rapidly recurring transitional cell carcinoma of the urinary tract following surgical treatment. J Urol 1996; 156:363–367.

105. Mohr DN, Offord KP, Owen RA, Melton J III. Asymptomatic microhematuria and urologic disease: a population-based study. JAMA 1986; 256:224–229.

106. Torti FM, Lum BL. The biology and treatment of superficial bladder cancer. J Clin Oncol 1983; 2:505–531.

107. Kalish LA, Garnick MB, Richie JP. Appropriate endpoints for superficial bladder cancer clinical trials. J Clin Oncol 1987; 5:2004–2008.

108. Esrig D, Elmajian D, Groshen S, Freeman JA, Stein JP, Su-Chiu C, Nichols PW Skinner DG, Jones PA, Cote RJ. Accumulation of nuclear p53 and tumor progression in bladder cancer. N Engl J Med 1994; 331:1259–1264.

109. Nseyo UO, Lamm DL. Therapy of superficial bladder cancer. Semin Oncol 1996; 23: 598–604.

110. Lamm DL. Carcinoma in situ. Urol Clin North Am 1992; 19:499–508.

111. Herr HW, Schwalb DM, Zhang ZF, Sogani PL, Fair WR, Whitmore Jr. WF, Oettger HF. Intravesical bacillus Calmette-Guerin therapy prevents tumor progression and death from superficial bladder cancer: ten-year follow-up of a prospective randomized trial. J Clin Oncol 1995; 13:1404–1408.

112. Lamm DL. Complications of bacillus Calmette-Guerin immunotherapy. Urol Clin North Am 1992; 19:565–572.

113. Glashan RW. A randomized controlled study of intravesical alpha-2b-interferon in carcinoma in situ of bladder. J Urol 1990; 144:658–661.

114. Sarosdy MF, Lamm DL, Williams R, Moon TD, Flanigan RC, Crawford ED, Wilks NE, Earhart RH, Merritt JA. Phase I trial of oral bropirimine in superficial bladder cancer. J Urol 1992; 147:31–36.

115. Nseyo UO. Photodynamic therapy. Urol Clin North Am 1992; 19:591–599.

116. Leung HY, Griffiths, Neal DE. Progress in the management of solid tumors: Bladder cancer. Postgrad Med J 1996; 72:719–724.

117. Freiha FS. Open bladder surgery. In: Walsh PC, Retik AB, Stamey TA, Vaughan ED Jr eds. Campbell's Urology. Philadelphia: Saunders, 1992:2750–2774.

118. Leibovitch I, Avigad I, Ben-Chaim J, Nativ O, Goldwasser B. Is it justified to avoid radical cystoprostatectomy in elderly patients with invasive transitional cell carcinoma of the bladder? Cancer 1993; 71:3098–3101.

119. Strombakis N, Herr HW, Cookson MS, Fair WR. Radical cystectomy in the octogenarian. J Urol 1997; 158:2113–2117.

120. Kock NG, Nilson AE, Nilsson LO, Norlen LJ, Philipson BM. Urinary diversion via a continent ileal reservoir: clinical results in 12 patients. J Urol 1982; 128:469–475.

121. Rowland RG, Mitchell ME, Bihrle P, Kahnoski RJ, Piser JE. Indiana continent urinary reservoir. J Urol 1987; 137: 1136–1139.

122. Vogelzang NJ, Moormeier JA, Awan AM, Weichselbaum RR, Farah R, Straus FH, Schoenberg HW, Chodak GW. Methotrexate, vinblastine, doxorubicin and cisplatin followed by radiotherapy or surgery for muscle invasive bladder cancer: the University of Chicago experience. J Urol 1993; 149:753–757.

123. Sternberg CN. Neoadjuvant and adjuvant chemotherapy in locally advanced bladder cancer. Semin Oncol 1996; 23:621–632.

124. Hall RR, for the MRC Advanced Bladder Cancer Working Party, EORTC GU Group, et al. Neo-adjuvant CMV chemotherapy and cystectomy or radiotherapy in muscle invasive bladder cancer. First analysis of MRC/EORTC intercontinental trial (abstr). Proc Am Soc Clin Oncol 1996; 15(Suppl):244.

125. Roosen JV, Geertsen U, Jahn H, Weinreich J, Nissen HM. Invasive, high grade transitional cell carcinoma of the bladder treated with transurethral resection. Scand J Urol Nephrol 1997; 31:39–42.

126. Bales GT, Kim H, Steinberg GD. Surgical therapy for locally advanced bladder cancer. Semin Oncol 1996; 23:605–613.

127. Nerstrom B on behalf of the Danish Bladder Cancer Group (DAVECA). Preoperative irradiation (40GY) and cystectomy versus radiotherapy (60GY) followed by salvage cystectomy in the treatment of advanced bladder cancer (T2-T4a). A randomized study (DAVECA 8201). Eur Urol 1990; 18(Suppl 1):5(Abstr 9).

128. Smith JA Jr, Crawford ED, Blumenstein B, et al. A randomized prospective trial of preoperative irradiation plus radical cystectomy versus surgery alone for transitional cell carcinoma of the bladder. A Southwest Oncology Group study (abstr). J Urol 1988; 139:266A(Abstr 416).

129. Bloom HJG, Hendry WF, Wallace DM, Skeet RG. Treatment of T3 bladder cancer: controlled trial of pre-operative radiotherapy and radical cystectomy versus radical radiotherapy. Br J Urol 1982; 54:136–151.

130. Phillips HA, Howard GCW. Split course radical radiotherapy for bladder cancer in

the elderly: nonsense or common sense? A report of 76 patients. Clin Oncol (Royal College of Radiologists) 1996; 8:35–38.

131. Rostom AY, Tahir S, Gershung AR, Kandil A, Folkes A, White WF. Once weekly irradiation for carcinoma of the bladder. Int J Radiat Oncol Biol Phys 1996; 35:289–292.

132. Coppin CML, Gospodarowicz MK, James K, Tannock IF, Zee B, Carson J, Pater J, Sullivan LD. Improved local control of invasive bladder cancer by concurrent cisplatin and preoperative or definitive radiation. J Clin Oncol 1996; 14:2901–2907.

133. McLaren DB, Morrey D, Mason MD. Hypofractionated radiotherapy for muscle invasive bladder cancer in the elderly. Radiother Oncol 1997; 43:171–174.

134. Kachnic LA, Kaufman DS, Heney NM, Atthausen AF, Griffin PP, Zietman AL, Shipley WU. Bladder preservation by combined modality therapy for invasive bladder cancer. J Clin Oncol 1997; 14:1022–1029.

135. Tester W, Porter A, Asbell S, Coughlin C, et al. Combined modality program with possible organ preservation for invasive bladder carcinoma: results of RTOG protocol 85-12. Int J Radiat Oncol Biol Phys 1993; 25:783–790.

136. Housset M, Maulard C, Chretien Y, Dufour B, et al. Combined radiation and chemotherapy for invasive transitional-cell carcinoma of the bladder: a prospective study. J Clin Oncol 1993; 11:2150–2157.

137. Sella A, Logothetis CJ, Dexeus FH, Amato R, Finn L, Fitz K. Cisplatin combination chemotherapy for elderly patients with urothelial tumors. Br J Urol 1991; 67:603–607.

138. Veronesi A, Lo Re G, Carbone A, Trovo MG, Dal Bo V, Talamini R, Santarossa S, Francini M, Monfardini S. Multimodal treatment of locally advanced transitional cell bladder carcinoma in elderly patients. Eur J Cancer 1994; 30A:918–920.

139. Segati R, Bari M, Azzarello G, Signorelli C, Marchini M, Finccavento G, Longo M, Pappagallo GL, Vinante O. Carboplatin monochemotherapy in elderly patients with nonoperable transitional cell carcinoma of the bladder: a two-stage, phase II study. Eur Urol 1996; 29:312–317.

140. Yagoda A. Chemotherapy of urothelial tract tumors. Cancer 1987; 60:574–585.

141. Natale RB, Yagoda A, Watson RC, Whitmore WF, Blumenreich M, Braun DW. Methotrexate: an active drug in bladder cancer. Cancer 1981; 47:1246–1250.

142. Roth BJ. Chemotherapy for advanced bladder cancer. Semin Oncol 1996; 23:633–644.

143. Sternberg CN, Yagoda A, Scher HI, Watson RC, Geller N, Herr HW, Morse MJ, Sogani PC, Vaughan ED, Bander N, Weiselberg L, Rosado K, Smart T, Lin SY, Penenberg D, Fair WR, Whitmore WF. Methotrexate, vinblastine, doxorubicin and cisplatin for advanced transitional cell carcinoma of the urothelium. Cancer 1989; 64:2448–2458.

144. Logothetis CJ, Dexeus FH, Finn L, Sella A, Amato RJ, Ayala AG, Kilbourn RG. A prospective, randomized trial comparing MVAC and CISCA chemotherapy for patients with metastatic urothelial tumors. J Clin Oncol 1990; 8:1050–1055.

145. Loehrer PJ, Einhorn LH, Elson PJ, Crawford ED, Kuebler P, Tannock I, Raghavan D, Stuart-Harris R, Sarosdy MF, Lowe EA, Blumenstein B, Trump D. A randomized comparison of cisplatin alone or in combination with methotrexate, vinblastine, and doxorubicin in patients with metastatic urothelial carcinoma: a cooperative group study J Clin Oncol 1992; 10:1066–1073.

146. Loehrer PJ, Elson P, Dreice R, Hahn R, Nichols CR, Williams R, Einhorn LH. Esca-

lated dosages of methotrexate, vinblastine, doxorubicin, and cisplatin plus recombinant human granulocyte colony-stimulating factor in advanced urothelial carcinoma: an Eastern Cooperative Oncology Group trial. J Clin Oncol 1994; 12:483–488.

147. Scher HI, Geller NL, Curley T, Tao Y. Effect of relative cumulative dose-intensity on survival of patients with urothelial cancer treated with M-VAC. J Clin Oncol 1993; 11:400–407.

148. Roth BJ, Dreicer R, Einhorn LH, Neuberg D, Johnson DH, Smith JL, Hudes GR, Schultz SM, Loehrer PJ. Significant activity of paclitaxel in advanced transitional-cell carcinoma of the urothelium: a phase II trial of the Eastern Cooperative Oncology Group. J Clin Oncol 1994; 12:2264–2270.

149. McCaffery JA, Hilton S, Mazumdar M, Sadan S, Kelly WK, Scher HI, Bajorin D. Phase II trial of docetaxel in patients with advanced or metastatic transitional cell carcinoma. J Clin Oncol 1997; 15:1853–1857.

150. Stadler WM, Kuzel T, Roth B, Raghavan D, Dorr FA. A phase II study of single agent gemcitabine in previously untreated patients with metastatic urothelial cancer. J Clin Oncol 1997; 15:3394–3398.

151. DeLena M, Gridelli C, Lorusso, et al. Gemcitabine activity (objective responses and symptom improvement) in resistant stage IV bladder cancer (abstr). Proc Am Soc Clin Oncol 1996; 15(Suppl):246.

152. Von der Maase H, Andersen L, Crino L, Weissbach L, Dogliotti L. A phase II study of gemcitabine and cisplatin in patients with transitional cell carcinoma (TCC) of the urothelium (abstr). Proc Am Soc Clin Oncol 1997; 16(Suppl):324a.

153. Stadler WM, Murphy B, Kaufman D, Raghavan D, Voi M. Phase II trial of gemcitabine (GEM) plus cisplatin (CDDP) in metastatic urothelial cancer (UC) (abstr). Proc Am Soc Clin Oncol 1997; 16(Suppl):323a.

154. Yu MC, Mack TM, Hanisch R, Cicioni C, Henderson BE. Cigarette smoking, obesity, diuretic use, and coffee consumption as risk factors for renal cell carcinoma. J Natl Cancer Inst 1986; 77:351–356.

155. Mandel JS, McLaughlin JK, Schlehofer B, et al. International renal-cell cancer study. IV. Occupation. Int J Cancer 1995; 61:601–605.

156. LaForgia S, Lasota J, Latif F, Boghosian-Sell L, Kastury K, Ohta M, Druck T, Atchison L, Cannizzaro LA, Barnea G. Detailed genetic and physical map of the 3p chromosome region surrounding the familial renal cell carcinoma chromosome translocation, t(3;8)(p14.2;q24.1). Cancer Res 1993; 53:3118–3124.

157. Linehan WM, Lerman MI, Zbar B. Identification of the von Hippel-Lindau gene: its role in renal carcinoma. JAMA 1995; 273:564–570.

158. Zbar B, Tory K, Merino M, Schmidt L, Glenn G, Choyke P, Walther MM, Lermann M, Linehan WM. Hereditary papillary renal cell carcinoma. J Urol 1994; 151:561–566.

159. Kiely JM. Hypernephroma—the internist's tumor. Med Clin North Am 1966; 50:1067–1083.

160. Ritchie AWS, Chisholm GD. The natural history of renal carcinoma. Semin Oncol 1983; 10:390–400.

161. Tsukamoto T, Kumamoto Y, Yamazaki K, Miyao N, Takahashi A, Masumori N, Satoh M. Clinical analysis of incidentally found renal cell carcinomas. Eur Urol 1991; 19:109–113.

162. Johnson CD, Dunnick NR, Cohan RH, Illescas FI. Renal adenocarcinoma: CT staging of 100 tumors. Am J Roentgenol 1987; 148:59–63.

163. Semelka RC, Shoenut JP, Magro CM. Renal cancer staging: comparison of contrast-enhanced CT and gadolinium-enhanced fat-suppressed spin-echo and gradient-echo MR imaging. J Magn Reson Imaging 1993; 3:597–602.

164. Horan JJ, Robertson CN, Choyke PL, Frank JA, Miller DL, Pass HI, Linehan WM. The detection of renal carcinoma extension into the renal vein and inferior vena cava: a prospective comparison of venacavography and magnetic resonance imaging. J Urol 1989; 142:943–948.

165. Robson CJ, Churchill BM, Anderson W. The results of radical nephrectomy for renal cell carcinoma. J Urol 1969; 101:297–301.

166. American Joint Committee on Cancer: Kidney. In: Fleming ID, Cooper JS, Henson DE, et al., eds. Cancer Staging Manual. 5th ed. Philadelphia: Lippincott, 1997: 231–232.

167. Guinan PD, Vogelzang NJ, Fremgen AM, Chmiel JS, Sylvester JL, Sener SF, Imperato JP. Renal cell carcinoma: tumor size, stage and survival. J Urol 1995; 153:901–903.

168. Guiliani L, Giberti L, Martorana G, Rovida S. Radical extensive surgery for renal cell carcinoma: long-term results and prognostic factors. J Urol 1990; 143:468–474.

169. Linehan WM, Shipley WU, Parkinson DR. Cancer of the kidney and ureter. In: DeVita VT Jr, Hellman S, Rosenberg SA. Cancer: Principles and Practice of Oncology. Philadelphia: Lippincott-Raven, 1997:1271–1300.

170. Kjaer M, Frederiksen PL, Engelholm SA. Postoperative radiotherapy in stage II and III renal adenocarcinoma. A randomized trial by the Copenhagen Renal Cancer Study Group. Int J Radiat Oncol Biol Phys 1987; 13:665–672.

171. Novick AC. Partial nephrectomy for renal cell carcinoma. Urol Clin North Am 1987; 14:419–433.

172. Novick AC. Current surgical approaches, nephron-sparing surgery, and the role of surgery in the integrated immunologic approach to renal-cell carcinoma. Semin Oncol 1995; 22:29–33.

173. Damhuis RAM, Blom JHM. The influence of age on treatment choice and survival in 735 patients with renal carcinoma. Br J Urol 1995; 75:143–147.

174. Samet J, Hunt WC, Key C, Humble CG, Goodwin JS. Choice of cancer therapy varies with age of patient. JAMA 1986; 255:3385–3390.

175. Maldazys JD, DeKernion JB. Prognostic factors in metastatic renal carcinoma. J Urol 1986; 136:376–379.

176. Yagoda A, Abi-Rached B, Petrylak D. Chemotherapy for advanced renal-cell carcinoma: 1983–1993. Semin Oncol 1995; 22:42–60.

177. Chapman AE, Goldstein LJ. Multiple drug resistance: biologic basis and clinical significance in renal-cell carcinoma. Semin Oncol 1995;22:17–28.

178. Rosenberg SA, Lotze MT, Muul LM, Chang AE, Avis FP, Leitman S, Linehan WM, Robertson CN, Rubin JT. A progress report on the treatment of 157 patients with advanced cancer using lymphokine-activated killer cells and interleukin-2 or high-dose interleukin-2 alone. N Engl J Med 1987; 316:889–897.

179. Rosenberg SA, Yang JC, Topalian SC, Schwartzentruber DJ, Weber JS, Parkinson DR, Seipp CA, Einhorn JH, White DE. Treatment of 283 consecutive patients with

metastatic melanoma or renal cell cancer using high-dose bolus interleukin-2. JAMA 1994; 271:907–913.

180. Law TM, Motzer RJ, Mazumdar M, Sell KW, Walther PJ, O'Connell M, Khan A, Vlamis V, Vogelzang NJ, Bajorin DF. Phase III randomized trial of interleukin-2 with or without lymphokine-activated killer cells in the treatment of patients with advanced renal cell carcinoma. Cancer 1995; 76:824–832.

181. Atkins MB, Sparano J, Fisher RI, Sunderland M, Margolin K, Ernest ML, Sznol M, Atkins MB, Dutcher JP, Micetich KC, Weiss GR. Randomized phase II trial of high-dose interleukin-2 either alone or in combination with interferon alpha-2b in advanced renal cell carcinoma. J Clin Oncol 1993; 11:661–670.

182. Stadler WM, Vogelzang NJ. Low-dose interleukin-2 in the treatment of metastatic renal-cell carcinoma. Semin Oncol 1995; 22:67–73.

183. Parkinson DR, Sznol M. High-dose interleukin-2 in the therapy of metastatic renal cell carcinoma. Semin Oncol 1995; 22:61–66.

184. Siegel JP, Puri RK. Interleukin-2 toxicity. J Clin Oncol 1991; 9:694–704.

185. Rackley R, Novick A, Klein E, Bukowski R, McLain D, Goldfarb D. The impact of adjuvant nephrectomy on multimodality treatment of metastatic renal cell carcinoma. J Urol 1994; 152:1399–1403.

186. Fleischmann JD, Kim B. Interleukin-2 immunotherapy followed by resection of residual renal cell carcinoma. J Urol 1991; 145:938–941.

187. Sella A, Swanson DA, Ro JY, Putman JB Jr., Amato RJ, Markowtiz AB, Logothetis CJ. Surgery following response to interferon-alpha-based therapy for residual renal cell carcinoma. J Urol 1993; 149:19–22.

188. Ershler WB, Longo DL. Aging and cancer: issues of basic and clinical science (review). J Natl Cancer Inst 1997; 89:1489–1497.

14
Gastrointestinal Cancer

Harold J. Burstein and Robert J. Mayer
Dana–Farber Cancer Institute and
Brigham and Women's Hospital,
Harvard Medical School
Boston, Massachusetts

I. INTRODUCTION

Gastrointestinal (GI) malignancies are common among the elderly. Age is a significant risk factor for most cancers, and particularly for those arising in the alimentary tract. Fig. 1 shows the striking relationship between cancer incidence and age for several major GI cancers (1). The incidence rises between 20- and 100-fold as the population ages from 40 to 70 years. The elderly—those older than age 65 years—comprise the vast majority of cases of colorectal, gastric, pancreatic, and esophageal cancers (Table 1) (2, 3). Indeed, to speak of the management of these tumors is to discuss their management in the elderly.

The diagnostic, staging, and therapeutic strategies for GI malignancies are independent of age. As is widely the case for most reports in the medical literature, the elderly are relatively underrepresented in clinical studies of gastrointestinal cancer (4). The results of cohort-control studies examining standard treatments for a variety of cancers, including colon and stomach cancers, suggest that the response rate to chemotherapy treatments is no different in patients over the age of 70 years than in younger patients (5). Relative underrepresentation of the elderly with GI cancers is a factor both in large, randomized trials and in smaller phase II studies despite the lack of evidence that older patients experience significantly more toxicity than younger patients in these trials (6). Despite the more limited available data, the lessons derived from studies of younger patients have become applicable to all patients, including the elderly. The treatments—usually relying on combinations of surgery, chemotherapy, and radiation therapy—can be associated with considerable

325

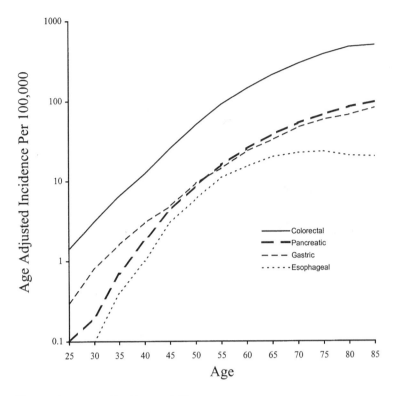

Figure 1 Age and incidence of GI cancers.

Table 1 Incidence and Mortality from Gastrointestinal
Cancers in the Elderly[a]

Anatomic site	No. of new cases	No. of deaths	% of cases over age 65 years
Colon	95,600	47,700	74
Rectum	36,000	8,800	66
Pancreas	29,000	28,900	72
Stomach	22,600	13,700	68
Esophagus	12,300	11,900	56

[a] SEER data for US population, 1998; see Ref. 3.

morbidity, and the risk of significant complications is higher in patients with more comorbid illness, advanced disease, and greater age (7, 8). In general, the presumption should be to treat patients with optimal therapy regardless of age, and then to adjust therapy based on the patient's individual preferences and specific medical condition. The multimodality care of patients with gastrointestinal cancers depends on the coordinated efforts of surgeons, radiation oncologists, medical oncologists, and primary care providers experienced in the care of the elderly.

II. COLON AND RECTAL CANCER

A. Screening and Chemoprevention

Primary care providers and geriatricians have an important role in detecting early-stage colorectal cancer. Screening tests for colorectal cancer have been shown to result in a survival benefit (9, 10). The American Cancer Society has endorsed (11) the published screening recommendations of a multidisciplinary expert panel (12), which recommended that patients with average risk and older than age 50 years undergo annual fecal occult blood testing with flexible sigmoidoscopy every 5 years, or total colon examination such as double-contrast barium enema every 5–10 years, or colonoscopy every 10 years. Any positive screening test should lead to colonoscopy with biopsy of suspicious lesions. Patients with a history of colon polyps or of known familial cancer syndromes, such as familial adenomatous polyposis or hereditary nonpolyposis colorectal cancer, merit more frequent and earlier evaluation.

Among the screening options, colonoscopy is probably the preferred test; it allows for inspection as well as biopsy of suspicious lesions and polyps. Polyps are a frequent problem in the elderly. The likelihood of polyps containing cancer increases with the size and number of polyps. Patients with greater than average risk by virtue of a family history of colon cancer or of adenomatous polyps merit screening at a younger age, beginning at 40 years old. These interventions can have significant impact on the health of the elderly population. The risk factors for colorectal cancer are listed in Table 2. Familial colon cancer syndromes are more likely to affect younger family members, and they are less common in the elderly population. Epidemiological data suggest that the regular use of nonsteroidal anti-inflammatory agents and aspirin is associated with a reduction in the incidence of colorectal cancer (13). It is thought that the benefits of anti-inflammatory agents on colon cancer require years of regular use. For patients with other indications for aspirin therapy such as heart disease or risk of stroke, aspirin can also be recommended for prevention of colorectal cancer. It is not yet clear whether everyone over the age of 50 years should be advised to take aspirin for colorectal cancer prevention.

B. Presenting Symptoms

The clinical presentation of colorectal cancer can vary depending on the site of the primary tumor. Tumors of the proximal colon—where the stool is relatively liquid—

Table 2 Risk Factors for Gastrointestinal Cancers

	Esophageal	Gastric	Colorectal	Pancreatic
Medical Conditions	Barrett's esophagus	Atrophic gastritis	Colon polyps, including familial	Diabetes
	Achalasia	Pernicious anemia	HNPCC	Chronic pancreatitis
	Plummer–Vinson syndrome	*Helicobacter pylori* infection	Inflammatory bowel disease	Peptic ulcer surgery
	Esophageal webs	Prior peptic ulcer surgery		
	Obesity	Menetrier's disease, gastric polyps, other stomach pathology		
	Gastro-esophageal reflux			
Behavioral/Social	Smoking	Occupational	Smoking	Smoking
	Alcohol	Socioeconomic status		Occupational exposures
	Caustic ingestions	Smoking?		
Dietary	Low fruit/vegetable	Low fruit/vegetable	High saturated fat	
	High fat	Salted/smoked/unrefrigerated foods	High meat	
M:F ratio	3:1	2:1	1.5:1	1.3:1

HNPCC, hereditary nonpolyposis colon cancer gene families.

often lead to iron-deficiency anemia from chronic blood loss. More distal lesions in the transverse or descending colon, where the stool is more formed, frequently come to medical attention because of crampy abdominal pain due to colonic obstruction. Rectal tumors are often associated with narrowing of stool caliber, tenesmus, or frank rectal bleeding (hematochezia), but they rarely are associated with anemia. During recent decades, there has been an unexplained proximal migration in the presenting location of colorectal cancers.

Presenting symptoms of colorectal cancer in the elderly tend to be similar to those for other age populations (14, 15). Symptoms in the elderly such as fatigue and bowel changes tend to be both insidious and common, and thus a thoughtful evaluation of these complaints is required to detect colorectal cancers. Older patients are sometimes less able to tolerate the physiological stress of anemia from colorectal cancer; conversely, they tend to be less attentive to problems such as constipation.

C. Prognostic Factors

Survival for all patients with colorectal cancer is dependent on stage. Staging for colorectal cancer is based on the extent of invasion through the bowel wall and the presence of metastatic disease in lymph nodes or systemically. Tumors that invade the colonic wall without penetration through the wall are considered stage I disease. These have an excellent prognosis with 85–90% survival at 5 years. Tumors that penetrate into but not through the muscularis propria (T2; Dukes Astler–Coller B1) have a more favorable prognosis than stage II tumors, which invade through the full depth of the colonic wall (T3; Dukes Astler–Coller stage B2). Patients with stage II disease have a 70–80% 5-year survival. Involvement of any regional lymph nodes with cancer is classified as stage III disease (TxN1-2M0; Dukes Astler–Coller stage C), which carries an approximately 40–50% 5-year survival in the absence of adjuvant therapy. Patients with metastatic disease (stage IV) have a poor prognosis, with only 5% survival at 5 years and 60% mortality in the first year alone.

For all stages, elderly patients (>60 years) tend to have a lower 5-year survival than younger patients, and this deleterious pattern is amplified with greater age. Studies suggest several reasons for this trend: competing causes of mortality, the presence of comorbid illnesses (16, 17), emergency presentations and worse outcomes after surgery, and, historically, less frequent utilization of appropriate therapy. In the past, elderly colorectal cancer patients have been less likely to receive chemotherapy (18–20) and radiation therapy (21). Definitive surgical care is routinely provided for older colorectal cancer patients, in contrast to the practice in other GI malignancies where the greater associated morbidity may discourage extensive surgery (22).

Series of surgical patients at single institutions suggest that elderly colorectal patients are more likely to present with acute abdominal symptoms requiring emergency surgery. However, the data from the National Cancer Data Base indicate that elderly patients are slightly less likely to present with stage IV (metastatic) disease

(23). Roughly 25% of patients less than 60 years old have metastatic disease on presentation versus less than 20% for those over the age of 60 years. This distinction may be somewhat artificial, however, since comprehensive staging studies may be performed less frequently in elderly patients.

D. Diagnostic Staging

Appropriate staging tests include a thorough physical examination, chest radiograph, and liver function tests. A full colonoscopy should be performed to exclude synchronous lesions, which occur in a small percentage of patients. The carcinoembryonic antigen (CEA) level should be measured preoperatively. Patients who have high CEA levels initially, or whose levels fail to return to normal after surgery, are more likely to develop recurrent disease (24, 25). The routine role of CT/MRI scans to assess the liver is controversial, but such imaging is indicated in patients whose symptoms (weight loss, liver tenderness, fever, anorexia) suggest the presence of metastatic disease. Patients with symptoms of tenesmus or physical findings of a perirectal lesion merit a pelvic CT scan prior to surgery.

E. Treatment

1. Surgery

The standard initial management of colorectal cancer remains en bloc resection of the tumor, with adequate surgical margins proximally and distally, and resection of the draining lymphatic regions (26). Even for patients with metastatic disease, surgical resection is often an important part of palliative treatment. Elderly patients are a distinctive population, and they require careful perioperative management of hemodynamic, fluid and electrolyte, respiratory, and endocrine and renal problems (27). The risks of colorectal surgery in the elderly population have been well studied. Data from Medicare claims suggest that mortality from colorectal surgery rises as a function of age; the increase in mortality seems most noticeable after age 75 years (28). The risk for perioperative mortality increases from less than 4% for those less than 75 years old to more than 8% for those 85 years old or more. Analyses of this trend have suggested that this increased risk is predominantly due to comorbid illness in the patient population and not to age per se. Large proportions of patients in this age group will have multiple medical problems, including cardiovascular and pulmonary disease, and are usually receiving multiple medications (29, 30). In one series of elderly patients requiring surgery for colorectal cancer, nearly 50% had nonlocalized disease at the time of diagnosis, the majority of patients had cardiac disorders, nearly 40% had chronic pulmonary disease, and many had neurological, vascular, renal, hepatic, and diabetic diseases (31). Multiple single-institutional reports regarding colorectal surgery in the elderly demonstrate rising rates of complications and mortality from surgery, growing higher in the very old population (32–

35). All these studies suggest that concurrent medical problems contribute significantly to the rising toxicity of surgery, but all conclude that the risk of surgery in the elderly is both justifiable and justified.

The principles of surgical management of rectal cancer differ somewhat from those of intraperitoneal colonic tumors (29, 30). The rectum lacks an adequate serosal layer, and local spread of tumor into pelvic structures is a more common problem than in colon cancer. For this reason, presurgical imaging of the pelvis with CT scan or MRI is often performed. In rectal cancers, sphincter-sparing operations are often feasible, but adequate resection may require an abdominoperineal resection (APR). For patients with low-lying rectal cancers, preoperative radiation therapy with or without chemotherapy may allow sphincter-sparing surgery in many cases that would have otherwise required APR and resultant colostomy (36). There is growing interest in the use of laparoscopic techniques of tumor resection for colon and rectal cancers. Laparoscopic surgery seems to be as safe as open surgery for elderly patients with colorectal cancers, although firm data on cancer outcomes between the two approaches await the results of an ongoing randomized trial.

Most patients destined to relapse after curative surgery for colorectal cancer do so within the first 2 years. Eighty percent of recurrences occur within 24 months, and there are very few recurrences after 5 years of disease-free follow-up. Up to 7% of patients will develop metachronous lesions (37). For this reason, all patients merit follow-up colonoscopy performed within the first year of resection and, if normal, every 3–5 years thereafter (12). The value of routine testing with CEA levels after surgical resection is controversial (38). A rising CEA level after surgery often heralds metastatic diseaes; however, it has not been shown that earlier detection by tumor marker analysis improves survival for patients with recurrent colorectal cancer. For patients who have isolated metastases to liver or lung, surgical resection of the metastatic lesion may confer a significantly prolonged disease-free survival. Thus, for patients who are potential candidates for these types of salvage metastatectomy operations, early detection may be more valuable, and routine testing of CEA is more justifiable. However, to be useful, the test ought to be performed every 2–3 months postoperatively. Testing can probably be discontinued after 3 years, as most recurrences will happen within that time interval.

2. Adjuvant Therapy

Patterns of failure after surgery for colon and rectal cancers differ (39). For colon cancer (tumors located above the peritoneal reflection), local recurrence rates are 3–12% whereas systemic tumor recurrences, particularly in the liver, develop in one third of patients. By contrast, local failure is far more common in rectal cancer (tumors located below the peritoneal reflection), occurring in roughly one quarter of stage II/B2 patients, and more than half of stage III/C patients. This difference is probably more a consequence of local anatomical features (more difficult resection, absence of serosal barrier in rectum) than of biological differences between the tumors. As a consequence of these different patterns of tumor recurrence, differing strategies for postsurgical treatment have evolved for colon and rectal cancers. For colon cancer, systemic chemotherapy alone is utilized, whereas in rectal cancer, radiation therapy to the pelvis combined with systemic chemotherapy is employed.

Multiple large, randomized studies have demonstrated a significant survival benefit for treating patients with stage C (stage III) colon cancer with adjuvant systemic chemotherapy. These regimens employ 5-fluorouracil, administered in several ways with such other agents as levamisole or leucovorin (39, 40). Such treatment has resulted in a 5–15% absolute reduction (or a 33% relative reduction) in the risk of death after 5 years. Retrospective analyses of subsets of patients with earlier stage disease suggest that chemotherapy may also be of benefit for "high-risk" stage B2 (stage II) patients, such as those with tumor adherent to other abdominal organs or who present with clinical obstruction or perforation. However, prospective randomized studies have shown no survival benefit when adjuvant therapy has been administered to patients with standard risk stage II (B2) cancers (41, 42). The principal toxicities of 5-fluorouracil–based chemotherapy are mucositis, diarrhea, skin irritation/dermatitis, and myelosuppression, with the pattern of these side effects being dependent on the dose schedule of chemotherapy selected.

Elderly patients tolerate chemotherapy (43, 44), although they are more predisposed to certain toxic side effects, such as gastrointestinal distress, mucositis, hematological toxicities, and cardiac toxicities than are younger patients (45, 46). For the 5-fluorouracil (5-FU) regimens commonly used in GI malignancies, mucositis and diarrhea are particularly more severe in treated elderly patients. In a population-based study of 5-FU therapy for adjuvant treatment of colon cancer, the incidence of toxicity requiring hospitalization rose dramatically with age (47). Thirty-five percent of patients over age 75 years required hospitalization for toxic side effects versus only 8% of those less than age 70 years. Slightly more than one half of the patients over age 75 years of age did not complete the course of adjuvant treatment versus 35% of those younger than 70 years old. Clinicians should expect more side effects in older patients receiving adjuvant chemotherapy; however, the mortality benefits are independent of age, and supportive management should enable most older patients to do well with adjuvant treatment.

For rectal cancer, postoperative chemoradiation therapy has become the standard of care in the adjuvant setting (39). Large randomized studies have demonstrated the benefit of 5040 cGy radiation therapy combined with chemotherapy in improving both local control and overall survival in patients with stages II and III rectal cancers. The optimal combination and delivery of the two modalities remains to be determined. Recent data suggest that continuous infusion of 5-FU administered concomitantly with radiation therapy may be superior to bolus 5-FU, presumably because of an enhanced radiation-sensitizing effect (48). There is interest in the possible use of chemotherapy and radiation therapy prior to surgery for certain patients in the hope of shrinking the tumor and allowing for sphincter preservation in patients who would otherwise require a colostomy (36). Pelvic radiation therapy can cause local mucosal irritation, diarrhea, and tenesmus. Irradiation of the pelvic bone marrow can rarely cause myelosuppression, especially in patients with limited hematopoietic reserve and in those receiving chemotherapy. Older patients are particularly at risk for more small bowel toxicity from radiation treatments (49). Again, comorbid conditions such as hypertension, peripheral vascular disease, diabetes, and prior surgery all contribute to small bowel toxicity in older cancer patients receiving pelvic/abdominal radiotherapy. A review of radiation therapy in patients older than 80 years old with a variety of cancers found that 40% of all patients at a single institution—and 53% of those being treated with curative intent—had unplanned interruptions in their treatment because of side effects or concurrent illnesses (50).

3. Treatment of Metastases

Metastatic disease is a common problem for patients with colorectal cancer, and it is usually incurable. Palliative treatments include systemic chemotherapy, focal radiation therapy, surgery for hepatic metastases, and hepatic artery infusional chemotherapy (51). These treatments need to be applied judiciously in the elderly population, with appropriate consideration of the realistic benefits and side effects of the therapy.

Systemic chemotherapy can palliate pain, reduce the tumor burden, and prolong life in patients who respond. Historically, 5-FU and 5-FU–based regimens have been the mainstay of systemic treatment, with response rates of 15–30% (52). A topoisomerase I inhibitor, irinotecan, has been shown to produce significant response rates even in patients previously treated with 5-FU, and it is quickly becoming the standard treatment for refractory metastatic colorectal cancer (53). The dose-limiting side effect is diarrhea, which can usually be managed with the use of loperamide. A preliminary analysis of the experience using irinotecan in elderly patients with colorectal cancer suggests that patients older than age 70 years will tolerate this drug (54). Although older patients had slightly more frequent diarrhea and neutropenia than did younger patients, these differences were not statistically significant, and the response rates to treatment were equivalent in patients over or under 70 years old.

The role of intrahepatic chemotherapy infusion in the management of patients with liver metastases is controversial. Meta-analyses of randomized trials of intrahepatic versus systemic chemotherapy have suggested higher response rates for intrahepatic infusion; however, this enhanced probability of disease regression has not resulted in prolonged overall survival (55, 56). In the elderly population, the need for surgery for the placement of an hepatic arterial catheter and the subcutaneous installation of an infusion pump raises additional concerns about the routine utilization of this treatment. Surgical resection of isolated liver metastates may confer survival benefit in carefully selected patients (57, 58). Operative mortality rates on the order of 5% have been reported in series of these highly selected patients. In a recent analysis, age greater than 60 years was found to be an adverse prognostic factor for patients undergoing liver metastasis resection (59). Nonetheless, a review of patients older than age 70 years undergoing liver resections for metastatic colorectal cancer showed no significant difference in perioperative morbidity or mortality, or in long-term survival, in the older patients compared to younger patients at the same institution (60).

III. GASTRIC CANCER

Stomach cancer has declined in incidence since the 1930s, when it was the leading cause of cancer death in American men and third for women. The reasons for the decline in incidence are unclear, although they may be related to changes in socioeconomic status, diet, and food storage and preservation. This change has been accompanied by a proximal migration of cancers within the stomach, with a greater proportion of lesions now originating in the cardia than previously when most arose in the antrum (61, 62). Gastric cancer remains a problem among the elderly; as seen in Fig. 1, the incidence rises steadily with age. Risk factors for gastric carcinoma are listed in Table 2. Widespread screening programs for gastric cancer are conducted in Japan, where the incidence of the disease is much higher. Perhaps because of these interventions, the frequency of early-stage gastric cancer detection is far higher in the Japanese population than in Americans.

A. Presenting Symptoms

Gastric cancer presents with insidious and nonspecific findings—weight loss, abdominal pain, nausea, and anorexia. Unfortunately, most of these are associated with more advanced stage disease. More localized, easily resectable cancers are usually asymptomatic. The great majority of patients undergo exploratory surgery once a diagnosis of gastric cancer is made. At the time of surgery, however, most patients will be found to have advanced disease (stage III or IV) with a 5-year survival rate of 13% or less. Because gastric cancers can cause significant local symptoms such as dysphagia, bleeding, or gastrointestinal obstruction, surgery is still recommended for most patients, and can be of significant palliative benefit even in those with known metastatic disease.

B. Treatment

Complete surgical resection of the stomach tumor and removal of associated lymph nodes remains the only curative modality for gastric cancer. Regardless of age, the perioperative mortality rate for resection of gastric cancer is roughly 7%. An analysis of gastric cancer patients over age 70 years operated on at Memorial Sloan–Kettering Cancer Center in New York found a similar mortality rate, although the older patients were more likely to have additional complications and to require longer hospitalizations (63). Reviews of other institutional experiences have shown considerable variability in the perioperative mortality rate, particularly in the elderly (64, 65). Stage-adjusted mortality rates for patients operated on with curative intention seem no worse in the elderly population (29, 64, 65). Older patients tend to present with disease in a similar stage distribution as the population as a whole (66). However, a smaller percentage of older patients is deemed appropriate for resection owing to comorbid disease or advanced disease and a reluctance to attempt exploratory surgery. In Japan, where early-stage disease is more common, it has been found that older patients (>70 years old) are more likely to have metastatic disease and less favorable histological and pathological features than younger (<40 years old) patients (67). This may reflect the different epidemiology of gastric cancer in the different societies.

Postoperative treatment recommendations for gastric cancer depend on the presence or absence of residual tumor. For patients who have undergone an incomplete surgical resection, and thus have locally advanced gastric cancer, combined modality therapy with radiation treatment and chemotherapy has been shown to confer a modest survival benefit (68, 69). However, for patients who have undergone a ''curative'' operation, neither adjuvant chemotherapy nor radiation therapy has been shown to prolong survival (70). Chemotherapy can be useful for palliation of symptoms, and it may prolong life in patients with advanced disease. Several studies comparing chemotherapy versus best supportive care have shown a survival benefit for treatment (71). Many chemotherapeutic agents in combination are effective (61, 72); such treatments have been given safely to older patients with gastric cancer (73). A published report of a randomized study in patients with advanced adenocarcinoma of the esophagus and stomach showed improved survival benefit, diminished toxicity, and better short-term quality of life scores for treatment with the ECF (epirubicin, cisplatin, 5-FU) regimen in comparison to the FAMTX (5-FU, doxorubicin, methotrexate) program (74). In this study, half the patients were more than 60 years old, although the majority of patients had a performance status of 0 or 1.

IV. PANCREATIC CANCER

Pancreatic cancer is more common among the elderly, as age is the primary risk factor for developing the disease. Other associated risks for pancreatic cancer are listed in Table 2. It is an ominous disease; virtually all patients diagnosed will eventually succumb to the cancer.

A. Presenting Symptoms and Diagnosis

The classic clinical presentation is of pain and weight loss, with jaundice occurring if the tumor arises in the pancreatic head. Diagnostic evaluation with CT scan usually reveals a pancreatic mass or diffuse enlargement of the gland. Histological diagnosis with CT guided fine-needle aspiration or other modality is necessary to distinguish pancreatic adenocarcinoma from lymphoma or islet cell tumor.

B. Treatment

1. Surgery

Most patients have advanced disease at the time of presentation; 50% will have overt metastases, and another 20% will have local lymph node involvement (75). A national survey of clinical practice revealed that only 14% of patients undergo a total resection of their pancreatic cancer (75). The mortality rates for pancreatic surgery have decreased with greater experience; much of this has been attributed to performance of the operation by fewer surgeons possessing greater experience (76). The precise role of surgery on the natural history of pancreatic cancer is not clear; even for patients with tumor confined to the pancreas (stage I), the 5-year survival is less than 10%. Although only a minority of patients (5–20%) have potentially resectable disease, many patients may benefit from surgical palliation to alleviate biliary obstruction. For patients with advanced cancer, endoscopic stent deployment for biliary drainage may offer adequate palliation with much less morbidity.

Pancreatic surgery is not commonly performed in the elderly. Nationally, only 10% of pancreatic cancer patients greater than the age of 70 years and 6% of those greater than 80 years old underwent resection. Thus, elderly patients undergoing pancreatic resection represent a carefully selected population. At centers with extensive experience in pancreatic surgery, the procedure can have as low as a 6% perioperative mortality rate for patients aged 70 years old or older (60, 77). These older patients have similar rates of complications, intensive care unit admissions, and hospital lengths of stay as younger patients.

2. Chemotherapy

Chemotherapy can offer palliative benefit for some patients with advanced pancreatic cancer. Historically, 5-FU has been the mainstay of therapy, although significant therapeutic responses are noted in less than one fifth of patients, and these are usually transient (78). A newer agent, the nucleoside analogue gemcitabine, has been shown to have similar activity, and it may offer a minimal survival advantage for patients when compared to 5-FU (79, 80). The principal toxicities of gemcitabine include nausea and vomiting, and bone marrow suppression with continued administration. Adjuvant 5-FU combined with radiation therapy is generally offered to patients who have undergone a complete resection for pancreatic cancer. This practice is based on a study which compared such treatment to surgery alone, and found a slight survival benefit for combined modality therapy (81).

V. ESOPHAGEAL CANCER

Esophageal cancer, like other GI malignancies, occurs with increasing frequency in the elderly (82). Predisposing factors for esophageal cancer are listed in Table 2. Over the past decade, there has been a dramatic rise in the incidence of adenocarcinoma of the esophagus and a slight decline in the incidence of squamous cell carcinoma (83, 84). The reasons for this change are not known. Patients with Barrett's esophagus are at greater risk for developing esophageal adenocarcinoma. Although these patients are often followed with regular endoscopic evaluation, there are little data as to whether this costly procedure improves clinical outcomes.

A. Presenting Symptoms

Most esophageal cancer patients present with dysphagia and weight loss, and many have a long-term history of gastro-esophageal reflux (i.e., heartburn) (84a). As with other cancers in the elderly, these complaints are non-specific and relatively common. Most patients have advanced disease at the time of diagnosis, making them noncandidates for radical surgical resection.

B. Treatment

Prior to attempted surgical resection, patients with esophageal cancer should undergo CT scans of the chest and abdomen and, if available, endoscopic ultrasonography. The findings from these studies can help select patients who will potentially benefit from total esophagectomy, and spare those with advanced disease from the morbidity of surgery. Some patients may benefit from surgery for palliation of dysphagia, although endoscopic dilatation and/or stenting are gaining increasing use as a palliative strategy, especially for patients with more advanced disease or worse prognosis.

Esophageal surgery has recently been associated with a 6–8% perioperative mortality rate, although morbidity can be much higher, affecting nearly one quarter of patients. For appropriate elderly candidates, surgical outcomes are no worse than those experienced by younger patients (77). Among the very elderly (those patients aged 80–90 years), major upper abdominal or thoracic surgery requires careful physiological monitoring and preoperative evaluation, but it has been successfully performed (85).

Several randomized studies have compared either combination chemotherapy and radiation therapy to radiation therapy alone (86) or preoperative chemotherapy and radiation therapy to surgery alone (87, 88) in patients with esophageal cancer. The nonsurgical study comparing chemoradiation to radiation alone for patients with either squamous cell or adenocarcinoma histological subtype of esophageal cancer demonstrated a survival benefit for the combined modality approach. The two studies comparing chemoradiation therapy with surgery had differing mortality outcomes. The larger study, conducted in patients with squamous cell esophageal cancer, showed no overall survival benefit (88), whereas the smaller study, performed in patients with esophageal adenocarcinoma, showed improved overall survival with combined modality therapy (87). Toxicities were considerable, including profound esophagitis and bone marrow suppression, as well as the risks of surgery. In all three studies, the chemotherapy and radiation therapy were significantly more toxic than either radiation therapy or surgery alone. Larger, hopefully more definitive, trials have been initiated to better define the value of preoperative treatment.

For the majority of patients with esophageal cancers whose tumors are unresectable, multimodality treatments offers the only opportunity for prolonged life and palliation. More intensive chemotherapy combinations (74) or the introduction of new agents (89) may prove to be useful in the future.

VI. CONCLUSIONS

Gastrointestinal malignancies are common in the elderly population, and they represent a significant and growing public health problem. Changes in diet, behavior, and primary care screening patterns could have major impacts on the frequency and mortality of these cancers. The nonspecific symptoms of gastrointestinal cancers make diagnosis difficult. Regrettably, many cases are discovered only after the cancer has spread beyond a point of curative treatment. A careful and prompt evaluation of gastrointestinal pain or bleeding, as well as of weight loss, is warranted given the prevalence of these diseases in the elderly.

Elderly patients diagnosed with gastrointestinal cancer merit extensive, minimally invasive staging studies to help in decisions for further treatment. Patients found to have locally advanced or metastatic disease can be spared larger operations, and care should focus on palliation. For those patients who are surgical candidates, careful assessment and treatment of comorbid medical problems can minimize the risk of subsequent oncological surgery. Since surgery remains the sine qua non of definitive care for GI cancers, every reasonable attempt should be made to prepare older patients for curative surgical resection. Since the elderly will experience more side effects from surgery, chemotherapy, and radiation therapy, careful consideration of tumor stage and available treatment options is critical. In addition, providers can anticipate more side effects, treatment delays and cessations, and more concurrent illness when treating older cancer patients.

There are little direct data bearing on the treatment of elderly patients with gastrointestinal cancers. The available information comes from limited series of highly selected elderly patient populations, characterized as having few comorbid illnesses and excellent performance status. Most treatment guidelines for gastrointestinal malignancies are extrapolated from studies of younger populations of patients. To improve on this situation, elderly patients should be sought more actively for inclusion in clinical trials, and more data should be presented that stratify patients by age. In the meanwhile, clinicians must carefully weigh the realistic benefits of treatment against potential side effects when offering cancer therapy to the elderly.

ACKNOWLEDGMENT

Supported in part by NIH grant 5T32CA09172-23.

REFERENCES

1. Kosary CL, Ries LAG, Miller BA, Hankey BF, Harras A, Edwards BK, eds. SEER cancer statistics review, 1973–1992: tables and graphs, National Cancer Institute. NIH Pub. No. 96-2789. Bethesda, MD, 1995.
2. Yancik R. Cancer burden in the aged. Cancer 1997; 80:1273–1283.
3. Landis SH, Murray T, Bolden S, Wingo PA. Cancer statistics, 1998. CA Cancer J Clin 1998; 48:6–30.
4. Trimble EL, Carter CL, Cain D, Freidlin B, Ungerleider RS, Friedman MA. Representation of older patients in cancer treatment trials. Cancer 1994; 74:2208–2214.
5. Cascinu S, Del Ferro E, Catalano G. Toxicity and therapeutic response to chemotherapy in patients aged 70 years or older with advanced cancer. Am J Clin Oncol 1996; 19: 371–374.
6. Giovanazzi-Bannon S, Rademaker A, Lai G, Benson AB. Treatment tolerance of elderly cancer patients entered onto phase II clinical trials: an Illinois Cancer Center study. J Clin Oncol 1994; 12:2447–2452.
7. McKenna RJ. Clinical aspects of cancer in the elderly. Cancer 1994; 74:2107–2117.
8. Crocker I, Prosnitz L. Radiation therapy of the elderly. Clin Geriatr Med 1987; 3:473–481.
9. Mandel JS, Bond JH, Church TR, Snover DC, Bradley GM, Schuman LM, Ederer F. Reducing mortality from colorectal cancer by screening for fecal occult blood. N Engl J Med 1993; 328:1365–1371.
10. Selby JV, Friedman GD. Sigmoidoscopy in the periodic health examination of asymptomatic adults. JAMA 1989; 261:595–601.
11. Byers T, Levin B, Rotheberger D, Dodd GD, Smith RA. American Cancer Society guidelines for screening and surveillance for early detection of colorectal polyps and cancer: update 1997. CA Cancer J Clin 1997; 47:154–160.
12. Winawer SJ, Fletcher RH, Miller L, Godless F, Stolar MH, Mulrow CD, Woolf SH, Glick SN, Ganiats TG, Bond JH, Rosen L, Zapka JG, Olsen Sj, Giardiello FM, Sisk JE, Van Antwerp R, Brown-Davis C, Marciniak DA, Mayer RJ. Colorectal cancer screening: clinical guidelines and rationale. Gastroenterology 1997; 112:594–692.
13. Giovannucci E, Egan KM, Hunter DJ, Stampfer MJ, Colditz GA, Willett WC, Speizer FE. Aspirin and the risk of colorectal cancer in women. N Engl J Med 1995; 333:609–14.
14. Curless R, French J, Williams GV, James OFW. Comparison of gastrointestinal symp-

toms in colorectal carcinoma patients and community controls with respect to age. Gut 1994; 35:1267–1270.

15. Curless R, French JM, Williams GV, James OFW. Colorectal carcinoma: do elderly patients present differently? Age Ageing 1994; 23:102–107.

16. Yancik R, Havlik RJ, Wesley MN, Ries L, Long S, Rossi WK, Edwards BK. Cancer and comorbidity in older patients: a descriptive profile. Ann Epidemiol 1996: 6:399–412.

17. Vercelli M, Simoni C, Venturino A, Biancardi V, Reggiardo G, D'Onofrio A, Modenesi M, Rosso R. Comorbidity among elderly patients with and without cancer (abstr). Proc Am Soc Clin Oncol 1994; 13:467.

18. Mor V, Masterson-Allen S, Golderg RJ, Cummings FJ, Glicksman AS, Fretwell MD. Relationship between age at diagnosis and treatments by cancer patients. J Am Geriatr Soc 1985; 33:585–589.

19. Newcomb PA, Carbone PP. Cancer treatment and age: patient perspectives. J Natl Cancer Inst 1993; 85:1580–1584.

20. Goodwin JS, Samet JM, Hunt WC. Determinants of survival in older cancer patients. J Natl Cancer Inst 1996; 88:1031–1038.

21. Guadagnoli E, Weitberg A, Mor V, Silliman RA, Glicksman AS, Cummings FJ. The influence of patient age on the diagnosis and treatment of lung and colorectal cancer. Arch Intern Med 1990; 150:1485–1490.

22. Samet J, Hunt WC, Kay C, Humble CG, Goodwin JS. Choice of cancer therapy varies with age of patient. JAMA 1986; 255:3385–3390.

23. Jessup JM, McGinnis LS, Steele GD, Mench HR, Winchester DP. The National Cancer Data Base Report on Colon Cancer. Cancer 1996; 78:918–926.

24. Moertel CG, O'Fallon JR, Go VLW, O'Connell MJ, Thynne GS. The preoperative carcinoembryonic antigen test in the diagnosis, staging, and prognosis of colorectal cancer. Cancer 1986; 58:603–610.

25. Wanebo HJ, Rao B, Pinsky CM, Hoffman RG, Stearns M, Schwartz MK, Oettgen HF. Preoperative carcinoembryonic antigen level as a prognostic indicator in colorectal cancer. N Engl J Med 1978; 299:448–51.

26. Cohen AM. Surgical considerations in patients with cancer of the colon and rectum. Semin Oncol 1991; 18:381–387.

27. Patterson WB. Surgical issues in geriatric oncology. Semin Oncol 1989; 16:57–65.

28. Whittle J, Steinberg EP, Anderson FG, Herbert R. Results of colectomy in elderly patients with colon cancer based on Medicare claims data. Am J Surg 1992; 163:572–576.

29. Berger DH, Roslyn JJ. Cancer surgery in the elderly. Clin Geriatr Med 1997; 13:119–141.

30. McGinnis LS. Surgical treatment options for colorectal cancer. Cancer 1994; 74:2147–2150.

31. Fitzgerald SD, Longo WE, Daniel GL, Vernava AM. Advanced colorectal neoplasia in the high-risk elderly patient: is surgical resection justified? Dis Colon Rectum 1993; 36:161–166.

32. Lewis AAM, Khoury GA. Resection for colorectal cancer in the very old: are the risks too high? BMJ 1988; 296:459–461.

33. Kingston RD, Jeacock J, Walsh S, Keeling F. The outcome of surgery for colorectal

cancer in the elderly: a 12 year review from the Trafford Database. Eur J Surg Oncol 1995; 21:514–516.

34. Hessman O, Bergkvist L, Strom S. Colorectal cancer in patients over 75 years of age— determinants of outcome. Eur J Surg Oncol 1997; 23:13–19.

35. Avital S, Kashtan H, Hadad R, Webin N. Survival of colorectal carcinoma in the elderly. Dis Colon Rectum 1997; 40:523–529.

36. Friedman GM, Coia LR. Adjuvant and neoadjuvant treatment of rectal cancer. Semin Oncol 1995; 22:611–624.

37. Welch JP, Donaldson GA. Detection and treatment of recurrent cancer of the colon and rectum. Am J Surg 1978; 135:505.

38. American Society of Clinical Oncology. Clinical practice guidelines for the use of tumor markers in breast and colorectal cancer. J Clin Oncol 1996; 10:2843–2877.

39. Fuchs CS, Mayer RJ. Adjuvant chemotherapy for colon and rectal cancer. Semin Oncol 1995; 22:472–487.

40. Machover D. A comprehensive review of 5-fluorouracil and leucovorin in patients with metastatic colorectal carcinoma. Cancer 1997; 80:1179–1187.

41. Moertel CG, Fleming TR, Macdonald JS, Haller DG, Lourie JA, Tanger CM, Unger- leider JS, Emerson WA, Tormey DC, Glick JH, Veeder MH, Mailliard JA. Intergroup study of fluorouracil plus levamisole as adjuvant therapy for stage II/Dukes' B2 colon cancer. J Clin Oncol 1995; 13:2936–2943.

42. International Multicentre Pooled Analysis of Colon Cancer Trials (IMPACT) Investiga- tors. Efficacy of adjuvant fluorouracil and folinic acid in colon cancer. Lancet 1995; 346:939–944.

43. Balducci L, Extermann M. Cancer chemotherapy in the older patient. Cancer 1997; 80: 1317–1322.

44. Schneider M, Thyss A, Ayela P, Gaspard MH, Otto J, Creisson A. Chemotherapy for patients aged over 80. In: Fentiman IS, Monfardini S, eds. Cancer in the Elderly. Oxford, UK: Oxford University Press, 1994:53–60.

45. Conti JA, Christman K. Cancer chemotherapy in the elderly. J Clin Gastroenterol 1995; 21:65–71.

46. Baker SD, Grochow LB. Pharmacology of cancer chemotherapy in the older person. Clin Geriatr Med 1997; 13:169–183.

47. Brower M, Asbury R, Kramer Z, Pandya K, Bennett JM. Adjuvant chemotherapy for colorectal cancer in the elderly: population-based experience. Proc Am Soc Clin Oncol (abstr) 1995; 12:195.

48. O'Connell MJ, Martenson JA, Wieand HS, Krook JE, Macdonald JS, Haller DG, Mayer RJ, Gunderson LL, Rich TA. Improving adjuvant therapy for rectal cancer by combining protracted-infusion fluorouracil with radiation therapy after curative surgery. N Engl J Med 1994; 331:502–507.

49. Farniok FE, Levitt SH. The role of radiation therapy in the treatment of colorectal can- cer. Implications for the older person. Cancer 1994; 74:2154–2159.

50. Wasil T, Rush S, Lichtman SM. Retrospective analysis of external beam radiation ther- apy in patients aged 80 and above. Proc Am Soc Clin Oncol (abstr) 1997; 16;74.

51. Lichtman SM, Bayer RL. Gastrointestinal cancer in the elderly. Clin Geriatr Med 1997; 13:307–326.

52. Mayer RJ. Chemotherapy for metastatic colorectal cancer. Cancer 1992; 70:1414–1424.

53. Rothenberg ML, Eckardt JR, Kuhn JG, Burriss HA, Nelson J, Hilsenbeck SG, Rodriguez GI, Thurman GM, Smith LS, Eckhardt G, Weiss GR, Elfring GL, Rinaldi DA, Schaaf LJ, Von Hoff DD. Phase II trail of irinotecan in patients with progressive or rapidly recurrent colorectal cancer. J Clin Oncol 1996; 14:1128–1135.

54. Pazdur R, Zinner R, Rothenberg ML, von Hoff DD, Hainsworth JD, Blanke CD, Cox JV, Elfring GL, Wolf DL, Mohrland JS, Schaaf LF, Petit RG. Age as a risk factor in irinotecan (CPT-11) treatment of 5-FU-refractory colorectal cancer. Proc Am Soc Clin Oncol (abstr) 1997; 16:260.

55. Meta-analysis Group in Cancer. Reappraisal of hepatic arterial infusion in the treatment of nonresectable liver metastases from colorectal cancer. J Natl Cancer Inst 1996; 88: 252–258.

56. Harmantas A, Rotsetin LE, Langer B. Regional versus systemic chemotherapy in the treatment of colorectal carcinoma metastatic to the liver. Is there a survival difference? Meta-analysis of the published literature. Cancer 1996; 78:1639–1645.

57. Cady B, Stone MD. The role of surgical resection of liver metastases in colorectal carcinoma. Semin Oncol 1991; 18:399–406.

58. Ballantyne GH, Quin J. Surgical treatment of liver metastases in patients with colorectal cancer. Cancer 1993; 71:4252–4266.

59. Nordlinger B, Guiguet M, Vaillant JC, Balladur P, Boudjema K, Bachellier P, Jaeck D. Surgical resection of colorectal carcinoma metastases to the liver. A prognostic scoring system to improve case selection, based on 1568 patients. Cancer 1996; 77:1254–1262.

60. Fong Y, Blumgart LH, Fortnre JG, Brennan MR. Pancratic or liver resection for malignancy is safe and effective for the elderly. Ann Surg 1995; 222:426–437.

61. Fuchs CS, Mayer RJ. Gastric carcinoma. N Engl J Med 1995; 333:32–41.

62. Wanebo HJ, Kennedy BJ, Chmiel J, Steele G, Winchester D, Osteen R. Cancer of the stomach. A patient care study by the American College of Surgeons. Ann Surg 1993; 216:583–592.

63. Schwarz RI, Karpeh MS, Brennan MF. Factors predicting hospitalization after operative treatment for gastric carcinoma in patients older than 70 years. J Am Coll Surg 1997; 184:9–15.

64. Damhuis RAM, Tilanus HW. The influence of age on resection rates and postoperative mortality in 2773 patients with gastric cancer. Eur J Cancer 1995; 31:928–931.

65. Winslet MC, Mohsen YMA, Powell J, Allum WH, Fielding JWL. The influence of age on the surgical management of carcinoma of the stomach. Eur J Surg Oncol 1996; 22: 220–224.

66. Javlik RJ, Yancik R, Long S, Ries L, Ewards B. The National Institute on Aging and the National Cancer Institute SEER collaborative study on comorbidity and early diagnosis of cancer in the elderly. Cancer 1994; 74:2101–2106.

67. Maehara Y, Emi Y, Tomisaki S, Oshiro T, Kakeji Y, Ichiyoshi Y, Sugimachi K. Age-related characteristics of gastric carcinoma in young and elderly patients. Cancer 1996; 77:1774–1780.

68. Moertel CG, Childs DS, Reitemeier RJ, Colby MY, Holbrook MA. Combined 5-fluorouracil and supervoltage radiation therapy of locally unresectable gastrointestinal cancer. Lancet 1969; 2:600–602.

69. Gastrointestinal Tumor Study Group. A comparison of combination chemotherapy and combined modality therapy for locally advanced gastric carcinoma. Cancer 1982; 49: 1771–1777.

70. Hermans J, Bonenkamp JJ, Boon MC, Bunt AMG, Ohyama S, Sasako M, Van de Velde CJH. Adjuvant therapy after curative resection for gastric cancer: meta-analysis of randomized trials. J Clin Oncol 1993; 11:1441–1447.

71. Wils J. The treatment of advanced gastric cancer. Semin Oncol 1996; 23:397–406.

72. Pelley RJ. Role of chemotherapy in the palliation of gastrointestinal malignancies. Semin Oncol 1995; 22(Suppl 3):45–52.

73. Maehara Y, Yamamoto M, Endo K, Baba H, Kusumoto H, Sugimachi K. Postoperative chemotherapy for gastric cancer in the elderly. Chemotherapy 1994; 40:279–286.

74. Webb A, Cunningham D, Scarffe JH, Harper P, Norman A, Joffe JK, Hughes M, Mansi J, Findlay M, Hill A, Oates J, Nicolson M, Hickish T, O'Brien M, Iveson T, Watson M, Underhill C, Wardly A, Meehan M. Randomized trial comparing epirubicin, cisplatin, and fluorouracil versus fluorouracil, doxorubicin, and methotrexate in advanced esophagogastric cancer. J Clin Oncol 1997; 15:261–267.

75. Niederhuber JE, Brennan MR, Menck HR. The National Cancer Data Base report on pancreatic cancer. Cancer 1995; 76:1671–1677.

76. Warshaw AL, Fernandez-del Castillo C. Pancreatic carcinoma. N Engl J Med 1992; 326:455–465.

77. Karl RC, Smith SK, Fabri PJ. Validity of major cancer operations in elderly patients. Ann Surg Oncol 1995; 2:107–113.

78. Schnall SF, Macdonald JS. Chemotherapy of adenocarcinoma of the pancreas. Semin Oncol 1996; 23:220–228.

79. Burris HA, Moore MJ, Andersen J, Green MR, Roethenberg ML, Modiano MR, Cripps MC, Portenoy RK, Storniola AM, Tarassoff P, Nelson R, Dorr FA, Stephens CD, von Hoff DD. Improvements in survival and clinical benefit with gemcitabine as first-line therapy for patients with advanced pancreas cancer: a randomized trial. J Clin Oncol 1997; 15:2403–2413.

80. Moore M. Activity of gemcitabine in patients with advanced pancreatic carcinoma. Cancer 1996; 78:633–638.

81. Kalser MH, Ellenberg SS. Pancreatic cancer. Adjuvant combined radiation and chemotherapy following curative resection. Arch Surg 1985; 120:899–903.

82. Daly JM, Karnell LH, Mench HR. National cancer data base report on esophageal carcinoma. Cancer 1996; 78:1820–1828.

83. Mayer RJ. Overview: the changing nature of esophageal cancer. Chest 1993; 103:404S–405S.

84. Blot WJ. Esophageal cancer trends and risk factors. Semin Oncol 1994; 21:403–410.

84a. Lagergren J, Bergstrom R, Lindgren P, Nyren D. Symptomatic gastroesophageal reflux as a risk factor for esophageal adenocarcinoma. N Engl J Med 1999; 340:825–831.

85. Alexander HR, Turnbull AD, Salamone J, Keefe D, Melendez J. Upper abdominal surgery in the very elderly. J Surg Oncol 1991; 47:82–86.

86. Al-Sarraf, M, Martz K, Herskovic A, Leichman L, Brindle JS, Vaitkevicius VK, Cooper J, Byhardt R, Davis L, Emami B. Progress report of combined chemoradiotherapy versus radiotherapy alone in patients with esophageal cancer: an Intergroup study. J Clin Oncol 1997; 15:277–284.

87. Walsh TN, Noonan N, Hollywood D, Kelly A, Keeling N, Hennessy TPJ. A comparison of multimodal therapy and surgery for esophageal adenocarcinoma. N Engl J Med 1996; 335;462–467.

88. Bosset JF, Gignoux M, Triboulet JP, Tiret E, Mantion G, Elias D, Lozach P, Ollier JC, Pavy JJ, Mercier M, Sahmoud T. Chemoradiotherapy followed by surgery compared with surgery alone in squamous-cell cancer of the esophagus. N Engl J Med 1997; 337: 161–167.

89. Ajani JA, Ilson Dh, Daugherty K, Pazdur R, Lynch PM, Lesen DP. Activity of taxol in patients with squamous cell carcinoma and adenocarcinoma of the esophagus. J Natl Cancer Inst 1994; 86:1086–1091.

15
Lung Cancer

Steven M. Grunberg and Samer E. Bibawi
University of Vermont
Burlington, Vermont

I. INTRODUCTION

Lung cancer holds a unique but contradictory position among the solid tumors. Although not the most common tumor in terms of incidence or prevalence, the tendency toward more advanced stage at presentation and the short median survival of patients with this tumor have made lung cancer a particularly lethal problem. In fact, lung cancer has long been the leading cause of cancer death in men and for the last 10 yeras has also been the leading cause of cancer death in women (1).

II. CAUSATION AND DETECTION

Lung cancer is predominantly related to chemical carcinogen exposure and has an extended period between first exposure and development of the tumor. Approaches to this tumor (including efforts at prevention, detection, and treatment) are therefore by necessity directed at different age groups. Most cases of lung cancer are related to smoking, and most chronic smokers have begun smoking before reaching adulthood. Efforts at prevention, including increased education and increased taxation (to reduce the affordability of cigarettes), are primarily directed at the young adult and preadult populations. Smoking cessation programs, which may include both pharmacological and behavioral interventions, are then aimed at the young adult and adult populations. However, since the appearance of lung cancer itself is directly related to carcinogen exposure as expressed in combined intensity and duration of smoking (pack-years), lung cancer screening, detection, and treatment become greater considerations as the population increases in age. In fact, more than half the patients diagnosed with lung cancer are more than 65 years of age (2).

Although the increased incidence of lung cancer in the elderly might therefore appear to be the natural endpoint of a continuum, certain unique features of lung cancer as observed in the older population may be important in terms of detection and treatment. Over the past several decades, adenocarcinoma has become the most common form of lung cancer. However, in the elderly population, squamous carcinoma continuous to be the most common histology and may account for more than 50% of the observed cases of lung cancer (3). Lung cancer also tends to be diagnosed more often at a localized stage in elderly populations as compared to younger populations. O'Rourke et al. (4) reviewed a database of 22,874 lung cancer cases contained in a centralized registry. Lung cancer was localized at the time of diagnosis in only 15.3% of patients under 55 years of age but was localized in 25.4% of patients over 74 years of age. The incidence of distant disease at time of presentation decreased from 48.7% in patients less than 55 years of age to 36.7% in patients over 74 years of age. The finding of a greater frequency of localized disease might be consistent with the increased frequency of squamous cell carcinoma. However, this would not explain the increase in frequency of squamous cell carcinoma itself in the older population. Other factors such as diet have been considered as possible contributors to the genesis of lung cancer. Shibata et al. (5) followed 5080 elderly male subjects for 8 years and found a reduced risk of lung cancer for subjects with a high consumption of beta-carotene. However, a strong inverse relationship was found between dietary beta-carotene and smoking status, and the dietary factor did not have an independent effect on lung cancer incidence when adjusted for smoking. Since squamous cell carcinoma has a predictably strong correlation with smoking, this factor deserves to be further examined. Hoffman et al. (6) noted a 30–50% decrease in the risk of developing lung cancer in subjects smoking filtered cigarettes as compared to nonfiltered cigarettes. Theoretically, the increased incidence of squamous cell carcinoma in the present elderly population could be explained by the fact that these patients began smoking before the introduction of filtered cigarettes and therefore had a more intense carcinogen exposure. If this particular facet of smoking behavior is indeed critical, then the increased incidence of squamous cell carcinoma of the lung in the elderly population should persist at least through the early decades of the 21st century. On the other hand, if the increased incidence of squamous cell lung cancer in the elderly population merely reflects the fact that older patients have smoked for a longer period of time and therefore generally have a greater overall (pack-year) exposure, then the increased incidence of squamous cell carcinoma in this population will be a continuing trend that will not be modified by present cigarette type or composition.

Since localized squamous cell carcinoma is most likely to be effectively addressed with curative therapy, the preponderance of this type and stage of disease in an elderly population raises important questions concerning screening and early detection. In general, screening using either chest radiograph or sputum cytology is not considered of value in lung cancer. The large-scale lung cancer detection trials sponsored by the National Cancer Institute in the 1970s at Johns Hopkins University in Baltimore, MD, (7), Memorial Sloan–Kettering Cancer Center in New York City (8), and the Mayo Clinic in Rochester, MN, (9) documented an increase in benchmark survival but not an increase in overall survival, and they therefore are considered to reflect lead-time bias and length-related sampling. However, the limitations of these studies may not apply as strongly to a highly selected (elderly) population at greater risk for localized disease in a central location. This target population can be further limited by consideration of pulmonary function tests and pulmonary symptomatology. DeMaria and Cohen (10) noted that dyspnea (a central symptom) is more common in an elderly population with lung cancer, whereas chest pain (a peripheral symptom) tends to be seen in a younger population. Identification of dyspnea as a particularly important symptom would also support the observation that abnormal spirometry (reduced airflow) is an even stronger predictor of development of lung cancer than either pack-years of smoking exposure or age (11). Petty (12) has therefore suggested an algorithm in which smokers with abnormal spirometry and symptoms of cough, wheeze, or dyspnea are considered at highest risk and therefore an appropriate target group for intensive lung cancer screening. The value of induced sputum cytology has been emphasized by Jack et al. (13), who noted a 58% sensitivity and 100% specificity for induced sputum cytology in the detection of lung cancer in an older population. The importance of better access to medical services for the detection of early-stage lung cancer has also been suggested by Grover et al. (14), who found an increased incidence of localized as compared to metastatic lung cancer in the older male population when comparing post-Medicare (1967–1975) data to pre-Medicare (1960–1965) data. Investigations of the possibility that screening a high-risk elderly population would detect localized lung cancer and thereby increase the cure rate and expected survival continue to be necessary.

III. TREATMENT

A. Surgery

Surgery remains the treatment of choice for non–small-cell lung cancer and is the modality most likely to result in cure. Major limitations for the use of this technique in the general population include the infrequency of detection of lung cancer at a localized stage (only approximately one fourth of lung cancer cases are detected while still resectable [15]) and the fact that the main environmental risk factor for lung cancer (smoking) also induces both cardiovascular and pulmonary comorbid conditions that independently increase the risk of surgery. In contrast, the demographics of lung cancer in the elderly are particularly favorable for the use of potentially curative surgery, since the frequency of localized lung cancer at presentation is higher (25.4%) in patients over 75 years of age as compared to 15.3% in patients under 54 years of age (4). However, Smith et al. (16), using data from the Virginia

Cancer Registry (1985–1989) and Medicare claims records, found that the elderly are still much less likely to be offered surgery as initial therapy. In reviewing 2812 cases, the use of surgery as all or part of the initial therapy was found to decrease from 44% in patients aged 65–69 years to 6% in those over 85 years old. This did not represent increased use of radiotherapy as a less aggressive alternative for primary treatment of lung cancer but rather the tendency to give no therapy at all. Patients receiving no therapy increased from 11% in the 65- to 69-year age group to 52.3% in patients over 85 years of age, whereas the use of radiotherapy alone as primary therapy remained at a relatively constant frequency throughout all the age groups considered.

The question, therefore, remains as to why the elderly are less likely to be offered surgery as primary therapy. The argument that curative surgery would not make a difference in overall survival due to the limited life expectancy of elderly patients must be rejected, since the average survival of older adults exceeds the average survival of patients with uncontrolled cancer (17). Comorbid conditions do tend to increase with age and might therefore increase the risk of surgery. However, increasing comorbidity and increasing age are not necessarily synonymous. These two factors must be separated to identify patient populations where surgery can be safely and successfully performed irregardless of advancing age.

The older surgical literature does indeed suggest increased risk for thoracic surgery in the elderly. Postoperative mortality rates as much six times higher have been reported in patients over 70 years old compared to patients under 60 years old (18). Whittle et al. (19) reviewed Medicare data on 1290 patients who underwent surgical resection for lung cancer between 1983 and 1985. The perioperative death rate in this group was 7.4%, with a 1-year survival of 69% and a 2-year survival of 54%. However, subset analysis revealed an increased perioperative death rate and decreased 1- and 2-year survival in male patients, older patients, and patients undergoing pneumonectomy. Sherman and Guidot (20) reviewed 139 cases of patients undergoing lung resection. Although younger patients (<70 years old) were more likely to undergo pneumonectomy (rather than a lesser surgical procedure), older patients were found to have an increased incidence of potentially serious medical problems. Operative mortality in the older group was 9.4% compared to 4.0% in the younger group. No statistically significant difference in postoperative complications, hospital stay, or actuarial survival was found, and cardiopulmonary status was considered to be the most important predictive factor for successful surgery. Damhuis and Schutte (21) reviewed 7899 cases of lung cancer between 1984 and 1992 to determine resection rate and 30-day postoperative mortality. Resection was more likely to be performed in patients under 70 years old (26%) than those over 70 years old (14%). However, multivariate analysis of this series revealed a significant risk due to increased age and increased extent of surgery, with perioperative mortality rising from 1.4% in patients under 60 years old to 4.0% in those over 70 years old. Pneumonectomies were performed in 27% of the patients over 70 years old as compared to 37% of the patients under 70 years old. This trend toward increased mortality for older patients was not considered to be striking, and the risk was considered to be acceptable for the types of surgery performed.

The majority of the surgical literature suggests that comorbid condition rather than age is the deciding factor as to whether surgical resection should be offered to patients with lung cancer. Knott-Craig et al. (22) pointed out that the mortality rate for aggressive lung resection in a general population can run from 3 to 6%, whereas notable morbidity may be seen in 15–30%. By comparison, their results of 4.8% mortality and 17.9% morbidity in 41 patients over 70 years old are quite reasonable. Namikawa et al. (23) reviewed the records of 128 patients over 75 years old undergoing pulmonary resection for lung cancer. Perioperative (30 day) mortality in this group was only 2.3%. An increase in the death rate 2–6 months later was attributed to non–cancer-related causes. Breyer et al. (24) reviewed 218 thoracotomies (166 for lung cancer) and noted a death rate of 3% and a complication rate of 34%. However, complications were related to amount of lung removed, congestive heart failure, and prior lung surgery with age and sex not considered to be significant factors. Roxburgh et al. (25) summarized a series of 370 patients referred for terminal lung cancer, 179 of whom were operable. Hospital mortality was increased in older (more than 70 years old) patients compared to younger patients, with a rate of 4.7% compared to 1.9% for patients undergoing lobectomy and 9.1% compared to 6.2% for patients undergoing pneumonectomy. However, 2- and 4-year survival rates adjusted for stage were equivalent between the two groups, and surgery was considered to be an acceptable primary therapy. Ishida et al. (26) reviewed 185 cases of patients over 70 years old undergoing resection for lung cancer. Operative mortality was 3% and the 5-year survival was 48%. Pulmonary complications were predicted by poor presurgical pulmonary function tests and by smoking history in both younger and older groups. Careful evaluation of pulmonary function tests for obstructive or restrictive defects was suggested as being the main factor in determining whether aggressive surgery would be feasible. Cangemi et al. (27) reported a similar postoperative death rate for older and younger patients (4.8% vs 3%), whereas Jie et al. (28) reviewed 920 cases of non–small-cell lung cancer who underwent surgery between 1969 and 1985 and noted no difference in survival based either on tumor histology or age.

Octogenarians might be considered to be at particular risk due to increased comorbidity. However, several series have not supported this idea. Shirakusa et al. (29) reported 32 patients over the age of 80 years, of whom 21 underwent lobectomy and 3 pneumonectomy. There were no perioperative deaths (within 30 days), whereas the 5-year survival for stage I patients was 79% and the 5-year survival for stage III patients was 31%. These investigators concluded that the surgical decision should be based on the stage of disease and cardiopulmonary status rather than on age. Pagni et al. (30) reported 54 octogenarians who underwent lung surgery. A lesser but appropriate resection (42 lobectomies and 1 pneumonectomy) was favored and 3.7% operative mortality and 11% major complications were reported. Survival for all 52 patients discharged from hospital was 86% at 1 year, 62% at 3 years, and

42% at 5 years. For the 39 patients with stage I disease, the 1-year survival was 97%, 3-year survival was 78%, and 5-year survival was 57%. An aggressive surgical approach (short of pneumonectomy) was therefore suggested for healthy octogenarian patients with stage I disease.

Santambrogio et al. (31) reported a prospective series of patients with stage I or II non–small-cell lung cancer who were treated between 1986 and 1991. There were 519 patients, of whom 54 were over 70 years old. Operative morbidity was only slightly worse in the older group (7.4 vs 6.9%) as was operative mortality (5.5 vs 1.3%). Two- and 5-year survival for stage I patients were comparable between groups. Newer techniques and more aggressive postoperative management can also contribute to improved survival. Knott-Craig et al. (22) described a perioperative protocol for patients undergoing resection for lung cancer that included preoperative digitalis, subcutaneous heparin, veno-occlusive stockings, and aggressive pulmonary toilet. This program resulted in a mortality rate of 4.8% and a morbidity rate of 17.9% in 41 patients over 70 years of age. Francini et al. (32) have suggested that quantitative perfusion lung scan can be used to accurately predict postoperative performance status in patients with compromised pulmonary status preoperatively and thereby allow surgery to be done more safely with better postoperative outcome. Roviaro et al. (33) and Knott-Craig et al. (22) have also suggested the value of limited access (video-assisted thoracoscopic) surgery for some patients, particularly those with small peripheral lesions who might not be able to tolerate lobectomy. The use of this procedure might also decrease postoperative pain and improve the speed of surgical recovery. The long-term efficacy of thoracoscopic resection as opposed to formal lobectomy remains to be determined.

B. Radiotherapy

Radiotherapy continues to be widely used for the treatment of non–small-cell lung cancer and can be used with palliative intent or for potential cure in patients with early-stage and localized lesions. Smith et al. (16) found that radiotherapy was the most commonly used primary treatment for lung cancer in all age groups 65–69 years old and older and was used with a similar frequency (40–50%) in all of the older groups. Radiotherapy tends to be used for patients considered *medically inoperable* (a term which may refer to cardiopulmonary status, age, or simple refusal to undergo surgery). However, multivariate analysis can separate the influence of these different factors. Graham et al. (34) analyzed the outcome of 103 patients with stage I or II non–small-cell lung cancer and a median age of 67 years. Survival of patients who received palliative radiotherapy was similar to that of patients who received no therapy at all. However, patients who received radical radiotherapy had a 2-year survival of 35% and a 5-year survival of 14%. Age greater than 70 years was not a significant factor in predicting survival although weight loss, tumor size, and time-dose factor were significant. Noordijk et al. (35) reviewed 50 inoperatable patients with stage I non–small-cell lung cancer, 40 of whom were over 70 years of age. Treatment with radiotherapy to a dose of 60 Gy resulted in a response rate of 90%, with a complete response rate of 50% for tumors less than 4 cm in size. Survival was dependent on tumor size but not on age and was similar to that of 86 patients over 70 years of age who had undergone surgery as primary treatment at the same hospital. It was therefore concluded that radiotherapy was a good alternative for patients with tumors under 4 cm in size.

Several additional series have had similar results. Furuta et al. (36) treated 32 patients over 75 years of age with stage I or II non–small-cell lung cancer using definitive radiotherapy (at least 60 Gy). The mean age of patients in this series was 79 years old with 11 patients over 80 years of age. No acute complications were seen specific to radiotherapy. The two-year survival was 57% and the 5-year survival was 36%. Most deaths in this series were due to heart disease rather than cancer. Gava et al. (37) reviewed 196 patients with lung cancer over 70 years of age, 182 of whom received radiotherapy. Of this group, 109 (60%) received radical radiotherapy, whereas 73 (40%) received palliative therapy. The full course of planned radiotherapy was completed by 163 patients (91%). Relief of symptoms of lung cancer was noted in approximately 80% and the quality of life remained stable before and after treatment, emphasizing the feasibility of radiotherapy in this age group. Katano et al. (38) reviewed the outcome for 86 patients over 75 years of age compared to 178 patients under 75 years of age receiving 60–70 Gy. The two- and 5-year survival rates were similar in both groups, although a trend to inferior survival of elderly patients with stage III disease was noted.

Questions concerning radiotherapy dose and concomitant use of radiotherapy and chemotherapy have also been examined. Lonardi et al. (39) reported 71 patients at least 70 years of age who received immediate radiotherapy for symptomatic relief. Half of the patients received more than 50 Gy and half less than 50 Gy. The higher dose group had a superior median survival (7 vs 4 months) as well as a superior 6-month survival (48 vs 39%) and 12-month survival (32 vs 11%). Toxicity was mild with good palliation of both pain and hemoptysis. It was therefore emphasized that patients should receive higher dose radiotherapy if possible because of the equivalent tolerance and improved outcome. Atagi et al. (40) used a combination of carboplatin and radiotherapy (50–60 Gy over 5 weeks) in 29 patients with non–small-cell lung cancer and a median age of 79 years. There were 1 complete and 14 partial responses (total response rate 54%). The major toxicity was hematological but was tolerable in all patients, again emphasizing the feasibility of such combined therapy even in an elderly patient population.

The use of cranial radiotherapy in an elderly population has raised some special concerns. Catell et al. (41) reported 23 patients over 80 years of age who received 30 Gy in 10 fractions for brain metastases. The full course of therapy was completed by 19 of these patients and median survival was 10 weeks. The investigators emphasized that cranial radiotherapy for lung cancer in elderly patients can provide benefit equivalent to that in younger patients. However, follow-up in this series was quite short. Several series reporting long-term follow-up after cranial radiotherapy have raised additional questions concerning the possibility of psychiatric deterioration. Laaksonen et al. (42) reported an elderly male with small-cell lung cancer who underwent cranial radiotherapy after 2 years of interferon treatment and developed a reversible dementia-like syndrome. Long-term follow-up of the NCI Navy series (43) of patients who received prophylactic cranial radiotherapy for small-cell lung cancer has also shown a steady and measurable decrease in neuropsychiatric function for many years following therapy. It is conceivable that this could be worsening of preexisting arteriosclerotic vascular disease. However, to minimize such risk prophylactic cranial radiotherapy might be reserved for younger patients with an excellent response to chemotherapy and an excellent performance status prior to initiation of cranial radiotherapy.

When radiotherapy is used as primary therapy for lung cancer, the question of radiation pneumonitis also arises. Koga et al. (44) reviewed the incidence and severity of radiation pneumonitis in 62 patients with lung cancer (33 below 70 years old and 29 above 70 years old) receiving 1.5–2.0 Gy per day for 3–5 weeks. The incidence of radiation pneumonitis was found to be proportionate to field size and radiation dose in both younger and older patients. However, severe radiation pneumonitis tended to be more common in older patients regardless of body size or chemotherapy administered.

Thus, the trend to use radical radiotherapy as a potentially curative modality for poor-prognosis patients with lung cancer is encouraging. However, gratification due to the success of this modality and control of both symptoms and tumor growth must be tempered by careful observation for potential late toxicities, including both radiation encephalitis and radiation pneumonitis.

C. Chemotherapy

The use of chemotherapy in lung cancer has been controversial. In limited-disease small-cell lung cancer, chemotherapy will result in an extremely high response rate, an increase in survival, and some cures. Even in extensive-disease small-cell lung cancer, a high response rate and an increase in survival will be achieved. Recent advances in the chemotherapy of non–small-lung cancer have also produced very good response rates and a modest increase in survival. However, aggressive systemic therapy is accompanied by the potential for significant toxicity, and careful consideration must be given to the question of whether benefits outweigh risks for patients with significant comorbid disease.

The same arguments apply to the elderly as apply to younger patients. If expected natural survival exceeds expected survival with advanced lung cancer, then therapy that can increase survival with an acceptable level of toxicity and with the maintenance of a good quality of life is reasonable. However, in the elderly, one must often take into consideration quantitatively and qualitatively greater levels of comorbid disease. In small-cell lung cancer, the large number of active agents has resulted in the design of numerous highly active combination chemotherapy regimens. Thus, regimens can easily be selected that will avoid corresponding comorbid disease (i.e., selection of nonnephrotoxic agents for the patient with renal insufficiency or noncardiotoxic agents for the patient with coronary artery disease). Until recently, the limited number of active agents in non–small-cell lung cancer did not allow such flexibility. However, the recent introduction of several new families of chemotherapeutic agents (taxanes, topoisomerase I inhibitors, nucleoside analogues) as well as the development of new chemoprotective agents now allow the design of regimens following similar principles.

The literature examining the effect of age on response and survival in small cell lung cancer is somewhat contradictory. Albain et al. (45) analyzed the Southwest Oncology Group database of 2580 patients participating in 10 small-cell lung cancer trials between 1976 and 1988 to identify significant prognostic factors and prognostic groups. Age greater than 70 years was found to be a negative prognostic factor for patients with limited disease but not extensive disease. Osterlind et al. (46), using a database of 874 patients, found advanced age to have a borderline negative prognostic effect in extensive disease. Siu et al. (47), reviewing 608 patients with limited-disease small-cell lung cancer who participated in two National Cancer Institute of Canada studies, found age to be a significant adverse factor in univariate but not multivariate analysis (since advanced age correlated with increased dose omissions). Ashley et al. (48), analyzing 674 patients with small-cell lung cancer treated at the Royal Marsden Hospital in London, found that the response rate was proportional to the performance status but not age in both univariate and multivariate analyses. Survival was highly dependent on the stage and performance status in both univariate and multivariate analyses, with advanced age having a marginally negative effect ($P = .03$) in the multivariate analysis. Shepherd et al. (49) examined the effect of advanced age on survival in small-cell lung cancer by analyzing the outcome for 123 patients over 70 years old divided into three subgroups by age (70–74, 75–80, and >80 years). Survival was not affected by increasing age. On the other hand, Nou (50), examining a database of 345 patients receiving chemotherapy and radiotherapy for small-cell lung cancer, noted a significant effect of both the stage and age on survival in multivariate analysis. However, survival was only marginally decreased in patients 70–75 years old. In spite of increased toxicity, aggressive chemotherapy could therefore still be recommended for this group. It would appear that although there is a trend toward advanced age being a negative prognostic factor for survival in small-cell lung cancer, age often has a marginal effect when compared with the stage of disease and performance status. Withholding chemotherapy for small-cell lung cancer strictly because of age, particularly in the patient with a good performance status and limited disease, is not reasonable.

The potential for increased toxicity when older patients are treated with chemotherapy could be a matter of concern. Both Oshita et al. (51), using a cisplatin-based regimen in patients over 75 years old, and Findlay et al. (52), using an intensive combination of cyclophosphamide, doxorubicin, and vincristine in patients over 70 years old, felt that the level of toxicity (particularly myelosuppression) observed was greater than anticipated. Kelly et al. (53), using a database of 96 patients treated with combination chemotherapy including vinca alkaloids, noted peripheral neuropathy to be more common in patients over 65 years old. These observations may be due to a generalized decrease in organ function reserve with advancing age. However, differences in the pharmacology of the agents involved must also be considered. Lind et al. (54) reported an increase in volume of distribution and elimination half-life of ifosfamide with advancing age that could have a potential clinical effect. Teramoto et al. (55) noted a decrease in chemotherapy induced generation of oxygen free radicals with increasing age which could be correlated with a decreased absolute granulocyte count. Since the mechanism of action of many chemotherapeutic agents depends on free radicals, both efficacy and toxicity could potentially be influenced. The effect of age on the pharmacokinetics and pharmacodynamics of chemotherapeutic agents is an area that deserves further investigation.

With the availability of an increasing range of chemotherapeutic agents, regimens have been designed with the specific purpose of decreasing toxicity. Several regimens have been adapted for use against small-cell lung cancer in the elderly. One of the most popular of these combinations is etoposide and carboplatin. Carboplatin is considered to be a less toxic alternative to cisplatin, with myelosuppression supplanting the neurotoxicity, nephrotoxicity, and emetogenicity of the parent compound. The hypothesis that carboplatin accompanied by either intravenous or oral etoposide can be easily administered owing to relatively low levels of acute toxicity has been tested by several investigators. Frasci et al. (56) and Berzinec et al. (57) both found the etoposide/carboplatin combination to be active and extremely well tolerated in patients over 70 years of age. However Shibata et al. (58), Evans et al. (59), and Raghavan et al. (60), although they considered the combination feasible in an older population, all noted a high level of myelosuppression. Etoposide has been administered as a single agent by both the oral and intravenous routes. Bork et al. (61), Carney et al. (62), and Smit et al. (63) have all reported single-agent etoposide to be active and well tolerated in the elderly. Teniposide, an alternative epipodophyllotoxin, also has activity against small-cell lung cancer. Although single-agent teniposide has an inferior complete response rate (64, 65), the combination of teniposide and carboplatin was reported by Michel (66) to be highly active and well tolerated in 24 patients with a median age of 72 years.

Chemotherapeutic regimens for non–small-cell lung cancer are still usually based on platinum family compounds. Newer regimens in this category include combinations of cisplatin or carboplatin with paclitaxel, docetaxel, gemcitabine, or vinorelbine (67). Many of these regimens therefore carry the potential for significant toxicity. Improved supportive care measures have had a major impact in improving feasibility and tolerability of such regimens for patients of all age groups. Development of modern antiemetics (particularly combinations of serotonin antagonists and dexamethasone [68]) has markedly decreased both the incidence and severity of chemotherapy-induced nausea and vomiting. Weight loss and poor appetite remain matters of particular concern. However, Niiranen et al. (69) treated 89 patients over 70 years of age receiving chemotherapy for lung cancer with medroxyprogesterone acetate and reported a marked increase in appetite and weight gain and a decrease in chemotherapy-related side effects.

Several chemotherapeutic regimens not containing platinum family compounds have also been developed to reduce toxicity. A combination of oral cyclophosphamide and oral etoposide has been shown to have reasonable efficacy in non–small-cell lung cancer with modest toxicity and can be given completely on an outpatient basis (70). Colleoni et al. (71) and Gridelli et al. (72) have examined the use of single-agent vinorelbine for the treatment of non–small-cell lung cancer. Response rates in the range of 15–25% with manageable myelosuppression were noted. In addition, Mattioli et al. (73) noted an increase in quality of life and psychosocial functioning in 9 of 15 patients (median age 70 years) treated for non–small-cell lung cancer with single-agent vinorelbine.

Age would definitely not appear to be a contraindication to chemotherapy in either small-cell or non–small-cell lung cancer in appropriately selected patients. In fact, Albain et al. (74), using the 2531-patient Southwest Oncology Group extensive-stage non–small-cell lung cancer database, identified age of at least 70 years as a positive predictive factor for survival. However, the choice of chemotherapeutic agents must be carefully adjusted for preexisting comorbid conditions, and modern supportive care measures should be aggressively employed. Standard guidelines for lung cancer chemotherapy (such as reevaluation for response after two cycles of chemotherapy) cannot be ignored, since increased toxicity can be expected in any age group if an extended course of treatment is undertaken. With appropriate care, increased survival due to chemotherapy with maintenance of good quality of life is possible for elderly patients with advanced lung cancer.

IV. CONCLUSIONS

Lung cancer is the result of a life-long behavior (smoking) pattern that culminates in an increased risk of disease for the elderly. However, patients who develop this disease at a more advanced age may have a greater chance of having a localized and more treatable presentation. Accurate and timely detection and evaluation for therapy are therefore of particular importance in this group. Improved techniques for both treatment and supportive care have increased the range of reasonable and tolerable therapies available to the aging population. These therapeutic options cannot be dismissed without a careful evaluation of the stage of disease, comorbid disease, and individual desires for therapy. Assuming that the elderly as a group will not benefit from aggressive treatment for lung cancer would be a significant disservice to these patients.

REFERENCES

1. Parker SL, Tong T, Bolden S, Wingo PA. Cancer Statistics, 1997. CA Cancer J Clin 1997; 47:5–27.
2. O'Rourke MA, Crawford J. Lung cancer in the elderly. Clin Geriatr Med 1987; 3:595–623.
3. North-Eastern Italian Oncology Group–Neoplasms of the Elderly Committee. Clinical characteristics, diagnosis and treatment of elderly patients with lung cancer at non-surgical institutions: a multicenter study. Tumori 1990; 75:429–433.
4. O'Rourke MA, Feussner JR, Feigl P, Laszlo J. Age trends of lung cancer stage at diagnosis. Implications for lung cancer screening in the elderly. JAMA 1987; 258:921–926.
5. Shibata A, Paganini-Hill A, Ross RK, Yu MC, Henderson BE. Dietary beta-carotene, cigarette smoking, and lung cancer in men. Cancer Causes Control 1992; 3:207–214.
6. Hoffmann D, Rivenson A, Chung FL, Wynder EL. Potential inhibitors of tobacco carcinogenesis. Ann NY Acad Sci 1993; 686:140–160.
7. Frost JK, Ball WC Jr., Levin ML, Tockman MS, Baker RR, Carter D, Eggleston JC, Erozan YS, Gupta PK, Khouri NF, Marsh BR, Stitik FP. Early lung cancer detection: results of the initial (prevalence) radiologic and cytologic screening in the Johns Hopkins Study. Am Rev Respir Dis 1984; 130:549–554.
8. Flehinger BJ, Melamed MR, Zaman MB, Heelan RT, Perchick WB, Martini N. Early lung cancer detection: results of the initial (prevalence) radiologic and cytologic screening in the Memorial Sloan-Kettering Study. Am Rev Respir Dis 1984; 130:555–560.
9. Fontana RS, Sanderson DR, Taylor WF, Woolner LB, Miller WE, Muhm JR, Uhlenhopp MA. Early lung cancer detection: results of the initial (prevalence) radiologic and cytologic screening in the Mayo Clinic Study. Am Rev Respir Dis 1984; 130:561–565.
10. DeMaria LC Jr, Cohen HJ. Characteristics of lung cancer in elderly patients. J Gerontol 1987; 42:540–545.
11. Tockman MS, Anthonisen NR, Wright EC, Donithan MG. Airways obstruction and the risk for lung cancer. Ann Intern Med 1987; 106:512–518.
12. Petty TL. Lung cancer and chronic obstructive pulmonary disease. Hematol Oncol Clin North Am 1997; 11:531–541.
13. Jack CI, Sheard JD, Lippitt B, Fromholtz A, Evans CC, Hind CR. Lung cancer in elderly patients: the role of induced sputum production to obtain a cytological diagnosis. Age Ageing 1993; 22:227–229.
14. Grover SA, Cook EF, Goldman L. The impact of Medicare on early cancer detection in the elderly. Am J Public Health 1988; 78:58–60.
15. Shields TW. Surgical therapy for carcinoma of the lung. Clin Chest Med 1993; 14:121–147.
16. Smith TJ, Penberthy L, Desch CE, Whittemore M, Newschaffer C, Hillner BE, McClish D, Retchin SM. Differences in initial treatment patterns and outcomes of lung cancer in the elderly. Lung Cancer 1995; 13:235–252.
17. Yellin A, Benfield JR. Surgery for bronchogenic carcinoma in the elderly. Am Rev Respir Dis 1985; 131:197.
18. Ginsberg RJ, Hill LD, Eagan RT, Thomas P, Mountain CF, Deslauriers J, Fry WA,

Butz RO, Goldberg M, Waters PF, Jones DP, Pairolero P, Rubinstein L, Pearson FG. Modern thirty-day operative mortality for surgical resections in lung cancer. J Thorac Cardiovasc Surg 1983; 86:654–658.

19. Whittle J, Steinberg EP, Anderson GF, Herbert R. Use of Medicare claims data to evaluate outcomes in elderly patients undergoing lung resection for lung cancer. Chest 1991; 100: 729–734.

20. Sherman S, Guidot CE. The feasibility of thoracotomy for lung cancer in the elderly. JAMA 1987; 258:927–930.

21. Damhuis RA, Schutte PR. Resection rates and postoperative mortality in 7,899 patients with lung cancer. Eur Respir J 1996; 9:7–10.

22. Knott-Craig CJ, Howell CE, Parsons BD, Paulsen SM, Brown BR, Elkins RC. Improved results in the management of surgical candidates with lung cancer. Ann Thorac Surg 1997; 63:1405–1409.

23. Namikawa S, Shimamoto A, Takao M, Yada I. Surgical treatment of lung cancer over 75 years old. Lung Cancer 1997; 18(Suppl 1): 115.

24. Breyer RH, Zippe C, Pharr WF, Jensik RJ, Kittle CF, Faber LP. Thoracotomy in patients over age seventy years. J Thorac Cardiovasc Surg 1981; 81:187–193.

25. Roxburgh JC, Thompson J, Goldstraw P. Hospital mortality and long-term survival after pulmonary resection in the elderly. Ann Thorac Surg 1991; 51:800–803.

26. Ishida T, Yokoyama H, Kaneko S, Sugio K, Sugimachi K. Long-term results of operation for non-small cell lung cancer in the elderly. Ann Thorac Surg 1990; 50:919–922.

27. Cangemi V, Volpino P, D'Andrea N, Puopolo M, Tomassini R, Cangemi R, Piat G. Lung cancer surgery in elderly patients. Tumori 1996; 82:237–241.

28. Jie C, Wever AM, Huysmans HA, Franken HC, Wever-Hess J, Hermans J. Time trends and survival in patients presented for surgery with non-small-cell lung cancer 1969–1985. Eur J Cardiothorac Surg 1990; 4:653–657.

29. Shirakusa T, Tsutsui M, Iriki N, Matsuba K, Saito T, Minoda S, Iwasaki T, Hirota N, Kuono J. Results of resection for bronchogenic carcinoma in patients over the age of 80. Thorax 1989; 44:189–191.

30. Pagni S, Federico JA, Ponn RB. Pulmonary resection for lung cancer in octogenarians. Ann Thorac Surg 1997; 63:785–789.

31. Santambrogio L, Nosotti M, Bellavita N, Mezzetti M. Prospective study of surgical treatment of lung cancer in the elderly patient. J Gerontol A Biol Sci Med Sci 1996; 51:M267–M269.

32. Francini A, Filosso PL, Podio V, Casalegno F, Oliaro A, Casadio C, Bisi G. Quantitative perfusion lung scanning in the surgery of the lung cancer in the elderly. Lung Cancer 1997; 18(Suppl 1):230.

33. Roviaro G, Varoli F, Rebuffat C, Vergani C, Maciocco M, Scalambra SM, Sonnino D, Gozi G. Videothoracoscopic staging and treatment of lung cancer. Ann Thorac Surg 1995; 59:971–974.

34. Graham PH, Gebski VJ, Langlands AO. Radical radiotherapy for early nonsmall cell lung cancer. Int J Radiat Oncol Biol Phys 1995; 31:261–266.

35. Noordijk EM, v.d.-Poest-Clement E, Hermans J, Wever AM, Leer JW. Radiotherapy as an alternative to surgery in elderly patients with resectable lung cancer. Radiother Oncol 1988; 13:83–89.

36. Furuta M, Hayakawa K, Katano S, Saito Y, Nakayama Y, Takahashi T, Imai R, Ebara T,

Mitsuhashi N, Niibe H. Radiation therapy for stage I-II non-small cell lung cancer in patients aged 75 years and older. Jpn J Clin Oncol 1996; 26:95–98.

37. Gava A, Bertossi, L, Zorat PL, Ausili-Cefaro G, Olmi P, Pavanato G, Mandoliti G, Polico C. Radiotherapy in the elderly with lung carcinoma: The experience of the Italian "Geriatric Radiation Oncology Group." Rays 1997; 22(Suppl):61–65.

38. Katano S, Hayakawa K, Mitsuhashi N, Saito Y, Nakayama Y, Furuta M, Suzuki Y, Nasu S, Niibe H. Radiation therapy for elderly patients with limited non-small cell lung cancer. Lung Cancer 1997; 18(Suppl 1):130.

39. Lonardi F, Pavanato M, Coeli M. Radiation therapy (RT) of symptomatic advanced non small cell lung cancer (NSCLC) in the elderly. Lung Cancer 1997; 18(Suppl 1): 127.

40. Atagi S, Furuse K, Kawahara M, Ogawara M, Matsui K, Kudoh S, Negoro S. Phase II trial of daily low-dose carboplatin (CBDCA) and radiotherapy (RT) in elderly patients with unresectable locally advanced non-small cell lung cancer (NSCLC). Lung Cancer 1997; 18(Suppl 1):138.

41. Catell D, Steinfeld A, Donahue B. Lung cancer metastic to brain in octogenarians. Lung Cancer 1997; 18(Suppl 1): 130.

42. Laaksonen R, Niiranen A, Iivanainen M, Mattson K, Holsti L, Farkkila M, Cantell K. Dementia-like, largely reversible syndrome after cranial irradiation and prolonged interferon treatment. Ann Clin Res 1988; 20:201–203.

43. Johnson BE, Becker B, Goff WB, Petronas N, Krehbiel MA, Makuch RW, McKenna G, Glatstein E, Ihde DC. Neurologic, neuropsychologic and computed cranial tomography scan abnormalities in 2-to-10 year survivors of small-cell lung cancer. J Clin Oncol 1985; 3:1659–1667.

44. Koga K, Kusumoto S, Watanabe K, Nishikawa K, Harada K, Ebihara H. Age factor relevant to the development of radiation pneumonitis in radiotherapy of lung cancer. Int J Radiat Oncol Biol Phys 1988; 14:367–371.

45. Albain KS, Crowley JJ, Leblanc M, Livingston RB. Determinants of improved outcome in small-cell lung cancer: An analysis of the 2,580-patient Southwest Oncology Group data base. J Clin Oncol 1990; 8:1563–1574.

46. Osterlind K, Hansen HH, Hansen M, Dombernowsky P, Andersen PK. Long-term disease-free survival in small-cell carcinoma of the lung: A study of clinical determinants. J Clin Oncol 1986; 4:1307–1313.

47. Siu LL, Shepherd FA, Murray N, Feld R, Pater J, Zee B. Influence of age on the treatment of limited-stage small-cell lung cancer. J Clin Oncol 1996; 14:821–828.

48. Ashley SE, O'Brien MER, Smith IE. Age is not an adverse predictive factor in the treatment of small cell lung cancer. Lung Cancer 1997; 18(Suppl 1): 22–23.

49. Shepherd FA, Amdemichael E, Evans WK, Chalvardjian P, Hogg-Johnson S, Coates R, Paul K. Treatment of small cell lung cancer in the elderly. J Am Geriatr Soc 1994; 42:64–70.

50. Nou E. Full chemotherapy in elderly patients with small cell bronchial carcinoma. Acta Oncol 1996; 34:399–406.

51. Oshita F, Kurata T, Kasai T, Fakuda M, Yamamota N, Ohe Y, Tamura T, Eguchi K, Shinkai T, Saijo N. Prospective evaluation of the feasibility of cisplatin-based chemotherapy for elderly lung cancer patients with normal organ functions. Jpn J Cancer Res 1995; 86:1198–1202.

52. Findlay MP, Griffin AM, Raghavan D, McDonald KE, Coates AS, Duval PJ, Gianoutsos

P. Retrospective review of chemotherapy for small cell lung cancer in the elderly: does the end justify the means? Eur J Cancer 1991; 27:1597–1601.

53. Kelly P, O'Brien AA, Daly P, Clancy L. Small-cell lung cancer in elderly patients: the case for chemotherapy. Age Ageing 1991; 20:19–22.

54. Lind MJ, Margison JM, Cerny T, Thatcher N, Wilkinson PM. The effect of age on the pharmacokinetics of ifosfamide. Br J Clin Pharmacol 1990; 30:140–143.

55. Teramoto S, Fukuchi Y, Shu CY, Orimo H. Influences of cisplatin combination chemotherapy on oxygen radical generation by blood in elderly and adult patients with lung cancer. Chemotherapy 1995; 41:222–228.

56. Frasci G, Comella P, DelGaizo F, DeCataldis G, Pozzo C, Panza N, Cioffi R, Bianco A, Della VM, Gravina A, Comella G. Carboplatin (CBDCA)-oral etoposide (VP16) personalized dosing in elderly or poor performance status NSCLC patients. Lung Cancer 1997; 18(Suppl 1):38.

57. Berzinec P, Arpasova M, Kuzmova H. Carboplatin and etoposide in patients aged 75 years or older with small cell lung cancer. Lung Cancer 1997; 18(Suppl 1):46.

58. Shibata K, Nakatsumi Y, Kasahara K, Bando T, Fujimura M, Matsuda T. Analysis of thrombocytopenia due to carboplatin combined with etoposide in elderly patients with lung cancer. J Cancer Res Clin Oncol 1996; 122:437–442.

59. Evans WK, Radwi A, Tomiak E, Logan DM, Martins H, Stewart DJ, Goss G, Maroun JA, Dahrouge S. Oral etoposide and carboplatin. Effective therapy for elderly patients with small cell lung cancer. Am J Clin Oncol 1995; 18:149–155.

60. Raghavan D, Bishop JF, Stuart-Harris R, Zalcberg J, Morstyn G, Kefford RF, Matthews JP. Carboplatin-containing regimens for small cell lung cancer: implications for management in the elderly. Semin Oncol 1992; 19(Suppl 2):12–16.

61. Bork E, Hirsch F, Jeppesen N, Lassen U, Vallentin S, Osterlind K, Mejer J, Ingeberg S, Bergman B, Dombernowsky P. Oral etoposide (VP-16) every 3 wks or continuously to elderly patients with small cell lung cancer (SCLC): preliminary results of a randomized study. Lung Cancer 1997; 18(Suppl 1):25.

62. Carney DN, Keane M, Grogan L. Oral etoposide in small cell lung cancer. Semin Oncol 1992; 19(Suppl 14):40–44.

63. Smit EF, Carney DN, Harford P, Sleijfer DT, Postmus PE. A phase II study of oral etoposide in elderly patients with small cell lung cancer. Thorax 1989; 44:631–633.

64. Tummarello D, Isidori P, Pasini F, Cetto G, Cellerino R. Teniposide as single drug therapy for elderly patients affected by small cell lung cancer. Eur J Cancer 1992; 28A: 1081–1084.

65. Cerny T, Pedrazzini A, Joss RA, Brunner KW. Unexpected high toxicity in a phase II study of teniposide (VM-26) in elderly patients with untreated small cell lung cancer (SCLC). Eur J Cancer Clin Oncol 1988; 24:1791–1794.

66. Michel G, Leyvraz S, Bauer J, Aapro M, Stahel R, Alberto P. Weekly carboplatin and VM-26 for elderly patients with small-cell lung cancer. Ann Oncol 1994; 5:369–370.

67. Edelman MJ, Gandara DR. Current status of new chemotherapeutic agents in non–small cell lung cancer. J Oncol Index Rev 1997; 1:3–6.

68. Grunberg SM, Hesketh PJ. Control of chemotherapy-induced emesis. N Engl J Med 1993; 329:1790–1796.

69. Niiranen A, Kajanti M, Tammilehto L, Mattson K. The clinical effect of medroxyprogesterone (MPA) in elderly patients with lung cancer. Am J Clin Oncol 1990; 13: 113–116.

70. Grunberg SM, Crowley J, Livingston R, Gill I, Williamson SK, O'Rouke T, Braum T, Marshall ME, Weick JK, Balcerzak SP, Martino RL. Extended administration of oral etoposide and oral cyclophosphamide for the treatment of advanced non-small cell lung cancer: A Southwest Oncology Group study. J Clin Oncol 1993; 11:1598–1601.

71. Colleoni M, Gaion F, Nelli P, Colmellere CM, Manente P. Weekly vinorelbine in elderly patients with non-small-cell lung cancer. Tumori 1994; 80:448–452.

72. Gridelli C, Perrone F, Gallo C, De Marinis F, Ianniello G, Cigolari S, Cariello S, Di Costanzo F, D'Aprile M, Rossi A, Migliorino R, Bartolucci R, Bianco AR, Pergola M, Monfardini S. Vinorelbine is well tolerated and active in the treatment of elderly patients with advanced non-small cell lung cancer. A two-stage phase II study. Eur J Cancer 1997; 33:392–397.

73. Mattioli R, Imperatori L, Casadei V, Manna G, Frausini G, Guidi F, Gattafoni P, Paggi P, Lonardo D, Consales D. The impact of vinorelbine in elderly (aged >70 years) with NSCLC: a preliminary report. Lung Cancer 1997; 18(Suppl 1):41.

74. Albain KS, Crowley JJ, LeBlanc M, Livingston RB. Survival determinants in extensive-stage non–small-cell lung cancer: the Southwest Oncology Group experience. J Clin Oncol 1991; 9:1618–1626.

16
Leukemias, Lymphomas, and Myelomas

Stuart M. Lichtman and Jonathan E. Kolitz
North Shore University Hospital,
New York University School of Medicine
Manhasset, New York

I. NON–HODGKIN'S LYMPHOMA

The non–Hodgkin's lymphomas (NHLs) consist of a heterogeneous group of disorders of the lymphoid system. Each of these entities are distinguished by specific clinical, histological, immunological, molecular, and genetic characteristics (1).

Non–Hodgkin's lymphomas are the sixth most common cause of cancer-related deaths in the United States (2). In 1995, more than 45,000 new NHLs were diagnosed and over 21,000 patients died of these diseases. The average age of aggressive lymphomas is 56 years (2). The incidence of non–Hodgkin's lymphoma increases with age, with 25–35% of all lymphomas occurring in this older age group (3). In addition, the worldwide incidence is increasing independent of the acquired immunodeficiency syndrome (AIDS) epidemic (3, 4). The aging of the population should dramatically increase the number of older patients with NHL.

Etiologies of NHL include inherited and acquired immunodeficiency disorders (including posttransplantation lymphoproliferative disorder), autoimmune disorders (Hashiomoto's thyroiditis, Sjögren's syndrome), and occupational and environmental exposures (1). Viruses such as EBV, HTLV-1, Kaposi's sarcoma–associated herpesvirus, and hepatitis C have been implicated (2, 5–9). *Helicobacter pylori* infection of the stomach can result in chronic gastritis and the associated development of MALT (mucosa associated lymphoid tissue) (2, 10, 11).

A. Presentation and Evaluation

Patients with NHL will often manifest the disease as an asymptomatic nodal enlargement. Patients should be questioned regarding B symptoms (fever, night sweats, pruritus). A thorough history should be obtained documenting the duration and rate of lymph node enlargement. In patients with indolent nodal lymphomas, this information may influence the choice of therapy and the decision of whether or not to initiate treatment. The history should also include the presence or absence of fevers, night sweats, and unexplained weight loss (B symptoms) and the presence of symptoms such as bone pain or gastrointestinal (GI) discomfort that might indicate extranodal involvement (2).

The physical examination should be directed toward node-bearing areas and sites of common extranodal involvement. Particular attention should be given to recording the site and size of all abnormal lymph nodes, including the epitrochlear and inguinal/femoral sites. The size of the liver and spleen should be noted. The physical examination and subsequent special studies are dictated, in part, by a specific disease entity and sites of disease at presentation. For example, patients with preauricular lymph node enlargement often have disease in Waldeyer's ring which can be identified only with indirect laryngoscopy. Waldeyer's ring involvement can also be associated with GI involvement, prompting contrast studies of the GI tract in patients who appear to have localized disease. Because patients with lymphoma of the skin often have multiple cutaneous lesions that may be remote from one another, the skin should be inspected carefully and suspicious lesions should be biopsied. Because patients with lymphoma of the paranasal sinuses, bone marrow, gonads, or eye have a high risk of central nervous system (CNS) involvement, radiographic studies of the CNS and analysis of the cerebrospinal fluid are appropriate (2). A suggested evaluation is listed in Table 1.

B. Staging

Currently, patients with NHLs are staged with the Ann Arbor system originally developed for Hodgkin's disease. This schema emphasizes the distribution of nodal disease sites, because Hodgkin's disease commonly spreads through contiguous lymph node groups. The Ann Arbor system, summarized in Table 2, is based on the number of sites of involvement, the presence of disease above or below the diaphragm, the existence of systemic symptoms, and the presence of extranodal disease.

C. Pathology

The Working Formulation (Table 3), which modified the Rappaport classification, established a uniform classification that has clinical relevance and has been useful in predicting survival and curability (12, 13). It is based on morphology and biological aggressiveness. However, it does not distinguish between tumors of B- or T-cell

Table 1 Staging and Diagnosis

1. Definitive diagnosis can only be made by biopsy of pathologic lymph nodes or tumor tissue. Ideally the tissue should be subjected to analysis including immunophenotyping, cytogenetics and molecular studies
2. Careful history
3. Physical examination including evaluation of lymph node bearing areas
4. Chest radiograph
5. CT scan of the chest, abdomen, and pelvis
6. Bone marrow biopsy (some advocate bilateral, particularly in low grade)
7. Gallium scan (selected patients)
8. CBC with differential, platelet count and evaluation of the peripheral blood smear
9. General blood chemistry evaluation, β_2-microglobulin
10. HIV serology depending on history and histology
11. CSF evaluation in selected patients (aggressive lymphoma with involvement of bone marrow, epidural, testicular, paranasal sinus, and nasopharyngeal areas)
12. UGI series in patients with head and neck primary
13. Ultrasound of opposite testis in testicular lymphoma
14. MRI of spine if clinically indicated

CT, computed tomography; CBC, complete blood cell count; HIV, human immunodeficiency virus; CSF, cerebrospinal fluid; UGI, upper gastrointestinal; MRI, magnetic resonance imaging.

lineage or recognize other subtypes of lymphoma that are defined by specific characteristics of immunophenotyping and genetic techniques (12). Because of these deficiencies, a revised European-American classification of lymphoid neoplasms has been proposed (14). It emphasizes currently available morphological, immunological, and genetic techniques (Table 4).

Table 2 Ann Arbor Staging of Non–Hodgkin's Lymphoma

Stage	Description
I	Involvement of a single lymph node region or lymphoid structure or single extralymphatic organ or site (IE)
II	Involvement of two or more lymph node regions on the same side of the diaphragm or involvement of an extralymphatic organ or site (IIE)
III	Involvement of lymph node regions on both sides of the diaphragm, which may be accompanied by involvement of the spleen (IIIS), or localized involvement of an extralymphatic organ or site (IIIE), or both (IIISE)
IV	Diffuse or disseminated involvement of one or more extranodal organs or tissues Identification of the presence or absence of symptoms should be noted with each stage designation. A = asymptomatic; B = fever, sweats, weight loss >10% of body weight

Table 3 Working Formulation and Rappaport Classification Equivalent for
Non–Hodgkin's Lymphoma

Working formulation	Rappaport equivalent
Low grade	
A. Small lymphocytic	Diffuse, well-differentiated, lymphocytic
B. Follicular, small cleaved	Nodular, poorly differentiated, lymphocytic
C. Follicular, mixed, small cleaved and large cell	Nodular, mixed
Intermediate grade	
D. Follicular, large cell	Nodular, histiocytic
E. Diffuse, small cleaved cell	Diffuse, poorly differentiated, lymphocytic
F. Diffuse, mixed small and large cell	Diffuse, mixed
G. Diffuse, large cell	Diffuse, histiocytic
High grade	
H. Immunoblastic	Diffuse, histiocytic
I. Lymphoblastic	Lymphoblastic
J. Diffuse, small noncleaved cell	Diffuse, undifferentiated (Burkitt's and non–Burkitt's types)

D. Prognosis

Age has been shown to be prognostic factor in the treatment of large-cell lymphoma.
Some studies have suggested that patients more than 65 years old have greater toxicity, lower complete response (CR), and decreased survival and that the therapy was
often complicated due to comorbid medical conditions (15–18). Shipp examined
the impact of age on the outcome of patients with aggressive NHL (18). Data from 16
single institutions and cooperative groups in the United States, Europe, and Canada
participating in the International Non–Hodgkin's Lymphoma Prognostic Factors
Project were reviewed (17, 18). The clinical characteristics of patients aged 60 years
of age and younger were compared with those older than 60 years of age. The
proportion of patients in both groups presenting with advanced-stage disease (III/
IV), elevated serum lactate dehydrogenase, extranodal disease, and a poor performance status were comparable, suggesting that the disease at diagnosis was similar
in the two groups. Based on those five clinical factors, an International Index was
developed (Table 5). Patients were categorized into four risk groups (low, low intermediate, high intermediate, and high) that predict the CR and 5-year survival. The
CR rates for the two patient groups were similar, but the older patients were much
less likely to maintain their CRs. The age-related differences in relapse rates trans-
lated into significant age-related differences in overall survival between these risk
groups. Survival in patients greater than 60 years of age in the high-risk group was
31% at 2 years and 21% at 5 years. This compares to 37 and 32%, respectively, in
the under 60 years age group. Although the International Index was developed for

Table 4 Revised European–American Classification

Working formulation	B-Cell neoplasms	T-Cell neoplasms
Low grade		
Small lymphocytic consistent with CLL	B-cell CLL/PLL/SLL Marginal zone/MALT Mantle cell	T-cell CLL/PLL LGL ATL/L
Plasmacytoid	Lymphoplasmacytic- immunocytoma zone Marginal zone/MALT B-cell CLL/PLL/SLL	
Follicular, small cleaved	Follicle center, follicular, grade I Mantle cell Marginal zone/MALT	
Follicular, mixed	Follicle center, follicular, grade II Marginal zone/MALT	
Intermediate grade		
Follicular, large cell	Follicle center, follicular, grade III	
Diffuse, small cleaved	Mantle cell Follicle center, diffuse small cell Marginal zone/MALT	T-cell CLL/PLL LGL ATL/L Angioimmunoblastic Angiocentric
Diffuse, mixed	Large B-cell lymphoma (rich in T cells) Follicle center, diffuse small cell Lymphoplasmacytoid Marginal zone/MALT Mantle cell	Peripheral T-cell, unspecified ATL/L Angioimmunoblastic Angiocentric Intestinal T-cell lymphoma
Diffuse, large	Diffuse large B-cell lymphoma	Peripheral T cell, unspecified ATL/L Angioimmunoblastic Angiocentric Intestinal T-cell lymphoma
High grade		
Large-cell immunoblastic	Diffuse large B-cell lymphoma	Peripheral T cell, unspecified ATL/L Angioimmunoblastic Angiocentric Intestinal T-cell lymphoma
Lymphoblastic	Precursor B-lymphoblastic	Precursor T lymphoblastic
Small noncleaved cell		
Burkitt's	Burkitt's	
Non–Burkitt's	High-grade B-cell, Burkitt- like diffuse large B cell	Peripheral T cell, unspecified

Source: Ref. 87.

Table 5 International Index

Risk group	Risk factors	CR rate (%)	2-yr survival (%)	5-yr survival (%)
All patients				
Low	0, 1	87	84	73
Low intermediate	2	67	66	51
High intermediate	3	55	59	43
High	4, 5	44	58	26
≤60 years				
Low	0	92	90	83
Low intermediate	1	78	79	69
High intermediate	2	57	59	46
High	3	46	37	32
>60 years				
Low	0	91	80	56
Low intermediate	1	71	68	44
High intermediate	2	56	48	37
High	3	36	31	21

CR, complete response.
Factors: age ≥60 years; LDH > normal; PS ≥2; extranodal sites >1; stage III or IV.
Source: Ref. 17.

aggressive lymphomas, it has also shown to be predictive of low-grade histology (19, 20).

A study to determine age-related differences in NHL has been completed. Nine hundred and fifty consecutive, human immunodeficiency virus–negative patients observed in the same institute were reported. Patients were grouped into six age groups and cross tabulated by Working Formulation categories and the Revised European-American Lymphoma classification. There was a tendency of the low-grade category to increase with increasing age (16.8% in the age group 15–34 years old to 32.4% in the age group 65–74 years old), although a subsequent decline was seen at age 75 years or older (23.2%). Also the intermediate-grade category was more frequent in the elderly (46.6 and 49.4% at 65–74 years and at 75 years or older, respectively). The relative excess of low-grade NHL in patients older than 55 years of age was accounted for by the high proportion of small lymphocytic lymphomas, which, however, somewhat declined at age 75 years or older. B- and T-cell lymphomas accounted for 85.9% and 9.0% of all cases, respectively. B- and T-cell and non–B-cell, non–T-cell, and histiocytic NHL accounted for the remaining 5.1%. A highly significant trend of an increase in the proportion of B-cell lymphomas with an age increase was noted to be chiefly attributable to the excess of a T-cell (15.1%) and an undetermined phenotype (18.6%) in patients younger than 35 years of age. An extranodal location was not significantly related to age groups.

Thus, the study showed some interesting differences in NHL morphology and cell phenotype according to age (21).

E. Treatment

1. Low-Grade Lymphoma (IWF A–C)

Only 15% of patients with indolent lymphoma present with stage I or II disease. Involved-field radiation therapy (RT) is the treatment of choice in localized low-grade NHL. A Stanford University study had a median follow-up duration which was 7.7 years. The longest follow-up duration was 31 years. Actuarial survival rates at 5, 10, 15, and 20 years were 82, 64, 44, and 35%, respectively. The median survival time was 13.8 years. At 5, 10, 15, and 20 years, 55, 44, 40, and 37% of patients, respectively, were relapse free (22). Combination chemotherapy regimens alone or combined with RT have no role in managing early-stage disease (2, 23). Therefore, in older patients presenting with early-stage disease, localized RT is highly curable, particularly if the patients have a limited life expectancy.

There is no curative treatment for advanced low-grade lymphoma. The median survival is more than 9 years in many series. One study of 147 patients followed for 15 years showed 53 of the 147 alive and 76 of the 94 patient deaths were from lymphoma (2, 24). Therefore, the benefits of treatment was be weighed against potential toxicities, particularly in elderly, debilitated patients. In this latter group of patients, a watch and wait approach may be appropriate. Most studies have shown that patients managed in this way will need chemotherapy within 2–4 years after diagnosis. Approximately 50% of patients will require therapy initially owing to symptomatic disease. The complete response rate of untreated patients with single-agent alkylating therapy (chlorambucil, cyclophosphamide) ranges from 30 to 60%, with a median response duration of 18–24 months (2). Another study randomized patients to chlorambucil, CVP (cyclophosphamide, vincristine, prednisone), CVP plus total lymphoid irradiation, and involved-field irradiation and low-dose total body irradiation. There was no significant difference in relapsed-free or overall survival (25, 26).

Other therapeutic measures include the nucleoside analogues fludarabine, 2′-deoxycoformycin, and 2-chlorodeoxyadenosine, interferon-α, and antibody-based therapy with a murine anti-CD20 antibody (27–33). These drugs should be relatively well tolerated in elderly patients and may be a reasonable option. The long-term benefits of these drugs, whether alone or in combination, remains to be determined.

2. Aggressive Lymphoma (IWF D–H)

a. Stages I and II

The original studies of early-stage aggressive lymphoma evaluated laparotomy-staged patients who were subsequently treated with large-field or total nodal irradiation. This yielded 5-year survival rates of stage I 73% and stage II 56% (12, 26). The addition of varying number of cycles of CHOP (see Table 6) or similar therapy yield improved outcomes. It is suggested that clinically staged patients with fewer than three sites of disease and no bulky masses receive short-course CHOP chemotherapy followed by involved-field radiotherapy (34). Patients with bulky disease (>10 cm) or other poor prognostic factors should be managed similarly to patients with advanced-stage disease. The high survival rates make this the appropriate treatment for older patients.

b. Stages III and IV

Age is a known risk factor for poor treatment outcome in advanced stage, aggressive NHL patients (18). Survival rates in older, poor-risk patients are as low as 21% at 5 years (13). A large intergroup trial compared the regimens MoM-BACOD (35), ProMACE-CytaBOM (36), and MACOP-B (37) with CHOP (Table 6). This trial established CHOP as standard therapy in all patients. However the overall 6-year survival of all patients in the CHOP group was only 33%. The main differences in the treatment arms were diminished toxicity with CHOP. There is a paucity of data on the true toxicity and overall efficacy of this regimen patients older than 70 years of age.

3. Clinical Trials in the Older Patient

a. Randomized Trials

There have been three randomized trials in older patients with advanced, aggressive lymphoma (Table 7). Sonneveld reported on a trial in which CNOP was compared to CHOP (Table 8). The results demonstrated a more favorable response to the CHOP regimen (CR 49 vs 31%). However, overall survival was equivalent. The schedule used was treatment every 4 weeks instead of the standard 3-week schedule. In the complete group of patients at 3 years, 17% of CHOP and 13% of CNOP

Table 6 Regimens for Aggressive Non–Hodgkin's Lymphoma

Regimen	Drugs	Reference
CHOP	Cyclophosphamide, doxorubicin, vincristine, prednisone	254
m-BACOD	Methotrexate, bleomycin, doxorubicin, cyclophosphamide, vincristine, dexamethasone	35
ProMACE-CytaBOM	Prednisone, doxorubicin, cyclophosphamide, etoposide, cytarabine, bleomycin, vincristine, methotrexate	36
MACOP-B	Methotrexate, doxorubicin, cyclophosphamide, vincristine, prednisone, bleomycin	37

Table 7 Randomized Trials

Author	No. of patients	Age	Therapy	CR (%)	Survival	Overall survival	Reference
Bastion et al., 1997	220	75	CVP	33	14	13 months	39
	233		CVP+ [a]THP-ADM	47	21		
Sonneveld et al., 1995	148	70.1	CHOP	49	42	17%	38
			CNOP	31	26		
Meyer et al., 1995	38	71	CHOP	68	74%	13%	40
			CHOP	74	51%		

[a]Epirubicin.

Table 8 Primary Chemotherapy of Advanced Aggressive Non–Hodgkin's Lymphoma

Drug regimen	Dose (mg/m^2)	Route	Days
CHOP			
Cyclophosphamide	750	iv	1
Doxorubicin	50	iv	1
Oncovin	1.4	iv	1
Prednisone	60	po	1–5
Repeat treatment every 21 days			
m-BACOD			
Methotrexate[a]	200	iv	8, 15
Blemycin	4 units	iv	1
Doxorubicin	45	iv	1
Cyclophosphamide	600	iv	1
Vincristine	1	iv	1
Dexamethasone	6	iv	1–5
Repeat treatment every 21 days			
MACOP-B			weeks
Methotrexate[a]	400	iv	2, 6, 10
Doxorubicin	50	iv	1, 3, 5, 7, 9, 11
Cyclophosphamide	350	iv	1, 3, 5, 7, 9, 11
Vincristine	1.4	iv	2, 4, 6, 8, 10, 12
Prednisone	75 mg total	po	Daily
Bleomycin	10 units	iv	4, 8, 12
ProMACE-CytaBOM			
Etoposide	120	iv	1
Cyclophosphamide	650	iv	1
Doxorubicin	25	iv	1
Prednisone	60	iv	1–14
Cytarabine	300	iv	8
Bleomycin	5	iv	8
Vincristine	1.4	iv	8
Methotrexate[a]	120	iv	1

[a]Leucovorin rescue.

patients were alive and disease free. Toxicity was similar and they importantly demonstrated that CHOP is tolerated by the majority of elderly patients. Progressive lymphoma, not toxicity, is the important cause of treatment failure (38). Bastion et al. demonstrated that anthracyclines were crucial to good outcome in the older patient population (39). Their study had a median survival time of 13 months. Death during chemotherapy occurred in 16 and 21% of patients on the CVP and CTVP (T = THP-doxorubicin; epirubicin) arms, respectively. Lymphoma progression was the primary cause of death. Meyer attempted to give CHOP in weekly one third divided doses. There was no difference in response or survival and the standard regimen was preferred (40). Therefore, CHOP should be the standard for good-performance status patients. These studies also emphasized that lymphoma failure, not comorbid illness, is the important factor in overall survival in older patients.

b. Single-Arm Studies

There remains the need for alternative regimens for treatment of NHL in the elderly population. Many practitioners are fearful of the CHOP regimen at full dose in the elderly patient population. However, there is no substantial information to confirm that this excess in toxicity exists. In fact, the randomized trials tend to refute this. However, in many large multicenter trials, the patients selected do not represent the poorer performance status patients often seen in general practice. A number of nonrandomized clinical trials in elderly patients with malignant lymphoma have been performed (15, 40, 41–65). The goals of these studies were to use different chemotherapeutic drugs to reduce toxicity as compared with the standard CHOP regimen. The hope was to deliver an effective regimen while maintaining quality of life by ameliorating side effects. Mitoxantrone often has been used to minimize cardiac toxicity, nausea, vomiting, mucositis, and alopecia. Oral etoposide, prednimustine, and other drugs have been incorporated to minimize side effects. Comparisons between trials are difficult because of differing entry requirements. In particular, there is a great difference in age ranges (and median ages) of patient. The 2-year disease-free survival rate ranges from 15 to 55%. In many studies to reduce side effects, dose reductions or treatment modifications may have compromised efficacy. Attempts to devise a less toxic regimen may have lead instead to tolerable, nontoxic, less effective regimens. However, they do fulfill the need of an alternative regimen for selected poor-performance status patients. Table 9 lists some of these regimens.

4. Treatment of Relapsed Aggressive Lymphoma

Most elderly patients who have relapsed or refractory lymphoma have poor performance scores and short survival. It is therefore usually inappropriate to pursue aggressive therapy. These patients can possibly be palliated with one of the less toxic regimens discussed previously or oral etoposide (62). Therapy of relapsed disease has traditionally excluded bone marrow transplantation as a modality for older patients. There has been increasing data to show that well-selected patients over the age of 60 years can tolerate and may benefit from the procedure (66–69). In addition, older patients do not have an increased risk of inadequate graft collection. The data imply no difference in hematopoiesis between older and younger patients (70). There is also no age-related delay of engraftment in older leukemic patients (71). But only a most extraordinary patient would be able to withstand reinduction therapy (Table 10) and the rigors of the transplantation process. Careful patient selection and evaluation are crucial. Interpretation of transplant data in the older patient must take into account this selection process (72).

Table 9 Alternative Regimens for Elderly Patients with Aggressive
Non–Hodgkin's Lymphoma

Drug regimen	Dose (mg/m^2)	Route	Days (or weeks)
P/DOCE			weeks
Doxorubicin	50	iv	1, 2, 7, 8
Vincristine	1.2	iv	1, 7
Cyclophosphamide	300	iv	1, 4, 7
Etoposide	50	iv	1, 4
Etoposide	100	po	1, 4 (days 2–5)
Prednisone	50 mg total	po	1, 4, 7 (10 days)
8-week regimen			
C-MOPP			
Cyclophosphamide	650	iv	1, 8
Oncovin (vincristine)	1.4	iv	1, 8
Procarbazine	100	po	2–15
Prednisone	40	po	2–15
Repeat treatment every 28 days			
CNOP			
Cyclophosphamide	750	iv	1
Novantrone (mitoxantrone)	10	iv	1
Oncovin	1.4	iv	1
Prednisone	60	po	1–5
Repeat treatment every 28 days			
TNOP			
Thiotepa	20	iv	1
Novantrone (mitoxantrone)	10	iv	1
Vincristine	1	iv	1
Prednisone	60	iv	1
Repeat treatment every 21 days			

Source: Refs. 64 and 65.

5. Special Situations

a. CNS Lymphoma

Primary CNS lymphoma (PCNSL) is rising in incidence in both the AIDS and non-AIDS populations (73–76). This may be partly due to increased detection using modern imaging techniques (77). Primary CNS lymphoma it affects all ages, but its peak incidence occurs in the sixth and seventh decade in immunocompetent patients, making it a problem in elderly patients. The pathology is usually of a large-cell lymphoma (78). It usually presents as a brain tumor, but the leptomeninges, eyes, and spinal cord also are frequently affected. Systemic lymphoma is not present, and comprehensive systemic staging is unnecessary, but appropriate neurological staging

Table 10 Salvage Chemotherapy of Non-Hodgkin's Lymphoma

Drug regimen	Dose (mg/m^2)	Route	Days
Etoposide	50	po	1–21
DHAP			
Cisplatin	100	24 h civ	1
Ara-C	2 g	3 h civ	Every 12 h for 2 days on day 2
Dexamethasone	40 mg total	iv	1–4
EPOCH/CHOPE			
Etoposide	50	24 h civ	1–5
Onvocin (vincristine)	4	24 h civ	1–5
Doxorubicin	10	24 h civ	1–5
Cyclophosphamide	750	iv	6
Prednisone	60	po	1–6
ESHAP			
Etoposide	40	iv	1–4
Solumedrol	250–500	iv	1–5
Ara-C	2 g	iv	5
Cisplatin	25 mg	24 h civ	1–4

civ, continuous intravenous.
Source: Refs. 249–253.

is imperative. Standard therapy has been whole-brain radiotherapy, giving a median survival of 12–18 months in non-AIDS patients but only 2–5 months in AIDS patients. However, a high local recurrence rate indicates that the addition of chemotherapy is warranted (79). In non-AIDS patients, the addition of chemotherapy to radiotherapy has improved the prognosis, with median survivals of 30–45 months. Deangelis has pioneered the use of chemotherapy in this disorder. The regimen she employs specifies that all patients have placement of an Ommaya reservoir and receive pre-RT systemic methotrexate, 1 g/m^2 plus six doses of intra-Ommaya methotrexate at 12 mg per dose. A full course of cranial RT (4000-cGy whole-brain RT plus a 1440-cGy boost) is followed by two cycles of high-dose cytarabine (ara-C), with each course consisting of two doses of 3 g/m^2 ara-C separated by 24 h and infused over 3 h. The pharmacokinetic analyses of this therapy has been extensively studied (80, 81). In elderly patients, a chemotherapy-alone regimen has been developed. Chemotherapy alone for PCNSL is effective in the elderly and eliminates the risk of RT-related neurotoxicity. Radiation therapy can salvage those who relapse after chemotherapy (82).

b. Mantle Cell Lymphoma

Mantle cell lymphoma was first described in the 1970s and accounts for 5% of non–Hodgkin's lymphomas (1). The malignant lymphoid cells are irregular to occasionally cleaved nuclei that occur in a nodular (mantle zone) or diffuse forms. It was previously classified as intermediate lymphocytic lymphoma. The neoplastic cells are thought to originate in CD^+ B cells of the mantle zone of lymphoid follicles. The histological patterns are diffuse, nodular, and mantle zone. The prognosis is poorer than in other small-cell NHL, which is indolent. In one review of 46 cases, the median age was 54 years with a slight male predominance. Generalized lymphadenopathy was the most common presentation, with abdominal involvement. Bone marrow involvement was uncommon in the mantle zone variety. The response to chemotherapy correlated with mantle zone histology. Three-year survival rates were 100, 50, and 55% for patients with mantle zone, nodular, and diffuse histologic patterns, respectively (1, 83, 84).

c. Mucosa-Associated Lymphoid Tissue–Derived Lymphomas

Mucosa-associated lymphoid tissue (MALT)–lymphomas was described in 1983. These lymphomas arise from a variety of extranodal sites, most frequently the gastrointestinal tract, in the setting of chronic local inflammatory disorders or autoimmune disorders. The cells are related to the marginal zone B cells. The characteristics and outcome of 108 patients with MALT lymphoma were analyzed according to the initial location of the lymphoma within or outside of the gastrointestinal tract of one hundred eight patients with MALT, 55 (51%) had GI involvement and 53 (49%) had another involved extranodal site: 13 orbit, 11 lung, 10 skin, 7 parotid, 6 thyroid, 3 Waldeyer's ring, 2 breast, and 1 pancreas involvement. At diagnosis, 35 patients (32%) had disseminated disease. No difference in the clinical or biological characteristics was observed between GI and non-GI patients. A complete response after the first treatment was reached in 76% of the patients, with no difference between the two subgroups. With a median follow-up of 52 months, median survival was not reached and was identical in the two subgroups, but GI MALT patients had a longer time to progression (8.9 years compared with 4.9 years in non-GI patients). The different non-GI locations seemed to have a similar outcome. The implication of *Helicobacter pylori* in the pathogenesis of MALT gastric lymphoma has changed treatment options (10, 11). Eradication with antibiotics plus an antacid induced a regression in a number of trials. All studies report a high rate of *H. pylori* eradication associated with total regression of the lymphoma. Long-term follow-up will be necessary to determine the best treatment strategy (85).

d. Aggressive Histology (IWF I–J)

These entities will discussed in Sec. IV. B.

II. HODGKIN'S DISEASE

Hodgkin's disease has been known since first described by Thomas Hodgkin in 1832. Its epidemiology has been well studied. In the United States, the incidence of Hodgkin's is 3 per 100,000 persons annually. In 1997, it was estimated that there would be 7500 cases and 1480 deaths (86). There has been a slight decrease in incidence in older patients in the past 15 years, which is felt to represent more accurate diagnosis of lymphomas (87). The disease has a bimodal age incidence pattern in economically advanced countries. There is an increased risk with an increasing educational level of the patient. The incidence is also higher in whites than blacks and higher in men than in women (87). The poorer prognosis in older patients may reflect an inherent biological difference in this group (88, 89).

Hodgkin's is diagnosed after detection of superficial lymph nodes. More than 80% of patients present with lymphadenopathy above the diaphragm, often involving the anterior mediastinum (90). About 40% of patients have systemic symptoms. These include fever, night sweats, or weight loss and chronic pruritus. These symptoms usually occur more frequently in older patients and are a negative prognostic factor (90).

A. Pathology (See Table 12)

In a lymph node biopsy, the Reed–Sternberg cells is the diagnostic tumor cell that must be identified (90). There has been much debate as to its etiology of the cell. Hodgkin's disease differs from almost every known malignancy in a unique cellular composition in which a minority of neoplastic cells are in an inflammatory background (87). The pathological classification of Hodgkin's disease has evolved from the original description of Jackson and Parker, and the subsequent Rye Conference Classifications and that of Lukes and Butler (87, 91). Currently, the Revised European American Lymphoma (REAL) classification is gaining prominence, particularly the realization of the unique characteristics of the nodular variant of lymphocyte predominant disease (92).

Lymphocyte-predominant Hodgkin's disease is an indolent disorder associated with a long survival which represents 5% of all cases. Its features include a small number of large, dysplastic cells, designated lymphocytic and histiocytic (L&Husband) cells, and numerous small lymphocytes. The L&Husband cells have been found to be a monoclonal expansion of B cells (93, 94). The nodular subtype, nodular lymphocyte-predominant Hodgkin's disease (NLPHD), comprises from 2.0 to 6.5% of most studies. They are know to have a higher risk of development of non–Hodgkin's lymphoma. In making a proper diagnosis of this subtype, immunophenotype analysis is critical, particularly the finding of B-cell–associated antigens and the lack of Hodgkin's disease–associated antigens and the Epstein-Barr virus (EBV). This suggests that NLPHD is not related to other types of Hodgkin's disease (87). The median age is in the mid-30, but NLPHD has been seen at all ages. The male to female ratio is >3:1. It usually involves palpable nodes without mediastinal involvement. Three fourths of patients with NLPHD present at an early stage. Greater than 90% of affected patients have a complete response and are alive at 10 years. Late relapses in NLPHD are more common than other subtypes. The occurrence of NLPHD in an older patient would make it a highly curable disease in that patient's expected lifetime.

Table 11 Comparison of Real and Rye Classifications of Hodgkin's Disease

REAL classification	Rye classification
Lymphocyte predominance, nodular (with or without diffuse)	Lymphocyte predominance, nodular
Classic disease	
Lymphocyte-rich classic disease	Lymphocyte predominance, diffuse
	Lymphocyte predominance, nodular
Nodular sclerosis	Nodular sclerosis
Mixed cellularity	Mixed cellularity
Lymphocyte depletion	Lymphocyte depletion

Source: Refs. 87 and 92.

Nodular sclerosis is the most common subtype, and it is typically seen in young adults with supradiaphragmatic presentations. Mixed cellularity is the second most common histology. This subtype of Hodgkin's disease is more often diagnosed in males, usually presenting with generalized lymphadenopathy or extranodal disease and with associated systemic symptoms (90). Lymphocyte depletion is rare, and with the advent of antigen markers, many of these patients have T-cell non–Hodgkin's lymphoma (90). The subtypes of classic Hodgkin's disease are listed in Table 11.

B. Evaluation

A suggested outline for evaluation of patients presenting with Hodgkin's disease is listed in Table 12. These studies are appropriate for the elderly patient. As the role for chemotherapy has become more prominent in recent years, there has been a decline in the incidence of staging laparotomies. Particularly in elderly patients, this

Table 12 Evaluation of Hodgkin's Disease

1. Careful pathological evaluation of lymph nodes
2. History with emphasis on B symptoms, weight loss, fever, sweats
3. Laboratory studies include complete blood count, examination of the peripheral blood smear, ESR, renal and hepatic function
4. Radiographic studies to include chest radiograph, CT scans of the chest, abdomen, and pelvis, gallium 67 scan, bipedal lymphangiogram (optional)
5. Bone marrow aspiration and biopsy
6. Laparotomy and/or liver biopsy in selected patients

ESR, erythrocyte sedimentation rate; CT, computed tomography.

Table 13 Cotswold Staging Classification of Hodgkin's Disease

Stage	Description
I	Involvement of a single lymph node region or lymphoid structure
II	Involvement of two or more lymph node regions on the same side of the diaphragm
III	Involvement of lymph node regions on both sides of the diaphragm, which may be accompanied by involvement of the spleen
III$_1$	With or without involvement of the splenic, hilar, celiac nodes
III$_2$	With involvement of paraaortic, iliac, and mesenteric nodes
IV	Diffuse or disseminated involvement of one or more extranodal organs or tissues
Designations applicable to all stages	
A	No symptoms
B	Fever, drenching night sweats, unexplained loss of >10% of body weight within the preceding 6 months
X	Bulky disease (a widening of the mediastinum by more than one third or the presence of a nodal mass with a maximal dimension greater than 10 cm)
E	Involvement of a single extranodal site that is contiguous or proximal to the known nodal site
CS	Clinical stage
PS	Pathological stage

invasive procedure has been shunned. More recently there has been an increase in the use of laparoscopic procedures in staging and splenectomy (95–99). This may be better tolerated for elderly patients, but it is not yet known whether this will change clinical practice. The staging is similar to the Ann Arbor staging of non–Hodgkin's lymphoma. The Cotswald Staging is more specific for Hodgkin's disease (Table 13).

C. Therapy

1. Treatment of Stages I and II

Irradiation of the mantle and para-aortic fields (subtotal lymphoid irradiation) is the standard for most patients with surgically confirmed early-stage Hodgkin's disease. Several series report a 15- to 20-year survival rates of 90% and relapsed free survivals of 75–80%. Most relapses occur within the first 3 years. Many patients relapsing after radiation therapy are curable with chemotherapy (87, 90, 100). High-risk patients may benefit from combined chemotherapy and radiation. Risk factors may include an elevated erythrocyte sedimentation rate, B symptoms, large mediastinal adenopathy, age 50 years or older, and four or more involved sites (87). Elderly patients should generally tolerate radiation therapy as well as younger patients (101–104). They may, however, be a some increased risk of small bowel damage (105).

Subdiaphragmatic presentations of stages I and II occur in older patients and have a poorer prognosis. Radiation is recommended for stage I and a combined modality approach for stage II (106, 107).

2. Treatment of Stages III and IV

Chemotherapy is the standard treatment of advanced disease (Table 14). MOPP has been the primary effective combination chemotherapy regimen for advanced disease since the 1960s. A randomized trial comparing MOPP, ABVD, and MOPP/ABVD was completed by the Cancer and Leukemia Group B (108). The overall response rate was 93%, with complete responses in 77%: 67% in the MOPP group, 82% in the ABVD group, and 83% in the MOPP–ABVD group. The rates of failure-free survival at 5 years were 50% for MOPP, 61% for ABVD, and 65% for MOPP-ABVD. Age, stage (III vs IV), and regimen influenced failure-free survival significantly. Overall survival at 5 years was 66% for MOPP, 73% for ABVD, and 75% for MOPP–ABVD. MOPP had more severe toxic effects on bone marrow than ABVD and was associated with greater reductions in the prescribed dose. Therefore, ABVD therapy for 6–8 months was as effective as 12 months of MOPP alternating with ABVD, and both were superior to MOPP alone. ABVD was less myelotoxic than MOPP or ABVD alternating with MOPP. ABVD should also be the standard for elderly patients.

There have been various combination chemotherapy regimens advocated for elderly patients with the theory that they cannot tolerate standard regimens. The ChlVPP, NOVP, or ''ABVD without D'' regimens are suggested (109). A small

Table 14 Combination Chemotherapy for Hodgkin's Disease

Drug regimen	Dose (mg/m^2)	Route	Days
MOPP			
Nitrogen mustard	6	iv	1, 8
Vincristine	1.4	iv	1, 8
Procarbazine	100	po	1–14
Prednisone	40	po	1–14
ABVD			
Doxorubicin	25	iv	1, 15
Bleomycin	10	iv	1, 15
Vinblastine	6	iv	1, 15
DTIC	375	iv	1, 15
ChlVPP			
Chlorambucil	6	po	1–14
Vinblastine	6	iv	1, 8
Procarbazine	100	po	1–14
Prednisone	40	po	1–14

trial of 25 patients over 65 years of age using CVP/CEB (chlorambucil, vinblastine, procarbazine, prednisone, cyclophosphamide, etoposide, bleomycin) has been reported (110). The investigators thought that this low-toxicity regimen may be appropriate for older patients. The Eastern Cooperative Oncology Group (ECOG) analyzed outcome by age (111). The complete remission percentages were identical in both studies (72%), with no significant difference between the three age groupings (<40, 40–59, and >60 years). This lack of difference is probably a result of the eligibility criteria for cooperative group trials which eliminates poor-risk patients. This was true as well for disease-free survival. Nevertheless, overall survival was significantly better for the under aged 40 group. This was accounted for by the poorer outcome of salvage treatment in the older age group. The M.D. Anderson group observed a CR rate of 87% and survival of 58%, with a median follow-up of 58 months. Their population consisted of only those entered on protocols. It suggests that patients whose condition is adequate enough to allow them to receive standard therapy with a curative intent have a similar outcome to that seen in younger patients (112).

Limited data regarding the cause of the age-related decrease in survival times in patients with Hodgkin's disease are available (113). In a retrospective study of a nonselected population of patients with Hodgkin disease, the investigators evaluated which factors contributed to the age-related prognostic effect in this disease. The survival curves of 182 patients were compared, and survival time was found to decrease markedly after the age of 50 years. Differences in disease characteristics between older and younger patients were small and not statistically significant. Significantly fewer older patients received adequate treatment (34 vs 2%), and they were less likely to have complete disease remission (61 vs 90%). However, the relapse-free survival time of patients with complete disease remission was not significantly different from that of younger patients: 50% of all patients being free of disease after 10 years. Intercurrent disease did not appear to be responsible for decreased survival times in the elderly (32 vs 26%). The investigators conclude that the inability to give adequate treatment seems to be the major determinant of the poorer overall survival time of older patients with Hodgkin's disease.

A Swedish study performed an outcome analysis on outcome of older patients (114). The younger patients had more intense screening evaluation. However, this did not affect survival. Patients treated with radiotherapy had survivals of 85%. The older patients receiving combination chemotherapy did poorly, with a 5-year survival of 33% as compared to 86% in the younger group. The main reason was a poor tolerance to therapy with many dose modifications. Another study emphasized the efficacy and tolerability of radiation therapy in older patients (115).

3. Toxicity of Therapy

There are a number of chronic toxicities which need to be considered in deciding therapy. Combined modality therapy may lead to the development of secondary malignancies. Table 15 lists some of these problems.

Table 15 Chronic Toxicities of Treatment for Hodgkin's Disease

Complication	Causes and risk factors	Management and prevention
Immunological dysfunction	Underlying disease, therapy	Vaccinations
Herpes zoster or varicella	Underlying disease, therapy	Systemic antiviral therapy, zoster immune globulin
Pneumococcal sepsis	Splenectomy, function asplenia after RT	Pretherapy pneumococcal vaccine, selected antibiotic prophylaxis, avoid splenectomy
Nonlymphocytic leukemia	Therapy	Avoid combined modality therapy
Myelodysplastic syndromes	Therapy	Avoid combined modality therapy
Non–Hodgkin's lymphoma	Therapy	Combination chemotherapy
Solid tumors	Direct or indirect RT exposure	Conventional management
Hypothyroidism	Direct or indirect RT exposure	Hormone replacement, thyroid suppression during therapy
Thyroid cancer	Direct or indirect RT exposure, chronic thyroid stimulation	Thyroid suppression
Male impotence	Underlying disease, therapy	Counseling, trial of testosterone
Female dyspareunia	Underlying disease, therapy	Counseling, cyclic estrogen replacement
Pericarditis, acute	Mediastinal RT, recall with chemotherapy after RT	Appropriate RT shielding and technique, avoid doxorubicin after RT, anti-inflammatory medication, pericardiocentesis
Pericarditis, chronic	Mediastinal RT	Appropriate RT shielding and technique, pericardiectomy
Cardiomyopathy	Mediastinal RT, doxorubicin, recall with chemotherapy after RT	Appropriate RT shielding and technique, avoid doxorubicin after RT, monitor for early signs of toxicity, limit cumulative doxorubicin dose, supportive medical management
Pneumonitis, acute	Direct or indirect RT, bleomycin, nitrosoureas, recall with chemotherapy after RT	Appropriate RT shielding and technique, monitor for early signs of toxicity, avoid known toxic drugs, avoid excessive Po$_2$
Pneumonitis, chronic	Same as above	Supportive management
Avascular necrosis	Steroid therapy	Anti-inflammatory medications, joint surgery
Dental caries	Salivary change after RT	Maintain good oral hygiene, daily fluoride treatments

RT, radiation therapy.
Source: Ref. 87.

4. Management of Relapsed Disease

Patients relapsing after initial therapy with radiation should have an excellent response to chemotherapy. Patients who relapse after a long (>12 month) disease-free interval have a high complete response rate to salvage therapy (87, 90). Some of these remissions are durable, but the curative potential is low (116). The only potentially curative treatment is bone marrow transplantation. This option is only available to a highly selected group of older patients similar to the non–Hodgkin's lymphomas (117).

III. MULTIPLE MYELOMA AND PLASMA CELL DYSCRASIAS

Plasma cell dyscrasias are a group of disorders characterized by the presence of a monoclonal serum immunoglobulin. There are a wide spectrum of disorders in this category (Table 16). In addition, Waldenström's macroglobulinema and amyloidosis are often included in this grouping (118, 119).

Multiple myeloma is widespread malignancy of monoclonal plasma cells. In 1995, there were an estimated 12,500 new cases with 10,300 deaths (119). There is a male/female ration of 1.3 to 1.0. The median age at presentation is 69.1 years of age (120). The frequency of the presence of a monoclonal protein in the population increases with age. Epidemiologically, multiple myeloma and monoclonal gammo-pathy of uncertain significance both have a rising incidence with advancing age with 14% of people over the age of 90 years having a monoclonal spike (120). The incident rate in African-Americans is double the frequency in the white population. No predisposing factors for the development of the disease has been elucidated.

A. Monoclonal Gammopathy of Uncertain Significance

Monoclonal gammopathy of uncertain significance (MGUS) is found in approximately 3% of persons older than 70 years and in 1% of those 50 years of age or

Table 16 Plasma cell Dyscrasias

Disorder	Marrow plasmacytosis	Ig peak	Background suppression	Lytic lesions	Renal disease	Calcium
Multiple myeloma	>15%	>3.0 g/dL	±	±	±	±
Asymptomatic myeloma	>15%	<4.5 g/dL	±	0	0	0
Solitary plasmacytoma	Normal	0	0	0	0	0
MGUS	<10%	<3.0 g/dL	0	0	0	0

MGUS, monoclonal gammopathies of undetermined significance.

older. During long-term follow-up, approximately one fourth of patients develop multiple myeloma (MM), amyloidosis, macroglobulinemia, or a similar malignant lymphoproliferative disorder. The actuarial rate of development of serious disease was 16% at 10 years, 33% at 20 years, and 40% at 25 years. The interval from recognition of the Mom-protein to the diagnosis of MM ranged from 2 to 29 years (median, 10 years) (121). There are no findings at the diagnosis of MGUS that reliably distinguish patients who will remain stable from those in whom a malignant condition will develop. Thus, a physician must perform serial measurements of the Mom-protein in the serum and periodic evaluation of the pertinent clinical and laboratory features to determine whether MM, macroglobulinemia, systemic amyloidosis, or related disorders have developed (121).

B. Solitary Plasmacytoma

Solitary plasmacytoma is characterized by the presence of a tumor consisting of monoclonal plasma cells identical to those in MM. In addition, skeletal radiographs must show no lytic lesions, a bone marrow aspirate must contain no evidence of MM, and immunoelectrophoresis or immunofixation of the serum and concentrated urine should show no Mom-protein. Exceptions to the presence of an Mom-protein occur, but therapy of the solitary lesion often results in disappearance of the Mom-protein. Tumoricidal irradiation (4000–5000 cGy) for approximately 4 weeks is the treatment of choice. Overt MM occurs in approximately 50% of patients with solitary plasmacytoma. Progression occurs in most patients within 3 years. The three patterns of failure are (a) development of MM, (b) local recurrence, and (c) development of new bone lesions in the absence of MM (121).

C. Amyloidosis

Primary systemic amyloidosis is an uncommon disease characterized by the accumulation in vital organs of a fibrillar protein consisting of monoclonal light chains. It can occur in 10% of patients with MM. The clinical features include the nephrotic syndrome, cardiomyopathy, heptomegaly, macroglossia, neuropathy, carpal tunnel syndrome, and periorbital purpura (122). To evaluate the efficacy of therapy, a randomized trial has been reported in 220 patients with biopsy-proved amyloidosis. The patients were randomly assigned to receive colchicine, melphalan, and prednisone or melphalan, prednisone, and colchicine. They were stratified according to their chief clinical manifestations. The median duration of survival was 8.5 months in the colchicine group, 18.0 months in the group assigned to melphalan and prednisone, and 17.0 months in the group assigned to melphalan, prednisone, and colchicine. Among patients who had a reduction in serum or urine monoclonal protein at 12 months, the overall length of survival was 50 months, whereas among those without a reduction at 12 months, the overall length of survival was 36 months. Thirty-four patients (15%) survived for 5 years or longer. Therefore, therapy with melphalan and prednisone results in objective responses and prolonged survival as compared with colchicine in patients with primary amyloidosis (123). A review details this disorder (124).

D. Indolent Multiple Myeloma

In approximately 20% of patients, MM presents in an asymptomatic patient. The diagnosis is confirmed by an analysis of the serum proteins. The clinical manifestations of this disease are consistent with a low tumor mass. These include lack of renal disease, hypercalcemia, or lytic bone lesions. It is recommended that chemotherapy not be instituted until there is a significant risk of complications. This is particularly true of elderly patients with significant comorbidity. An analysis of 101 consecutive, asymptomatic patients attempted to identify risk factors for progression. Serum myeloma globulin >30 g/L, IgA protein type, and Bence Jones excretion >50 mg/d were found to be significant independent variables (125). The presence of two or more of these features signified high-risk disease with early progression (median 17 months), whereas the absence of any variable was associated with prolonged stability (median 95 months) (125).

E. Multiple Myeloma

Multiple myeloma (MM) is a malignancy of monoclonal plasma cells that accounts for 10% of all hematological cancers. The 5-year survival rate for all patients is approximately 25–30%. The five-year survival is lower among patients 65 years old or older (20–25%) than in those less than 65 years of age (30–35%) (119). Tumor mass correlates with survival. This ranges from 7 months in unresponsive patients with a high tumor mass to 59 months in patients with a low tumor mass and responsive disease (119) (Table 17). The clinical features are variable. Findings which suggest the diagnosis include lytic bone lesions, anemia, azotemia, hypercalcemia, and infections (119). The clinical manifestations of MM are a result of direct tumor growth causing replacement of normal structures, accumulation of the immunoglobulin chains, and bone resorption (120). These manifestations and diagnostic studies are listed (Tables 18 and 19).

In patients who felt to have active MM and require treatment, commonly used regimens are listed (Table 20). Melphalan and prednisone remains the standard for newly diagnosed patients with low or intermediate tumor mass, particularly in older patients. Approximately 40% of patients will respond with a median remission of 2 years and an overall survival of 3 years. VAD (see Table 20) regimens are frequently used for high-risk (high tumor mass, hypercalcemia, renal insufficiency) disease. The survival advantage of VAD is unknown. Single-agent high-dose dexamethasone has also shown efficacy (126). Radiotherapy is frequently used in the palliation of painful bone lesions or in the treatment of spinal cord compression.

Interferon-α may prolong remission of MM in comparison to no treatment in patients who have responded to therapy. There is a question whether this provides

Table 17   Durie–Salmon Staging System

Stage	Criteria	Estimated cell mass
I	Hemoglobin >10 g/dL	Low
	Serum calcium ≤12 mg/dL	
	Normal bone or solitary plasmacytoma	
	Low M-component production rate:	
	IgG <5 g/dL	
	IgA <3 g/dL	
	Bence Jones protein <4 g/24 h	
II	Not fitting stage I or III	Intermediate
III	Hemoglobin >8.5 g/dL	Low
	Serum calcium >12 mg/dL	
	Multiple lytic bone lesions on radiograph	
	High M-component production rate:	
	IgG >5 g/dL	
	IgA >3 g/dL	
	Bence Jones protein >12 g/24 h	
A	Normal renal function	
B	Abnormal renal function	

Source: Ref. 119.

Table 18   Diagnostic Evaluation

Initial evaluation may include:
  Complete blood cell count with differential and platelets
  Routine chemical screen
  Bone marrow aspirate to assess plasmacytosis
  Serum protein electrophoresis and immunofixation to define
      protein type
  24-Hour urine protein and electrophoresis
  Quantitative immunoglobulins
  Skeletal survey (bone scans not effective since radioisotope
      uptake low in purely lytic disease other possible tests:
  β_2-Microglobulin
  LDH
  Plasma cell labeling index
  Ploidy

Table 19 Clinical Manifestions of Multiple Myeloma

System	Manifestation
Skeletal	Bone pain, fractures of the vertebrae or ribs, lytic lesions in 70% at diagnosis
Hematopoietic	Normocytic, normochromic anemia present in 60% of patients at diagnosis
Endocrine	20% of newly diagnosed patients have hypercalcemia (>11.5 mg/dL) secondary to bone destruction
Renal	20% of patients present with renal insufficiency and another 20% develop during the course of their illness. Bence Jones proteinuria is the most common cause; amyloidosis, hypercalcemia or light chain deposition may also contribute
Infections	Patients with myeloma develop bacterial infections; recently, gram-negative organisms have been the most common pathogens surpassing the gram-positive organisms

a survival advantage (127–130). Dexamethasone and interferon have been combined (131). Maintenance therapy with prolonged alkylating treatment does not lengthen remission and survival times. The continuation of this treatment may result in the development of a secondary myeloid leukemia.

Age has been studied as a prognostic variable in MM. There are conflicting results in this analysis. Studies which indicate that age is a poor prognostic indicator are community based and may have accepted patients with poor-performance scores and increased comorbidity. In trials from tertiary centers in which patient selection may have been more careful, no effect of age was noted (120). From an analysis among 26 different single prognostic variables, the following factors are listed in order of importance: β_2-microglobulin; bone marrow plasma cell percentage, hemoglobinemia, degree of lytic bone lesions, serum creatinine, and serum albumin. By analysis of these variables a prognostic index (PI) was obtained, making it possible to separate the whole patient group into three stages: stage I, stage II, and stage III, with a median survivals of 68, 36 and 13 months, respectively. Also, the responses to therapy and the survival curves presented significant differences among the three subgroups (132).

The presentation of active MM does not vary with age (133). There is no specific therapy for elderly patients with symptomatic MM. Standard regimens such as melphalan/prednisone (MP) and VAD should be well tolerated by elderly patients. Clavio et al. reviewed 113 consecutive patients with MM over the age of 64 years. The median age was 71 years. Stage IA, IIA, IIIA, and IIIB patients numbered 28, 33, 45 and 7, respectively. The M component was IgG in 73 patients (65%), IgA in 30 (26%), IgD in 3 (3%), and light chain in 5 (4%); no monoclonal component was detected in 2 patients (2%) cases. Sixty-three patients showed symptomatic

Table 20 Treatment of Multiple Myeloma

Disease	Regimen	Schedule
Untreated multiple myeloma	MP: melphalan (8 mg/m^2/d po) + prednisone (100 mg/d po) days 1–4	4 weeks
	VAD: vincristine (0.4 mg/d iv) + doxorubicin (9 mg/m^2/d iv) with both drugs given by continuous infusion on days 1–4 and dexamethasone 40 mg/d po on days 1–4; 9–12; 17–20	
	Dexamethasone 40 mg/d po on days 1–4; 9–12; 17–20	4 weeks
	VBMCP (M2): vincristine 0.03 mg/kg iv day 1; BCNU 0.5 mg/kg iv day 1; melphalan 0.25 mg/kg po days 1–4; cyclophosphamide 10 mg/kg iv day 1; prednisone 1 mg/kg po days 1–7	5 weeks
	VMCP: vincristine 1.0–1.5 mg iv day 1; melphalan 5–6 mg/m^2 po day 1–4; cyclophosphamide 100–125 mg/m^2 po days 1–4; prednisone 60 mg/m^2 po days 1–4	3 weeks
	VCAP: vincristine 1.0–1.5 mg iv day 1; doxorubicin 25–30 mg/m^2; cyclophosphamide 100–125 mg/m^2 po days 1–4; prednisone 60 mg/m^2 po days 1–4	3 weeks
	VBAP: vincristine 1.0–1.5 mg iv day 1; doxorubicin 25–30 mg/m^2; BCNU 25–30 mg/m^2; prednisone 60 mg/m^2 po days 1–4	3 weeks

Source: Refs. 120 and 255.

skeletal disease. Melphalan/prednisone was the first-line treatment in 84 patients (74%). Seventy-eight cases (69%) showed a sizable reduction in the tumor mass; objective and partial response was achieved in 57 (50%) and 21 (19%) patients, respectively. Patients with stages I–II disease fared significantly better than stage III patients (median survival: 70 vs 38 months; $P = .017$). Response to first-line treatment correlated with overall survival; patients with responsive or refractory disease had median survival rates of 64 and 20 months, respectively ($P = .0001$). Neither patients above nor below 75 years of age showed any difference in presentation features or in response to treatment. These results suggest that advanced age should not be considered a major obstacle to active treatment (134). Bladé et al. analyzed a subset of 178 patients over the age of 70 years of a group of 487 consecutive patients. All of the patients were randomized to receive MP versus alternating cycles of vincristine, cyclophosphamide, melphalan, and prednisone (VCMP) and vincristine, BCNU, Adriamycin (doxorubicin), and prednisone (VBAP). The presenting features and response to chemotherapy of older patients were no different to those of the younger population. However, the survival of elderly patients was significantly shorter (median 23.4 vs 33.5 months, $P < .001$). The overall response rate to MP in older patients was 50% (28% objective plus 22% partial response) compared with 61% (44% objective plus 17% partial response) to combination chemotherapy (P = not significant). Myelosuppression was moderate in both arms, although MP produced a higher degree of thrombocytopenia. There were no significant differences in survival between patients given MP versus VCMP/VBAP (median, 20 vs 27 months, $P = .2$). Response to treatment was associated with a significantly longer survival. Older patients with symptomatic myeloma tolerate chemotherapy and should be offered treatment.

1. Transplantation

Owing to the increased recognition of drug tolerance of older patients and the improved safety of autologous transplantation, patients with MM over the age of 60 years are being considered for this treatment (135, 136). A retrospective analysis consisting of 57 of 225 patients over 60 years of age who underwent an autotransplant after peripheral stem cell mobilization showed no difference in either the median number of CD34$^+$ cells collected or time to engraftment (137). Palumbo treated 50 patients over the age of 55 years, with a median age of 63 years, with high-dose melphalan and infusion of peripheral stem cells. The clinical outcome of these patients was compared to that of two different historical control groups. The first control group consisted of 160 patients (median age 62 years, range 54–71 years) treated with MP at diagnosis. The second control group consisted of 50 patients (median age 50 years, range 38–58 years) treated at diagnosis with a single or double transplant (for 29 patients, treatment was melphalan 140 mg/mom^2 plus total-body irradiation (TBI); for 21 patients, treatment was melphalan 200 mg/m^2, and treatment was melphalan 180 mg/m^2 + mitoxantrone 60 mg/m^2). After treatment, response >50% was 87% and complete remission 43%. After transplantation, response >50% was 86% and complete remission 50%. After MP, response >50% was 49% and complete remission 5%. In the transplanted group, the median follow-up of survivor was 28 months, with a median event-free survival of 30.9 months. In the transplanted and MP group, median event-free survival was 30.3 and 17 months, respectively. Both high-dose therapy and transplantation had a significantly longer event-free ($P < .0002$) than the MP group. Survival was not analyzed since the median follow-up was too short for the study group. The complete remission rate was similar to that obtained with transplantation in younger patients (median age 63 vs 50 years). The impact on the clinical outcome was encouraging but longer follow-up will be mandatory to draw definitive conclusions (135).

2. Other Therapy in Multiple Myeloma

Skeletal complications are a serious problem in this disease. Osteoporosis, pain, and fracture are devastating complications. These complications are caused by soluble factors that stimulate osteoclasts to resorb bone. Pamidronate has been approved to prevent these complications (138–144). The treatment of chronic anemia may be helped by the administration of erythropoietin (145, 146). Infectious complications of neutropenia may be reduced by the administration of colon-stimulating factors. Patients who receive high-dose dexamethasone may benefit from Pneumocystis prophylaxis with trimethoprim-sulfamethazole.

IV. LEUKEMIAS

A. Myelodysplastic Syndromes

The myelodysplastic syndromes (MDS) encompass five diagnostic entities: refractory anemia (RA), refractory anemia with excess blasts (RAEB), RAEB in transformation (RAEB-T), refractory anemia with ringed sideroblasts (RARS), and chronic myelomonocytic leukemia (CMMoL) (147). These diseases tend primarily to affect elderly patients, with the incidence of 5.3 per 100,000 during the sixth decade of life increasing two- to threefold per decade thereafter (148). Characteristic findings are bone marrow failure usually leading to anemia and often to bilineage and trilineage cytopenias. The main biological features of MDS are that they are clonal diseases marked by the frequent presence of nonrandom cytogenetic changes (149) and a reduced capacity to proliferate in tissue culture (150).

The clinical course of MDS can range between months and years, and it can be somewhat approximated by prognostic indices such as the Lille score, which factors in bone marrow blast percentage and karyotype at presentation along with the peripheral blood counts (151). The Lille score can predict a likelihood of evolution into acute myelogenous leukemia (AML) of 8–68% depending on prognostic findings.

Clonal cytogenetic abnormalities are observed in the majority of patients with MDS, and these findings have important prognostic value (149, 151). These abnormalities are especially prevalent in AML which develops following MDS associated with prior therapy with antineoplastic agents, with unbalanced aberrations involving chromosomal loss or gain (e.g., monosomy 5/5q-, monosomy 7/7q-, trisomy 8) predominating (152).

1. Therapy

Depending on a patient's clinical needs and physical condition, therapy for MDS can range from supportive care primarily involving transfusions of blood products and treatment of infection to conventional and experimental therapies utilizing hematopoietic growth factors and/or cytotoxic agents. Earlier strategies have frequently applied therapy with androgens. A large retrospective report demonstrated minimal to no activity on the part of danazol, a frequently used semisynthetic androgen in MDS (153).

Granulocyte colony-stimulating factor (G-CSF) (154) and low-dose granulocyte-macrophage colony-stimulating factor (GM-CSF) (155) can induce sustained reversal of neutropenia in a significant percentage of patients with MDS. Higher doses of *Escherichia coli*–derived GM-CSF were studied in a randomized phase II, crossover trial in which significant neutrophilic responses and decrease in infections were associated with use of this cytokine (156). With respect to other lineages, therapy with G-CSF and GM-CSF has been associated with either no or modest effects on hemoglobin. Some multilineage effects have been observed in patients with MDS receiving interleukin-3 (157). Anemia has been primarily treated with erythropoietin, with favorable responses being associated with low baseline serum erythropoietin (158) and tumor necrosis factor-α (159) levels. Changes in plasma transferrin receptor protein have not been predictive (160). Responses to erythropoietin are seen in up to 50% of patients, with attendant reductions in transfusion requirements and improvement in the quality of life. Addition of G-CSF to erythropoietin therapy may have synergistic effects and induce responses in some patients refractory to single-agent erythropoietin (161). Increases in platelet counts were noted in 27% of patients with MDS and severe thrombocytopenia in those receiving Interleukin-6, but toxicity limited long-term use of this agent (162). Interleukin-11, another platelet growth factor which has shown activity in patients with solid tumors receiving chemotherapy, may have a limited role to play in MDS by virtue of its ability to stimulate leukemia cell growth in vitro (163).

Two cytokines going through preclinical evaluation in MDS are mast cell growth factor (c-*kit* ligand), which stimulates the growth of very early progenitors (164), as well as thrombopoietin, a major growth factor involved in platelet production about which some concern exists regarding its possible stimulatory effect on myeloid blasts (165). One recent in vitro study focusing on MDS bone marrows did not demonstrate this liability on the part of thrombopoietin (166).

The use of the clinically available cytokines has to be individualized in MDS. There is consensus regarding the utility of erythropoietin in symptomatic patients with MDS. The role of the myeloid growth factors remains unclear, with its use generally being reserved for patients with recurrent infections. No survival advantage has yet to be documented with growth factor use, probably because of the crossover design of most randomized trials.

Growth factors may act by promoting maturation of leukemic clones or normal progenitors. Agents which have been applied primarily as maturational therapies include 13-*cis* retinoic acid, which was shown to be ineffective in a randomized trial (167), and all-*trans* retinoic acid (ATRA), which exerts modest bilineage- and trilineage effects, both when used alone and in combination with G-CSF (168). Attempts to counter apoptotic mechanisms in MDS have included trials of amifostine (169) and pentoxifylline, ciprofloxacin, and dexamethasone (170) resulting in preliminary evidence of tolerability and activity. Modest clinical activity was reported in a trial of hexamethylene bisacetamide (HMBA), another putative differentiating agent (171).

Chemotherapy has been used to treat MDS, with again the primary emphasis being to effect maturational changes in the leukemic population. Although about one third of patients treated with low-dose cytosine arabinoside (LDAC) responded in a phase III randomized study, no survival advantage or significant delay in progression to acute leukemia was noted (172). One small study suggested that LDAC may have striking activity in the 5q- syndrome, an MDS variant which primarily affects elderly women (173). Cytotoxicity rather than differentiation appeared to account for the clinical responses. More recently, 5-azacytidine has demonstrated activity in MDS (174), which is being further tested in a randomized, crossover study. Significant activity (54% overall response) was marred by a high toxic death rate (17%) with 5-aza-2' deoxycytidine (175).

Selected older patients with high-risk MDS have received intensive chemotherapy using fludarabine and ara-C, with (FLAG) and without G-CSF, with 50–60% of patients achieving CR and no indication that G-CSF increased the CR rate or reduced infectious complications (176). It appears that the minority of patients with MDS and normal cytogenetics treated with intensive AML-type chemotherapy are more likely to have increased relapse-free survival (177).

B. Acute Leukemia

Although intensive combination chemotherapy regimens for the treatment of acute leukemia can induce durable remissions, less than half of adults treated for acute lymphoblastic leukemia (ALL) and less than one quarter treated for acute myelogenous leukemia (AML) enjoy prolonged survival. When the analysis is confined to elderly patients, the outcome is even more dismal. These poor results are underscored by the realization that elderly patients enrolled in clinical trials reflect selection bias, with substantial numbers of elderly patients, particularly those with comorbid physical and cognitive conditions, being offered only supportive and palliative care. The significant underrepresentation of elderly patients in clinical trials has been described (178).

In addition to the obvious physical impediments of age, multiple biological, pharmacological, and pharmacodynamic factors present unique and troublesome obstacles to the success of available antileukemia therapies. The cardiac, pulmonary, and renal toxicities associated both with chemotherapy and with the antibiotics needed for the intensive support of the compromised, myelosuppressed patient are magnified in elderly patients. Because of this, intensive postremission therapies designed to prolong remission duration and increase the cure fraction are prohibitively toxic in most older patients. Cytogenetic abnormalities, multidrug resistance phenotypic expression, and age-specific variances in cytotoxic drug disposition conspire to reduce greatly the efficacy and increase the toxicity of treatment. Overall, unlike younger patients, in whom innate drug resistance is the major element in treatment failure, the elderly patient with acute leukemia is not only more likely to harbor resistant persistent leukemia following therapy but is far more likely to succumb to therapy-related complications.

1. Acute Myelogenous Leukemia

The vast majority of cases of AML, irrespective of age, are sporadic and unrelated to known environmental or genetic risk factors (179). A 10-fold increase in incidence occurs with age, with the incidence exceeding 10 in 100,000 individuals after age 70 years (180). Biological differences related to the nature of the leukemic progenitor cell and its molecular and cytogenetic underpinnings accompany this increase in incidence.

a. Biological Features

At the cellular level, the available data point to the progenitor cell in elderly patients with AML as originating earlier in the hierarchy of myeloid development, so that stem cell features are more likely to be displayed (181). Although aging also affects the proliferative capacity of normal stem cells, the clinical consequences of this are less clear (71). Studies of clonality using methods such as assays for specific glucose-6-phosphate dehydrogenase isoenzymes in female heterozygotes have shown that clonal hematopoiesis is more likely to be established following attainment of complete remission in older than younger patients with AML (181). Ultimately, the higher likelihood of the derivation of leukemia from the hematopoietic stem cell in elderly patients rather than a more committed progenitor with higher replicative capacity and susceptibility to cytotoxic therapy may defeat the best chemotherapeutic efforts.

The clonal cytogenetic abnormalities found in elderly patients with AML tend to be less favorable than those of younger patients, and they are frequently identical to those highly prevalent in MDS (182). These findings are also similar to those observed in secondary leukemia following chemotherapy with alkylating agents. A useful paradigm for categorizing the chromosomal findings in acute leukemia assigns poor risk to karyotypes displaying a net gain or loss of genetic information (152). Such leukemias involve quantitative shifts in the number of putative regulatory and tumor suppressor sequences and are especially prevalent in the older patient with AML displaying such typical poor-risk cytogenetics as deletions of all or part of the long arm of chromosomes 5 and 7 and trisomies 8 and 21. These poor-risk cytogenetic features tend to predominate in the elderly and correlate with CD34 (stem cell) and p-glycoprotein (multidrug resistance-1, MDR-1) expression (183, 184). Conversely, balanced translocation such as t(8;21) seen in AML with maturation (M2), pericentric inversion of chromosome 16 and variants and t(15;17) in acute promyelocytic leukemia (APL, M3) tend to be associated with an improved outcome (185) and younger age (186). In all the favorable-risk karyotoypes, there occurs neither gain nor loss of genetic information but rather splicing of nucleic acid sequences which result in the manufacture of distinct regulatory elements germane to leukemogenesis. Of note, the secondary leukemias associated with epidophyllotoxin exposure tend to display balanced cytogenetic findings involving 11q23 (6) which, when seen in de novo AML, are significantly less common in elderly patients (187).

Expression of MDR-1 appears significantly to correlate with inferior CR rates, whereas elderly patients negative for MDR-1 have CR rates to contemporary induction regimens similar to that of younger patients (188). The CR incidence may be inversely related to the presence of multidrug-resistant cells with a high proliferative capacity in vitro (189). The extrusion of anthracyclines, epidophyllotoxins, and vinca alkaloids by transmembrane (MDR-1, MRP) and intracellular (lung resistance protein; LRP) proteins contributes to the inability of conventional therapies to eradicate the acute leukemias.

Functional measures of drug efflux have shown correlations both with CD34 and MDR-1 expression, with some measure of independence between the two variables such that efflux may be observed in CD34$^+$ AML, which does not express MDR-1 (190). In addition, more recently appreciated drug-resistance mediators such as the major vault protein LRP may be at least as important to clinical outcome as MDR-1 (191).

b. Therapy

Combination chemotherapy using an anthracycline with cytosine arabinoside (ara-C) has been the standard by which all contemporary induction regiments for AML are gauged. Depending on patient age and dose of anthracycline utilized, CR incidences have ranged widely. Idarubicin, aclarubicin, and mitoxantrone have been shown to be superior to daunorubicin in several randomized trials with respect to the CR incidence, but these findings may be due to dosing differences (reviewed in (Ref. 192). Equitoxic or myelosuppressive doses of the two agents may not have been used. A clear dose response for daunorubicin has not been established in randomized trials, although reducing dose may be deleterious (193). Intensification of the induction regimen with the addition of etoposide (194) or escalation of the ara-C dose (high-dose ara-C, or HiDAC [195]) appears to improve disease-free survival, whereas not increasing CR rates, illustrating the potential impact of higher dose regimens on the "quality" of remissions.

Despite conflicting results from randomized studies comparing palliative or supportive care with standard or dose-attenuated induction chemotherapy, the weight of the evidence suggests that good-performance status older patients fare better, with longer survival and fewer disease-related complications and hospitalizations when treated. In particular, two European studies comparing standard anthracycline/ara-C induction with a "watch and wait" approach (196) and with LDAC (197) demonstrated superiority for initial conventional induction therapy both with respect to the CR incidence and survival.

Less toxic regimens of moderate intensity have also proven their worth in randomized comparisons: The Finnish Leukemia Group demonstrated a higher CR incidence, reduced toxicity, and longer survival in older patients randomized to receive on oral induction regimen of etoposide, 6-thioguanine, and idarubicin as compared with a daunorubicin/ara-C induction which included 6-thioguanine (198). That study may have exploited the distinct pharmacokinetics of idarubicin in the elderly, which is associated with significant prolongations of the terminal half-life of the active metabolite idarubicinol as compared with younger patients (199). Similar findings showing a trend in favor of a dose-attenuated standard anthracycline/ara-C induction regimen versus full-dose therapy was reported by ECOG in a group of patients with an older median age (>70 years) (200).

An attempt to modulate the activity of LDAC by adding hydroxyurea and calcitriol led to a 45% CR incidence and a median survival of 12 months (201). Only a randomized comparison will clarify whether this combination represents an advance over LDAC alone. With the exception of acute promyelocytic leukemia, in which all-*trans* retinoic acid alone can induce CR by itself in most patients (202), no putative differentiation-inducing agent has demonstrated efficacy in AML outside of case reports.

Several novel regimens for the treatment of AML have been explored in the last several years in older patients (Table 21). Two of the regimens either omit ara-C altogether (mitoxantrone and etoposide) (203) or omit the anthracycline and combine fludarabine with ara-C with and without G-CSF (176). These regimens appear to be reasonably well tolerated, but they have not had substantial impacts on the outcome in patients with adverse features such as stem cell phenotype (CD34+) or poor-risk cytogenetics. In relapsed elderly patients, modest activity (28% CR, median survival 4 months) and moderate toxicity has been noted in a trial of continuous-infusion daunorubicin and carboplatin (204). On the higher end of the dosing scale, high-dose mitoxantrone plus HiDAC has been shown to be

Table 21 Newer Induction Regimens for AML in the Elderly

N	Regimen	CR (%)	Survival	Reference
28	High-dose mitoxantrone + HiDAC		9	205
67	Mitoxantrone + etoposide	55	9.2	203
112	Fludarabine + ara-C ± G-CSF	53–63[a]		176
39	Continuous-infusion daunorubicin + carboplatin	28[b]	4	204
29	Low-dose ara-C, hydroxyurea + calcitrol	45[c]	12	201

AML, acute myelocytic leukemia; HiDAC, high-dose acytosine arabinose; ara = c, acytosine arabinose; G-CSF, granulocyte colony-stimulating factor, MDS, myelodysplastic syndrome.
[a] Includes patients with high-risk MDS.
[b] Limited to prior treated and secondary AML.
[c] Includes antecedent MDS.

tolerable in older patients (205). HiDAC in that regimen is given once daily for 5 days, with the mitoxantrone given as a single large dose of 80 mg/m^2. No further therapy was given in that regimen, with survival outcomes being similar to those seen in studies including postremission therapy. Such an approach may offer a better quality of life with less impatient care.

Many studies have evaluated the role of hematopoietic growth factors in reducing toxicity related to induction therapy and evaluating the impact of these factors on relevant remission and survival endpoints. Both G-CSF and GM-CSF have been used before, during, and after remission induction therapy in patients in all age groups (reviewed in Ref. 206). In older patients, it appears that both growth factors can reduce days of neutropenia. Almost all studies fail to show major improvements in the CR incidence, and only one (207) showed a modest survival advantage. Attempts to take clinical advantage of the observation that the percentage of blasts in S phase may be increased by treatment with myeloid growth factors by concurrent administration of growth factors and cell cycle–active agents have been negative. Most clinical trials have not shown that available myeloid growth factors can foster deleterious effects by stimulating blast proliferation. On the other hand, the only positive trial of a myeloid growth factor in previously untreated older patients with AML required demonstration of marrow aplasia prior to initiating therapy with GM-CSF (207), unlike a comparable negative trial in which GM-CSF was started prior to performing the first postinduction bone marrow (208). However, the two trials utilized different GM-CSF preparations, further clouding any comparisons.

How best to maintain remission once it occurs remains open to question and represents a major area for future advances. The favorable effects of HiDAC consolidation in patients with good-risk cytogenetics (209) are largely outweighed by the significant toxicity of this therapy in the elderly, and transplantation approaches are generally limited to patients under the age of 70 years. The CALGB comparison favoring HiDAC over lower doses of ara-C (100 and 400 mg/m^2) as postremission therapy does not settle the question of whether a HiDAC regimen in the 1- to 2 g/m^2 range offers similar efficacy with reduced toxicity. Such a regimen has not been evaluated as postremission therapy in older patients with the good-risk karyotypes that respond favorably to 3 g/m^2 HiDAC regimens.

Ongoing areas of investigation include attempts to improve available remission induction treatments by overcoming intrinsic drug resistance mediated by p-glycoprotein and to reduce the toxicity and increase the efficacy of postremission therapies by exploring the utility of biological therapies (Table 22).

2. Acute Lymphoblastic Leukemia

Acute lymphoblastic leukemia (ALL) has a bimodal distribution with an early childhood peak followed by a marked increase after the age of 60 years, with the elderly predominating among adults with this diagnosis (210). Overall, the disease is quite rare, with an incidence of 1 per 100,000 in adults over age 60 years old (211).

Table 22 Novel Approaches to Treatment of AML in the Elderly

Therapy	Rationale	Example	Reference
MDR-1 modulation	Increase intracellular retention of natural products: anthracyclines, epidophyllotoxins	PSC-833	256
Monoclonal antibodies	Potentially non–cross resistant, less toxic, and specific means of targeting leukemia, either with native or radiolabeled antibodies	M195	257
Cytokines	Stimulate cellular cytotoxicity (natural or lymphokine-activated killer cells, cytotoxic T cells).	Interleukin-2	258

Despite treatment programs that are generally associated with less acute toxicity than those used to treat AML, prolonged disease-free survival for elderly patients with ALL is rare. Perhaps even more powerfully than in AML, biological features override all other considerations with respect to dictating treatment outcome. Most important among these biological features is that Philadelphia chromosome–positive ALL, which is uniformly incurable using conventional chemotherapy, may account for almost half of the cases of ALL in patients over 50 years old (212). Furthermore, t(4;11), another poor-risk karyotype, is more common in the elderly with ALL than in younger patients (212), and the poorer risk B-cell phenotype more and the favorable T-cell phenotype less common (211). Adverse prognostic factors in adult ALL are listed in Table 23.

Two large intensive multidrug combination chemotherapy programs centered on induction therapy with cyclophosphamide, an anthracycline, vincristine, and prednisone with (213) and without (214) 1-asparaginase have treated substantial numbers of adults, but less than 10% of the treated patients were over 60 years old. For the small number of reported elderly patients, the CR rates were 39 and 58%, respectively, and the remission durations and survivals were very brief. In both

Table 23 Adverse Prognostic Factors in Adult ALL

Age
Cytogenetics: t(9;22), t(8;14), t(2;8), t(8;22), t(4;11)
Absence of mediastinal mass
L3 (Burkitt's) morphology/mature B phenotype
High white blood cell count
Failure to achieve CR by day 28

ALL, acute lymphocytic leukemia.

series, the probability of survival beyond 3 years in CR patients was less than 20%. Elderly patients with ALL receiving an intensive induction chemotherapy regimen did have a significant reduction in therapy-related mortality with the introduction of G-CSF (215). An infusional regimen of vincristine, doxorubicin, and dexamethasone (VAD) has not substantially improved upon these results (216).

Given these dismal results, strategies need to be developed to overcome the drug resistance which the poor-risk karyotypes confer. Agents aimed at overcoming MDR-mediated mechanisms of resistance may be less effective in ALL than AML because of the relatively reduced expression of p-glycoprotein in ALL (217). Younger patients with the poor-risk karyotypes are being offered transplantation, an impossibility for the elderly patients with ALL. A theoretically more promising and attractive approach involves the use of monoclonal antibodies, which may impact on minimal residual disease with substantially reduced toxicity as compared with cytotoxic therapies. An initial attempt to eliminate minimal residual disease in ALL using the murine anti-CD19 immunotoxin anti-B4–blocked ricin and molecular monitoring showed no consistent benefit (218). Modest clinical effects were seen in a refractory group of ALL patients treated with the anti-CD52 humanized monoclonal CAMPATH-1H (219). These approaches will continue to amplify and hopefully bear fruit as newer biologics enter clinical trials.

C. Chronic Lymphocytic Leukemia

Chronic lymphocytic leukemia (CLL) is the most common leukemia in adults in the United States and most of western Europe. It accounts for approximately 30% of all leukemias. The median age at diagnosis is 65–70 years, and it is rarely seen before the age of 35 years. There is a male to female ratio of 2:1. There has been a trend toward a higher median age at diagnosis in recent years, particularly among patients with early-stage disease (220). Therefore, there will be an increased number of patients with this disorder owing to the aging of the population (221).

There is no known etiology for CLL; however, some factors have been associated. There is a high familial risk, with family members having a two to seven times risk of developing the disease. There is no known association with exposure to radiation, alkylating agents, or leukemogenic chemicals (221).

1. Laboratory Features

CLL is characterized by marked lymphocytosis with a mean value of $30-50 \times 10^9/L$. The lymphocytes are small and mature with little cytoplasm and clumped chromatin. Some larger nucleolated cells, which may represent prolymphocytes, may be seen, but should compromise no more than 10% of the cells. The diagnostic criteria have been established by the National Cancer Institute–Sponsored Working Group (NCI–WG) (Tables 24 and 25) (222).

Table 24   NCI–WG Diagnostic Criteria of CLL

Absolute lymphocytosis consisting of mature appearing cells of at least 5000/mm³
Phenotypes of the lymphocytes should reveal:
  1. Predominance of B cells which are CD19⁺, CD20⁺, CD23⁺, and CD5⁺
  2. Monoclonality with respect to either κ or λ
  3. Low-density surface immunoglobulin expression
Bone marrow evaluation:
  1. Not an absolute necessity if the above criteria are met
  2. More necessary when the absolute lymphocyte count is relatively low
  3. Bone marrow aspirate must show ≥30% of all nucleated cells to be lymphoid with
       normal cellularity or hypercellularity
  4. Pattern of lymphoid infiltration in bone marrow biopsy has prognostic importance:
       a. diffuse involvement correlates with progressive or advanced disease
       b. nondiffuse (nodular or interstitial) patterns predict better response

NCI–WG, National Cancer Institute Working Group; CLL, chronic lymphocytic leukemia.
Source: Ref. 222.

2.   Differential Diagnosis

There are other chronic lymphoproliferative disorders which can be similar in presentation and morphology to CLL. Prolymphocytic leukemia has >55% prolymphocytes in the peripheral blood smear and/or greater than 15,000/mm³ absolute count of prolymphocytes. These lymphocytes are CD5⁻ in approximately 50% of cases and usually are bright staining surface immunoglobulin. Mantle cell lymphoma in the leukemia phase has cells which are CD5⁺ but are CD23⁻. The lymph node architecture is characteristic of this disorder. The other chronic disorders include hairy cell leukemia, splenic lymphoma with villous lymphocytes, large granular lymphocytosis, Sézary cell leukemia, leukemic phase of follicular center cell lymphoma, and adult T-cell leukemia/lymphoma (223).

Table 25   Diagnostic Criteria for CLL According to the National Cancer Institute (NCI) and International Workshop on CLL (IWCLL)

Cells	NCI	IWCLL
Lymphocytes	≥5 × 10⁹/L + ≥ 1 B-cell marker (CD19, CD20, CD23)	≥10 × 10⁹/L + B-phenotype or bone marrow involvement
Atypical cells	<55%	—
Bone marrow lymphocytes	≥30%	>30%

CLL, chronic lymphocytic leukemia.
Source: Ref. 221.

Table 26   Staging System for CLL

Rai stage	Modified Rai stage	Clinical characteristics	Median survival (yr)
0	Low	Lymphocytosis in peripheral blood and bone marrow only	>10
I	Intermediate	Lymphocytosis and enlarged nodes	6
II		Lymphocytosis and enlarged spleen and/or liver	
III	High	Lymphocytosis and anemia (Hgb <10 g/dL)	2
IV		Lymphocytosis and thrombocytopenia (platelets <100 × 10^9/L)	

CLL, chronic lymphocytic leukemia.
Source: Ref. 221.

3. Staging

The two most common and valuable staging systems for CLL are those of Rai and Binet (Tables 26 and 27). The NCI-WG recommends modification of the five-stage Rai system by using the three-risk group (see Table 25) (222, 223). In addition, the low and high β$_2$-microglobulin levels are associated with good- and poor-survival times, respectively (224). The lymphocyte doubling time (longer than 1 year is better) and bone marrow biopsy lymphocytic infiltration patterns are also important predictors (225). There are very good-prognosis patients who are in the low-risk, or Binet A, groups who may be classified as smoldering CLL. This includes a blood lymphocyte count of less than 30,000/mm^3, lymphocyte doubling time of greater than 12 months, hemoglobin >12g%, and bone marrow biopsy showing a nondiffuse lymphocytic infiltration pattern (223, 226).

Table 27   Binet System for CLL

Binet stage	Clinical characteristics	Median survival (yr)
A	Hemoglobin ≥10 g/dL, platelets ≥100 × 10^9/L, and <3 areas involved	>1
B	Hemoglobin ≥10 g/dL, platelets ≥100 × 10^9/L, and ≥3 areas involved	6
C	Hemoglobin <10 g/dL, platelets <100 × 10^9/L, or both (independent of areas involved)	2

CLL, chronic lymphocytic leukemia.
Source: Ref. 221.

4. Treatment

The NCI–WG recommends initiating therapy for CLL if criteria of active disease are met (222, 223). These criteria include the presence of disease-related symptoms (weight loss, fatigue, poor performance score, fever without infection, or night sweats), progressive anemia or thrombocytopenia, autoimmune anemia or thrombocytopenia not responding to corticosteroids, massively enlarged nodes or spleen, progressive or rapid rate of increase in blood lymphocyte count, and repeated infections with or without hypogammaglobulinemia.

Radiation to an enlarged spleen and bulky lymphadenopathy may also help selected patients with CLL. Splenectomy may be reasonable when the spleen is enlarged and there is evidence of hypersplenism, particularly if chemotherapy and/ or radiation therapy has not been effective (227).

The standard treatment of CLL has been chlorambucil (228). The drug is most commonly used on an intermittent schedule with a single dose of 0.4 mg/kg every 2 weeks. There are, however, many variations on this. The response rate to single-agent therapy is approximately 75% with two thirds of patients responding to second and subsequent courses. Cyclophosphamide has been also used as a single agent, but it is more commonly incorporated in combination with vincristine and prednisone. The response rates to this combination (CVP) has varied from 44 to 77%, with higher response rates in previously untreated patients. Many regimens combine chlorambucil with prednisone (228, 229). However, there are dangers to prolonged corticosteroid therapy, particularly in the elderly. Corticosteroids are used for the treatment of autoimmune phenomena such as autoimmune thrombocytopenia and hemolytic anemia. No survival advantage is seen with any one permutation of the scheduling of chlorambucil and/or the addition of corticosteroids.

There have been trials comparing chlorambucil to combination regimens in CLL, particularly CVP (230). In one study, no significant difference in survival was observed with median values of 4.8 years for chlorambucil and prednisone and 3.9 years for CVP. Median survival for the Rai stage III and IV patients was 4.1 years. There is some question whether an increased dose intensity of chlorambucil is associated with a prolonged survival (228).

In the French Cooperative Group, Binet stage A patients were randomized to immediate versus delayed continuous oral chlorambucil. Survival was slightly higher in the delayed-treatment group. Other studies have shown no survival advantage for immediate treatment. In Binet stage B, there was no difference when oral chlorambucil was compared to CVP. The median survival was 5 years. There is some data that anthracyclines may improve survival (231–234). However, some of these studies have been criticized, and multiagent regimens containing anthracyclines have not been frequently utilized (228).

a. Nucleoside Analogues

Fludarabine is a fluorinated derivative of 9-β-arabinofuranosyladenine (ara-A) which is relatively resistant to rapid deamination by adenosine deaminase. This compound, 9-β-arabinofuranosyl-2-fluoroadenine monophosphate (F-araAMP, fludara-bine) also has improved aqueous solubility (235). It has shown significant activity in low-grade lymphoproliferative malignancies, including chronic lymphocytic leu-kemia, Waldenström's macroglobulinemia, hairy cell leukemia, and non–Hodgkin's lymphoma (27, 236). Its response rate of up to 80% in previously untreated patients make it the most active drug in CLL (237). The addition of prednisone does not improve the response rate but is associated with an increased incidence of opportu-nistic infections, including *Pneumocystis carinii* pneumonia and *Listeria* sepsis or meningitis (238–241). This complication is partially due to the suppression of the CD4 lymphocytes. With therapy, CD4 levels were uniformly depressed from a me-dian 1015/μL pretreatment to a median 159/μL after 3 months of fludarabine therapy (239). Fludarabine has also been associated with an increased incidence of autoim-mune hemolytic anemia. The cause of autoimmune phenomena in CLL is not known, but some findings reinforce the view that they are caused by a disturbance in immu-noregulatory T cells (242–244).

Other nucleoside analogues have activity in CLL. Cladribine (2-chlorodeoxya-denosine, 2-CDA) is active at doses of 0.1 mg/kg/day for 7 days (221). The clinical experience with 2-CDA in CLL is limited, but the preliminary results suggest a similar efficacy as FAMP, whereas DCF (pentostatin; 2′-deoxycoformycin) seems to be less effective (221, 245, 246). Whether FAMP-treated patients have any advan-tage for overall or progression-free survival has to be answered by ongoing random-ized trials. Presently, the position of FAMP and 2-CDA as two extremely active single agents in CLL is that of second-line therapy. Their appropriate indication in the first-line strategy of CLL has, however, still to be defined.

Although fludarabine is being increasingly used as front-line treatment for CLL, its efficacy has only been proven as a second-line agent after oral alkylating drugs. A study of the Cancer and Leukemia Group B has shown a higher complete response and longer duration of remission and progression-free survival of fludara-bine as a compared to chlorambucil. There is no evidence of significant improvement in survival.

The efficacy of fludarabine as initial therapy for CLL has been demonstrated in a large cooperative group study which randomly assigned patients to therapy with fludarabine versus pulse chlorambucil (247). A third arm which combined fludara-bine and chlorambucil was closed, because it was associated with unacceptable he-matological toxicity and was not more effective than fludarabine alone (248). A significantly higher response incidence (70% vs 43%) and duration (33 vs 17 months) was seen in patients receiving fludarabine. Progression-free survival was also significantly better in the fludarabine arm. Because the study had a crossover design, no conclusions can be drawn regarding overall survival, which was similar in both arms. As a result, the strongest inference that can be drawn is that initial therapy with fludarabine is clearly associated with a superior initial outcome. Planned studies will address the question as to whether the addition of a monoclonal antibody variably reactive with CLL cells (Rituximab) can enhance the efficacy of fludarabine in previously untreated patients.

In deciding which therapy to use in elderly patients with CLL, there are a number of issues to considered. In early-stage patients, a period of observation is warranted (227). Chlorambucil is a safe initial treatment option for most patients. The combination of other drugs must be assessed on an individual basis. Prednisone may have significant complications in the elderly. It can exacerbate diabetes mellitus, osteoporosis, and cataracts. They may also manifest neuropsychiatric disturbances while on corticosteroids. The drug may also increase the risk of infection, particularly opportunistic infection. Vincristine neuropathy is particularly disabling in an elderly person. It may affect gait and motor function. Fludarabine can be used, but the risks of opportunistic infection must be considered and the use of prophylactic antifungal and antipneumocystis treatments should be administered. Growth factors and erythropoietin may be particularly beneficial to avoid treatment complications. CLL is not a curable disease, but patients can be maintained with an adequate quality of life with the appropriate use of drug therapy (227).

REFERENCES

1. Skarin AT, Dorfman DM. Non-Hodgkin's lymphomas: current classification and management. CA Cancer J Clin 1997; 47:351–372.
2. Shipp MA, Mauch PM, Harris NL. Non-Hodgkin's Lymphoma. In: DeVita VT Jr, Hellman S, Rosenberg SA, eds. Cancer: Principles and Practice of Oncology. Vol 1. 5th ed. Philadelphia: Lippincott, 1997; 2165–2219.
3. Preti A, Cabanillas F. Lymphoma in the elderly. Cancer Bull 1995; 47:192–196.
4. Devesa SS, Fears T. Non-Hodgkin's lymphoma time trends: United States and international data. Cancer Res 1992; 52:5432–5440.
5. Cesarman E, Chang Y, Moore PS, Said JW, Knowles DM. Kaposi's sarcoma-associated herpesvirus-like DNA sequences in AIDS-related body-cavity-based lymphomas. N Engl J Med 1995; 332:1186–1191.
6. Wang CY, Snow JL, Su WP. Lymphoma associated with human immunodeficiency virus infection. Mayo Clin Proc 1995; 70:665–672.
7. Penn I, Porat G. Central nervous system lymphomas in organ allograft recipients. Transplantation 1995; 59:240–244.
8. Penn I. The problem of cancer in organ transplant recipients: an overview. Transplant Sci 1994; 4:23–32.
9. Penn I. Cancers complicating organ transplantation. N Engl J Med 1990; 323:1767–1769.
10. Parsonnet J. Helicobacter pylori in the stomach—a paradox unmasked. N Engl J Med 1996; 335:278–280.
11. Weisenburger DD. Epidemiology of non-Hodgkin's lymphoma: recent findings regarding an emerging epidemic. Ann Oncol 1994; 5(suppl):519–524.
12. Molina A, Pezner RD. Non-Hodgkin's lymphoma. In: Pazdur R, Coia LR, Hoskins WJ, Wagman LD, eds. Cancer Management: A Multidisciplinary Approach. Huntington, NY: PRR, 1996: 226–256.
13. The Non-Hodgkin's Lymphoma Pathologic Classification Project. National Cancer Institute sponsored study of classifications of non-Hodgkin's lymphomas: summary

and description of a working formulation for clinical usage. Cancer 1982; 49:2112–2135.

14. Harris NL, Jaffe ES, Stein H, Banks PM, Chan JK, Cleary ML, Delsol G, De Wolf-Peeters C, Falini B, Gatter KC, et al. A revised European-American classification of lymphoid neoplasms: a proposal from the International Lymphoma Study Group. Blood 1994; 84:1361–1392.

15. Vose JM, Armitage JO, Weisenburger DD, Bierman PJ, Sorensen S, Hutchins M, Moravec DF, Howe D, Dowling MD, Mailliard J, et al. The importance of age in survival of patients treated with chemotherapy for aggressive non-Hodgkin's lymphoma. J Clin Oncol 1988; 6:1838–1844.

16. Dixon DO, Neilan B, Jones S, Lipschitz DA, Miller TP, Grozea PN, Wilson HE. Effect of age on therapeutic outcome in advanced diffuse histocytic lymphoma: the Southwest Oncology Group experience. J Clin Oncol 1986; 4:295–305.

17. A predictive model for aggressive non-Hodgkin's lymphoma. The International Non-Hodgkin's Lymphoma Prognostic Factors Project. N Engl J Med 1993; 329:987–994.

18. Shipp MA. Prognostic factors in aggressive non-Hodgkin's lymphoma: who has "high risk" disease? Blood 1994; 83:1165–1173.

19. Hermans J, Krol AD, van Groningen K, Kluin PM, Kluin-Nelemans JC, Kramer MH, Noordijk EM, Ong F, Wijermans PW. International Prognostic Index for aggressive non-Hodgkin's lymphoma is valid for all malignancy grades. Blood 1995; 86:1460–1463.

20. Bastion Y, Berger F, Bryon PA, Felman P, Ffrench M, Coiffier B. Follicular Lymphomas: assessment of prognostic factors in 127 patients followed for 10 years. Ann Oncol 1991; 2:123–129.

21. Carbone A, Franceschi S, Gloghini A, Russo A, Gaidano G, Monfardini S. Pathological and immunophenotypic features of adult non-Hodgkin's lymphomas by age group. Hum Pathol 1997; 28:580–587.

22. MacManus MP, Hoppe RT. Is radiotherapy curative for stage I and II low-grade follicular lymphoma? Results of a long-term follow-up study of patients treated at Stanford University. J Clin Oncol 1996; 14:1281–1290.

23. Yahalom J, Varsos G, Fuks Z, Myers J, Clarkson BD, Straus DJ. Adjuvant cyclophosphamide, doxorubicin, vincristine, and prednisone chemotherapy after radiation therapy in stage I low-grade and intermediate-grade non-Hodgkin lymphoma. Results of a prospective randomized study. Cancer 1993; 71:2342–2350.

24. Lister Ta. The management of follicular lymphoma. Ann Oncol 1991; 2:131–135.

25. Rosenberg SA. Karnofsky memorial lecture. The low-grade non-Hodgkin's lymphomas: challenges and opportunities. J Clin Oncol 1985; 3:299–310.

26. Hoppe R. The role of radiation therapy in the management of the non-Hodgkin's lymphomas. Cancer 1985; 55:2176.

27. Chun HG, Leyland-Jones B, Cheson BD. Fludarabine phosphate: a synthetic purine antimetabolite with significant activity against lymphoid malignancies. J Clin Oncol 1991; 9:175–188.

28. Cheson BD. The purine analogs—a therapeutic beauty contest (editorial). J Clin Oncol 1992; 10:868–87 (corrected and republished editorial originally printed in J Clin Oncol 1992; 10:352–355.)

29. Grossbard ML, Nadler LM. Monoclonal antibody therapy for indolent lymphomas. Semin Oncol 1993; 20:118–135.

30. Davis TA, Maloney DG, Liles TM, Czerwinski D, Levy R. Long-term remissions in patients treated with anti-idiotype monoclonal antibodies for non-Hodgkin's lymphoma (meeting abstract). Proc Annu Meet Am Soc Clin Oncol 1996; (abstr. 1383), 15.

31. Grillo-Lopez AJ, Maloney DG, Bodkinu D, Schilder RI, White C, Foon K, Janakiraman N, Neidhart J, Rosenberg J, Shen CD, et al. IDEC-C2B8: initial phase II results in patients with B-cell lymphoma (meeting abstract). Ninth Annual Scientific Meeting of the Society for Biological Therapy: Biological Therapy of Cancer IX, October 1995, Napa, California.

32. White CA, Grillo-Lopez AJ, Maloney D, Bodkin D, Schilder R, Foon K, Neidhart J, Janakiraman N, Dallaire B, Shen D, et al. IDEC-C2B8: Improved tolerance correlated with pharmacodynamic effects in patients with B-cell NHL (meeting abstract). Proc Annu Meet Am Assoc Cancer Res 1995; (abstr. 3799), 36.

33. Grillo-Lopez AJ, Maloney DG, Bodkin D, Schilder RI, White C, Foon K, Janakiraman N, Neidhart J, Rosenberg J, Shen CD, et al. IDEC-C2B8: initial phase II results in patients with B-cell lymphoma (meeting abstract). J Immunother 1994; 16.

34. Glick JH, Kim K, Earle J, O'Connell MJ. An ECOG randomized Phase III trial of CHOP vs CHOP + radiotherapy (XRT) for intermediate grade early stage non-Hodgkins's lymphoma (NHL) (meeting abstract). Proc Annu Meet Am Soc Clin Oncol 1995; 14.

35. Shipp MA, Harrington DP, Klatt MM, et al. Identification of major prognostic subgroups of patients with large cell lymphoma treated with m-BACOD or M-BACOD. Ann Intern Med 1986; 104:757–765.

36. Fisher RI, DeVita DT, Hubbard SM, et al. Randomized trial of ProMACE-MOPP vs. ProMACE-CytaBOM in previously untreated, advanced stage, diffuse aggressive lymphomas. Proc Annu Meet Am Soc Clin Oncol 1984; 3:242.

37. Klimo P, Connors JM. MACOP-B chemotherapy for the treatment of diffuse large-cell lymphoma. Ann Intern Med 1985; 102:596–602.

38. Sonneveld P, de Ridder M, van der Lelie H, Nieuwenhuis K, Schouten H, Mulder A, van Reijswould I, Hop W, Lowenberg B. Comparison of doxorubicin and mitoxantrone in the treatment of elderly patients with advanced diffuse non-Hodgkin's lymphoma using CHOP versus CNOP chemotherapy. J Clin Oncol 1995; 13:2530–2539.

39. Bastion Y, Blay JY, Divine M, Brice P, Bordessoule D, Sebban C, Blanc M, Tilly H, Lederlin P, Deconinck E, et al. Elderly patients with aggressive non-Hodgkin's lymphoma: disease presentation, response to treatment, and survival—a Groupe d'Etude des Lymphomes de l'Adulte study on 453 patients older than 69 years. J Clin Oncol 1997; 15:2945–2953.

40. Meyer RM, Browman GP, Samosh ML, et al. Randomized phase II comparison of standard CHOP with weekly CHOP in elderly patients with non-Hodgkin's lymphoma. J Clin Oncol 1995; 13:2386–2393.

41. Tirelli U, Carbone A, Zagonel V, Veronesi A, Canetta R. Non-Hodgkin's lymphomas in the elderly: prospective studies with specifically devised chemotherapy regimens in 66 patients. Eur J Cancer Clin Oncol 1987; 23:535–540.

42. Tirelli U, Carbone A, Zagonel V, Veronesi A, Canetta R. Non-Hodgkin's lymphomas in the elderly: prospective studies with specifically devised chemotherapy regimens in 66 patients. Eur J Cancer Clin Oncol 1987; 23:535–540.

43. Sonneveld P, Michiels JJ. Full dose chemotherapy in elderly patients with non-Hodgkin's lymphoma: a feasibility study using a mitoxantrone containing regimen. Br J Cancer 1990; 62:105–108.

44. Zagonel V, Tirelli U, Carbone A, Errante D, Morassot S, Sorio R, Monfardini S. Combination chemotherapy specifically devised for elderly patients with unfavorable non-Hodgkin's lymphoma. Cancer Invest 1990; 8:577–582.

45. O'Reilly SE, Klimo P, Connors JM. Low-dose ACOP-B and VABE: Weekly chemotherapy for elderly patients with advanced-stage diffuse large-cell lymphoma. J Clin Oncol 1991; 9:741–747.

46. Tirelli U, Zagonel V, Errante D, Serraino D, Talamini R, DeCicco M, Carbone A, Monfardini S. A prospective study of a new combination chemotherapy regimen in patients older than 70 years with unfavorable non-Hodgkin's lymphoma. J Clin Oncol 1992; 10:228–236.

47. Salvagno L, Contu A, Bianco A, Endrizzi L, Schintu GM, Olmeo N, Aversa SML, Chiarion-Sileni V, Soraru M, Fiorentino MV. A combination of mitoxantrone, etoposide and prednisone in elderly patients with non-Hodgkin's lymphoma. Ann Oncol 1992; 3:833–837.

48. Inanc SE, Onat H. Brief weekly chemotherapy for elderly patients with intermediate-grade or high-grade non-Hodgkin's lymphoma. J Natl Cancer Inst 1993; 85:1088–1089.

49. Caracciolo F, Petrini M, Capochiani F, Papineschi F, Grassi B. Third generation chemotherapy with P-VABEC for aggressive non-Hodgkin's lymphoma of the elderly. Leuk Lymphoma 1993; 11:115–118.

50. Liang R, Todd D, Chan TK, Chiu E, Lie A, Ho F. COPP chemotherapy for elderly patients with intermediate and high grade non-Hodgkin's lymphoma. Hematol Oncol 1993; 11:43–50.

51. Martelli M, Guglielmi C, Coluzzi S, Avvisati G, Amadori S, Giovannini M, Torromeo C, Mandelli F. P-VABEC: a prospective study of a new weekly chemotherapy regimen for elderly aggressive non-Hodgkin's lymphoma. J Clin Oncol 1993; 11: 2362–2369.

52. O'Reilly SE, Connors JM, Howdle S, Hoskins P, Klasa R, Klimo P, Stuart DS. In search of an optimal regimen for elderly patients with advanced-stage diffuse large-cell lymphoma: results of a phase II study of P/DOCE chemotherapy. J Clin Oncol 1993; 11:2250–2257.

53. Young WA, Greco FA, Greer JP, Hainsworth JD. Aggressive non-Hodgkin's lymphoma in the elderly: treatment regimen containing extended-schedule etoposide. J Natl Cancer Inst 1994; 86:1346–1347.

54. Bessell EM, Coutts A, Fletcher J, Toghill PJ, Moloney AJ, Ellis IO, Hulman G, Jenkins D. Non-Hodgkin's lymphoma in elderly patients: a phase II study of MCOP chemotherapy in patients aged 70 years or over with intermediate- or high-grade histology. Eur J Cancer 1994; 9:1337–1341.

55. Goss PE, Burkes R, Rudinskas L, King M, Chow W, Myers R, Davidson M, Poldre P, Crump M, Sutton D, et al. Prednisone, oral etoposide, and novantrone for treatment of non-Hodgkin's lymphoma: a preliminary report. Semin Hematol 1994; 31:23–29.

56. Bertini M, Freilone R, Vitolo U, Botto B, Pizzuti M, Gavarotti P, Levis A, Orlandi E, Orsucci L, Pini M, et al. P-VEBEC: a new 8-weekly schedule with or without rG-CSF

for elderly patients with aggressive non-Hodgkin's lymphoma (NHL). Ann Oncol 1994; 5:895–900.

57. Caracciolo F, Petrini M, Capochiani E, Papineschi F, Carulli G, Grassi B. Alternating chemotherapy regimen (P-VABEC) for intermediate and high-grade non-Hodgkin's lymphoma of the middle aged and elderly. Hematol Oncol 1994; 12:185–192.

58. Epelbaum R, Haim N, Leviov M, Ben-Shahar M, Ben-Arie Y, Dror Y, Faraggi D. Full dose CHOP chemotherapy in elderly patients with non-Hodgkin's lymphoma. Acta Oncol 1995; 34:87–91.

59. Novitzky N, King HS, Johnson C, Jacobs P. Treatment of aggressive non-Hodgkin's lymphoma in the elderly. Am J Hematol 1995; 49:103–108.

60. Goss P, Burkes R, Rudinskas L, King M, Chow W, Myers R, Davidson M, Poldre P, Crump M, Sutton D, et al. A phase II trial of prednisone, oral etoposide, and novantrone (PEN) as initial treatment of non-Hodgkin's lymphoma in elderly patients. Leuk Lymphoma 1995; 18:145–152.

61. Coiffier B, Biron P, Bastion Y, Haioun C, Bordessoulle D, Sebban C, Blanc M, Tilly H, Salles B, Bouabdallah R, et al. Elderly lymphoma patients have a long survival if treated with curative intent. A study from the G.E.L.A. on 453 patients older than 69 years (abstract 1279). Proc Annu Meet Am Soc Clin Oncol 1996; 417.

62. Niitsu N, Umeda M. Evaluation of long-term daily administration of oral low-dose etoposide in elderly patients with relapsing or refractory non-Hodgkin's lymphoma. Am J Clin Oncol 1997; 20:311–314.

63. Lichtman SM, Fusco D, Kolitz J, et al. Treatment of elderly patients with intermediate and high grade non-Hodgkin's lymphoma. A trial of thiotepa, Novantrone (mitoxantrone), Oncovin and prednisone (T-NOP). Blood 1994; 84(suppl 1):643a.

64. O'Reilly S, Connors JM, Macpherson N, Klasa R, Hoskins P. Malignant lymphomas in the elderly. Clin Geriatr Med 1997; 13:251–263.

65. Lichtman SM. Lymphoma in the older patient. Semin Oncol 1995; 22:25–28.

66. Vose JM. The effect of age on bone marrow transplantation (meeting abstract). Third International Conference: Clinical Application of Cytokinin and Growth Factors in Hematology of Oncology, 1995; Atlanta, GA, p 46.

67. Fields KK, Ballester OF, Goldstein SC, Hiemenz JW, Perkins JB, Machesney LD, Elfenbein GJ. Age effects in patients undergoing autologous bone marrow or peripheral blood stem cell transplantation (meeting abstract). Proc Annu Meet Am Soc Clin Oncol 1996; 1621A.

68. Miller CB, Piantadosi S, Vogelsang GB, Marcellus DC, Grochow L, Kennedy MJ, Jones RJ. Impact of age on outcome of patients with cancer undergoing autologous bone marrow transplant. J Clin Oncol 1996; 14:1327–1332.

69. Stewart D, Bierman P, Anderson J, Vose J, Bishop M, Pierson J, Kessinger A, Armitage J. High dose chemotherapy (HDC) with autologous hematopoietic rescue in patients (pts) age 60 and over (meeting abstract). Proc Annu Meet Am Soc Clin Oncol 1994; A1260.

70. Berkahn LC, Simpson DR, Stewart AK, Crump M, Keating A. Hematopoiesis in the elderly: age is no obstacle to the collection of an adequate autograft. San Diego: American Society of Hematology, 1997; 90(10; Suppl 1).

71. Keating A. The hematopoietic stem cell in elderly patients with leukemia. Leukemia 1996; 10.

72. Kusnierz-Glaz CR, Schlegel PG, Wong RM, Schriber JR, Chao NJ, Amylon MD,

Hu WW, Negrin RS, Lee Y, Blume KG, et al. Influence of age on the outcome of 500 autologous bone marrow transplant procedures for hematologic malignancies. J Clin Oncol 1997; 15:18–25.

73. Deangelis LM. Current management of primary central nervous system lymphoma. Oncology 1995; 9:63–71.

74. Phuphanich S, Werner M, Lyman G. Increasing incidence of primary central nervous system lymphoma (PCNSL) in the elderly: Florida Cancer Data Systems (FCDS) Proc Annu Meet Am Soc Clin Oncol (meeting abstract). 1995; 14:A421.

75. Williams CK. Primary central nervous system lymphoma (PCNSL) in Saskatchewan (SK): A 30-year trend (meeting abstract). Proc Annu Meet Am Soc Clin Oncol 1994.

76. Forsyth PA, DeAngelis LM. Biology and management of AIDS-associated primary CNS lymphomas. Hematol Oncol Clin North Am 1996; 10:1125–1134.

77. Krogh-Jensen M, d'Amore F, Jensen MK, Christensen BE, Thorling K, Pedersen M, Johansen P, Boesen AM, Andersen E. Incidence, clinicopathological features and outcome of primary central nervous system lymphomas. Population-based data from a Danish lymphoma registry. Danish Lymphoma Study Group, LYFO. Ann Oncol 1994; 5:349–354.

78. DeAngelis LM, Yahalom J. Primary central nervous system lymphoma. In: DeVita VT Jr, Hellman S, Rosenberg SA, eds. Cancer: Principles and Practice of Oncology. Vol 1. 5th ed. Philadelphia: Lippincott, 1997; 2233–2242.

79. Nelson DF, Martz KL, Bonner H, Nelson JS, Newall J, Kerman HD, Thomson JW, Murray KJ. Non-Hodgkin's lymphoma of the brain: can high dose, large volume radiation therapy improve survival? Report on a prospective trial by the radiation therapy oncology group: RTOG 8315. Int J Radiat Oncol Biol Phys 1992; 23:9–17.

80. DeAngelis LM, Kreis W, Chan K, Dantis E, Akerman S. Pharmacokinetics of Ara-C and Ara-U In Plasma and Csf after high-dose administration of cytosine arabinoside. Cancer Chemother Pharmacol 1992; 29:173–177.

81. Kreis W, Lesser M, Budman DR, Arlin Z, DeAngelis L, Baskind P, Feldman EJ, Akerman S. Phenotypic Analysis of 1-B-D-arabinofuranosylcytosine deamination in patients treated with high doses and correlation with response. Cancer Chemother Pharmacol 1992; 30:126–130.

82. Freilich RJ, Delattre JY, Monjour A, DeAngelis LM. Chemotherapy without radiation therapy as initial treatment for primary CNS lymphoma in older patients. Neurology 1996; 46:435–439.

83. Weisenburger DD, Armitage JO. Mantle cell lymphoma—an entity comes of age. Blood 1996; 87:4483–4494.

84. Majlis A, Pugh WC, Rodriguez MA, Benedict WF, Cabanillas F. Mantle cell lymphoma: correlation of clinical outcome and biologic features with three histologic variants. J Clin Oncol 1997; 15:1664–1671.

85. Thieblemont C, Bastion Y, Berger F, Rieux C, Salles G, Dumontet C, Felman P, Coiffier B. Mucosa-associated lymphoid tissue gastrointestinal and nongastrointestinal lymphoma behavior: analysis of 108 patients. J Clin Oncol 1997; 15:1624–1630.

86. Parker SL, Tong T, Bolden S, Wingo PA. Cancer Statistics, 1997. CA Cancer J Clin 1997; 47:5–27.

87. DeVita VT, Jr, Mauch PM, Harris NL. Hodgkin's disease. In: DeVita VT Jr, Hellman S, Rosenberg SA, eds. Cancer: Principles and Practice of Oncology. Vol 1. 5th ed. Philadelphia: Lippincott, 1997; 2242–2283.

88. Kennedy BJ, Loeb V, Jr, Peterson V, Donegan W, Natarajan N, Mettlin C. Survival in Hodgkin's disease by stage and age. Med Pediatr Oncol 1992; 20:100–104.

89. Salminen EK. The outcome of > or = 70-year-old non-Hodgkin's lymphoma patients. Int J Radiat Oncol Biol Phys 1995; 32:349–353.

90. Yahalom J, von Mehren M, Schilder RJ. Hodgkin's disease. In: Pazdur R, Coia LR, Hoskins WJ, Wagman LD, eds. Cancer Management: A Multidisciplinary Approach. Huntington, NY: PRR, 1996; 205–225.

91. Lukes R, Butler J, Hicks E. Natural history of Hodgkin's disease as related to its pathological picture. Cancer 1966; 26:317.

92. Harris NL, Jaffe ES, Stein H, Banks PM, Chan JK, Cleary ML, Delsol G, De Wolf-Peeters C, Falini B, Gatter KC, et al. A revised European-American classification of lymphoid neoplasms: a proposal from the International Lymphoma Study Group. Blood 1994; 84:1361–1392.

93. Marafioti T, Hummel M, Anagnostopoulos I, Foss HD, Falini B, Delsol G, Isaacson PG, Pileri S, Stein H. Origin of nodular lymphocyte-predominant Hodgkin's disease from a clonal expansion of highly mutated germinal-center B cells. N Engl J Med 1997; 337:453–458.

94. Ohno T, Stribley JA, Wu G, Hinrichs SH, Weisenburger DD, Chan WC. Clonality in nodular lymphocyte-predominant Hodgkin's disease. N Engl J Med 1997; 337:459–465.

95. Childers JM, Balserak JC, Kent T, Surwit EA. Laparoscopic staging of Hodgkin's lymphoma. J Laparoendosc Surg 1993; 3:495–499.

96. Emmermann A, Zornig C, Peiper M, Weh HJ, Broelsch CE. Laparoscopic splenectomy. Technique and results in a series of 27 cases. Surg Endosc 1995; 9:924–927.

97. Lefor AT, Flowers JL, Heyman MR. Laparoscopic staging of Hodgkin's disease. Surg Oncol 1993; 2:217–220.

98. Phillips EH, Carroll BJ, Fallas MJ. Laparoscopic splenectomy. Surg Endosc 1994; 8: 931–933.

99. Terrosu G, Donini A, Silvestri F, Petri R, Anania G, Barillari G, Baccarani U, Risaliti A, Bresadola F. Laparoscopic splenectomy in the management of hematological diseases. Surgical technique and outcome of 17 patients. Surg Endosc 1996; 10:441–444.

100. Roach M, Brophy N, Cox R, Varghese A, Hoppe RT. Prognostic factors for patients relapsing after radiotherapy for early-stage Hodgkin's disease. J Clin Oncol 1990; 8: 623–629.

101. Zietman AL, Linggood RM, Brookes AR, Convery K, Piro A. Radiation therapy in the management of early stage Hodgkin's disease presenting in later life. Cancer 1869; 68:1869–1873.

102. Scalliet P. Radiotherapy in the elderly. Eur J Cancer 1991; 27:3–5.

103. Peschel RE, Wilson L, Haffty B, Papadopoulos D, Rosenzweig K, Feltes M. The effect of advanced age on the efficacy of radiation therapy for early breast cancer, local prostate cancer and grade III–IV gliomas. Int J Radiat Oncol Biol Phys 1993; 26:539–544.

104. Pignon T, Horiot J-C, van den Bogaert W, van Glabbeke M, Scalliet P. No age limit for radical radiotherapy in head and neck cancer. Eur J Cancer 1996; 32A:2075–2081.

105. Farniok KE, Levitt SH. The role of radiation therapy in the treatment of colorectal cancer. Implications for the older patient. Cancer 1994; 74:2154–2159.

106. Liew KH, Ding JC, Cruickshank D, Quong GG, Wolf MM, Cooper IA. Infradiaphrag-

matic Hodgkin's disease, long term follow-up of a rare presentation. Aust NZJ Med 1991; 21:16–21.

107. Enrici RM, Osti MF, Anselmo AP, Banelli E, Cartoni C, Sbarbati S, Padovan FS, Zurlo A, Biagini C. Hodgkin's disease stage I and II with exclusive subdiaphragmatic presentation. The experience of the Departments of Radiation Oncology and Hematology, University "La Sapienza" of Rome. Tumori 1996; 82:48–52.

108. Canellos GP, Anderson JR, Propert KJ, Nissen N, Cooper MR, Henderson ES, Green MR, Gottlieb A, Peterson BA. Chemotherapy of advanced Hodgkin's disease with MOPP, ABVD, or MOPP alternating with ABVD. N Engl J Med 1992; 327:1478–1484.

109. Fiorentino MV. Lymphomas in the elderly. Leukemia 1991; 1:79–85.

110. Levis A, Depaoli L, Bertini M, Botto B, Ciravegna G, Freilone R, Gallamini A, Gavarotti P, Ricardi U, Scalabrini DR, et al. Results of a low aggressivity chemotherapy regimen (CVP/CEB) in elderly Hodgkin's disease patients. Haematologica 1996; 81: 450–456.

111. Bennett JM, Andersen JW, Begg CB, Glick JH. Age and Hodgkin's disease: the impact of competing risks and possibly salvage therapy on long term survival: an E.C.O.G. study. Leuk Res 1993; 17:825–832.

112. Diaz-Pavon JR, Cabanillas F, Majlis A, Hagemeister FB. Outcome of Hodgkin's disease in elderly patients. Hematol Oncol 1995; 13:19–27.

113. Erdkamp FL, Breed WP, Bosch LJ, Wijnen JT, Blijham GB. Hodgkin's disease in the elderly: a registry-based analysis. Cancer 1992; 70:830–834.

114. Enblad G, Glimelius B, Sundstrom C. Treatment outcome in Hodgkin's disease in patients above the age of 60: a population-based study. Ann Oncol 1991; 2:297–302.

115. Glimelius B, Enblad G, Kalkner M, Gustavsson A, Jakobsson M, Branehog I, Lenner P, Bjorkholm M. Treatment of Hodgkin's disease: the Swedish national care programme experience. Leuk Lymphoma 1996; 21:71–78.

116. Longo DL, Duffey PL, Young RC, Hubbard SM, Ihde DC, Glatstein E, Phares JC, Jaffe ES, Urba WJ, DeVita VT Jr. Conventional-dose salvage combination chemotherapy in patients relapsing with Hodgkin's disease after combination chemotherapy: the low probability for cure. J Clin Oncol 1992; 10:210–218.

117. Linch DC, Winfield D, Goldstone AH, Moir D, Hancock B, McMillan A, Chopra R, Milligan D, Hudson GV. Dose intensification with autologous bone-marrow transplantation in relapsed and resistant Hodgkin's disease: results of a BNLI randomised trial. Lancet 1993; 341:1051–1054.

118. Cohen HJ. Monoclonal gammopathies: a model for neoplasia in older persons. In: Balducci L, Lyman GH, Ershler WB, eds. Geriatric Oncology. Philadelphia: Lippincott, 1992; 92–96.

119. Weber DM. Multiple myeloma and other plasma cell dyscrasias. In: Pazdur R, Coia LR, Hoskins WJ, Wagman LD, eds. Cancer Management: A Multidisciplinary Approach. Huntington, NY: PRR, 1996; 257–270.

120. Gautier M, Cohen HJ. Multiple myeloma in the elderly. J Am Geriatr Soc 1994; 42: 653–664.

121. Kyle RA. Monoclonal gammopathy of undetermined significance and solitary plasmacytoma. Implications for progression to overt multiple myeloma. Hematol Oncol Clin North Am 1997; 11:71–87.

122. Kyle RA, Gertz MA. Primary systemic amyloidosis: clinical and laboratory features in 474 cases. Semin. Hematol 1995; 32:45–59.
123. Kyle RA, Gertz MA, Greipp PR, Witzig TE, Lust JA, Lacy MQ, Therneau TM. A trial of three regimens for primary amyloidosis: colchicine alone, melphalan and prednisone, and melphalan, prednisone, and colchicine. N Engl J Med 1997; 336:1202–1207.
124. Falk RH, Comenzo RL, Skinner M. The systemic amyloidoses. N Engl J Med 1997; 337:898–909.
125. Weber DM, Dimopoulos MA, Moulopoulos LA, Delasalle KB, Smith T, Alexanian R. Prognostic features of asymptomatic multiple myeloma. Br J Haematol 1997; 97: 810–814.
126. Alexanian R, Dimopoulos MA, Delasalle K, Barlogie B. Primary dexamethasone treatment of multiple myeloma. Blood 1992; 80:887–890.
127. Abrahamson GM, Bird JM, Newland AC, Gaminara E, Giles C, Joyner M, Kelsey SM, Lewis D, McCarthy DM, Roques AW, et al. A randomized study of VAD therapy with either concurrent or maintenance interferon in patients with newly diagnosed multiple myeloma. Br J Haematol 1996; 94:659–664.
128. Samson D, Volin L, Schanz U, Bosi A, Gahrtron G. Feasibility and toxicity of interferon maintenance therapy after allogeneic BMT for multiple myeloma: a pilot study of the EBMT. Bone Marrow Transplant 1996; 17:759–762.
129. Capnist G, Vespignani M, Spriano M, Damasio E, Craviotto L, Rizzoli V, Contu A, Olmeo N, Tedeschi L, Fabris P, et al. Impact of interferon at induction chemotherapy and maintenance treatment for multiple myeloma. Preliminary results of a multicenter study by the Italian non-Hodgkin's Lymphoma Cooperative Study Group (NHLCSG). Acta Oncol 1994; 33:527–529.
130. Anonymous. Interferon-alpha 2b added to melphalan-prednisone for initial and maintenance therapy in multiple myeloma. A randomized, controlled trial. The Nordic Myeloma Study Group. Ann Intern Med 1996; 124:212–222.
131. Dimopoulos MA, Weber D, Delasalle KB, Alexanian R. Combination therapy with interferon-dexamethasone for newly diagnosed patients with multiple myeloma. Cancer 1993; 72:2589–2592.
132. Pasqualetti P, Collacciani A, Maccarone C, Casale R. Prognostic factors in multiple myeloma: selection using Cox's proportional hazard model. Biomed Pharmacother 1996; 50:29–35.
133. Blade J, Munoz M, Fontanillas M, San Miguel J, Alcala A, Maldonado J, Besses C, Moro MJ, Garcia-Conde J, Rozman C, et al. Treatment of multiple myeloma in elderly people: long-term results in 178 patients. Age Ageing 1996; 25:357–361.
134. Clavio M, Casciaro S, Gatti AM, Spriano M, Bonanni F, Poggi A, Vallebella E, Pietrasanta D, Prencipe E, Goretti R, et al. Multiple myeloma in the elderly: clinical features and response to treatment in 113 patients. Haematologica 1996; 81:238–244.
135. Palumbo A, Pileri A, Triolo S, et al. Intensified therapy with stem cell support for elderly myeloma patients. Blood 1997; 90 (Suppl 1):1015a.
136. Vesole DH, Jagannath S, Tricot G, Vaught L, Barlogie B. High-dose intensive therapy with autologous transplantation in multiple myeloma patients over age 60. Proc Am Soc Clin Oncol 1994; 13:1400a.

137. Guba SC, Vesole DH, Jaggannath S, Bracy D, Barlogie B, Tricot G. Peripheral stem cell mobilization and engraftment in patients over age 60. Bone Marrow Transplant 1997; 20:1–3.

138. Berenson JR, Lichtenstein A, Porter L, Dimopoulos MA, Bordoni R, George S, Lipton A, Keller A, Ballester O, Kovacs MJ, et al. Efficacy of pamidronate in reducing skeletal events in patients with advanced multiple myeloma. Myeloma Aredia Study Group. N Engl J Med 1996; 334:488–493.

139. Jantunen E, Laakso M. Bisphosphonates in multiple myeloma: current status; future perspectives. Br J Haematol 1996; 93:501–506.

140. Laakso M, Jantunen E. Bisphosphonate therapy in multiple myeloma. Acta Oncol 1996; 5:55–56.

141. Jantunen E, Lahtinen R, Laakso M. Use of clodronate in multiple myeloma. Leuk Lymphoma 1995; 19:207–211.

142. Adam Z, Prokes B, Hajek D, Vorlicek J. Increasing bone density in myeloma patients after the administration of clodronate. Acta Med Austriaca 1995; 22:9–12.

143. Roux C, Ravaud P, Cohen-Solal M, de Vernejoul MC, Guillemant S, Cherruau B, Delmas P, Dougados M, Amor B. Biologic, histologic and densitometric effects of oral risedronate on bone in patients with multiple myeloma. Bone 1994; 15:41–49.

144. Clemens MR, Fessele K, Heim ME. Multiple myeloma: effect of daily dichloromethylene bisphosphonate on skeletal complications. Ann Hematol 1993; 66:141–146.

145. Osterborg A, Boogaerts MA, Cimino R, Essers U, Holowiecki J, Juliusson G, Jager G, Najman A, Peest D. Recombinant human erythropoietin in transfusion-dependent anemic patients with multiple myeloma and non-Hodgkin's lymphoma—a randomized multicenter study. The European Study Group of Erythropoietin (Epoetin Beta) Treatment in Multiple Myeloma and Non-Hodgkin's Lymphoma. Blood 1996; 87:2675–2682.

146. Barlogie B. Treatment of the anemia of multiple myeloma: the role of recombinant human erythropoietin. Semin Hematol 1993; 30:25–27.

147. Bennett JM. Classification of the myelodysplastic syndromes. Clin Haematol 1986; 15:909–923.

148. Williamson PJ, Kruger AR, Reynolds PJ, Hamblin TJ, Oscier DG. Establishing the incidence of myelodysplastic syndrome. Br J Haematol 1994; 87:743–745.

149. Yunis JJ, Lobell M, Arnesen MA, Oken MM, Mayer MG, Rydell RE, Brunning RD. Refined chromosome study helps define prognostic subgroups in most patients with primary myelodysplastic syndrome and acute myelogenous leukaemia. Br J Haematol 1988; 68:189–194.

150. Greenberg PL, Mara B. The preleukemic syndrome: correlation of in vitro parameters of granulopoiesis with clinical features. Am J Med 1979; 66:951–958.

151. Morel P, Hebbar M, Lai JL, Duhamel A, Preudhomme C, Wattel E, Bauters F, Fenaux P. Cytogenetic analysis has strong independent prognostic value in de novo myelodysplastic syndromes and can be incorporated in a new scoring system: a report on 408 cases. Leukemia 1993; 7:1315–1323.

152. Pedersen-Bjergaard J, Rowley JD. The balanced and the unbalanced chromosome aberrations of acute myeloid leukemia may develop in different ways and may contribute differently to malignant transformation. Blood 1994; 83:2780–2786.

153. Chabannon C, Molina L, Pegourie-Bandelier B, Bost M, Leger J, Hollard D. A review of 76 patients with myelodysplastic syndromes treated with danazol. Cancer 1994; 73: 3073–3080.

154. Negrin RS, Haeuber DH, Nagler A, Kobayashi Y, Sklar J, Donlon T, Vincent M, Greenberg PL. Maintenance treatment of patients with myelodysplastic syndromes using recombinant human granulocyte colony-stimulating factor. Blood 1990; 76:36–43.

155. Rose C, Wattel E, Bastion Y, Berger E, Bauters F, Coiffier B, Fenaux P. Treatment with very low-dose GM-CSF in myelodysplastic syndromes with neutropenia. A report on 28 cases. Leukemia 1994; 8:1458–1462.

156. Schuster MW, Allen SL, Lichtman SM, Schulman P, DeMarco L, Buman DR, Muuse WT. The use of erythropoietin in the treatment of myelodysplastic syndrome and myelofibrosis. Proc Am Soc Clin Oncol 1990; 9:789a.

157. Ganser A, Ottmann OG, Seipelt G, Lindemann A, Hess U, Geissler G, Maurer A, Frisch J, Schulz G, Mertelsmann R, et al. Effect of long-term treatment with recombinant human interleukin-3 in patients with myelodysplastic syndromes. Leukemia 1993; 7:696–701.

158. Stone RM, Bernstein SH, Demetri G, Facklam DP, Arthur K, Andersen J, Aster JC, Kufe D. Therapy with recombinant human erythropoietin in patients with myelodysplastic syndromes. Leuk Res 1994; 18:769–776.

159. Stasi R, Brunetti M, Bussa S, Conforti M, Martin LS, La Presa M, Bianchi M, Parma A, Pagano A. Serum levels of tumour necrosis factor-alpha predict response to recombinant human erythropoietin in patients with myelodysplastic syndrome. Clin Lab Haematol 1997; 19:197–201.

160. Adamson JW, Schuster M, Allen S, Haley NR. Effectiveness of recombinant human erythropoietin therapy in myelodysplastic syndromes. Acta Haematol 1992; 87 Suppl 1:20–24.

161. Negrin RS, Stein R, Doherty K, Cornwell J, Vardiman J, Krantz S, Greenberg PL. Maintenance treatment of the anemia of myelodysplastic syndromes with recombinant human granulocyte colony-stimulating factor and erythropoietin: evidence for in vivo synergy. Blood 1996; 87:4076–4081.

162. Gordon MS, Nemunaitis J, Hoffman R, Paquette RL, Rosenfeld C, Manfreda S, Isaacs R, Nimer SD. A phase I trial of recombinant human interleukin-6 in patients with myelodysplastic syndromes and thrombocytopenia. Blood 1995; 85:3066–3076.

163. Lemoli RM, Fogli M, Fortuna A, Amabile M, Zucchini P, Grande A, Martinelli G, Visani G, Ferrari S, Tura S. Interleukin-11 (IL-11) acts as a synergistic factor for the proliferation of human myeloid leukaemic cells. Br J Haematol 1995; 91:319–326.

164. Backx B, Broeders L, Lowenberg B. Kit ligand improves in vitro erythropoiesis in myelodysplastic syndrome. Blood 1992; 80:1213–1217.

165. Matsumura I, Ikeda H, Kanakura Y. The effects of thrombopoietin on the growth of acute myeloblastic leukemia cells. Leuk Lymphoma 1996; 23:533–538.

166. Tokunaga Y, Miyamoto T, Gondo H, Okamura T, Niho Y. Effect of thrombopoietin on proliferation of CD7-positive blasts from acute myelogenous leukemia. Blood 1997; 90(Suppl 1):69a.

167. Koeffler HP, Keitjan D, Mertelsmann R, et al. Randomized study of 13-cis-retinoic acid v placebo in the myelodysplastic disorders. Blood 1988; 71:703–708.

168. Ganser A, Seipelt G, Verbeek W, Ottmann OG, Maurer A, Kolbe K, Hess U, Elsner S, Reutzel R, Wormann B, et al. Effect of combination therapy with all-trans-retinoic acid and recombinant human granulocyte colony-stimulating factor in patients with myelodysplastic syndromes. Leukemia 1994; 8:369–375.

169. List AF, Heaton R, Glinsmann-Gibson B, Brasfield F, Crook L, Taetle R, Kurman M. Phase I/II clinical trial of amifostine in patients with myelodysplastic syndrome: promotion of multilineage hematopoiesis. Proc Annu Meet Am Soc Clin Oncol 1997; 16:21a.

170. Raza A, Gezer S, Venugopal P, Kaizer H, Hines C, Thomas R, Alvi S, Mundle S, Shetty V, Borok R, et al. Hematopoiesis and cytogenetic responses to novel anti-cytokine therapy in myelodysplastic syndromes. Proc Annu Meet Am Soc Clin Oncol 1997; 16:22a.

171. Andreeff M, Stone R, Michaeli J, Young CW, Tong WP, Sogoloff H, Ervin T, Kufe D, Rifkind RA, Marks PA. Hexamethylene bisacetamide in myelodysplastic syndrome and acute myelogenous leukemia: a phase II clinical trial with a differentiation-inducing agent. Blood 1992; 80:2604–2609.

172. Miller KB, Kim K, Morrison FS, Winter JN, Bennett JM, Neiman RS, Head DR, Cassileth PA, MJ OC. The evaluation of low-dose cytarabine in the treatment of myelodysplastic syndromes: a phase-III intergroup study. Ann Hematol 1992; 65:162–168 (published erratum appears in Ann Hematol 1993; 66:164.)

173. Juneja HS, Jodhani M, Gardner FH, Trevarthen D, Schottstedt M. Low-dose ARA-C consistently induces hematologic responses in the clinical 5q-syndrome. Am J Hematol 1994; 46:338–342.

174. Silverman LR, Holland JF, Weinberg RS, Alter BP, Davis RB, Ellison RR, Demakos EP, Cornell CJJ, Carey RW, Schiffer C, et al. Effects of treatment with 5-azacytidine on the in vivo and in vitro hematopoiesis in patients with myelodysplastic syndromes. Leukemia 1993; 7(Suppl 1):21–29.

175. Wijermans PW, Krulder JW, Huijgens PC, Neve P. Continuous infusion of low-dose 5-Aza-2'-deoxycytidine in elderly patients with high-risk myelodysplastic syndrome. Leukemia 1997; 11:1–5.

176. Estey E, Thall P, Andreeff M, Beran M, Kantarjian H, S OB, Escudier S, Robertson LE, Koller C, Kornblau S, et al. Use of granulocyte colony-stimulating factor before, during, and after fludarabine plus cytarabine induction therapy of newly diagnosed acute myelogenous leukemia or myelodysplastic syndromes: comparison with fludarabine plus cytarabine without granulocyte colony-stimulating factor. J Clin Oncol 1994; 12:671–678.

177. de Witte T, Suciu S, Peetermans M, Fenaux P, Strijckmans P, Hayat M, Jaksic B, Selleslag D, Zittoun R, Dardenne M, et al. Intensive chemotherapy for poor prognosis myelodysplasia (MDS) and secondary acute myeloid leukemia (sAML) following MDS of more than 6 months duration. A pilot study by the Leukemia Cooperative Group of the European Organisation for Research and Treatment in Cancer (EORTC-LCG). Leukemia 1995; 9:1805–1811.

178. Trimble EL, Carter CL, Cain D, Freidlin B, Ungerleider RS, Friedman MA. Representation of older patients in cancer treatment trials. Cancer 1994; 74:2208–2214.

179. Sandler DP, Ross JA. Epidemiology of acute leukemia in children and adults. Semin Oncol 1997; 24:3–16.

180. Groves FD, Linet MS, Devesa SS. Patterns of occurrence of the leukaemias. Eur J Cancer 1995; 6:941–949.

181. Fialkow PJ, Singer JW, Raskind WH, Adamson JW, Jacobson RJ, Bernstein ID, Dow LW, Najfeld V, Veith R. Clonal development, stem-cell differentiation, and clinical remissions in acute nonlymphocytic leukemia. N Engl J Med 1987; 317:468–473.

182. Pedersen-Bjergaard J, Philip P. Two different classes of therapy-related and de-novo acute myeloid leukemia? Cancer Genet Cytogenet 1991; 55:119–124.

183. te Boekhorst PA, de Leeuw K, Schoester M, Wittebol S, Nooter K, Hagemeijer A, Lowenberg B, Sonneveld P. Predominance of functional multidrug resistance (MDR-1) phenotype in CD34+ acute myeloid leukemia cells. Blood 1993; 82:3157–3162.

184. Sonneveld P, van Rens GL, de Goevere MJ, Schoester M, Scheper R, Smit E. Molecular and functional analysis of multidrug resistance phenotypes in poor-risk AML with -7/7q- karyotype. Blood 1995;86(Suppl 1):517a.

185. Arthur DC, Berger R, Golomb HM, Swansbury GJ, Reeves BR, Alimena G, Van Den Berghe H, Bloomfield CD, de la Chapelle A, Dewald GW, et al. The clinical significance of karyotype in acute myelogenous leukemia. Cancer Genet Cytogenet 1989; 40:203–216.

186. Dastugue N, Payen C, Lafage-Pochitaloff M, Bernard P, Leroux D, Huguet-Rigal F, Stoppa AM, Marit G, Molina L, Michallet M, et al. Prognostic significance of karyotype in de novo adult acute myeloid leukemia. The BGMT group. Leukemia 1995; 9: 1491–1498.

187. Bloomfield CD, Goldman A, Hassfeld D, de la Chapelle A. Fourth International Workshop on Chromosomes in Leukemia 1982: clinical significance of chromosomal abnormalities in acute nonlymphoblastic leukemia. Cancer Genet Cytogenet 1984; 11:332–350.

188. Willman CL. Immunophenotyping and cytogenetics in older adults with acute myeloid leukemia: significance of expression of the multidrug resistance gene-1 (MDR1). Leukemia 1996; 10: Suppl 533–535.

189. te Boekhorst PA, Lowenberg B, van Kapel J, Nooter K, Sonneveld P. Multidrug resistant cells with high proliferative capacity determine response to therapy in acute myeloid leukemia. Leukemia 1995; 9:1025–1031.

190. Leith CP, Chen IM, Kopecky KJ, Appelbaum FR, Head DR, Godwin JE, Weick JK, Willman CL. Correlation of multidrug resistance (MDR1) protein expression with functional dye/drug efflux in acute myeloid leukemia by multiparameter flow cytometry: identification of discordant MDR−/efflux+ and MDR1+/efflux− cases. Blood 1995; 86:2329–2342.

191. List AF, Spier CS, Grogan TM, Johnson C, Roe DJ, Greer JP, Wolff SN, Broxterman HJ, Scheffer GL, Scheper RJ, et al. Overexpression of the major vault transporter protein lung-resistance protein predicts treatment outcome in acute myeloid leukemia. Blood 1996; 87:2464–2469.

192. Rowe JM, Tallman MS. Intensifying induction therapy in acute myeloid leukemia: has a new standard of care emerged? Blood 1997; 90:2121–2126.

193. Yates J, Glidewell O, Wiernik P, Cooper MR, Steinberg D, Dosik H, Levy R, Hoagland C, Henry P, Gottlieb A, et al. Cytosine arabinoside with daunorubicin or adriamycin for therapy of acute myelocytic leukemia: a CALGB study. Blood 1982; 60:454–462.

194. Bishop JF, Lowenthal RM, Joshua D, Matthews JP, Todd D, Cobcroft R, Whiteside MG, Kronenberg H, Ma D, Dodds A, et al. Etoposide in acute nonlymphocytic leukemia. Australian Leukemia Study Group. Blood 1990; 75:27–32.

195. Bishop JF, Matthews JP, Young GA, Szer J, Gillett A, Joshua D, Bradstock K, Enno A, Wolf MM, Fox R, et al. A randomized study of high-dose cytarabine in induction in acute myeloid leukemia. Blood 1996; 87:1710–1717.

196. Lowenberg B, Zittoun R, Kerkhofs H, Jehn U, Abels J, Debusscher L, Cauchie C, Peetermans M, Solbu G, Suciu S, et al. On the value of intensive remission-induction chemotherapy in elderly patients of 65+ years with acute myeloid leukemia: a randomized phase III study of the European Organization for Research and Treatment of Cancer Leukemia Group. J Clin Oncol 1989; 7:1268–1274.

197. Tilly H, Castaigne S, Bordessoule D, Casassus P, Le Prise PY, Tertian G, Desablens B, Henry-Amar M, Degos L. Low-dose cytarabine versus intensive chemotherapy in the treatment of acute nonlymphocytic leukemia in the elderly. J Clin Oncol 1990; 8: 272–279.

198. Ruutu T, Almqvist A, Hallman H, Honkanen T, Jarvenpaa E, Jarventie G, Koistinen P, Koivunen E, Lahtinen R, Lehtinen M, et al. Oral induction and consolidation of acute myeloid leukemia with etoposide, 6-thioguanine, and idarubicin (ETI) in elderly patients: a randomized comparison with 5-day TAD. Finnish Leukemia Group. Leukemia 1994; 8:11–15.

199. Leoni F, Ciolli S, Giuliani G, Pascarella A, Caporale R, Salti F, Cervi L, Rossi Ferrini P. Attenuated-dose idarubicin in acute myeloid leukaemia of the elderly: pharmacokinetic study and clinical results. Br J Haematol 1995; 90:169–174.

200. Kahn SB, Begg CB, Mazza JJ, Bennett JM, Bonner H, Glick JH. Full dose versus attenuated dose daunorubicin, cytosine arabinoside, and 6-thioguanine in the treatment of acute nonlymphocytic leukemia in the elderly. J Clin Oncol 1984; 2:865–870.

201. Slapak CA, Desforges JF, Fogaren T, Miller KB. Treatment of acute myeloid leukemia in the elderly with low-dose cytarabine, hydroxyurea, and calcitriol. Am J Hematol 1992; 41:178–183.

202. Frankel SR, Eardley A, Heller G, Berman E, Miller WH, Jr., Dmitrovsky E, Warrell RP, Jr. All-trans retinoic acid for acute promyelocytic leukemia. Results of the New York Study. Ann Intern Med 1994; 120:278–286.

203. Bow EJ, Sutherland JA, Kilpatrick MG, Williams GJ, Clinch JJ, Shore TB, Rubinger M, Schacter BA. Therapy of untreated acute myeloid leukemia in the elderly: remission-induction using a non-cytarabine-containing regimen of mitoxantrone plus etoposide. J Clin Oncol 1996; 14:1345–1352.

204. Archimbaud E, Troncy J, Devaux Y, Sebban C, Assouline D, Fiere D. Continuous-infusion daunorubicin and carboplatin for high-risk acute myeloid leukemia in the elderly. Proc Annu Meet Am Assoc Cancer Res 1992; 33:A1264.

205. Feldman EJ, Seiter K, Damon L, Linker C, Rugo H, Ries C, Case DC, Jr., Beer M, Ahmed T. A randomized trial of high- vs standard-dose mitoxantrone with cytarabine in elderly patients with acute myeloid leukemia. Leukemia 1997; 11:485–489.

206. Schiffer CA. Hematopoietic growth factors as adjuncts to the treatment of acute myeloid leukemia. Blood 1996; 88:3675–3685.

207. Rowe JM, Andersen JW, Mazza JJ, Bennett JM, Paietta E, Hayes FA, Oette D, Cassileth PA, Stadtmauer EA, Wiernik PH. A randomized placebo-controlled phase III study of granulocyte-macrophage colony-stimulating factor in adult patients (>55 to 70 years of age) with acute myelogenous leukemia: a study of the Eastern Cooperative Oncology Group (E1490). Blood 1995; 86:457–462.

208. Stone RM, Berg DT, George SL, Dodge RK, Paciucci PA, Schulman P, Lee EJ, Moore JO, Powell BL, Schiffer CA. Granulocyte-macrophage colony-stimulating factor after initial chemotherapy for elderly patients with primary acute myelogenous leukemia. Cancer and Leukemia Group B. N Engl J Med 1995; 332:1671–1677.

209. Bloomfield CD, Lawrence D, Arthur DC, Berg DT, Schiffer CA, Mayer RJ. Curative impact of intensification with high-dose cytarabine in acute myeloid leukemia varies by cytogenetic group. Blood 1994;84 (suppl 1):111a.

210. Linet MS, Devesa SS. Descriptive epidemiology of the leukemias. In: Wiernik PH, Cannelos G, Kyle RA, Schiffer C, eds. Neoplastic Diseases of the Blood. New York: Churchill Livingstone, 1991; 207–212.

211. Taylor PR, Reid MM, Proctor SJ. Acute lymphoblastic leukaemia in the elderly. Leuk Lymphoma 1994; 13:373–380.

212. Secker-Walker LM, Craig JM, Hawkins JM, Hoffbrand AV. Philadelphia positive acute lymphoblastic leukemia in adults: age distribution, BCR breakpoint and prognostic significance. Leukemia 1991; 5:196–199.

213. Larson RA, Dodge RK, Burns CP, Lee EJ, Stone RM, Schulman P, Duggan D, Davey FR, Sobol RE, Frankel SR, et al. A five-drug remission induction regimen with intensive consolidation for adults with acute lymphoblastic leukemia: cancer and leukemia group B study 8811. Blood 1995; 85:2025–2037.

214. Clarkson B, Ellis S, Little C, Gee T, Arlin Z, Mertelsmann R, Andreeff M, Kempin S, Koziner B, Chaganti R, et al. Acute lymphoblastic leukemia in adults. Semin Oncol 1985; 12:160–179.

215. Larson RA, Linker CA, Dodge RK, George SL, Davey FR, Frankel SR, Powell BL, Schiffer CA. Granulocyte-colony stimulating factor (filgrastim; G-CSF) reduces the time to neutrophil recovery in adults with acute lymphoblastic leukemia receiving intensive remission induction chemotherapy: Cancer and Leukemia Group B study 9111. Proc Am Soc Clin Oncol 1994; 13:995a.

216. Kantarjian HM, S OB, Smith T, Estey EH, Beran M, Preti A, Pierce S, Keating MJ. Acute lymphocytic leukaemia in the elderly: characteristics and outcome with the vincristine-Adriamycin-dexamethasone (VAD) regimen. Br J Haematol 1994; 88:94–100.

217. Ludescher C, Eisterer W, Hilbe W, Gotwald M, Hofmann J, Zabernigg A, Cianfriglia M, Thaler J. Low frequency of activity of P-glycoprotein (P-170) in acute lymphoblastic leukemia compared to acute myeloid leukemia. Leukemia 1995; 9:350–356.

218. Szatrowski TP, Larson RA, Dodge R, Sklar J, Reynolds C, Westbrook CA, Hurd D, Kolitz J, Velez-Garcia E, Frankel SR, et al. The effect of anti-B4-blocked ricin on minimal residual disease in adults with B-lineage acute lymphoblastic leukemia. Blood 1996; 88(Suppl 1):669a.

219. Kolitz JE, O'Mara V, Willemze R, Poynton CH, Jaeger U, Brody J, Schulman P. Treatment of acute lymphoblastic leukemia with CAMPATH-1H: initial observations. Blood 1994;84(Suppl 1):301a.

220. Call TG, Phyliky RL, Noel P, Habermann TM, Beard CM, O'Fallon WM, Kurland LT. Incidence of chronic lymphocytic leukemia in Olmsted County, Minnesota, 1935 through 1989, with emphasis on changes in initial stage at diagnosis. Mayo Clin Proc 1994; 69:323–328.

221. Cortes JE, Kantarjian H. Chronic leukemias. In: Pazdur R, Coia LR, Hoskins WJ, Wagman LD, eds. Cancer Management: A Multidisciplinary Approach. 2nd ed. Huntington, NY: PRR, 1998; 306–328.

222. Cheson BD, Bennett JM, Grever M, Kay N, Keating MJ, O'Brien S, Rai KR. National Cancer Institute-sponsored Working Group guidelines for chronic lymphocytic leukemia: revised guidelines for diagnosis and treatment. Blood 1996; 87:4990–4997.

223. Rai KR, Kipps TJ, Barlogie B. Chronic lymphocytic leukemia and myeloma: Update

on the biology and management. Educational Book of the American Society of Hematology 1996; 62–73.

224. Keating MJ, Lerner S, Kantargian H, Freireich EJ, O'Brien S. The serum β2M level is more powerful than stage in predicting response and survival in CLL. Blood 1995; 86(Suppl 1):606a.

225. Axdorph U, Nilsson BI, Nilsson BR, Bjorkholm M. Leucocyte doubling time is a useful predictor of progression-free survival in chronic lymphocytic leukaemia. J Intern Med 1995; 237:205–209.

226. Montserrat E, Rozman C. Chronic lymphocytic leukaemia: prognostic factors and natural history. Baillieres Clin Haematol 1993; 6:849–866.

227. Rai KR. Chronic lymphocytic leukemia in the elderly population. Clin Geriatr Med 1997; 13:245–249.

228. Deisseroth AB, Kantarjian H, Andreeff M, Talpaz M, Keating MJ, Khouri I, Champlin RB. Chronic leukemias. In: DeVita VT Jr, Hellman S, Rosenberg SA, eds. Cancer: Principles and Practice of Oncology. 5th ed. Philadelphia: Lippincott, 1997: 2321–2343.

229. Raphael B, Andersen JW, Silber R, Oken M, Moore D, Bennett J, Bonner H, Hahn R, Knospe WH, Mazza J, et al. Comparison of chlorambucil and prednisone versus cyclophosphamide, vincristine, and prednisone as initial treatment for chronic lymphocytic leukemia: long-term follow-up of an eastern cooperative oncology group randomized clinical trial. J Clin Oncol 1991; 9:770–776.

230. Montserrat E, Alcala A, Parody R, Domingo A, Garcia-Conde J, Bueno J, Ferran C, Sanz MA, Giralt M, Rubio D, et al. Treatment of chronic lymphocytic leukemia in advanced stages. A randomized trial comparing chlorambucil plus prednisone versus cyclophosphamide, vincristine, and prednisone. Cancer 1985; 56:2369–2375.

231. French Cooperative Group on Chronic Lymphocytic Leukemia. Is the CHOP regimen a good treatment for advanced CLL? Results from two randomized clinical trials. Leuk Lymphoma 1994; 13:449–456.

232. French Cooperative Group on Chronic Lymphocytic Leukaemia. Natural history of stage A chronic lymphocytic leukaemia untreated patients. Br J Haematol 1990; 76: 45–57.

233. The French Cooperative Group on Chronic Lymphocytic Leukemia. A randomized clinical trial of chlorambucil versus COP in stage B chronic lymphocytic leukemia. Blood 1990; 75:1422–1425.

234. The French Cooperative Group on Chronic Lymphocytic Leukemia. Effects of chlorambucil and therapeutic decision in initial forms of chronic lymphocytic leukemia (stage A): results of a randomized clinical trial on 612 patients. Blood 1990; 75:1414–1421.

235. Hande KR, Garrow GC. Purine antimetabolites. In: Chabner BA, Longo DL, eds. Cancer Chemotherapy and Biotherapy: Principles and Practice. Philadelphia: Lippincott-Raven, 1996:235–252.

236. Puccio CA, Mittelman A, Lichtman SM, Silver RT, Budman DR, Chun HG, Ahmed T, Feldman EJ, Coleman M, Arnold PM, et al. A loading dose/continous infusion schedule of fludarabine phosphate in chronic lymphocytic leukemia. J Clin Oncol 1991; 9:1562–1569.

237. Keating MJ, Kantarjian H, S OB, Koller C, Talpaz M, Schachner J, Childs CC, Frei-

reich EJ, McCredie KB. Fludarabine: a new agent with marked cytoreductive activity in untreated chronic lymphocytic leukemia. J Clin Oncol 1991; 9:44–49.

238. Sudhoff T, Arning M, Schneider W. Prophylactic strategies to meet infectious complications in fludarabine-treated CLL. Leukemia 1997; 11(Suppl 2):S38–41.

239. O'Brien S, Kantarjian H, Beran M, Smith T, Koller C, Estey E, Robertson LE, Lerner S, Keating M. Results of fludarabine and prednisone therapy in 264 patients with chronic lymphocytic leukemia with multivariate analysis-derived prognostic model for response to treatment. Blood 1993; 82:1695–1700.

240. Bergmann L, Fenchel K, Jahn B, Mitrou PS, Hoelzer D. Immunosuppressive effects and clinical response of fludarabine in refractory chronic lymphocytic leukemia. Ann Oncol 1993; 4:371–375.

241. Hequet O, de Jaureguiberry JP, Jaubert D, Gisserot O, Muzellec Y, Brisou P. Listeriosis after fludarabine treatment for chronic lymphocytic leukemia. Hematol Cell Ther 1997; 39:89–91.

242. Di Raimondo F, Giustolisi R, Cacciola E, S OB, Kantarjian H, Robertson LB, Keating MJ. Autoimmune hemolytic anemia in chronic lymphocytic leukemia patients treated with fludarabine. Leuk Lymphoma 1993; 11:63–68.

243. Tsiara S, Christou L, Konstantinidou P, Panteli A, Briasoulis E, Bourantas KL. Severe autoimmune hemolytic anemia following fludarabine therapy in a patient with chronic lymphocytic leukemia. Am J Hematol 1997; 54.

244. Myint H, Copplestone JA, Orchard J, Craig V, Curtis D, Prentice AG, Hamon MD, Oscier DG, Hamblin TJ. Fludarabine-related autoimmune haemolytic anaemia in patients with chronic lymphocytic leukaemia. Br J Haematol 1995; 91:341–344.

245. Saven A, Lemon RH, Kosty M, Beutler E, Piro LD. 2-Chlorodeoxyadenosine activity in patients with untreated chronic lymphocytic leukemia. J Clin Oncol 1995; 13:570–574.

246. Bergmann L. Present status of purine analogs in the therapy of chronic lymphocytic leukemias. Leukemia 1997; (11 Suppl 2):S29–34.

247. Rai KR, Peterson B, Elias L, Shepherd L, Hines J, Nelson D, Cheston B, Kolitz J, Schiffer CA. A randomized comparison of fludarabine and chlorambucil for patients with previously untreated chronic lymphocytic leukemia: a CALGB, CTG/NCI-C and ECOG Intergroup study. Blood 1997; 88(Suppl 1):141a.

248. Rai KR, Peterson B, Kolitz J, Elias L, Shepherd L, Hines J, Cheson B, Schiffer C. Fludarabine induces a high complete remission rate in previously untreated patients with active chronic lymphocytic leukemia: a randomized intergroup study. Blood 1995; 86(Suppl 1):607a.

249. Velasquez WS, Cabanillas F, Salvador P, McLaughlin P, Fridrik M, Tucker S, Jagannath S, Hagemeister FB, Redman JR, Swan F, et al. Effective salvage therapy for lymphoma with cisplatin in combination with high-dose Ara-C and dexamethasone (DHAP). Blood 1988; 71:117–122.

250. Velasquez WS, McLaughlin P, Tucker S, Hagemeister FB, Swan F, Rodriguez MA, Romaguera J, Rubenstein E, Cabanillas F. ESHAP—an effective chemotherapy regimen in refractory and relapsing lymphoma: a 4-year follow-up study. J Clin Oncol 1994; 12:1169–1176.

251. Wilson WH, Bryant G, Bates S, Fojo A, Wittes RE, Steinberg SM, Kohler DR, Jaffe ES, Herdt J, Cheson BD, et al. EPOCH chemotherapy: toxicity and efficacy in relapsed and refractory non-Hodgkin's lymphoma. J Clin Oncol 1993; 11:1573–1582.

252. Niitsu N, Umeda M. Evaluation of long-term daily administration of oral low-dose etoposide in elderly patients with relapsing or refractory non-Hodgkin's lymphoma. Am J Clin Oncol 1997; 20:311–314.

253. Lichtman SM, Niedzwiecki D, Carlisle T, Cooper MR, Johnson J, Peterson BA. Phase II study of infusional chemotherapy with doxorubicin, vincristine and etoposide plus cyclophosphamide and prednisone (I-CHOPE) in resistant diffuse aggressive non-hodgkin's lymphoma: CALGB 9255. Proc Annu Meet Am Soc Clin Oncol 1998; 17:1179.

254. Fisher RI, Gaynor ER, Dahlberg S, Oken MM, Grogen TM, Mize EM, Glick JH, Coltman CAJ, Miller TP. Comparison of a standard regimen (CHOP) with three intensive chemotherapy regimens for advanced non-Hodgkin's lymphoma. N Engl J Med 1993; 328:1002–1006.

255. Weber DM. Multiple myeloma and other plasma cell dyscrasias. In: Pazdur R, Coia LR, Hoskins WJ, Wagman LD, eds. Cancer Management: A Multidisciplinary Approach. Huntington, NY: PRR, 1996:257–270.

256. Lee E, George S, Caligiuri M, Dodge R, Smith R, Szatrowski T, Schiffer CA. A phase I study of induction chemotherapy for older patients with acute leukemia using ara-C, daunorubicin and etoposide with and without the MDR modulator PSC-833: Cancer and Leukemia Group B study 9420. Blood 1997; 90(Suppl 1):506a.

257. Caron PC, Schwartz MA, Co MS, Queen C, Finn RD, Graham MC, Divgi CR, Larson SM, Scheinberg DA. Murine and humanized constructs of monoclonal antibody M195 (anti-CD33) for the therapy of acute myelogenous leukemia. Cancer 1994; 73:1049–1056.

258. Foa R. Does interleukin-2 have a role in the management of acute leukemia? J Clin Oncol 1993; 11:1817–1825.

17

Treatment of Melanoma and Sarcoma

Jeffrey Scott Stephens and William G. Kraybill
Roswell Park Cancer Institute
Buffalo, New York

I. MELANOMA

In the United States, it was estimated that there would be 40,300 cases and 7300 deaths from melanoma in 1997 (1). No tumor is increasing at a faster rate than malignant melanoma (2–3). Age is an independent negative prognostic factor for survival in melanoma patients (3–5). The estimated percentage of patients with melanoma which are elderly is between 8 and 37% (3–6). The SEER (Surveillance, Epidemiology, and End Results [Program]) registry has reported that 16% of its melanoma patients were greater than 70 years of age (7). Reasons suggested for poorer survival of elderly patients with melanoma include a delay in diagnosis, lack of education in prevention and surveillance, increase in the incidence of more aggressive lesions, decrease in the immune function, and thinner skin leading to early invasion. In this section, we will discuss the current presentation, classification, staging, and treatment of cutaneous melanoma, focusing on how these issues affect the elderly patient.

A. Histological Types

Superficial spreading melanoma is the most common type of melanoma, accounting for an estimated 70% of melanoma cases (8). Nodular melanoma accounts for 15–30% of cases, whereas lentigo maligna melanoma accounts for an estimated 4–10% of cases. Lentigo maligna is seen most commonly on the face of the elderly patient, is less aggressive, and is associated with a lower incidence of metastasis (8). Histological subtypes of melanoma which have a worse prognosis are found more commonly in the elderly patient. A study of melanoma patients comparing patients 30–39 years of age and those greater than 70 years of age showed a higher incidence of acral lentigenous melanoma and nodular melanoma in the older population (3). A Scottish review of patients greater than 65 years of age with melanoma also demonstrated an increase of nodular and acral lentigenous melanoma (4).

B. Staging and Prognostic Factors

Current staging in melanoma follows the system adopted by the American Joint Committee on Cancer (AJCC) in 1992 and is based on the TNM (tumor, nodes, metastasis) system reflecting tumor thickness/level of invasion, in-transit metastasis, nodal involvement, and distant spread (9) (Table 1). Factors that have been shown to have prognostic value are Breslow's thickness, Clark's level, sex, ulceration, age, location of the primary, and the presence of clinically positive lymph nodes (10). Although Breslow's thickness is felt to be a more powerful predictor of recurrence and survival than Clark's level of invasion, a retrospective analysis demonstrated that both carried significant prognostic power when corrected for each other (11). The older patient population has an increased incidence of thick melanomas, which is increased in all histological subtypes of melanoma and may partially explain the worse survival seen in the elderly (12).

Lack of education may result in elderly patients presenting with thicker melanomas. Education programs in Scotland have resulted in a decrease in lesion thickness in all patients less than 65 years old (4). In the United States, a decrease in thickness of melanoma at presentation has been attributed to education programs (2, 13). Education and earlier detection and treatment may lead to improved survival in the older patient. Many elderly patients are followed by primary care physicians. Early detection of melanomas could be further enhanced by education of primary care physicians in the fundamentals of skin examination and reemphasis of the importance of this examination in the elderly (14). Tumor ulceration is an independent negative predictive factor and is more common in the elderly (2, 5, 8, 10, 15). This may also be a contributing factor in the worse prognosis of older patients with melanoma (3, 4, 13). Female melanoma patients have a better prognosis than their male counterparts (15–17). However, this advantage is found only in younger patients. In males and females greater than 70 years of age, survival is the same (3). Tumor site is an important prognostic factor, with tumors of the extremities carrying a better prognosis than lesions of the head and neck and trunk. Melanoma patients with upper extremity lesions carry an improved prognosis compared to lesions of the lower extremity. Elderly patients with melanoma present with more head and neck lesions as well as more lesions of the lower extremity. Other factors associated with advanced age thought to lead to a worse prognosis are a decreased ability to repair DNA and a decreased immune function (18–19).

Table 1 American Joint Committee on Cancer Staging System for
Cutaneous Melanoma

Primary Tumor (T)	
Tx	Primary tumor cannot be assessed
T0	No evidence of primary tumor
Tis	Melanoma in situ (atypical melanotic hyperplasia, severe melanotic dysplasia) Clark's level I
T1	Tumor <0.75 mm, Clark's II (invades papillary dermis)
T2	Tumor 0.75–1.5 mm, Clark's III (invades to reticular dermal interface)
T3	Tumor 1.5–4 mm, Clark's IV (invades reticular dermis)
T3a	Tumor 1.5–3 mm
T3b	Tumor 3–4 mm
T4	Tumor >4 mm, Clark's V (invades into subcutaneous tissue and/or satellites)
T4a	Tumor >4 mm
T4b	Satellites within 2 cm of primary tumor
Lymph Node (N)	
Nx	Regional lymph nodes cannot be assessed
N0	No regional lymph node metastasis
N1	Metastasis in regional lymph node <3 cm in size
N2	Metastasis in regional lymph node >3 cm in size and/or in-transit metastasis
N2a	Metastasis in regional lymph node >3 cm
N2b	In-transit metastasis
N2c	Both N2a and N2b
Distant Metastasis (M)	
Mx	Presence of distant metastasis cannot be assessed
M1	Distant metastasis
M1a	Metastasis in lymph nodes, skin, or subcutaneous tissue beyond regional lymph nodes
M1b	Visceral metastasis

Stage Grouping			
I	T1 or T2	N0	M0
II	T3 or T4	N0	M0
III	Any T	N1 or N2	M0
IV	Any T	Any N	M1

C. Biopsy

As with most other tumors, the biopsy technique is important in the management of melanoma. Excisional biopsy with 1- to 2-mm margins should be used for most lesions. Shave biopsy should not be used for pigmented lesions. In large lesions where excisional biopsy is impractical, an incisional or punch biopsy directed to

Table 2 NIH Consensus Conference on Diagnosis
and Treatment of Melanoma: Essential and Suggested
Factors in the Pathological Report

Diagnosis
Measured thickness in millimeters
Margins
Subtype (SSM, NM, LMM, ALM, melanoma in situ)
Level (Clark's levels I through IV)
Ulceration (present/absent)
Regression (present/absent)
Precursor lesion (present/absent: type)
Satellitosis (present/absent)
Angiolymphatic invasion (present/absent)
Mitotic activity
Host response (lymphocyte infiltrate)
Radial vs vertical growth phase

the portion of larger lesions which is most elevated or darkest should be performed. Large pigmented lesions on the face, which are common in the elderly population, should have an incisional biopsy. Factors felt to be essential to the pathological report were listed by the National Institues of Health (NIH) consensus conference on the diagnosis and treatment of early melanoma (20) (Table 2). Accurate reporting of all of these parameters allow the clinician appropriately to select therapy.

D. Treatment

Treatment of melanoma can be separated into three areas of concern. First, treatment of the primary tumor site following diagnostic confirmation consists of wide local excision. Second, is the status of the regional nodal drainage basin which may include observation, elective node dissection, sentinel lymph node dissection, or therapeutic node dissection. The ability to detect and demonstrate the presence of regional metastasis may lead to the use of adjuvant therapy with interferon-α-2b. Third, treatment of advanced and metastatic disease may be addressed with surgical resection, regional perfusion, chemotherapy, immunotherapy, or radiation therapy.

1. Primary Lesion

a. Wide Local Excision

Historically, the excision of a melanoma was performed with a 5-cm margin. Recently, more conservative margins have been shown to be safe. In the World Health Organization (WHO) prospective randomized trial of 1-cm versus 3-cm resection, patients with melanomas less than 1 mm thick showed no significant difference in local recurrence or in disease-free or overall survival when treated with 1-cm margins (21). A second prospective randomized trial by the Melanoma Intergroup evaluated the use of 2-cm versus 4-cm margins in lesions between 1 and 4 mm thick (22). There was no difference in local recurrence or survival. Fewer patients in the 2-cm–margin group required skin grafting, which resulted in a decrease in the length of hospital stay. Current NIH recommendations for the treatment of the primary melanoma site are a 0.5-cm margin for melanoma in situ, 1-cm margin for lesions less than 1 mm thick, and 2-cm margins for lesions between 1 and 4 mm thick (20). Unfortunately, there are no prospective data that address the margin necessary for a lesion more than 4 mm thick. Most experienced melanoma surgeons will manage these patients with 2- to 3-cm margins.

2. Primary Radiation Therapy

Radiation therapy techniques which limit the penetration of the energy beam can be used for patients with lentigo maligna melanoma (23). Local control rates in patients with thin lesions are as high as 90%. In elderly patients with lentigo maligna melanoma who are not candidates for surgical therapy, radiation therapy may be an effective alternative.

E. Therapy of Regional Disease

1. Elective Lymph Node Dissection

The value of elective lymph node dissection (ELND) in the treatment of melanoma patients is controversial. In patients with intermediate-thickness lesions (1–4 mm), retrospective series have shown both benefit and no benefit of ELND with regard to survival (24, 25). Data from a recent report of the Melanoma Intergroup Trial showed no survival benefit with ELND. However, subset analysis demonstrated a survival benefit in patients less than 60 years old and in patients with lesions between 1 and 2 mm in thickness (26).

2. Sentinel Lymph Node Biopsy

Because adjuvant interferon-α-2b therapy has recently shown a significant survival benefit in node-postitive melanoma patients, the examination of the regional lymph nodes becomes important in the planning of adjuvant therapy (27). Although older patients have no proven benefit from ELND, they may still be candidates for adjuvant therapy based on the presence or absence of nodal metastasis.

In patients with clinically negative lymph nodes, an alternative method to evaluate the lymph node basin draining a particular primary site was introduced by Morton et al. (28). The ''sentinel lymph node'' is described as the first lymph nodes to receive drainage from a given cutaneous site. Biopsy of the sentinel lymph node has been shown to be predictive of the status of the remaining lymph nodes. Lymphoscintigraphy can identify which nodal areas are at risk for metastasis. Initial techniques used vital blue dye alone to map the draining of the lymphatics, isolate the sentinel node and remove it. This technique has been refined with the use of radiolabeled sulfur colloid and an intraoperative gamma counter to identify the sentinel node (29). Following removal, the sentinel lymph node is sent for permanent pathological examination. If the sentinel node contains metastatic melanoma, a full therapeutic nodal dissection is done. The decision to employ sentinel lymph node biopsy in the elderly patient must be based on two questions. If the patient were to have occult nodal metastasis, would he or she be medically able to withstand adjuvant therapy or a therapeutic nodal dissection? If patients are unable to tolerate these therapies, sentinel lymph node biopsy should not be done. If the patient is thought to be a candidate for adjuvant therapy and/or is able to undergo a therapeutic lymph nodal dissection, then the biopsy of the sentinel node should be done. Currently, we employ sentinel node biopsy in all patients with lesions greater than 1 mm in thickness who are either candidates for interferon-α-2b or therapeutic lymph node dissections.

3. Therapeutic Nodal Dissection

Patients may present with clinically apparent nodal metastasis either synchronously with a primary melanoma or some time after treatment of the primary melanoma. The majority of delayed nodal metastasis occur within 1–3 years of primary diagnosis (30). Factors that predict the development of nodal metastasis after definitive primary therapy are increasing Breslow thickness and the presence of primary tumor ulceration (31).

Surgical removal of lymph nodes in the axilla should include all three levels of axillary nodes and the supra-axillary fat pad (37). In a retrospective review, the nodal tissue above the axillary vein contained positive nodes in 17 of 104 patients (16%) (38). Surgical removal of clinically positive groin lymph nodes should include superficial, obturator, deep inguinal, and iliac nodes (37, 39). Superficial dissection only is associated with a slightly lower rate of morbidity, a higher local recurrence, and no improvement in overall survival (36). Long-term survival has been shown in patients with iliac node dissections demonstrating metastatic nodes (39). Occasionally, frail patients with clinically positive lymph nodes may benefit from a superficial nodal dissection for palliation of symptoms and regional control.

Factors predictive of survival in patients with nodal metastasis are ulceration of the primary tumor, the number of positive lymph nodes, the size of clinically palpable disease, the presence of extracapsular spread, and fixation (30–35). Although recurrence in the nodal basin is uncommon following therapeutic lymph node dissection; in patients with bulky disease, regional recurrence has been reported in between 10 and 46% of patients (32–35). Because of the significant regional recurrence rate in patients with bulky disease following therapeutic nodal dissection (TLND), postoperative radiation therapy has been evaluated. In patients with postoperative radiation following neck dissections, the 2-year regional control rate was 83%, an improvement over previously reported control rates of surgery alone (40). These results have not been confirmed in sites outside of the head and neck.

F. Adjuvant Therapy

Melanoma patients who are felt to have a high risk of recurrence may be considered for adjuvant therapy. Those with a significant risk of recurrence include patients with primary lesions greater than 4 mm in thickness, patients with nodal metastasis, patients with in-transit metastasis, and patients with complete surgical resection of distant metastasis. The risk of relapse following surgical therapy, ability effectively to treat local, regional, or distant relapse, and the effectiveness and toxicity of the adjuvant therapy should be considered prior to any adjuvant treatment (43). Interferon-α-2b (INF-α-2b) is the only proven adjuvant therapy for malignant melanoma (27, 43). A prospective randomized compared INF-α-2b to observation in melanoma patients with stages IIB, IIIA, and recurrent nodal disease (27). There was a significant increase in disease-free and overall survival in patients with nodal metastasis. Treatment with high-dose INF-α-2b in this study was associated with significant toxicity resulting in a dose reduction or a delay in therapy in 50% of patients. In other studies of INF-α-2b, a dose reduction and shorter lengths of therapy have not been effective (43). One randomized trial using a lower dose did show a significant reduction in recurrence, but the small number of patients in this series did not demonstrate an improvement in survival (44). Although anecdotally some elderly patients are less able to tolerate INF-α-2b, there is no direct evidence to suggest that older patients have a poorer response or that the toxicity should preclude consideration for adjuvant INF-α-2b. Indeed, half of the patients in the Eastern Cooperative Oncology Group Trial of INF-α-2b were over 50 years of age (27). Decisions concerning the use of this adjuvant therapy should be based on clinical evaluation of the patient.

Other forms of adjuvant therapy include vaccine therapy, immunomodulation, and intravenous chemotherapy (43, 45). Vaccine therapy and immunomodulation with interleukin-2 (IL-2), monoclonal antibodies, bacillus Calmette-Guérin (BCG) injection, and INF-α have shown activity in phase II trials, but no conclusive improvement in survival has been shown when used in the adjuvant setting (43, 45). Multidrug chemotherapy based on dacarbazine (DTIC) and cisplatin have also shown activity in the advanced disease setting with no improvement in survival when used in the adjuvant setting (43, 45). These adjuvant treatments are felt to be less well tolerated in the elderly patient, but few of these studies have looked directly at toxicity in older patients.

G. Advanced Disease

Prognostic factors in patients with metastatic disease include the number of metastatic sites, anatomical location of disease, and the disease-free interval (46–49).

Options for treatment of advanced disease include regional hyperthermic chemotherapy perfusion for disease limited to an extremity, systemic chemotherapy, immunotherapy, radiation, and surgery. Complete surgical resection of stage IV melanoma has been shown to improve survival in properly selected cases (46–49). Incomplete resection or debulking of tumor has no survival benefit. Advanced age and an inability to tolerate surgical intervention will lessen the role of this treatment in the elderly population. Isolated limb perfusion techniques have been shown to be effective in the treatment of advanced disease limited to the extremity and have decreased the amputation rate in patients with locally advanced disease of the extremity (50, 51). Although regional therapy is felt to be well tolerated in the elderly, these patients may have significant peripheral vascular disease and significant comorbid conditions that may limit the ability to tolerate therapy.

The treatment of advanced melanoma with systemic chemotherapy has shown limited success (45, 52). The most active agent in the treatment of metastatic melanoma is DTIC, both alone and in combination with other agents. Other chemotherapeutic agents show a low response rate. Although cisplatin was not effective as a single agent, it has been shown to improve response rates in combination therapy. Treatment of metastatic disease with INF-α-2b alone has a low response rate, but when added to multidrug regimens, the response improves to as high as 73%. The most effective regimen contains IL-2, INF-α, dacarbazine, carmustine (BCNU), cisplatin (DDP), and tamoxifen. Current recommended first-line therapy of advanced melanoma includes a combination of dacarbazine, carmustine, cisplatin, and tamoxifen with INF-α and IL-2 to be used as second- and third-line therapies (45).

The ability of elderly patients to tolerate these regimens has not been specifically assessed. Although physical condition and the ability to tolerate therapy rather than chronological age should be used in the decision to judge what is appropriate therapy, many older patients will have difficulty with many of these regimens. Some elderly patients may benefit from single-agent or less toxic regimens for palliation.

II. SOFT–TISSUE SARCOMA

It was estimated that there would be 6600 soft-tissue sarcomas (STSs) in 1997, with an estimated 4100 deaths (1). The age-adjusted risk of sarcoma is highest in the elderly (53). Sarcomas arise from connective tissue and can appear anywhere in the body. The majority of sarcomas arise in the extremities, with the thigh being the most common site. Successful treatment of (STS) depends on the adequate surgical resection of the primary tumor. Factors that affect local recurrence and survival include tumor size, tumor grade, tumor depth, adequate surgical resection, and advanced age. Historically, sarcomas of the extremity were treated with amputation above the joint most proximal to the tumor. Less radical surgical excision was later combined with external beam radiation which resulted in limb salvage, but without a decrease in disease-free or overall survival. The current standard of care in extremity and truncal wall sarcomas is the complete surgical removal of tumor combined with radiation therapy. Retroperitoneal sarcomas are treated with wide surgical excision alone. The addition of radiation therapy to the management of retroperitoneal sarcoma is being assessed in some sarcoma centers. Modern radiotherapy techniques may be beneficial in selected cases. In this chapter, we will discuss the current staging, diagnosis, treatment, and rehabilitation of STS patients with an emphasis on their management in the elderly patient.

A. Histological Types

Histological subtypes of sarcomas depend on their tissue of origin. The most common sarcomas are malignant fibrous histiocytoma (MFH), liposarcoma, leiomyosarcoma, fibrosarcoma, and rhabdomyosarcoma (53–57). Variation in the incidence of each of these subtypes is seen in different age groups. Malignant fibrous histiocytoma occurs more commonly in older patients (54). At Roswell Park Cancer Institute (RPCI), MFH accounts for 38% of sarcomas in patients greater than 65 years of age and only 19% of sarcomas in patients less than 65 years of age. Table 3 shows the incidence of histological type by age seen at RPCI. Recently, increased attention has been given to Kaposi's sarcoma owing to its prevalence in patients infected with the human immunodeficiency virus (HIV). Prior to the HIV epidemic, Kaposi's sarcoma was relatively rare and seen most commonly in older male patients. Other sarcomas such as embryonal rhabdomyosarcoma, extraskeletal Ewing's sarcoma, and extraskeletal osteosarcoma are seen in younger patients (54).

Table 3 Histological Subtype and Age of Sarcoma

Histology	Age <65(%) (n = 449)	Age >65(%) (n = 139)
Liposarcoma	110 (24)	36 (26)
Malignant fibrous histiocytoma (MFH)	84 (19)	53 (38)
Leiomyosarcoma	63 (14)	25 (18)
Synovial sarcoma	35 (8)	3 (2)
Unclassified	24 (5)	5 (4)
Rhabdomyosarcoma	21 (5)	1 (1)
Fibrosarcoma	20 (5)	3 (2)
Hemangiopericytoma	20 (5)	1 (1)
Spindle cell sarcoma	16 (4)	1 (1)
Malignant schawnoma	11 (2)	2 (1)
Clear cell sarcoma	6 (1)	0
Chondrosarcoma	6 (1)	0
Angiosarcoma	4 (1)	3 (2)
Others	29 (6)	6 (4)

Table 4 American Joint Committee on Cancer Staging System for Soft-Tissue Sarcoma

Primary Tumor (T)

T1	Tumor <5 cm
T2	Tumor >5 cm

Histological Grade of Tumor (G)

G1	Low grade
G2	Moderate grade
G3	High grade

Regional Lymph Nodes (N)

N0	Negative regional lymph nodes
N1	Positive regional lymph nodes

Distant Metastasis (M)

M0	No distant metastasis
M1	Distant metastasis

Tumor Stage

IA	G1	T1	N0	M0
IB	G1	T2	N0	M0
IIA	G2	T1	N0	M0
IIB	G2	T2	N0	M0
IIIA	G3	T1	N0	M0
IIIB	G3	T2	N0	M0
IVA	G1, G2, G3	T1, T2	N1	M0
IVB	G1, G2, G3	T1, T2	N0, N1	M1

B. Staging

The AJCC staging system for STS is based on the GTNM system (Table 4) (11). This system incorporates tumor grade, tumor size, nodal status, and the presence of metastasis in the staging system. The stage is dependent on the tumor grade, with low grade, intermediate grade, and high grade defining stages I through III. Stage IV disease designates sarcomas with nodal and/or distant metastasis. Enneking has proposed a staging system based on tumor grade and the tumor's occurrence superficially or deep to the investing fascia (Table 5) (58). Both of these systems reflect the importance of tumor grade on the prognosis of soft-tissue sarcoma.

C. Prognostic Factors

Tumor grade in the most powerful predictive factor (55–57, 59–61) for STS. Review of retrospective databases has identified risk factors for local recurrence, risk of distant metastasis, and risk for death from disease. Factors leading to an increase in the local recurrence include age greater than 50 years, positive margins, histological subtype of liposarcoma or peripheral nerve sheath tumor, presentation with recurrent disease, and treatment with limb-sparing surgery (56, 60–62). Factors that increase

Table 5 Enneking Staging System for Soft-Tissue
and Bone Sarcoma

Stage I (low grade)
IA   Within an anatomical compartment
IB   Extracompartmental
Stage II (high grade)
IIA   Within an anatomical compartment
IIB   Extracompartmental
Stage III (any grade with nodal or distant metastasis)

the risk of distant metastasis include increasing tumor size, grade, and depth (56, 62). Disease-free survival of extremity STS is adversely affected by increasing tumor size, higher tumor grade, increasing tumor depth, presentation with recurrent disease, positive margins, age greater than 50 years, female sex, the presence of necrosis, proximal site, positive lymph node metastasis, and the presence of local symptoms (55, 56, 59–61). A review retroperitoneal STS found the disease-free survival was worse with high-grade tumors and tumors resected with positive margins (63, 64).

D. Evaluation and Biopsy

The evaluation of patients with large masses consistent with the diagnosis of STS begins with a careful history and physical examination. This should include routine blood work and a chest radiograph. Prior to biopsy, careful imaging of the primary tumor should be done (65). For tumors of the body torso wall and retroperitoneum, computerized tomography (CT) is the imaging modality of choice. This may lead to other imaging studies. In patients with large tumors of the extremities, magnetic reasonance imaging (MRI) is the appropriate modality. Biopsy or excision of tumors prior to imaging disrupts tissue planes and can complicate the interpretation of subsequent imaging efforts. Small superficial lesions less than 3–5 cm in size at sites which can be reresected if necessary may be removed with an excisional biopsy (66, 67). This should only be done when it is the opinion of the surgeon that the lesion is benign; should it prove to be malignant, the site can be reresected. Other lesions should be biopsied prior to removal. Biopsy may be done by fine-needle aspiration (FNA), core needle biopsy, or incisional biopsy. The method chosen will depend on the expertise available in the institution. In all circumstances, the biopsy should be done or directed by the experienced oncological surgeon who will be performing the surgical resection. Although FNA is increasingly popular in the evaluation of some tumors, most institutions do not have sufficient experience with STS to use this biopsy technique in these uncommon tumors. Large soft-tissue tumors may be biopsied successfully with core needle biopsy in the outpatient area or under CT or ultrasound guidance in the radiology suite (68, 69). Biopsy under CT guidance helps identify the portion of the tumor most likely to be viable. More frequent use of CT guidance at the time of biopsy will improve the frequency of successful needle biopsy. When core needle biopsy is not possible or is nondiagnostic, incisional biopsy should be done with the incision along the long axis of the limb. Planning and performance of the biopsy of large soft-tissue masses is best done by the surgeon who will perform the definitive surgical resection. Complete staging of STSs includes a CT of the chest to evaluate the patient for evidence of pulmonary metastasis. This may be done prior to biopsy or following biopsy. Definitive treatment should be planned with the aid of a multidisciplinary approach.

E. Treatment

1.   Sarcoma of the Extremity and Trunk

a.   *Primary Radiation Therapy*

For large high-grade STSs of the extremity and trunk, the standard of care is surgical excision with adjuvant radiation. Treatment with radiation alone has been reported. Sarcoma patients most commonly treated with primary radiation are patients with unresectable disease, those whose comorbid conditions preclude surgery, and those who refuse amputation. Successful local control can be achieved with radiation alone depending on the size of the tumor and the amount of radiation given (70). Higher doses of radiation and smaller sarcomas will increase the likelihood of achieving local control (71). In patients who are not candidates for surgical resection or refuse amputation, primary radiation therapy may be considered.

b.   *Surgery*

Except for very large tumors, most low-grade STSs many be managed with wide surgical excision alone. Radiation may benefit large, low-grade tumors.

Local control and survival of extremity and truncal high-grade STSs is dependent on tumor size, grade, and obtaining an adequate surgical margin (55, 56, 59–62). Small superficial lesions are adequately treated with wide excision with negative margins (66, 67). Small superficial lesions excised with positive or unknown margins should have wide reexcision of the tumor bed. Even with adjuvant radiation therapy, intracapsular and marginal excisions are suboptimal and can result in a high local recurrence rate (66). Wide excisions have a lower risk of local recurrence and may include en bloc resection of adjacent muscle, nerve, and blood vessels (66). Compartment resection is based on the knowledge that the sarcoma does not usually invade the fascia which separates muscle compartments. Compartment resection represented the first formal effort at achieving limb salvage with surgery alone. Amputations are used less frequently for the treatment of primary disease and are more common in patients with bulky lesions, recurrent lesions, and those with involvement of large neurovascular bundles. Wide excision with radiation has decreased the need for these more aggressive surgical procedures, yet they are still occasionally necessary. Modern surgical and anesthetic techniques will allow appropriately aggressive surgical procedures to be performed in almost all elderly patients. In some situations, longer and more tedious dissections with limb salvage will improve posttreatment function. The addition of appropriately dosed radiation therapy will optimize the opportunity for local control and rehabilitation in these patients.

c. Surgery with Radiation

Adjuvant radiation therapy has been shown to improve local control following wide local excision in large high-grade extremity and truncal STSs (72–74). Radiation may be given preoperatively or following surgical excision of the primary tumor. Radiation therapy may include external beam radiation, brachytherapy, or a combination of these two modalities. Advantages of preoperative radiation include the use of smaller radiation treatment fields and treatment with lower doses resulting in shrinkage of the tumor leading to easier surgical removal and limb salvage (74). Preoperative external beam radiation has been associated with a modest increase in wound problems (73–77). Postoperative radiation allows for the complete assessment of the tumor prior to treatment with radiation. However, postoperative complications may delay or preclude radiation and larger doses and fields are necessary. Advantages of brachytherapy include localized treatment directly to the tumor bed and a shorter time to completion of adjuvant therapy. However, brachytherapy has been associated with a modest increase in wound problems (72, 73, 76). In the elderly population, shortening treatment time is sometimes very helpful. A lack of mobility and the difficulty of transportation in elderly patients with STS can make daily travel to and from the hospital for external beam radiation difficult. Wide surgical excision with high-dose brachytherapy can complete therapy within 2 weeks. A randomized trial has shown that postoperative brachytherapy improves local control in high-grade sarcomas, but no difference was seen in patients with low-grade tumors (72). No direct comparison of external beam radiation and high-dose brachytherapy has been done. However it is given, the use of radiation in combination with surgery allows limb preservation in most patients with STS.

d. Adjuvant Chemotherapy

The role of adjuvant chemotherapy in preventing systemic recurrence and improving survival in patients with high-risk STS remains unclear. Adriamycin (doxorubicin), DTIC, and ifosfamide are the most active drugs. Adriamycin has been used in combination with DTIC with good response rates (78). Trials using mesna uroprotective agent with ifosfamide, Adriamycin, and DTIC have shown good response rates in phase II trials and an improved response compared to the two-agent combination (79, 80). However, the three-agent therapy was associated with a significant number of treatment-related deaths, all of which were in patients greater than 50 years of age (80). A meta-analysis of 15 prospective randomized trials using Adriamycin and Adriamycin-based regimens showed an improvement in local control, disease-free survival, and a 4% increase in overall survival (81). The decision to place patients on adjuvant therapy is a difficult one. If possible, they should be placed on randomized clinical trials. Adequate surgical resection with radiation remains the mainstay of therapy of STS.

e. Recurrent Disease

Local recurrences of extremity and truncal STSs are treated in a manner similar to that of the primary tumor. Surgical excision with negative margins is necessary for local control, with the use of adjuvant therapy being dictated by the type and extent of prior therapy. In patients with limb recurrence where reexcision for limb salvage is not possible, then amputation may be necessary. Elderly patients with limited survival expectations may be best treated with conservative local measures allowing continued ambulation.

2. Retroperitoneal Sarcoma

Retroperitoneal STSs (RSTS) are uncommon tumors which account for 15% of STSs (82). Half of all retroperitoneal solid-tissue tumors are sarcomas, with the majority of the remainder being lymphomas or urogenital tumors (82). Patients present most commonly with an abdominal mass and increasing abdominal girth (82, 85–88). The median resected tumor size in RSTS is 15 cm (64, 83). Surgical resection with negative margins is the mainstay of therapy, with no proven benefit of adjuvant radiation or chemotherapy (63, 64, 84–88).

a. Surgery

Biopsy of RSTS can be obtained either with an open incisional biopsy or pre-operatively by CT-guided core biopsy (82). Care should be taken to avoid tumor spillage. Complete surgical resection is the primary treatment for RSTS and is possible in 50–100% of cases, with most series reporting resectability rates of 60–70% (63, 84, 86, 88). To assure a wide margin of resection, adjacent abdominal organs must commonly be resected. The most common organs removed are the kidney, colon, small bowel, pancreas, major vascular structures, and spleen (85). Care must be taken prior to surgery to assure contralateral kidney function should nephrectomy be required. Of patients who require resection of adjacent organs, 38% will require resection of two or more organs (85). Factors that influence the rate of local recurrence and survival are tumor grade, the extent of resection, and the presence of positive margins (63, 64, 85, 86). The 5-year survival rate following surgical removal of tumor has been reported between 23 and 74% (82, 83, 86, 87). The surgical management of a large RSTS represents challenging surgical and anesthetic problems in all patients. However, this is especially so for the elderly patient. Yet modern surgical and anesthetic techniques will allow most elderly patients to receive optimal surgical resections. The postoperative functionality of the patient, especially the elderly patient, should be taken into consideration preoperatively and treatment planning done accordingly.

b. Radiation Therapy and Chemotherapy

With the high incidence of local recurrence in RSTS, there has been interest in the addition of other treatment modalities. Although there have been single-institution reports of improved local control with radiation therapy, its effectiveness has not been proven in a prospective controlled trial. The limiting factor with radiation is the toxic effect on normal adjacent structures (82, 84). Preoperative radiation has the advantage of requiring a lower total dose of radiation, but it has not demonstrated lower rates of local recurrence. Brachytherapy and intraoperative radiation therapy have not conclusively shown improved local control (85). As with radiation therapy, there is no proven benefit to the addition of chemotherapy to the treatments of RSTS (82, 85, 88). At present, the treatment of RSTS is the surgical removal of the primary tumor with negative margins. When available, these patients should be placed on clinical trials.

c. Recurrence and Treatment

Recurrence following complete surgical removal of RSTS is variable and ranges between 39 and 90% (63, 82, 84–86). Local recurrence is a common problem in patients with RSTS, accounting for 75% of recurrences; they are more commonly associated with positive margins and high-grade tumors (85). Surgical treatment of local recurrences of RSTS has been shown to increase survival when complete excision of the recurrent tumor can be achieved. Resectability rates of locally recurrent RSTS are 44–64% (83, 85, 86). However, this is associated with a second recurrence in 49–90% of patients. In one series of patients with disseminated intra-abdominal sarcoma, complete resection of all gross tumor was accomplished in 64%. There was a significant survival advantage over those with incomplete resection (83). The median number of operations in this series was two, with long-term survivors receiving a median of two operations per year. There were no long-term survivors in patients with high-grade tumors, and time to recurrence was dependent on tumor grade. High-grade tumors recurred at a median of 15 months and low-grade tumors recurred at a median of 41 months. With modern anesthetic and surgical techniques, elderly patients with retroperitoneal sarcomas who are adequate surgical risks for removal of tumor are likely to benefit from resection with significant palliation of symptoms and prolonged survival. Distant recurrences in patients with retroperitoneal STSs are less common than local recurrence and show an equal distribution between the lung and liver. Although elderly patients are likely to benefit from initial aggressive resection of RSTS, plans for multiple laporatomies for repeat resection must take into consideration the patient's comorbidities.

3. Advanced Disease

Treatment of advanced STS depends on the location and extent of the recurrence. Except for RSTSs, which metastasize to the lung and liver, the most common site of distant metastases is the lung. Prognostic factors in patients with metastatic disease include the number and location of lesions, the disease-free interval, and the grade of the lesion. Surgical resection of lung metastasis is associated with a 5-year survival rate of 20–40% (89–91). Prognostic factors associated with improved survival following complete resection of pulmonary metastases include patients with fewer than two lesions, lesions less than 2 cm in diameter, longer disease-free interval, resection with negative margins, age less than 40 years, and grade I and II tumors (89, 90). The use of video-assisted thoracoscopic resection of metastatic sarcoma to the lung can be done with low morbidity and mortality, making it an attractive option in appropriately selected older patients.

4. Rehabilitation of the Elderly Patient

The development of limb-salvage techniques combining wide excision and radiation has improved the rehabilitation potential for all patients, but especially the elderly. Elderly patients are unlikely to adjust to major amputations. It is important to emphasize that sometimes longer and more tedious efforts to preserve function at the time of surgical resection may, along with appropriate adjuvant radiation, improve the opportunity for subsequent rehabilitation in the elderly patient. Physical disability of an older patient is associated with significant morbidity and mortality. Rehabilitation in the elderly patient is more difficult, less successful, and takes longer than in younger patients. The presence and complications of comorbid conditions is the most common cause of cessation of rehabilitation (92). Elderly patients have more comorbid conditions, which limit the success of rehabilitation (92–95). Careful control and treatment of comorbid medical conditions can lead to more successful rehabilitation of elderly patients. We as physicians must optimize our efforts at giving the elderly patient with STS the very best opportunity for rehabilitation with well-planned local therapies as well as appropriate management of associated comorbid conditions.

REFERENCES

1. Parker SL, Tong T, Bolden S, Wingo PA. Cancer statistics, 1997. CA Cancer J Clin 1997; 47:5–26.
2. Balch CM, Reintgen DS, Kirkwood JM, Houghton A, Peters L, Ang KK. Cutaneous melanoma. In: DeVita VT Jr, Hellman S, Rosenberg SA, eds. Cancer: Principles and Practice of Oncology. 5th ed. Philadelphia: Lippincott-Raven, 1997:1947–1979.
3. Loggie B, Ronan SG, Bean J, Das Gupta TK. Invasive cutaneous melanoma in elderly patients. Arch Dermatol 1991; 127:1188–1193.

4. McHenry PM, Hole DJ, MacKie RM. Melanoma in people aged 65 and over in Scotland, 1979–89. BMJ 1992; 304:746–749.

5. Austin PF, Cruse CW, Lyman G, Schroer K, Glass F, Reintgen DS. Age as a prognostic factor in the malignant melanoma population. Ann Surg Oncol 1994; 1:487–494.

6. Cohen HJ, Cox E, Manton K, Woodbury M. Malignant melanoma in the elderly. J Clin Oncol 1987; 5:100–106.

7. Young JL, Percy CL, Asire AJ, Berg JW, Cusano MM, Gloeckler LA, Horm JW, Lourie WI Jr, Pollack ES, Shambaugh EM. Cancer incidence and mortality in the United States, 1973–1977. Natl Cancer Inst Monogr 1981; 57:1–187.

8. Evans GRD, Manson PN. Review and current perspectives of cutaneous malignant melanoma. J Am Coll Surg 1994; 178:523–540.

9. American Joint Committee on Cancer. Manual for Staging of Cancer. 4th ed. Philadelphia: Lippincott-Raven, 1992:143–148.

10. Meyskens FL, Berdeaux DH, Parks B, Tong T, Loescher L, Moon TE. Cutaneous malignant melanoma (Arizona Cancer Center Experience). Cancer 1988; 62:1207–1214.

11. Morton DL, Davtyan DG, Wanek LA, Foshag LJ, Cochran AJ. Multivariate analysis of the relationship between survival and the microstage of primary melanoma by Clark level and Breslow thickness. Cancer 1993; 71:3737–3743.

12. Levine J, Kopf AW, Rigel DS, Bart RS, Hennessey P, Friedman RJ, Mintzis MM. Correlation of thickness of superficial spreading malignant melanomas and ages of patients. J Dermatol Surg Oncol 1991; 7:311–316.

13. Koh HK, Geller AC, Miller DR, Lew RA. The early detection of and screening for melanoma, international status. Cancer 1995; 75(Suppl):674–683.

14. Wender RC. Barriers to effective skin cancer detection. Cancer 1995; 75:691–698.

15. Drzewiecki KT, Andersen PK: Survival with malignant melanoma. A recessive analysis of prognostic factors. Cancer 1982; 49:2414–2419.

16. Shaw HM, McGovern VJ, Milton GW, Farago GA, McCarthy WH. Histologic features of tumors and the female superiority in survival from malignant melanoma. Cancer 1980; 45:1604–1608.

17. Balch CM, Murad TM, Soong S-J, Ingalls AL, Halpern NB, Maddox WA. A multifactorial analysis of melanoma: prognostic histopathological features comparing Clark's and Breslow's staging methods. Ann Surg 1978; 188:732–742.

18. Walford RL: Immunology and aging. Am J Clin Pathol 1980; 74:247–253.

19. Crawford J, Cohen HJ: Aging and neoplasia. Ann Rev Gerontol Geriatr 1984; 4:3–32.

20. NIH Consensus Conference. Diagnosis and Treatment of Early Melanoma. JAMA 1992; 268:1314–1319.

21. Veronesi U, Cascinelli N. Narrow excision (1-cm margins): A safe procedure for thin cutaneous melanoma. Arch Surg 1991; 126:438–441.

22. Balch CM, Urist MM, Karakousis CP, Smith TJ, Temple WJ, Drzewiecki K, Jewell WR, Bartolucci AA, Mihm MC, Barnhill R, Wanebo HJ. Efficacy of 2-cm surgical margins for intermediate thickness melanomas (1 to 4 mm); Results of a multi-institutional randomized surgical trial. Ann Surg 1993; 218:262–269.

23. Peters LJ, Byers RM, Ang KK: Radiotherapy for melanoma. In: Balch CM, ed. Cutaneous Melanoma. 2nd ed. Philadelphia: Lippincott-Raven, 1996:509–521.

24. McCarthy WH, Shaw HM, Cascinelli N, Santinami M, Belli F. Elective lymph node dissection for melanoma: two perspectives. World J Surg 1992; 16:203–213.

25. Coates AS, Ingvar CI, Peterson-Schaefer K, Shaw HM, Milton GW, O'Brien CJ, Thompson JF, McCarthy WH. Elective lymph node dissection in patients with primary melanoma of the trunk and limbs treated at the Sydney melanoma unit from 1960 to 1991. J Am Coll Surg 1995; 180:402–409.

26. Balch CM, Soong SJ, Bartolucci AA, Urist MM, Karakousis CP, Smith TJ, Temple WJ, Ross MI, Jewell WR, Mihm MC, Barnhill RL, Wanebo HJ. Efficacy of an elective regional lymph node dissection of 1 to 4 mm thick melanomas for patients 60 years of age and younger. Ann Surg 1996; 224:255–266.

27. Kirkwood JM, Strawderman MH, Ernstoff MS, Smith TJ, Borden EC, Blum RH. Interferon alpha-2b adjuvant therapy of high risk resected cutaneous melanoma: the Eastern Cooperative Oncology Group trial EST 1684. J Clin Oncol 1996; 14:7–17.

28. Morton DL, Wen DR, Wong JH, Economou US, Cagle LA, Storm FK, Foshag LJ, Cochran AJ. Technical details of intraoperative lymphatic mapping for early stage melanoma. Arch Surg 1992; 127:392–399.

29. Reintgen D, Balch CM, Kirkwood J, Ross M. Recent advances in the care of the patient with malignant melanoma. Ann Surg 1997; 225:1–14.

30. Balch CM, Soong SJ, Murad TM, Ingalls AL, Maddox WA. A multifactorial analysis of melanoma III.: Prognostic factors in melanoma patients with lymph node metastases (stage II). Ann Surg 1981; 191:377–388.

31. Berdeaux DH, Meyskens FL, Parks B, Tong T, Loescher L, Moon TE. Cutaneous malignant melanoma: the natural history and prognostic factors influencing the development of stage II disease. Cancer 1989; 63:1430–1436.

32. Calabro A, Singletary SE, Balch CM. Patterns of relapse in 1001 consecutive patients with melanoma nodal metastases. Arch Surg 1989; 124:1051–1055.

33. Monsour PD, Sause WT, Avent JM, Noyes RD. Local control following therapeutic nodal dissection for melanoma. J Surg Oncol 1993; 54:18–22.

34. Gadd MA, Coit DG. Recurrence patterns and outcome in 1019 patients undergoing axillary and inguinal lymphadenectomy for melanoma. Arch Surg 1992; 127:1412–1416.

35. Singletary SE, Shallenberger R, Guinee VF, McBride CM. Melanoma with metastasis to regional axillary or inguinal lymph nodes: Prognostic factors and results of surgical treatment in 714 patients. South Med J 1988; 81:5–9.

36. Singletary SE, Shallenburger R, Guinee VF. Surgical management of groin nodal metastases from primary melanoma on the lower extremity. Surg Gynecol Obstet 1992; 174:195–200.

37. Karakousis CP. Technique of lymphadenectomy for melanoma. Surg Oncol Clin North Am 1992; 1:157–193.

38. Karakousis CP, Goumas W, Rao U, Driscoll DL. Axillary node dissection in malignant melanoma. Am J Surg 1991; 162:202–207.

39. Karakousis CP, Driscoll DL, Rose B, Walsh D. Groin dissection in malignant melanoma. Ann Surg Oncol 1994; 1:271–277.

40. Ang KK, Byers RM, Peters LJ, Maor MH, Wendt CD, Morrison WH, Hussey DH, Goepfert H. Regional radiotherapy as an alternative or adjuvant to nodal dissection for high risk co-laneous malignant melanoma of the head and neck. Arch Otolaryngol Head Neck Surg 1990; 116:169–172.

41. Strom EA, Ross MI. Adjuvant radiation therapy after axillary lymphadenectomy for metastatic melanoma: toxicity and local control. Ann Surg Oncol 1995; 2:445–449.

42. Creagan ET, Cupps RE, Ivins JC, Pritchard DJ, Sim FH, Soule EH, Ofallaw JR. Adjuvant radiation therapy for regional nodal metastases for malignant melanoma: a randomized prospective study. Cancer 1978; 42:2206–2210.

43. Dickler MN, Coit DG, Meyers ML. Adjuvant therapy of malignant melanoma. Surg Oncol Clin North Am 1997; 6:793–812.

44. Rusciani L, Petraglia S, Alotto M, Calvieri S, Vezzoni G. Postsurgical adjuvant therapy for melanoma: Evaluation of a 3-year randomized trial with recombinant interferon-alpha after 3 and 5 years of follow-up. Cancer 1997; 79:2354–2360.

45. Nathan FE, Berd D, Mastrangelo MJ. Chemotherapy of melanoma. In: The Chemotherapy Source Book. Perry MC, ed. Baltimore: Williams & Wilkins, 1996: 1043–1069.

46. Barth A, Wanek LA, Morton DL. Prognostic factors in 1521 melanoma patients with distant metastases. J Am Coll Surg 1995; 181:193–201.

47. Hena MA, Emrich LJ, Nambisan RN, Karakousis CP. Effect of surgical treatment on stage IV melanoma. Am J Surg 1987; 153:270–275.

48. Karakousis CP, Moore R, Holyoke ED. Surgery in recurrent malignant melanoma. Cancer 1983; 52:1342–1345.

49. Overett TK, Shiu MH. Surgical treatment of distant metastatic melanoma: Indications and results. Cancer 1985; 56:1222–1230.

50. Krementz ET, Carter RD, Sutherland CM, Muchmore JH, Ryan RF, Creech O. Regional chemotherapy for melanoma; A 35-year experience. Ann Surg 1994; 220:520–535.

51. Thom AK, Alexander HR, Andrich MP, Barker WC, Rosenberg SA, Fraker DL. Cytokine levels and systemic toxicity in patients undergoing isolated limb perfusion with high-dose tumor necrosis factor, interferon gamma, and melphalan. J Clin Oncol 1995; 132:264–273.

52. Coates AS. Systemic chemotherapy for malignant melanoma. World J Surg 1992; 16: 277–281.

53. Storm HH. Cancers of the soft tissues. Cancer Surv 1994; 19/20:197–217.

54. Enzinger FM, Weiss SW. General considerations. In: Enzinger FM, Weiss SW, eds. Soft Tissue Tumors. 3rd Ed. St. Louis: Mosby, 1995:1–16.

55. Collin C, Godbold J, Hajdu S, Brennan M. Localized extremity soft tissue sarcoma: An analysis of factors affecting survival. J Clin Oncol 1987; 5:601–612.

56. Pisters PWT, Leung DHY, Woodruff J, Shi W, Brennan MF. Analysis of prognostic factors in 1041 patients with localized soft tissue sarcomas of the extremities. J Clin Oncol 1996; 14:1679–1689.

57. Gustafson P. Soft tissue sarcoma; epidemiology and prognosis in 508 patients. Acta Orthop Scand 1994; 65(Suppl):259:1–31.

58. Enneking WF, Spainer SS, Malawer MM. A system for the surgical staging of musculoskeletal sarcoma. Clin Orthop Rel Res 1980; 153:106–120.

59. Ueda T, Aozasa K, Tsujimoto M, Hamada H, Hayashi H, Ono K, Matsumoto K. Multivariate analysis for clinical prognostic factors in 163 patients with soft tissue sarcoma. Cancer 1988; 62:1444–1450.

60. Cakir S, Dincbas FO, Uzel O, Koca SS, Okkan S. Multivariate analysis of prognostic factors in 75 patients with soft tissue sarcoma. Radiother Oncol 1995; 37:10–16.

61. Collin CF, Friedrich C, Goldbald J, Hajdu S, Brennan MF. Prognostic factors for local recurrence and survival in patients with localized extremity soft-tissue sarcoma. Semin Surg Oncol 1998; 4:30–37.

62. LeVay J, O'Sullivan B, Catton C, Bell R, Fornasier V, Cummings B, Hao Y, Warr D, Quirt I. Outcome and prognostic factors in soft tissue sarcoma in the adult. Int J Radiat Oncol Biol Phys 1993; 27(5):1091–1099.

63. Singer S, Corson JM, Demetri GD, Healy EA, Marcus K, Eberlein TJ. Prognostic factors predictive of survival for truncal and retroperitoneal soft-tissue sarcoma. Ann Surg 1995; 221:185–195.

64. Bevilacqua RG, Rogatko A, Hajdu SI, Brennan MF. Prognostic factors in primary retroperitoneal soft-tissue sarcomas. Arch Surg 1991; 126:328–334.

65. Munk PL, Vellet AD, Bramwell V, Bell R, Hammond A, Beauchamp C. Soft tissue sarcomas: a plea for proper management. Can J Surg 1993; 36(2):178–180.

66. Chang EC, Sondak VK. Clinical evaluation and treatment of soft tissue tumors. In: Eds Enzinger FM, Weiss SW, eds. Soft Tissue Tumors. St. Louis: Mosby 1995:17–38.

67. Geer RJ, Woodruff J, Casper ES, Brennan MF. Management of small soft tissue sarcoma of the extremity in adults. Arch Surg 1992; 127:1285–1289.

68. Ball AB, Fisher C, Pittam M, Watkins RM, Westbury G. Diagnosis of soft tissue tumours by true cut biopsy. Br J Surg 1990; 77:756–758.

69. Barth RJ Jr., Merino MJ, Solomon D, Yank JC, Baker AR. A prospective study of the value of core needle biopsy and fine needle aspiration in the diagnosis of soft tissue masses. Surgery 1992; 112:536–543.

70. Yang JC, Glatstein EJ, Rosenburg SA, Antman KH. Sarcomas of soft tissues. In: DeVita VT Jr, Hellman S, Rosenburg SA, eds. Cancer: Principles of Practice and Oncology. Philadelphia: Lippincott, 1993; 1436–1488.

71. Tepper JE, Suit HD. Radiation therapy in soft tissue sarcomas. Cancer 1985; 55:2273–2277.

72. Pisters PWT, Harrison LB, Leung DHY, Woodruff JM, Casper ES, Brennan MF. Long-term results of a prospective randomized trial of adjuvant brachytherapy in soft tissue sarcoma. J Clin Oncol 1996; 14:859–868.

73. Spiro IJ, Rosenburg AE, Springfield D, Suit H, Phil D. Combined surgery and radiation therapy for limb preservation in soft tissue sarcoma of the extremity: The Massachusetts General Hospital Experience. Cancer Invest 1995; 13:86–95.

74. Lewis JJ, Benedetti F. Adjuvant therapy for soft tissue sarcomas. Surg Oncol North Am 1997; 6:847–862.

75. Brant TA, Parsons JT, Marcus RB, Spainer SS, Heare TC, Van Der Griend RA, Enneking WF, Million RR. Preoperative irradiation for soft tissue sarcomas of the trunk and extremities in adults. Int J Radiat Oncol Biol Phys 1990; 19:899–906.

76. Bujko K, Suit HD, Springfield DS, Convery K. Wound healing after preoperative radiation for sarcoma of soft tissues. Surg Gynecol Obstet 1993; 1176:124–134.

77. Rosenthal HG, Terek RM, Lane JM. Management of extremity soft-tissue sarcomas. Clin Orthop Rel Res 1993; 289:66–72.

78. Gottlieb JA, Baker LH, Quagliana JM, Luce JK, Whitecar JP, Sinkovics JG, Rivkin SE, Frei E. Chemotherapy of sarcomas with a combination of adriamycian and dimethyl triazeno imidazole carboximide. Cancer 1972; 30:1632–1638.

79. Elias A, Ryan L, Sulkes A, Collins J, Aisner J, Antman KH. Response to mesna, doxirubicin, ifosfamide, and dacarbizine in 108 patients with metastatic or unresectable sarcoma and no prior chemotherapy. J Clin Oncol 1989; 9:1208–1216.

80. Antman K, Crowley J, Balcerzak SP, Rivkin SE, Weiss GR, Elias A, Natale RB, Cooper RM, Barlogie B, Trump DL. An intergroup phase III randomized study of doxorubicin

and dacarbizine with or without ifosfamide and mesna in advanced soft tissue and bone sarcomas. J Clin Oncol 1993; 11:1276–1285.

81. Tierney JF, Stewart LA, Parmar MKB. Adjuvant chemotherapy for localized resectable soft-tissue sarcoma of adults; meta-analysis of individual data. Lancet 1997; 350:1647–1654.

82. Storm FK, Mahvi DM. Diagnosis and management of retroperitoneal soft-tissue sarcoma. Ann Surg 1991; 214:2–10.

83. Karakousis CP, Blumenson LE, Canavese G, Rao U. Surgery for disseminated abdominal sarcoma. Am J Surg 1992; 163:560–564.

84. Clark JA, Tepper JE. Role of Radiation therapy in retroperitoneal sarcomas. Oncology 1996; 10:1867–1874.

85. Jaques DP, Coit DG, Hajdu SI, Brennan MF. Management of primary and recurrent soft-tissue sarcoma of the retroperitoneum. Ann Surg 1990; 212:51–59.

86. Karakousis C, Velez AF, Gerstenbluth R, Driscoll DL. Resectability and survival in retroperitoneal sarcomas. Ann Surg Oncol 1996; 3:150–158.

87. Shiloni E, Szold A, White D, Freund HR. High-grade retroperitoneal sarcomas: role of an aggressive palliative approach. J Surg Oncol 1993; 53:197–203.

88. Glenn J, Sindelar WF, Kinsella T, Glatstein E, Tepper J, Costa J, Baker A, Sugarbaker P, Brennan MF, Seipp C, Wesley R, Young RC, Rosenburg SA. Results of multimodality therapy of resectable soft-tissue sarcomas of the retroperitoneum. Surgery 1985; 97:316–324.

89. Choong PF, Prithcard DJ, Rock MG, Frassica FJ. Survival after pulmonary metastasectomy in soft tissue sarcoma. Prognostic factors in 214 patients. Acta Orthop Scan 1995; 66:561–568.

90. Van Geel AN, Pastorino U, Jauch KW, Judson IR, Van Coevorden F, Buesa JM, Nielson OS, Boudinet A, Tursz T, Schmitz PI. Surgical treatment of lung metastases: The European Organization for Research and Treatment of Cancer-Soft tissue and bone sarcoma group study of 255 patients. Cancer 1996; 77:675–682.

91. Gadd MA, Casper ES, Woodruff JM, McCormack PM, Brennan MF. Development and treatment of pulmonary metastases in adult patients with extremity soft tissue sarcoma. Ann Surg 1993; 218:705–712.

92. Johnson VJ, Kondziela S, Gottschalk F. Pre- and post-operative mobility of trans-tibial amputees: correlation to medical problems, age and mortality. Prosthet Orthat Int 1995; 19:159–164.

93. Cutson TM, Bongiorni DR. Rehabilitation of the older lower limb amputee: a brief review. J Am Geriatr Soc 1996; 44:1388–1393.

94. McMurtry CT, Rosenthal A. Predictors of 2-year mortality among older male veterans on a geriatic rehabilitation unit. J Am Geriatr Soc 1995; 43:1123–1126.

95. Weiss GN, Gorton TA, Read RC, Neal LA. Outcomes of lower extremity amputations. J Am Geriatr Soc 1990; 38:877–883.

18
Oncology and Geriatrics: Overlapping but Not Congruent Spheres of Practice and Scientific Inquiry: Geriatric Oncology Defined as the Domain of Overlap

William R. Hazzard and Paul E. McGann
Wake Forest University School of Medicine
Winston–Salem, North Carolina

I. INTRODUCTION

As the United States approaches the 21st century, the demographic imperative of its progressively aging population is driving evermore intense scrutiny of the health and health care implications of that shift. And especially as the bulge of post–World War II Baby Boomers, who tend to dominate the contemporary U.S. scene, themselves enter the second half of middle age (defined by us as 50–75 years), the economic implications of the cost of Social Security and Medicare for their parents now and themselves in the future progressively preoccupy our socioeconomic and political landscape. This preoccupation is appropriate because of the inevitable association between advancing chronological age and predisposition to the multiple, chronic, often progressive, and frequently disabling diseases of advanced middle and old age carries portentous implications for the viability of these publicly funded health and economic systems for retired Americans in the 21st century.

This demographic imperative is fueling increased interest in the still underdeveloped discipline of geriatrics (the social and health care of the elderly). This discipline includes, but is not limited to, geriatric medicine (medical care of the elderly). However, as currently conceived, geriatric medicine in the U.S. health care system will not emerge as a "specialty" in the classic sense nor as a subspecialty by the U.S. model as defined within internal medicine by the subspecialties that include medical oncology, cardiology, nephrology, gastroenterology, infectious diseases, allergy and immunology, pulmonary medicine, endocrinology, diabetes, and metabolism, and rheumatology, which are all under the umbrella of internal medicine and certified as such by the American Board of Internal Medicine (ABIM). Instead, in the United States, geriatrics is conceived of as a "supraspecialty," perhaps dominated by internal medicine and its subspecialties and family medicine but also importantly bridging across to surgery and its subspecialties and other nonsurgical specialties that play substantive roles in appropriate health care of the elderly (notably rehabilitation medicine, psychiatry, neurology, dermatology, general surgery, urology, ophthalmology, orthopedics, plastic surgery, otorhinolaryngology, and cardiothoracic surgery). The true definition of geriatrics also embraces numerous other allied health professions, including nursing, social work, dentistry, the rehabilitation therapies, nutrition, psychology, and pharmacy. In ABIM parlance, geriatrics is thus a domain of "added qualifications." Since 1994 a "certificate of added qualifications (CAQ)" is granted to board-certified internists and family practitioners who have completed a minimum of 12 months of full-time clinical training in a program accredited by the Residency Review Committees of those two generalist disciplines and who pass an examination developed and administered jointly by the ABIM and the American Board of Family Practice (ABFP). (However, consistent with previous board practice, certified internists and family physicians with "substantial geriatric practice" were permitted to take the geriatric CAQ examination during its first four biennial offerings between 1988 and 1994 via the "grandfather" pathway without such fellowship training; and hence the vast majority [over 90%] of presently certified U.S. geriatricians have not had fellowship training.) Given the broad overlap between the bodies of knowledge and domains of practice germane to appropriate health care of the elderly shared in common by generalists (notably general internists and family physicians), nonmedical specialists such as neurologists, psychiatrists, general surgeons, and surgical subspecialists, and—the focus of this chapter—medical subspecialists, a definition of those bodies of shared and separate knowledge and practice represents a contemporary exercise of increasing importance.* Within the medical subspecialties, the relationship between progressive aging of the population and the incidence, prevalence, and burden of the diseases of late middle and old age underscores the importance of this exercise. And

---

* This exercise is the subject of an initiative sponsored by the American Geriatrics Society and administered through the Wake Forest University (formerly Bowman Gray) School of Medicine under a grant from the John A. Hartford Foundation entitled, "Integrating Geriatrics into the Subspecialties of Internal Medicine." The principal vehicle for this exercise has been a series of Geriatric Educational Retreats (GERs), 5-day intensive meetings for each of the subspecialties of internal medicine wherein leaders from a given subspecialty and geriatricians have defined the bodies of knowledge and practice and the research and educational agendas necessary to achieve this integration. That for medical oncology took

nowhere more than in medical oncology has this review more clearly underscored the powerful association between advancing age and the incidence of most forms of disease (in this instance, malignancy) and the mortality attributed thereto. Within other chapters in this volume, these associations are delineated malignancy by malignancy, and these correlations will not be repeated here. Suffice it to emphasize at this juncture, however, that of all the risk factors for morbidity and mortality from cancer, none is more powerful than the association with age per se (and this will likely only increase as the population burden of cigarette smoking–related morbidity and mortality wanes).

Thus, it was both timely and gratifying that medical oncologists from leading academic health centers and professional organizations identified population aging as a critical focus in planning for cancer research, education, and health care in the 21st century at the GER for medical oncology (the conference which was a progenitor for this volume). As with the other GERs, review of the appropriate clinical and academic domains for geriatrics and the subspecialty of medical oncology identified areas of training, research, and clinical competence distinctive to each but also a substantial common ground, which might be defined as "geriatric oncology." Therefore, in this chapter, we shall attempt to define the consensus emerging from that review as to those shared and separate domains but also what each specific discipline may gain from the other in forging its future.

II. WHAT GERIATRICIANS CAN LEARN FROM ONCOLOGISTS

Ever since the personal migration of the senior author (W.R.H.) over two decades ago from the subspecialty of endocrinology and metabolism to the "supraspecialty" of gerontology and geriatric medicine at the University of Washington (with a sabbatical year as a bridge between the two to learn the British approach to geriatrics at Oxford University and the St. Thomas's Medical School of London), I have continued to be impressed with the special insights of medical oncologists that in many ways form the template on which programs in academic and clinical geriatrics can be best modeled. First of all, many of my personal role models in the care of chronic progressive disease have been specialists in the care of patients with cancer. Medical oncologists are by virtue of the innate personality characteristics that attracted them to this field dedicated to the care of persons who are often sick and dying and for whom comfort and preservation of dignity are of paramount importance. As a corollary to this focus, medical oncologists are among the most effective "principal" caregivers among physicians, simultaneously managing increasingly sophisticated

---

place in Puerto Rico in February 1997, and a number of articles reflecting presentations and discussions there were published in the journal *Cancer* in an issue devoted to geriatric oncology in October 1997; 80(7):1267–1356.

technology and an exploding information base even as they deal with the social, psychological, and deepest emotional needs of patients who are facing their own mortality (there is still no more emotionally charged word in the English language in my experience than *cancer*; hence even the patient with nonprogressive skin cancer is transfixed by the revelation of their diagnosis and not easily reassured of its functionally benign nature). Second, the most effective medical oncologists in my experience are those who can effectively lead a multidisciplinary team and are not constrained by the conventional boundaries that might define the medical and nonmedical caring disciplines. Indeed, the most effective and compassionate oncologist is one who takes into account all aspects of the patient, their family, other caregivers, and their environment in molding a unique and dynamic care plan that addresses all of the needs of the patient and his or her supporters. It is hard to imagine a better role model for geriatricians than that. Third, in like fashion, effective medical oncologists have learned to communicate and collaborate with physician colleagues in related disciplines outside of internal medicine, notably surgical and radiation oncologists, a skill mirroring the effective care of frail elderly patients by medical geriatricians in concert with their fellow physicians in, for example, psychiatry, neurology, and rehabilitation medicine. Fourth, medical oncologists have led the way in crafting sensitive and common-sense care plans for dying patients given the often terminal nature of the primary illness. Indeed, I have for decades been heard to proclaim, "If I am old, frail, sick and dying, I hope I will be dying from cancer!" Why do I take this position? Because once that death is accepted as inevitable by both patient and caregivers, an effective palliative care plan can be designed and implemented, one centered around the patient's emotional, spiritual, and comfort needs rather than directed toward a curative process bound to be futile and only to prolong the agony of dying. Indeed in the mind of most persons, the terms *hospice* and *terminal cancer* care are synonymous (would that cardiologists, pulmonologists, nephrologists, and other specialists dealing with equally ill patients who are dying from disorders within their domain could be as insightful and sensitive in designing hospice programs for their patients in the last phase of their lives).

Moreover, geriatricians have much to learn from their colleagues in medical oncology per se. Not only the above attributes and practices totally germane to the general care of elderly patients defined under the supraspecialty of geriatrics but also the focus, scientific curiosity, and dedication to the understanding of the etiology, pathogenesis, and treatment of specific diseases should equally inform the practice of the geriatrician as they do the medical oncologist. Thus, from the medical oncologist, the geriatrician can learn never to stop asking why and what might be done to alleviate suffering even while recognizing that all too often the fundamental final common pathway toward decline, disability, and death has been entered by the elderly patient. Thus, as with both disciplines, acceptance of death (with dignity) is an essential attribute of the caring professional. However, in neither discipline is a lack of intellectual curiosity or "doing nothing" an excuse for professional or scientific laziness, indifference, or a cynical negative fatalism.

III. WHAT THE MEDICAL ONCOLOGIST CAN LEARN FROM THE GERIATRICIAN

Geriatrics is by definition the most general of specialties, more general than general internal medicine and family practice (with both of which, however, it shares major domains), more general than rehabilitation with all of its inter- and multidisciplinary, patient-centered assessment and management, and more general than any medical subspecialty even when caring for its oldest patients. Thus, the ability to think simultaneously in multiple dimensions of physical, social, psychological, environmental, and multidisciplinary professional assessment and practice and to do so dynamically through time defines the effective geriatrician. The difference between geriatrics and medical oncology here, however, is more one of degree than of kind. The geriatrician is at her or his best when dealing simultaneously with as many as a dozen or more problems in a given patient, some social, some psychological, some (all too often) iatrogenic, some classically organ system disease based, some other organ system based but outside the usual domains of the medical subspecialist (e.g., losses of function in the various systems of the special senses below the threshold defining them as disabilities or diseases), or, frequently, some or all of the above.

IV. SETTING THE STAGE: THE CASE OF MR. J

A 77-year-old man was admitted to the hematology/oncology service at the North Carolina Baptist Hospital, the teaching hospital of the Wake Forest University School of Medicine, because of the rapid onset of bilateral lower extremity weakness and left upper extremity weakness severe enough to prevent ambulation and function of the left upper extremity.

The patient had been diagnosed with non–Hodgkin's lymphoma of the gastrointestinal tract 5 months earlier. Staging laparotomy had been completed and the patient had completed two courses of chemotherapy and radiotherapy. He had been reasonably functional, quite cognitively intact, and he had been living at home with his wife of 52 years for the last 4 months. Past medical history was significant for hypertension, coronary artery disease, cardiac dysrhythmias, and a previous skin cancer removed from his face. In the acute care hospital, Mr. J. received a complete oncological and neurological evaluation, which included both spinal and cranial magnetic resonance imaging (MRI), a peripheral electromyelogram (EMG) and nerve condition study, a computed tomographic (CT) myelogram, and a lumbar puncture (LP). No discrete mass lesion or evidence of spinal cord compression was seen on the neuroimaging, but the radiologist did comment on two subtle areas of "enhancement" on the MRI of the spine, one in the thoracic spine and one at the level of the cauda equina. The significance of these findings was not known, but except for the patient's neurogenic bladder causing urinary retention, overflow incontinence, and necessitating placement of an indwelling Foley catheter, these two

MRI findings were not thought to be causally related to the patient's presenting focal neurological deficits.

Cytological examination of the cerebrospinal fluid (CSF) was positive for lymphoma, and the tumor cells demonstrated a predominance of CD20 cell surface markers. Lymphomatous involvement of the meninges, mediastinum, retroperitoneum, and spleen was diagnosed. An Ommaya CSF reservoir was surgically placed, and the patient received both intrathecal and systemic chemotherapy (according to the EPOCH* protocol), with only mild improvement in the patient's paraparesis and left upper extremity monoparesis. Functional improvement was insufficient to permit the patient to return home.

Mr. J. was transferred from the acute care hospital to the hospital-based Medicare-certified transitional (subacute) care unit (TCU) for a trial of rehabilitation. The patient's poor functional status, underlying diagnosis (advanced malignancy), and high degree of medical complexity would have excluded him from admission to a standard rehabilitation unit. The TCU is staffed by geriatricians and a team of rehabilitation professionals who are accustomed to high medical complexity and are not constrained by the rigid rehabilitation admission and outcome criteria demanded in facilities certified by the Commission on Accreditation of Rehabilitation Facilities (CARF) as "level 1" acute rehabilitation facilities.

Two days after admission to the TCU, the patient developed a neutropenic fever with no obvious source of infection. Treatment began on the TCU with penicillin, ceftazidime (Fortaz), and acyclovir, but owing to the life-threatening nature of the infection, the presence of the Ommaya reservoir, and the patient's requirement for acute care nursing, he was transferred back to the hematology/oncology acute care service. The oncologist added filgrostim (Neupogen) to the treatment regimen, and over the next 2 weeks both the patient, his neutrophil count, and his fever improved. No source of infection was ever identified. Three weeks after the initial attempt at rehabilitation, Mr. J. was transferred back to the TCU for a second attempt at rehabilitation.

On readmission to the TCU, the patient was observed to be a pleasant, thin, ill-appearing older man in no acute distress. Vital signs were stable. He was pale and had no hair and an Ommaya reservoir visible under the scalp. He had poor dentition and a black staining of his mouth.

General physical examination was remarkable for a slight resting tachycardia with occasional premature beats and runs of tachycardia. Hepatosplenomegaly was noted. A Foley catheter and peripheral iv were in situ. The patient had several pressure sores resulting from his prolonged acute care admission, including a stage III sacral pressure sore and stage I pressure sore on the left heel.

Neurological examination was remarkable for nearly total paraplegia. The patient was unable to move his legs or his toes. As well, there was total absence of grip strength in the left hand and only grade 1–2/5 power in most other muscles of the left upper extremity. Light touch sensation was normal throughout. Deep

---

* E, etoposide; P, prednisone; O, vincristine (neovin); C, cyclophosphamid; H, doxorubicin.

tendon reflexes were 0.25 in the right upper extremity but absent in the remaining three extremities. Cranial nerves, speech, swallowing, cognition, coordination (within the limitations imposed by the profound weakness), and affect were all thought to be normal. The patient was unable to walk or bear any weight, unable to transfer, and unable to use a wheelchair.

A comprehensive geriatric and rehabilitation assessment was performed and treatment plans devised and implemented. Admission Folstein mini-mental status examination (FMMSE) was 29/30 with an educational level of 9 years. Braden skin score was 13. Admission functional independence measure (FIM) was 57/133. The patient was placed in a Kin-air (or air-fluidized) bed to assist with pressure sore healing, and the rehabilitation goals were set to correspond to a FIM of 75/133. The patient's motivation was very high. The patient's sentence on his FMMSE was, "I want to go home."

The patient's medications were reviewed at admission team conference with a consulting pharmacist. The oncologists had done well avoiding polypharmacy in this patient with multiple complex, life-threatening conditions. He was only taking six nontopical, non-prn, nonnutritional supplement medications, and the only change that was made was to recommend long-acting morphine sulfate (MS Contin) for pain relief in place of the hydromorphone hydrochloride (Dilaudid) q3h which had been prescribed on the oncology service.

Mr. J. progressed well with daily rehabilitation. In keeping with the multidisciplinary spirit on the geriatric TCU, the oncologists continued to follow the patient. The patient initially received intrathecal methotrexate for his central nervous system (CNS) lymphoma. This was later changed to the experimental agent rituxan at a dose of 325 mg/m^2 with acetaminophen (Tylenol) and diphenhydramine hydrochloride (Benadryl) premedication, because this agent is thought to be more active in cells with the CD20 surface marker. Because of the patient's significant cardiac history and his history of tachydysrhythmias, currently treated with procainamide, the oncologist advised administration of the first dose of rituxan in the coronary care unit (CCU). This was accomplished without incident, and the patient was returned to the TCU the next day to complete his rehabilitation program.

Six weeks after his second admission to the TCU, Mr. J. was delighted to be discharged home. Although his neurological function had not returned to normal and he was still unable to walk, he could now move his feet, perform a sliding board transfer from bed to wheelchair, and use his left arm well enough to operate the remote control for a television or other home appliance. A "projection" modification of his wheelchair was made by the occupational therapist (Fig. 1). This allowed the patient to propel himself independently a distance of 300 ft (whereas prior to the rehabilitation admission, he was bed bound). The combination of bladder retraining and chemotherapy was successful in enabling the Foley catheter to be removed with maintenance of continence. The pressure sores improved, allowing discontinuation of the air-fluidized bed, which in turn led to further improvement in bed mobility. A home care occupational therapist visited the patient's home prior to discharge and recommended appropriate modifications to help the patient and his family cope

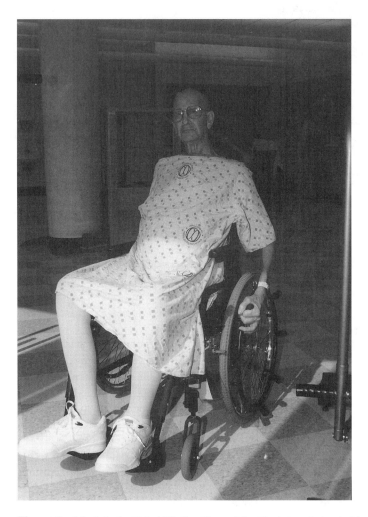

Figure 1   Mr. J. in the Rehabilitation Gym of the Center on Aging in his specially adapted wheelchair with the ''projections'' modification.

with his new wheelchair existence. Mr. J. met or exceeded all rehabilitation goals set for him by the Comprehensive Geriatric Team assessment on admission.

V.   COMPREHENSIVE GERIATRIC ASSESSMENT: THE "PROCEDURE" OF THE GERIATRICIAN

The epitome of the craft of the geriatrician is the practice of comprehensive geriatric assessment. At its most elaborate, the comprehensive geriatric assessment is composed of a several hour–long serial assessment (often spread over several encounters) by the geriatrician. The geriatrician is generally a member of a multidisciplinary team that almost always includes nursing and social work but also frequently extends to other health care professionals, notably rehabilitation therapists, non–profession-specific case managers, dietitians/nutritionists, dentists, recreational, occupational, physical, or speech therapists, and perhaps others. Such a detailed assessment by the geriatrician and her or his team is most often triggered by a request from a concerned patient (or, more often, spouse, child, or other supporter) but also occasionally by another physician perplexed by the problems presented by a frail elderly patient.

A. How A Complete Geriatric Assessment Is Done

Comprehensive geriatric assessment is a process and philosophy more than it is a body of knowledge (1). It is a way of approaching the complex interacting medical problems of frail older adults such that the difficulties which are troubling to them and their caregivers are adequately tabulated, appropriate patient and family education is delivered, and, most importantly, a plan is developed to enable the patient and caregivers to cope as best as possible with multiple, chronic, often progressive and irreversible illness.

It is important to acknowledge that comprehensive geriatric assessment, like so much of medical oncology, can only be accomplished as part of a multidisciplinary team. The four basic steps which are part of this team process are shown in Table 1. Although all members of the team are encouraged to contribute to all four steps, clearly some team members focus more on one step than on others. For example, the main contributors to step 3 (Medication Review) are consulting pharmacists and physicians, but clearly nurses, dieticians, physical therapists, and even family members are all able to make meaningful contributions to the reduction of polypharmacy in older patients.

Geriatricians themselves, in addition to participating in the group process described above, often analyze and synthesize large amounts of data collected by parsing the information into four identifiable domains. These domains interrelate in complex ways with essential interpersonal team dynamics (including the patient and his or her caregivers), resulting in an individualized human dimension to the treatment

Table 1 Four Basic Steps in Geriatric Assessment

1. Multisystem problem identification
2. Functional assessment
3. Medication review (for potential medication revision and possible elimination)
4. Coordinated, multidisciplinary plan construction

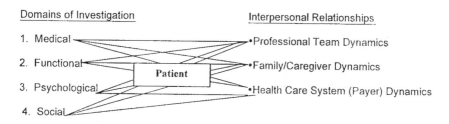

Figure 2 The domains of investigation during geriatric assessment, shown together with important interactive human relationship considerations.

plan which is at the core of the value of this process. The scheme shown in Fig. 2 attempts to outline some of these conceptual relationships.

We have compartmentalized the assessment process for education purposes. In real life, it is the synthesis of the multidimensional data with the interpersonal dynamics of the "patient-team-system entity" which has the most impact on the patient outcome.

As we further dissect the four principal domains of the geriatric investigations below, it is important to layer considerations of team dynamics, family dynamics, system dynamics, and individual patient characteristics on top of the technical skills of each domain (as Fig. 2 attempts to show.) Even the four domains themselves are not crisply defined. There is considerable overlap among all permutations of the medical–functional–psychological–social continuum. The classic geriatric example of such overlap is the assessment of cognitive function. Although we have classified it within the "psychological" domain, cognitive impairment as a patient state dramatically influences all aspects of the care planning in all three other domains, including collection of basic data, the first step in assessment.

1. Medical Domain

The collection of medical data on the elderly patient with cancer presenting to the physician for a comprehensive geriatric assessment should properly focus on all aspects of examination in which the oncologist acquired skills during the course of internal medicine residency and medical oncology fellowship training. There are five additional areas of expertise that have particular relevance to the complete understanding of the elderly patient with malignant disease:

1. An analysis of gait and transfers
2. Examination of the neurological system
3. Examination of visual function
4. Examination of hearing function
5. Nutritional assessment

The oncologist of the 21st century caring for patients of ever-increasing age should be familiar with basic methods to collect physical examination data in these areas despite the fact that they do not necessarily directly impinge on disease of the system in which a malignancy has presented. The knowledge base of the oncologist in this area should be that of a manager of complex medical illness rather than that of an organ system–or disease-focused subspecialist. The specific geriatric knowledge base acquired during fellowship training (mandated by the 1998 revision of listed requirements by the Residency Review Committee–Internal Medicine [RRC-IM]) should include awareness of the major causes of disability in elderly people related to these five medical areas (examples can be seen in Table 2).

More importantly, the oncologist must also have knowledge of how other members of a multidisciplinary health care team might be able to help in the detection and screening of disability in these areas, as well as the management of the disability which might be uncovered by such examinations. This is particularly evident when discussing common clinical methods for screening for visual and hearing impairment in elderly people. These screening techniques can be easily incorporated into an office practice by nonphysician health care professionals.

Table 2 Major Causes of Disability in Five Domains of Geriatric Medicine, Both General and Oncology Specific

	Examples of major causes of disability in the elderly	
Medical domain	In general population	In oncological population
1. Gait and transfer dysfunction	Osteoarthritis of knee and hip Deconditioning from prolonged hospitalization Postural hypotension	Deconditioning/malnutrition Pain due to bony metastases Neurological dysfunction caused by malignancy
2. Neurological dysfunction	Dementia Delirium Peripheral neuropathy	Delirium/metabolic disturbance CNS and cord lesions Paraneoplastic cerebellar dysfunction Chemotherapy toxicity
3. Visual dysfunction	Cataracts Macular degeneration Glaucoma	CNS tumors, primary and secondary Medication toxicity
4. Hearing dysfunction	Presbycusis Conductive hearing loss (cerumen impaction) Medication toxicity	Acoustic neuroma Medication toxicity
5. Malnutrition	Dementia Delirium Depression Medication toxicity Swallowing disorders	Cachexia Delirium Depression Medication toxicity

CNS, central nervous system.

Many physicians find the neurological/muscular examination difficult as it relates to function, and it is unlikely that sufficiently detailed and accurate neurological data will be collected by nonphysician health care professionals. Therefore, it behooves the oncologist who treats geriatric patients to become proficient during fellowship training in the rapid assessment of neurological function in the elderly patient, especially disorders of attention (such as delirium) and the various paraneoplastic neurological disorders and medication neurotoxicities, as illustrated by our case history above. Analysis of difficulties in gait and transfer ability also relates to a good neurological examination, but here physiotherapists are invaluable, especially in the therapeutic aspects of gait retraining.

a. Nutrition.

Assessment and treatment of poor nutritional status of older patients is absolutely critical to the successful rehabilitation of patients in geriatric oncology, and the topic of malnutrition should occupy a central place in any curriculum. The authors have observed a decline in the ability of postgraduate trainees in internal medicine systematically to assess patients for both micronutrient and protein-energy deficiencies. Such bedside clinical skills are essential to any geriatric assessment, and hence acquisition of those skills during fellowship training may be required.

2. Functional Domain

Functional assessment of all geriatric patients, no matter what the organ system of principal focus and attention, is a mandatory part of understanding the impact of the illness on the patient's quality of life. All practicing physicians, including medical oncologists, should have a working familiarity with the terminology and methods of assessing the categories of human functional performance as described by the acronyms BADL, IADL, and AADL. These categories are explained in Table 3. Again, it may not necessarily be the case that the physician will be the person who will collect the functional data from the patient or the family, but the health care delivery system must be developed in such a way that these functional data are available in at least a synopsis form to the physician as he or she incorporates the treatment plan into the lives of patients and their families. Nonphysician health care professionals, or in this case even non–health care professional secretarial or administrative staff, can be trained to collect simple functional data in a reliable fashion.

3. Psychological Domain

In dealing with the geriatric patient with malignant disease, the psychological and often psychiatric assessment is of the utmost importance. Detailed multiaxial *Diagnostic and Statistical Manual of Mental Disorders*, 4th edition (DSM-IV) diagnostic interviews by the oncologist are neither practical nor desirable when dealing with the geriatric patient with malignant disease unless specifically required for manage-

Table 3 Categories of Human Functional Performance of Importance to Geriatric Medicine

Categories (abbreviation)	Examples	Consequences of serious deficits	Published methods of assessing (Reference)
Basic activities of daily living (BADL)	Feeding Bathing Toileting/continence Dressing Transfers	Puts patient at risk for institutional placement	Katz ADL Scale (2) Barthel ADL Scale (3)
Instrumental activities of daily living (IADL)	Shopping Driving Telephoning Financial management Housework Taking medication	Patient requires weekly support to remain independent at home	Lawton IADL Scale (4) Fillenbaum IADL Scale (5)
Advanced activities of daily living (AADL)	Booking complex travel itinerary Executive-level work or consultation Lecturing Complex or intellectually demanding hobbies Participating in exercise program	Interferes with quality of life Problems are generally "early-warning indicators" for cognitive loss or depression	Guttman Scale for Elderly (6) Reuben AADL Scale (7)

Source: Ref. 1.

ment; here geropsychiatric consultation may be indicated. Psychological aspects of the evaluation with which all oncologists must be familiar and in which skills must be developed are detection of the major disorders of cognition and affect. The two principal cognitive disorders that oncologists will encounter in their practice are delirium and dementia. The most significant disorder of affect, one which is very common in geriatric oncology practice, is depression. Depression is a treatable disease with a known biological basis and is very common in medically ill elderly patients and notably in those with cancer. The treatment of depression has been revolutionized recently with the introduction of new classes of therapeutic agents (8–10). The practicing oncologist must be quite familiar with the recognition and identification of depression in elderly patients as well as with the full repertoire of treatment modalities for this illness. The reason it is so important that the oncologist understand depression in elderly patients is because the disease may be completely reversible in such patients, including those with cancer, and proper treatment of depression can have a dramatic, positive impact on the patient's quality of life. Any of the psychological disorders of old age, specifically delirium, dementia, or depression, when present in a patient with malignant disease, can have a dramatic impact on the compliance and response of a patient to standard oncological treatment, be it medical, surgical, or radiation therapy. The oncologist must be aware of the potential for delirium, dementia, and depression to cause treatment failure in his elderly patients, especially via noncompliance, so that proper corrective actions can be taken to ensure that patients receive the oncological treatment that is being prescribed for them. In the absence of such an assessment, even the most advanced oncological knowledge base will not result in optimal clinical outcomes.

4. Social Domain

Although the practicing oncologist might not have sufficient time to collect all the primary social information on geriatric patients, these data are equally as important as the psychological data in terms of the ultimate management of the patient. Proper treatment cannot be delivered to frail elderly patients without extensive knowledge of living arrangements, financial security, and the social support network. Office staff can be trained to collect this information for physicians so it is available at the time of the development of a treatment plan. Moreover, such information tends to be relatively stable over time (the death of a spouse or a change in living circumstances are notable exceptions) and hence need not be elicited at frequent intervals other than for changes.

Two other social issues are of great importance to the care of the geriatric patient with malignant disease. The first is the identification and treatment of caregiver stress, and the second is the development of advance directives, hopefully before the onset of critical illness. Currently, however, oncologists may often encounter geriatric patients in whom advance directives have not been established prior to critical illness. In this situation, the oncologist must skillfully elicit advance directive information at the time of critical illness. This is considerably more challenging than obtaining this information in advance of the onset of the crisis.

Caregiver stress is also important to assess during comprehensive assessment, because it diminishes both patient and caregiver quality of life and frequently also interferes with the ability to deliver appropriate medical treatment to the geriatric patient and his or her family. Caregiver stress also transmits conflict and disruption to the health care team and causes anxiety and nonproductive, nonhealing interactions during the course of hospitalizations and other encounters with the health care system. Germane to the specter of malpractice allegations, severe caregiver stress can also result in litigious behavior on the part of the family, the majority of which should be preventable.

Advance directives is a complex topic, the complete discussion of which is beyond the scope of this chapter (see Chap. 22). The superior medical oncologist, because of his or her extensive experience and training in the care of the dying and symptom control (palliative care), has always been a leader in advance directive knowledge and practice among all the medical subspecialties. There are many good guides available to the entire spectrum of decisions related to advance directives in the elderly to which the interested reader is referred (11–17). A more complex area which has less developed literature is the determination of advance directive information during the crisis situation of an acute hospital or intensive care admission.

B. Bringing It All Together

The most essential step in the complex process of comprehensive geriatric assessment is the synthesis of data and other information and its translation into an effective management plan by the multidisciplinary team as led or at least facilitated by the geriatrician. In this exercise, the role of the geriatrician as consummate integrationist, common sense planner, and listener is critical, as is her or his ability to follow up assiduously with details in the execution (and continual remodeling) of the plan developed. The previously mentioned factors of team, family, and system dynamics as well as patient preferences (see Fig. 2) figure prominently in this integrative process. Finally, it must be made clear that such a detailed, exhaustive assessment is neither necessary nor appropriate on every occasion for every geriatric patient. Quite to the contrary, a 20-min miniassessment is more frequently indicated, and triage of requests between those especially requiring medical assessment by a skilled geriatrician versus those warranting an exhaustive multidisciplinary assessment and follow-up is a critical first step in the process. These steps are also necessary for the cost-effective use of expensive personnel resources.

What underlies this process are the values, sensitivities, and attitudes of the effective geriatrician. These are based principally in sound ethics; the ability to weigh the risks, benefits, and costs of each contemplated step in the diagnosis or treatment with appropriate consideration of tradeoffs but at all times with the desires and best interests of the patient uppermost; and dedication to preservation of the dignity and quality of life of the afflicted as a first priority. To put it another way, the emphasis is on the welfare of the patient as a whole with primary attention to the quality rather than the quantity of life of that patient. Modern demographics have now shifted such that it is not unusual to encounter an elderly frail patient with dementia, depression, failing vision and hearing, anorexia and weight loss, progressive cardiovascular, pulmonary, and renal insufficiency, diabetes, and colon cancer, together with the social disruption associated with the recent death of a spouse and an impending move to an LTC facility. The geriatrician's approach to such a patient emphasizes detailed assessment, planning, and management of all problems—medical and social—rather than consideration of the patient as a "case of colon cancer" who also happens to have multiple co-existing morbidities (although often times the distinction between the two approaches is subtle). Thus (and as clearly reflected in the consensus among oncologists attending the GER in Puerto Rico in 1997), the ability to place the diagnosis and management of malignancy in the context of an elderly patient with a sometimes daunting number of real or potential comorbidities and social problems, as illustrated in the case above, is the nub of what might be called geriatric oncology.

What the oncologist may also perhaps learn from the geriatrician is keener grace and equanimity in accepting the limitation of a care plan in a patient who is frail and in the process of dying, a scenario with which both oncologists and geriatricians are perhaps altogether too familiar. In this circumstance, the medical oncologist is perhaps at risk for focusing too much on treatment options, recruitment into protocols, and, yes, at times, prescription of standard oncological therapy in one too frail or too close to death to benefit in any real sense. This includes the imperatives of securing appropriate advance directives as a matter of course early rather than late during treatment, communicating sensitively at all times with the patient, caregivers, and fellow professionals about these issues of respect for the patient's wishes (team, family, patient, and system dynamics; see Fig. 2) and of compulsively assuring that no patient will be taken by surprise or be otherwise unprepared for their diagnosis and its implications for the quality of the remainder of their life. Perhaps especially in the tertiary/quaternary academic health center with its historic preoccupation with state of the art diagnosis and treatment and care by successions (and often to the patient seemingly hoards) of nurses, medical students, residents, attending physicians, and other consultants is the risk of a lack of communication or unwanted surprises greatest.

VI. GERIATRIC ONCOLOGY: A CHALLENGE TO BETTER INFORMED PRACTICE

Also evident in the deliberations of the Oncology GER was the real lack of solid practice guidelines derived in a classic evidence-based medical fashion from randomized, controlled clinical trials as to the efficacy and cost effectiveness of the treatment of various forms of cancer in those who are truly old (defined chronologically as above the age 75-year threshold, which for many geriatricians defines [on average] the beginning of old age). And especially daunting is the dearth of information regarding such treatment in typical elderly patients with cancer (and multiple morbidities) as opposed to those highly selected persons free of disease or limitation in other organ systems (the ''elite elderly'' who comprise but a small percentage of those in their 80s, 90s, and above). Thus, the research imperative to enroll elderly patients in formal randomized clinical trials was laid out clearly by the investigators assembled in Puerto Rico and constitutes a challenge to the National Cancer Institute (NCI) and other supporting agencies (including Medicare!) to conduct such real-world trials.

A. So What Is Geriatric Oncology?

Thus, the considerable concordance between the attitudes, skills, and behaviors of geriatricians and oncologists can be readily identified. Cross training of all future medical oncologists in the appropriate care of the elderly in general but especially the frail elderly thus represents a proximate challenge to fellowship training program directors, Residency Review Committee–Internal Medicine bodies, and the ABIM. Proceeding from this imperative identified at each of the subspecialty GERs, the RRC-IM has mandated in the 1998 revision of its guidelines for requirements for accreditation of subspecialty training programs that *all* medical subspecialties must include experience in the diagnosis and management of a substantial number of patients over the age of 70 years as well as the development of subspecialty-specific guidelines for the training of future fellows in that discipline. For medical oncology, this should focus on those aspects of the diagnoses and management of the frailest patients in a true interdisciplinary mode parallel to that described above for comprehensive and minigeriatric assessment. It also must include management of the many, especially chronic, diseases whose incidence and prevalence, like that of cancer, increases with age (recalling experiences to diseases in each of the organ systems and diseases to which the medical oncologist was previously exposed during residency training in internal medicine). Thus, for example, the diagnosis and management of cardiovascular disease, diabetes, hypertension, renal insufficiency, and the multiply-afflicted and vulnerable elderly patient with one or more of the "geriatric syndromes" (urinary and/or fecal *i*ncontinence, falls and fractures, [*i*nstability], mental *i*ncompetence, *i*mpaired metabolic homeostasis, and *i*atrogenesis [notoriously including polypharmacy]—the "fives Is" of geriatrics) must be areas with which the oncologist caring for the elderly is familiar and with whose management she or he is competent and comfortable. This appropriately also includes cross consultation and collaboration with nononcologists and geriatricians and coordination of care across these disciplines when appropriate.

Whether such cross and additional training takes the form of geriatric fellows consulting in oncology clinics or vice versa (or both), didactic and seminar teaching, and/or comanagement of elderly patients with cancer in the home, long-term care facility, or clinic is clearly a matter of local adaptation and preference at this juncture. And whether a "subsubspecialty" of geriatric oncology indeed does or does not develop (as appears to be becoming the case, for instance, with geriatric cardiology) remains to be determined in the future. Suffice it to say here that a limited number of oncology fellowship training programs are beginning to develop tracks in geriatric oncology to allow special local added competence to be gained in the management of the frailest and most elderly patients with cancer by medical oncologists with a special interest and experience in this area of increasing importance.

But the central message of this chapter should be the preponderance of synchrony in attitudes, behaviors, and practices for the care of older patients by geriatricians and by medical oncologists with their common dedication to patient-centered diagnosis and management and a common commitment to ongoing, unflagging care of the most vulnerable in the population—the ever-growing number of old and oldest. Although the spheres of influence and activity of geriatricians and medical oncologists overlap, they will not be congruent. However, we would predict the emergence of the domain defined by that overlap as the care of the increasing number of very old patients with cancer, the domain of geriatric oncology.

REFERENCES

1. Applegate WB, Blass JP, Williams TF. Instruments for the functional assessment of older patients. N Engl J Med 1990; 322:1207.
2. Katz S. Progress in development of the index of ADL. Gerontologist 1970; 1(Part I): 20–30.
3. Maloney FI, Barthel DW. Functional evaluation: the Barthel Index. MD St Med J 1965; 61–65.
4. Lawton MP, Brody EM. Assessment of older people: self-maintaining and instrumental activities of daily living. Gerontologist 1969; 9:179.
5. Fillenbaum GG. Screening the elderly: a brief instrumental activities of daily living measure. J Am Geriatr Soc 1985; 33:698.
6. Rosow I, Breslau N. A Guttman Health Scale for the aged. J Gerontol 1966; 21:556.
7. Rueben DB, Laliberte L, Hiris J, Mor V. A hierarchical exercise scale to measure function at the advanced activities of daily living (AADL) level. J Am Geriatr Soc 1990; 38:855.
8. Dunbar GC. Paroxetine in the elderly: a comparative metanalysis against standard antidepressant pharmacotherapy. Pharmacology 1995; 51:137–144.
9. Preskorn SH. Recent pharmacologic advances in antidepressant therapy for the elderly. Am J Med 1993; 94:2S–11S.
10. Salzman C. Pharmacologic treatment of depression in the elderly. J Clin Psychiatry 1993; 54:23–28.
11. Jonsen AR, Cassel C, Lo B, Perkins HS. The ethics of medicine: an annotated bibliography of recent literature. Ann Intern Med 1980; 92:136.
12. Jonsen AR, Siegler M, Winslade WJ. Clinical Ethics: A Practical Approach to Ethical Decisions in Clinical Medicine. New York: McGraw-Hill. 1992.
13. Perkins HS. Ethics at the end of life: practical principles for making resuscitation decisions. J Gen Intern Med 1986; 1:170.
14. Mahowald MB. So many ways to think: an overview of approaches to ethical issues in geriatrics. Clin Geriatr Med 1994; 10:403–418.
15. Deon M, Sach GA. Advance directives and the patient self-determination act. Clin Geriatr Med 1994; 10:431–444.
16. Annas GJ. The Health Care Proxy and the Living Will. N Engl J Med 199; 321:1210–1213.
17. Uhlman RF, Clark H, Pearlman RA, et al. Medical management decisions in nursing home patients: principles and policy recommendations. Ann Intern Med 1987; 106: 879–885.

19
International Issues of Cancer

Martine Extermann
H. Lee Moffitt Cancer Center and University of South Florida
Tampa, Florida

Matti S. Aapro
Clinique de Genolier
Genolier, Switzerland

I. INTRODUCTION

Given the importance of the problem of cancer in the elderly, an international effort is needed to address this question. The goal of this chapter will be to address two questions related to this issue: (a) To what extent are older cancer patient populations comparable between different areas in the world? and (b) What is presently done as a research in various countries, and what could be done to obtain a broad transferability of the results?

II. ARE OLDER CANCER PATIENTS COMPARABLE THROUGHOUT THE WORLD?

As discussed in detail in Chapter 1 of this book, most cancers occur beyond the age of 65 years in developed countries. In developing countries, the elderly population is still small, but it is expected to more than double over the next 30 years. There is also a worldwide trend toward cancer being more and more frequently the cause of death in patients beyond the age of 65 years (1). The prevalence of the various cancers and their respective importance in the elderly population are discussed in the epidemiological section of this book. Most cancer studies have involved patients below 65–70 years old. In recent years, effort has been made to expand studies beyond that age range. However, these studies often restrict their accrual to otherwise healthy patients. Although this category is largely representative of the general population in younger patients, it is less and less the case as age advances. Around the age of 80 years, this portion of the population is usually estimated to be around 10% of the population. In an American setting, over 90% of older oncological patients present with some level of comorbidity (2). Is the prevalence of comorbidity the same in different areas of the world? Is the tolerance to treatment the same in different countries? Another characteristic of treatment in older cancer patients is that the focus gradually shifts from prolonging survival to quality of life endpoints, notably prolonging the period during which the patient is independent, which is also called active life expectancy. What data do we have about the achievability of this goal? Another key to the approach of older cancer patients is the role played by the social network of the individual. Geriatric studies have shown that a good support network increases survival (3). What is its weight compared to other elements such as tumor stage, comorbidity, functional status, or nutrition? And how can we compare a Florida golfer traveling North each summer to an Italian grandmother with all her family within 50 km?

Some data can give us a preliminary insight into the problem. These data belong to five categories: (a) epidemiological studies on aging; (b) patients enrolled in geriatric cohort studies; (c) patients enrolled in cooperative oncological studies; (d) patients treated in cancer centers, more specifically geriatric oncology programs; and (e) epidemiological studies on cancer patients.

A. Epidemiological Studies

Several epidemiological studies have assessed the evolution of active life expectancy in populations from different countries. It is interesting to note that although the life expectancy at birth of Americans is shorter than that of Japanese (76.0 vs 79.6 years [4]), the contrary is true for the life expectancy of elderly people. The life expectancy of 80-year-old American women is 2 years longer than that of a Japanese woman of the same age. The life expectancy of Japanese women is comparable to that of Swedish, French, and English women. For men, the difference is around 1.5 years (5). A Japanese study, using a decision analysis approach, concluded that 60-year-old Japanese individuals are expected to spend about 18.7 years (81%) in functional independence and about 4.4 years (19%) in disability in their future (6). When the authors compared the life expectancy of a 70-year-old Japanese person and estimates made for American people (7), they found a life expectancy of 14.7 years for Japanese people versus 13.3 years for Americans. Active life expectancy was 10.52 years (72%) versus 9.7 years (73%), respectively. Therefore, despite a more than 1-year difference in longevity, the proportion of active life expectancy was the same. Does this mean that the dependence period is incompressible? Some models seem to predict that enhancing recovery from disability can have a significant impact on active life expectancy (7). A very interesting study has been published that analyzes the incidence of chronic disabilities among older Americans (8). This incidence is lower than it would have been expected on the incidence rates of 1982. Although this study does not allow us to discern the cause of this improvement, nor the time at which this cause occurred, it demonstrates that the incidence of disability can be influenced. Interestingly, these results parallel a decrease in the prevalence of morbidity from several diseases (9). Further data from a worldwide survey also support the hypothesis of compression of disability. A 60-year-old sub-Saharan African male is expected to spend 53% of his remaining lifetime with a disability, whereas this proportion was 22% in an established market economy country (10).

B. Longitudinal Geriatric Studies

Several national longitudinal studies have been launched in recent years to address the issue of aging, notably its impact on self-reported health and on functional status. Their results are beginning to be systematically compared. One of them is the Seven Countries Study, which started with middle-aged men and now has cohorts in their 70s and 80s. The countries involved are the United States, Finland, the Netherlands, Italy, Croatia/Serbia, Greece, and Japan. A comparison between the survivors aged 70 years or more from the Finnish, the Dutch, and the Italian cohort was presented at the World Congress of Gerontology in Adelaide, Australia, August 1997 (11). Even in a subset of a relatively homogeneous European population, several differences could be seen. The most striking is on self-perceived health: 10–22% of Finnish men reported feeling healthy versus 72–86% of Italians and 89% of Dutch ($P < .001$). This number is 80% for Japanese. Activities of daily living (ADL) were good in 65–72% of Finnish, 63–78% of Italians, and 84% of Dutch ($P < .001$). Mean Mini-Mental State (MMS) score was 23.8–24.5 in Finland, 23.1–23.3 in Italy, and 26.2 in the Netherlands ($P < .001$). In an Australian study of people of similar age, 66.3–70.4% of men and women rated their health as good, very good, or excellent (no difference between sexes) (12). In that study, 69.3% of men and 68.1% of women were independent in the six basic ADL. In two studies of Americans of the same age range, the prevalence of independence in ADL and instrumental activities of daily living (IADL) was 77.3–81.1% (13). Most interestingly, 13.3% of the subjects who were disabled recovered over a period of 2 years in these American studies. Parallel results were obtained in another Dutch study exploring the impact of seven comorbidities on functional status. Some 20% of men and 12% of women were recovering from disability within 2 years. In the analysis by comorbidity type, cancer was the only disease that had a significant association with a potential for recovery (in women) (14). These are gross preliminary comparisons, but they highlight the fact that, for example, people with a similar functional status living on a same continent can rate their subjective health very differently. This should prompt the use of appropriate controls when designing, for example, an international quality of life study. The above studies also suggest a significant possibility of recovering from disability, especially in cancer patients.

C. Cooperative Oncological Trials

Patients enrolled in cooperative oncological studies represent a healthy subset of elderly patients. Trimble et al. (15) have tried to determine the importance of the selection bias in older patients by comparing patients accrued in sponsored by the National Cancer Institute (NCI) studies and the (SEER) (Surveillance, Evaluation, and End-Results [Program]) epidemiological data. Some differences are striking. For example, the mean age for leukemia in the general U.S. male population is 59.4 years, whereas it is 20.2 years in the NCI-sponsored studies. Breast cancer patients aged more than 75 years represent 22.8% of breast cancers but only 2.7% of the study patients. This leads to a major selection bias that impairs comparison between studies. However, these patients are treated according to rigorous protocols and therefore can be compared with good data quality to younger patients. So far, very few elderly patients have been included in dose-escalation studies. Patients above 70 years old were representing only 4% of such patients in a review of the European Organization for Research on Treatment of Cancer (EORTC) phase I trials (16). In a review of U.S. phase II trials, the healthy elderly seemed to tolerate one to two drug regimens as well as young patients (17). However, in the EORTC phase II single-agent trials, elderly patients were more likely to experience treatment delays and dose reductions (18). They were also more likely to be lost to follow-up or to refuse to continue treatment. Again, only 8% of the patients were 70 years old or older. In a review of phase II and III trials in metastatic breast cancer, the Piedmont Oncology Association in the southeastern United States did not find any significant difference in response and tolerance between patients 70–84 years old (median age 74 years) and younger patients (19). In ECOG studies of advanced diseases treated with multidrug chemotherapy regimens, patients 70 years old and older experienced toxicities globally similar to younger patients except for hematological toxicity, which was higher, notably with certain drugs, such as methotrexate and methyl-CCNU (methyl-N-(2-chloroethyl)-N'-cyclohexyl-N-nitrosourea) (20). The authors later demonstrated that this was also true for actinomycin D, doxorubicin hydrochloride (Adriamycin), vinblastine, and etoposide (21). The general conclusion that can be drawn from these cooperative studies in various countries is that a selected population of elderly patients can tolerate chemotherapy quite as well as their younger counterparts with the exception of an increased hematological toxicity and a greater likelihood to experience dose reductions and delays. The unanswered question is: Is this transferable to the average older patient with cancer? Another element that may be underestimated in cooperative studies is late toxicities, for example, cardiac or pulmonary toxicities, which appear to increase with age (22, 23).

D. Geriatric Oncological Programs

Early data from cohort studies of comprehensive geriatric assessment in cancer centers have recently become available. They offer a first insight into the general characteristics of the older cancer patients who actually present for specialized treatment. As these represent a subset of older persons with cancer, it is important to determine whether they represent a very healthy subset of the general population or if they present multiple ailments that should be taken into account when designing therapeutic approaches or clinical trials. One cohort is American: patients seen since 1994 by the Senior Adult Oncology Program (SAOP) at the H. Lee Moffitt Cancer Center & Research Institute in Tampa, Florida (2, 24). These patients are comprehensively evaluated by a multidisciplinary oncogeriatric team as part of their first visit to the program. The other cohort is Italian and includes data from several centers where oncologists made a geriatric evaluation (25). Patients in both cohorts are evaluated for mental status with the Folstein Mini-Mental Status (26), depression with the Geriatric Depression Scale (27), independence with ECOG performance status (PS) (28), activities of daily living (29), instrumental activities of daily living (30), and comorbidity with different methods (see below). In the American cohort, patients are evaluated by a multidisciplinary geriatric team; in the Italian cohort, evaluation is made by the oncologist.

The results of the initial examination in the two cohorts of patients are shown in Table 1. Patients had comparable levels of independence in functioning, according to ADL and IADL, but the Italians had a somewhat poorer ECOG performance status. These two observations are compatible, as the correlation between ECOG

Table 1 Comparison of Oncogeriatric Patients Between an American and an Italian Outpatient Cohort[a]

	Tampa		Italy
Median age	75 years	Mean age	72.7 years
ECOG/WHO PS 0-1	83.2%		68%
ADL independence	78.8%		83.2%
IADL independence	43.8%	IADL independent or 1 dependence	62%
GDS positive	26%		44.6%
MMS <26	25%	MMS <24	33.3%
Charlson 0	64%		
CIRS-G 0	6%		

PS, performance status; ADL, activities of daily living; IADL, instrumental activities of daily living; GDS, Geriatric Depression Scale; MMS, Mini-Mental Status; Charlson, Charlson Comorbidity Scale; CIRS-G, Cumulative Illness Rating Scale—Geriatric.
[a] See text for references.
Source: Compiled from Refs. 2, 24, and 25.

PS and ADL/IADL is moderate in older cancer patients (2). The American population was in better mental and emotional shape than the Italian one. Older patients seen at a geriatric oncological outpatient clinic are in worse functional condition than the average community-dwelling population. In Moffitt's SAOP clinic, 56.2% of the patients are dependent in the IADL, whereas only around 20% of the older community-dwelling American population presents a dependence (13).

Comorbidity is also an important problem in older cancer patients. The above-mentioned cancer clinics' cohort studies already allow some comparisons of comorbidities. One should nevertheless be aware that the two groups did not use the same definition. The Italian group used a classification per a list of disease types, whereas at Tampa, comorbidities were rated according to the Charlson Scale (31) and the Cumulative Illness Rating Scale–Geriatric (CIRS-G) (32). With these cautions in mind, the comparison is presented in Table 2. The results of the two studies on a few diseases are also compared in Table 3 with data from two American studies and one European epidemiological study. They are (a) the National Institute on Aging (NIA)/SEER Registry study, where data were obtained by chart review, which focuses on hospitalized older cancer patients (33); (b) the National Health Interview Survey, which used self-reported data in the general U.S. population, and has age subgroups (referred to in Ref. 33); and (c) in the Netherlands, the Eindhoven

Table 2 Comparison of Comorbidity Between American and Italian Cancer Patients[a]

Tampa		Italy	
Diseases	Prevalence (%)	Diseases	Prevalence (%)
Heart	29.6	Heart	20.4
Vascular	36	Vascular	21
		Hypertension	27.5
Hematological	2.5		
Respiratory	25.1	Bronchopneumopathy	14.1
Eyes + ENT	18.7		
Upper digestive	16.3	Digestive	21.6
Lower digestive	26.6		
Liver	16.3		
Renal	3.9		
Genitourinary	31	Urinary incontinency	4.8
Musculoskeletal/tegumment	43.3	Arthrosis, arthritis	30.2
		Osteoporosis	10.5
Neurological	10.8		
Endocrine/breast	29.1	Metabolic diseases	8.7
Psychological	18.2	Depression	14.4

[a] American patients are evaluated with the CIRS-G scale. Italian patients are evaluated by disease categories (2, 25). See text for details.

Table 3 Comorbidity in Various Cohorts of Older Cancer Patients

Diseases	Tampa (2) (%)	Italy (25) (%)	NIA/SEER (33) (%)	NHIS (33) (%)	Eindhoven (37) (%)
Heart diseases	30[a]	20	40–50		14–16 (+vascular)
Hypertension/vascular diseases	36[a]				
Hypertension		28	35–55	10–25	10–11
Vascular diseases		21			
Locomotive problems	43(+skin)[a]	41			
Arthritis		30	35–50	15–40	
Diabetes	7[b]	9	15–18	5–10	6.3–8.3

Tampa: outpatients from a geriatric oncology clinic. Italy: elderly outpatients from cancer clinics. NIA/SEER: analysis of the SEER registry (USA). NHIS: National Health Interview Survey (USA): assesses the general population. Eindhoven: population study by a cancer registry (NL). In the Tampa cohort, the comorbidity was measured by CIRS-G[a] and Charlson[b] scales. In the Italian and SEER studies, they were categorically defined by medical team and in the NHIS they were reported by patients. The Dutch study used a modified Charlson scale. In the epidemiological studies, data are pooled from various subgroups. See text for details.

Cancer Registry study where data on comorbidity from cancer registry cases were prospectively collected from medical records. In both American studies, the definition of diseases is categorical with no precise grading, but there is a distinction between a current problem and a past problem. The data used for the comparisons include patients 65 years old and above. The European study is using a modified Charlson Scale.

E. Epidemiological Cancer Studies

Evidence from epidemiological cancer studies is limited. The only study focusing on older cancer patients is the American NIA/SEER study cited above, which results are preliminary (33). It focuses on hospitalized patients. Another study evaluating data from one of the SEER contributors (Detroit) for breast cancer in a general population aged 40–84 years demonstrated a large difference in the cause of death with an increasing number of comorbidities (34). Patients with no comorbidity were four times more likely to die from their breast cancer than from their other diseases. Patients with three comorbid diseases (myocardial infarction, other heart diseases, diabetes, other cancer, respiratory, gallbladder, or liver disorder) were three times more likely to die from their other diseases than from breast cancer. However, the mean age of each subgroup of comorbidities was increasing too (from 59.7 years for the disease-free group to 70.4 years for the three comorbidities group). Nevertheless, decision analysis modeling allows us to conclude that the level of comorbidity outweighs the role of age in such patients (35). In an adaptation of their comorbidity scale, Charlson et al. found that each comorbidity unit (CU) (e.g., a myocardial infarction weighs 1 CU, whereas the acquired immunodeficiency syndrome [AIDS] weighs 6 CU) had a relative risk of death equivalent to a decade of age (36). On the European side, the Eindhoven Cancer Registry recently conducted a prospective registry-based study in southeast Netherlands using a modified Charlson scale (notably by adding hypertension and autoimmune diseases) (37). In the subset of patients aged 60–74 years, the global prevalence of comorbidity was 46%, and for 75 years and above, 56%. These numbers are higher than those encountered in a U.S. oncological center: 36% on the Charlson scale without addition of hypertension and autoimmune diseases (see Tables 2 and 3).

III. INSTRUMENTATION ISSUES IN INTERNATIONAL STUDIES

In order to allow international comparisons, one should therefore take into account the wide variety of the elderly population both within a country and between countries. Strong attention needs to be paid to an adequate description of the study population. The use of validated scales should be generalized. If the studies use patient-generated answers to questionnaires, these need to have been specifically validated for cross-lingual and cross-cultural validity. The questionnaires most sensitive to this issue are the quality of life (QOL) questionnaires.

A. Quality of Life and Translation of Questionnaires

The QOL tools are being developed in various languages and the equivalency of these tools is being tested (Table 4). The use of a QOL tool in several languages can encounter several pitfalls. The first one being at the translational level, the second at the statistical level, and the third at the implementation within trials level.

Several methods exist for the translation of QOL scales. The methods ensuring best semantic and content equivalence tend to be using a forward-back-forward scheme (38, 39). For example, the approach used by Cella and his group for Functional Assessment of Cancer Therapy (FACT) uses professional translators in a first step, a reconciliatory translation, a back translation into English, and finally a review by bilingual health professionals. The scale is then field tested with patients from the target country before being finalized for study use (38). The source document should not be idiomatic—It should be as clear as possible. The target document should be validated in several cultural groups speaking the same language (e.g., for French in France, Canada, Switzerland, and Western Africa).

The statistical analysis has to address the question: Are the differences in rating between translations due to flaws in the translation, to differences in the sample populations, or to true intercultural differences? Most groups use "sample-free" methods derived from the Rash model (38, 39). The principle of this method is to

Table 4 Some Frequently Used Oncological Quality of Life Scales Available in Several Languages[a]

Scale	Reference	Languages	Comments
CARES	69	English, Spanish	
EORTC-QLQ-C30 v.2.0	70, 71	Chinese, Czech, Danish, Dutch, English, Finnish, French, German, Greek, Hebrew, Hungarian, Italian, Japanese, Norwegian, Polish, Portuguese, Russian, Slovak, Slovenian, Spanish, Swedian, Turkish	In preparation: Afrikaans, Croatian, Lithuanian, Romanian, Serbian, Sotho. Cancer-specific modules
FACT	72	Afrikaans, Bulgarian, Chinese, Czech, Danish, Dutch, English, French, German, Greek, Hebrew, Hungarian, Italian, Japanese, Malay, Norwegian, Pedi, Polish, Protuguese, Russian, Slovak, Spanish, Swedish, Thai, Tswana, Zulu	Validated in older cancer patients (Overcash 96) Cancer-specific and other (e.g., HIV, fatigue) specific modules
FLIC	73	Chinese, Danish, Dutch, English, Flemish, French, German, Greek, Italian, Japanese, Luganda, Malay, Ndebele, Portuguese, Shona, Spanish, Swedish	
SF-36	74	English, German, Spanish, Swedish	Age-specific norms and population-based norms. Several other translations in testing.

[a] Some of these scales adaptations for dialectal changes (e.g., France vs Canadian French or European vs South American Spanish). Given the rapid evolution of the number of translations available for these scales, this table has no pretention to exhaustivity.

compare the rating of each item by a patient to the global rating of the scale by each patient. This allows us to evaluate independently the performance of the patients and of each item within the sample. This allows us to identify possibly biased items. These items can be then reviewed and either retranslated, discarded, or kept as "doubled items" for a particular pair of language comparisons (38).

Once a well-designed established translation is used, standard QOL analysis methods can be used, as the hypothesis can be made that the QOL scale will be predominantly unbiased for language, culture, literacy, or mode of administration. This gives highly consistent results across cultures (40).

The mode of administration and compliance is the third major pitfall in which such studies can fall, as any QOL studies. The amount of missing data can vary a lot according to center, especially if the QOL analysis is not part of the initial design (41). This is only magnified by cross-cultural problems, and careful attention should be paid to ensure adequate collection of the QOL data. Missing data are a major source of flaws in QOL studies. The QOL scales should either be included in the core of the study or tested in a well-defined subset of institutions with a precisely defined responsible personnel. The documentation should be as lean and user-friendly as possible. A centralized control personnel should be easily available for questions and tracking of data. Some groups, such as the International Breast Cancer Study Group, have dealt with the problem of compliance in large-scale studies by using single-items scales in each dimension of QOL. This resulted in a very short questionnaire with acceptable validity when compared with more complex scales (42, 43).

The development and testing of translations of QOL scales is, as one can deduct from the above comments, demanding in means and personnel. Therefore, geriatric oncologists planning international studies should plan to validate an already available scale in older cancer patients rather than creating one from scratch. The SAOP program in Tampa has conducted such a validation for the FACT-G, as compared to the SF-36, in a Floridian population (24). The reader interested in more details about the general principles of cross-lingual and cross-cultural evaluation of quality of life scales can find a more comprehensive review elsewhere (43a).

B. Comorbidity

Comorbidity weighting has been a challenge in geriatrics (44), as well as its relation with functional status. Various ways of measuring comorbidity have been used in oncological studies from global clinician assessment (light, moderate, severe) (45, 46), qualitative description (25, 33, 34), or the use of comorbidity scales (2, 31, 47–49). This can lead to highly variable estimates of the prevalence of comorbidity in oncological populations and poor reproducibility. A strict comparison of two well-defined comorbidity scales, the Charlson scale and the CIRS-G scale, gave a prevalence of comorbidity of 36 versus 94% in the same patient population (2). The Charlson scale focuses only on diseases that influence mortality. The CIRS-G permits a comprehensive record of comorbidities, minor and major, in a way similar to the WHO/ECOG/NCI common toxicity scale for treatment-related toxicity. It is presently unknown which comorbidities are key for treatment tolerance, QOL, or cancer prognosis in older patients. In order to help answer this question, comorbidity should be carefully defined with validated scales in international studies. Both the Charlson and the CIRS-G scales have proven reliable when validated in older cancer patients (2). The Charlson scale has also demonstrated similar predictive power across races in breast cancer patients (49).

C. Other Scales

A variable that is also strongly influenced by cultural differences is the *social support and network*. Little is known on this aspect for older cancer patients. We know that proxy estimation of quality of life and willingness to undertake treatment is unreliable (50–54). Reliable tools to estimate the support received from social network need to be developed and tested in older cancer patients. There is a wide potential for intercultural comparisons in the willingness to receive treatment and the role of social support in its tolerance.

Coping is another dimension that can be influenced by culture. In a comparison of two coping scales: the Herschbach coping inventory (FBBK) and the Perceived Adjustment to Chronic Illness Scale (PACIS), Hürny et al. (55) found a better correlation for Italian-Swiss than for German-Swiss patients.

Certain detailed *functional scales*, such as the Sickness Impact Profile, are also sensitive to translation (56). Even simpler functional scales are not exempt from difficulties. Gender and cross-cultural issues have long been recognized for an item such as preparing meals on Lawton's IADL and various attempts have been designed to solve this (30, 57, 58).

D. Comprehensive Geriatric Assessment

In order to take into account the multidimensional aspects that can influence the outcome of an older cancer patient, the Rolls Royce approach is to use a multidisciplinary team Comprehensive Geriatric Assessment (CGA). This may, however, only be possible in a few centers. For a large multicentric trial, a set of well-validated scales covering the various aspects of a CGA can be used by a trained rater (e.g., oncologist, geriatrician, nurse practitioner, or research nurse). The scales should cover at minimum: functional status, comorbidity, and nutritional and mental status. If QOL is a consideration, depression and social support should also be included. All these elements have been shown to be independent predictors of survival in cancer patients or in the elderly (3, 34, 59–64). Not accounting for these predictors can lead to systemic biases between the countries involved in the study. Our program in Tampa and the Italian groups have demonstrated a comprehensive approach is feasible in the setting of an oncological outpatient clinic. The level of patient acceptance and satisfaction is very high with our team approach (unpublished data). Actually, a multidisciplinary administration of the CGA seems better tolerated by the patients than a lengthy session with one examiner. Programs on the model of the one in Tampa are beginning to develop in other countries (e.g., in Tel-Aviv, Israel, and Lyon, France). In geriatric studies, a CGA has been shown to improve the independence and the survival of elderly persons in many settings (65). This is also true for patients with a severe illness such as cardiac insufficiency (66). The key conditions for success are a comprehensive follow-up (a one-time consultation type of approach does not seem effective) and overseeing by a physician (65). Whether the same is true in cancer patients remains a question to be explored.

IV. MATHEMATICAL METHODS

As we have emphasized earlier, the diversity of aging is a major obstacle to the recruitment of a representative sample of older individuals into clinical trials and the major limit to the use of clinical studies in clinical practice and across countries. This diversity represents also a major therapeutic challenge as it mandates individualized treatment plans, which cannot be tested in large clinical trials. Furthermore, the ability of the human mind to integrate complex prognostic data has limits (67). Recruiting large collectives of patients with particular risk profiles can be very difficult in geriatric oncology, especially when one steps out of the "healthy elderly" subgroup. Meta-analysis of different clinical trials may allow firmer conclusions of the value of prognostic factors and the effectiveness of therapeutic interventions in older persons with cancer. Decision analysis models may help estimate individual benefits and risks of different courses of action and to calculate the cost effectiveness of specific interventions. We should emphasize, however, that the reliability of mathematical methods is predicated on the reliability of clinical data. Thus, a uniform and comprehensive evaluation of the older patient across trials is essential to the applications of these methods and should be generalized even for trials in a single country.

V. INTERNATIONAL PROTOCOLS

Several international cooperative groups are developing studies in elderly cancer patients. However, as noted above, these studies are presently limited to healthy elderly. These groups are, for example, the International Breast Cancer Study Group, or the EORTC. National cooperative groups such as the Eastern Cooperative Oncology Group or the Swiss Group for Clinical Cancer Research (SAKK) have subgroups focused on elderly patients. Focus groups also exist, such as the Italian Geriatric Radiation Oncology Group (GROG) and the Gruppo Italiano di Oncologia Geriatrica (GIOG). The challenge that cooperative groups will face in the years to come is to develop adequate comparative means that will allow them to take into international studies patients more representative of the general population of their country and to describe adequately their status in order to enable international comparisons.

Most of the oncological research, and almost all of the geriatric oncology research, is presently conducted in developed countries. Among the various reasons for this are that: cancer is a disease of old age, the age pyramid is younger in developing countries, and many competing diseases are easier and cheaper to treat in developing countries. However, the life expectancy of the population is increasing rapidly in these countries and cancer, including cancer in the elderly, will become more and more a public health problem. Research in these countries is feasible, including comprehensive assessment of patients, including quality of life, and methodologies have been developed to optimize the results (68).

VI. CONCLUSIONS

Older cancer patients represent a highly heterogeneous population. The designer of an international study will have to give serious consideration to evaluation of the comorbidity and to functional, psychosocial, and cultural biases that may alter the relevance of the study results. They should be carefully assessed, ideally by a multidisciplinary CGA, and well-validated scales should be used. Population selection issues should be discussed in publications of the results. The clinicians reading the study results should find in the article the elements that will enable them to determine whether these results can be directly transferred to their population of patients, or if they should be adjusted for one or several of the variables mentioned above.

ACKNOWLEDGMENTS

The authors wish to thank Dr. Carol Moinpour of the SWOG data center, Seattle, WA, and Lauren Lent of Northwestern University, Evanston, IL, for providing many data and advice used in the quality of life section (Sec. III.A).

REFERENCES

1. Levi F, La Vecchia C, Lucchini F, Negri E. Worlwide trends in cancer mortality in the elderly, 1955–1992. Eur J Cancer 1996; 32A:652–672.
2. Extermann M, Overcash J, Lyman GH, Parr J, Balducci L: Comorbidity and functional status are independent in older cancer patients. J Clin Oncol 1998; 16:1582–1587.
3. Ell K, Nishimoto R, Mediansky L, Mantell J, Hamovitch M. Social relations, social support and survival among patients with cancer. J Psychosomat Res 1992; 36:531–541.

4. Statistical Abstract of the United States 1996. U.S. Department of Commerce, Economics and Statistics Administration, Bureau of the Census, Washington, DC.

5. Manton KG, Vaupel JW. Survival after the age of 80 in the United States, Sweden, France, England, and Japan. N Engl J Med 1995; 333:1232–1235.

6. Liu X, Liang J, Muramatsu N, Sugisawa H. Transitions in functional status and active life expectancy among older people in Japan. J Gerontol 1995; 50B:S383–394.

7. Rogers A, Rogers RG, Belanger A. Longer life but worse health? Measurement and dynamics. Gerontologist 1990; 30:640–649.

8. Manton KG, Corder L, Stallard E. Chronic disability trends in elderly United States populations: 1982–1984. Proc Natl Acad Sci: Med Sci 1997; 94:2593–2598.

9. Manton KG, Stallard E, Corder L. Changes in morbidity and chronic disability in the U.S. elderly population: evidence from the 1982, 1984, and 1989 national long term care surveys. J Gerontol 1995; 50B:S194–204.

10. Murray CJL, Lopez AD. Regional patterns of disability-free life expectancy and disability-adjusted life expectancy: Global Burden of Disease Study. Lancet 1997; 349: 1347–1352.

11. Dontas AS, Nissinen A, Kromhout D, Menotti A, Koga Y. A thirty years study of healthy middle-aged men: The Seven Countries Study. Symposium S020, Abstr. 468–473. World Congress of Gerontology, Adelaide Australia, August 1997.

12. Clarke MS, Andrews GS. Transitions in health status from the Australian Longitudinal Study on Aging. Abstr. 1888. World Congress of Gerontology, Adelaide Australia, August 1997.

13. Crimmins EM, Saito Y, Reynolds SL. Further evidence on recent trends in the prevalence and incidence of disability among older Americans from two sources: the LSOA and the NHIS. J Gerontol 1997; 52B:S59–S71.

14. Kriegsman DMW, Deeg DJH, van Eijk JTM. Influence of chronic diseases and partner status on changes in physical functioning among older men and women in the Netherlands. Abstr. 1216. World Congress of Gerontology, Adelaide Australia, August 1997.

15. Trimble EL, Carter CL, Cain D, Freidlin B, Ungerleider RS, Friedman MA. Representation of older patients in cancer treatment trials. Cancer 1994; 74:2208–2214.

16. Monfardini S, Sorio R, Kaye S. Should elderly cancer patients be entered in dose-escalation studies? Ann Oncol 1994; 5:964–965.

17. Giovanazzi-Bannon S, Rademaker A, Lai G, Benson AB. Treatment tolerance of elderly cancer patients entered onto phase II clinical trials: an Illinois Cancer Center study. J Clin Oncol 1994; 12:2447–2452.

18. Monfardini S, Sorio R, Hoctin Boes G, Kaye S, Serraino D. Entry and evaluation of elderly patients in European Organization for Research and Treatment of Cancer (EORTC) new-drug development studies. Cancer 1995; 76:633–638.

19. Christman K, Muss HB, Case D, Stanley V. Chemotherapy of metastatic breast cancer in the elderly. JAMA 1992; 268:57–62.

20. Begg CB, Carbone PP. Clinical trials and drug toxicity in the elderly. The experience of the Eastern Cooperative Oncology Group. Cancer 1983; 52:1986–1992.

21. Walsh SJ, Begg CB, Carbone PP. Cancer chemotherapy in the elderly. Semin Oncol 1989; 16:66–75.

22. Ginsberg SJ, Comis RL. The pulmonary toxicity of antineoplastic agents. Semin Oncol 1982; 9:34–51.

23. Von Hoff DD, Layard MW, Basa P, Davis HL, Von Hoff AL, Rozencweig M, Muggia FM. Risk factors for doxorubicin-induced congestive heart failure. Ann Intern Med 1979; 91:710–717.

24. Overcash J, Parr J, Perry J, Extermann M, Balducci L. Validity and reliability of the FACT-G scale for use in the older person with cancer. 3rd International Conference on Geriatric Oncology, Tampa, FL, November 1996.

25. Repetto L. For the GIOG (Gruppo Italiano Oncologia Geriatrica), Evaluation of the older person with cancer. 3rd International Conference on Geriatric Oncology, Tampa, FL, November 1996.

26. Folstein MF, Folstein SE, McHugh PR. "Mini Mental State." A practical method for grading the cognitive status of patients for the clinician. J Psychiatr Res 1975; 12: 189–198.

27. Yesavage J, Brink T, Rose T, Lum O, Huange O, Adey V, Leirer V. Development and validation of a geriatric depression screening scale: A preliminary report. J Psychiatr Res 1983; 7:37–49.

28. Zubrod CG, Schneiderman M, Frei E III, Brindley C, Gold GL, Shnider B, Oviedo R, Gorman J, Jones R, Jonsson U, Colsky J, Chalmers T, Ferguson B, Dederick M, Holland J, Selawry O, Regelson W, Lasagna L, Owens AH Jr. Appraisal of methods for the study of chemotherapy in man: comparative therapeutic trial of nitrogen mustard and triethylene thiophosphoramide. J Chron Dis 1960; 11:7–33.

29. Katz S, Ford AB, Moskowitz RW, Jackson BA, Jaffe MW. Studies of illness in the aged. The index of ADL: a standardized measure of biological and psychosocial function. JAMA 1963; 185:94–99.

30. Lawton MP, Moss M, Fulcomer M, Kleban MH. A research and service oriented multilevel assessment instrument. J Gerontol 1982; 37:91–99.

31. Charlson ME, Pompei P, Ales K, MacKenzie CR. A new method of classifying prognostic comorbidity in longitudinal studies: development and validation. J Chron Dis 1987; 40:373–383.

32. Miller MD, Paradis CF, Houck PR, Mazumdar S, Stack JA, Rifai H, Mulsant B, Reynolds III CF. Rating chronic medical illness burden in geropsychiatric practice and research: application of the Cumulative Illness Rating Scale. Psychiatry Res 1992; 41: 237–248.

33. Yancik R, Havlik RJ, Wesley MN, Ries L, Long S, Rossi WK, Edwards B. Cancer and comorbidity in older patients: a descriptive profile. Ann Epidemiol 1996; 6:399–412.

34. Satariano WA, Ragland DR. The effect of comorbidity on 3-year survival of women with primary breast cancer. Ann Intern Med 1994; 120:104–110.

35. Extermann M, Balducci L, Lyman GH. Optimal duration of adjuvant tamoxifen treatment in elderly breast cancer patients: influence of age, comorbidities and various effectiveness hypotheses on life-expectancy and cost. Breast Dis 9:327–339, 1996.

36. Charlson M, Szatrowski TP, Peterson J, Gold J. Validation of a combined comorbidity index. J Clin Epidemiol 1994; 47:1245–1251.

37. Coebergh JWW, Janssen-Heijnen MLG, Razenberg PPA. Prevalence of co-morbidity in newly diagnosed patients with cancer: a population-based study. Crit Rev Oncol Hematol 1998; 27:97–100.

38. Cella DF, Lloyd SR, Wright BD. Cross-cultural instrument equating: current research

and future directions. In: Bert Spilker, ed. Quality of Life and Pharmacoeconomics in Clinical Trials. 2nd Ed. Philadelphia: Lippincott-Raven, 1996:707–715.

39. Ware JE, Gandek BL, Keller SD, and the IQOLA Project Group. Evaluating instruments used cross-nationally: methods from the IQOLA Project. In: Bert Spilker, ed. Quality of Life and Pharmacoeconomics in Clinical Trials. 2nd Ed. Philadelphia: Lippincott-Raven, 1996:681–692.

40. Aaronson NK, Ahmedzai S, Bergman B, Bullinger M, Cull A, Duez NJ, Filiberti A, Flechtner H, Fleishman SB, de Haes JCJM, Kaasa S, Klee M, Osoba D, Razavi D, Rofe PB, Schraub S, Sneeuw K, Sullivan M, Takeda F. For the European Organization for Research and Treatment of Cancer Study Group on Quality of Life. The European Organization for Research and Treatment of Cancer QLQ-30: a quality-of-life instrument for use in international clinical trials in oncology. J Natl Cancer Inst 1993; 85: 365–376.

41. Hürny C, Bernhard J, Joss R, Willems Y, Cavalli F, Kiser J, Brunner K, Favre S, Alberto P, Glaus A, Senn H, Schatzmann E, Ganz PA, Metzger U. Feasibility of quality of life assessment in a randomized phase III trial of small cell lung cancer. Ann Oncol 1992; 3:825–831.

42. Hürny C, Bernhard J, Gelber RD, Coates A, Castiglione M, Isley M, Dreher D, Peterson H, Goldhirsch A, Senn HJ. Quality of life measures for patients receiving adjuvant therapy for breast cancer: an international trial. Eur J Cancer 1992; 28:118–124.

43. Hürny C, Bernhard J, Coates AS, Castiglione-Gertsch M, Peterson HF, Gelber RD, Forbes JF, Rudenstam CM, Simoncini E, Crivellari D, Goldhirsch A, Senn HJ. Impact of adjuvant therapy on quality of life in women with node-positive operable breast cancer. Lancet 1996; 347:279–284.

43a. Spilker B, ed. Quality of life and Pharmacoeconomics in Clinical Trials. 2nd ed. Philadelphia: Lippincott-Raven, 1996.

44. Guralnik JM. Assessing the impact of comorbidity in the older population. Ann Epidemiol 1996; 6:376–380.

45. Bergman L, Dekker G, van Kerkhoff EHM, Peterse HL, van Dongen JA, van Leeuwen FE. Influence of age and comorbidity on treatment choice and survival in elderly patients with breast cancer. Breast Cancer Res Treat 1991; 18:189–198.

46. Guadagnoli E, Shapiro C, Gurwitz JH, Silliman RA, Weeks JC, Borbas C, Soumerai SB. Age-related patterns of care: evidence against ageism in the treatment of early-stage breast cancer. J Clin Oncol 1997; 15:2338–2344.

47. Greenfield S, Blanco DM, Elashof RM, Ganz P. Patterns of care related to age of breast cancer patients. JAMA 1987; 257:2766–2770.

48. Bennett CL, Greenfield S, Aronow H, Ganz P, Vogelzang NJ, Elashoff RM. Patterns of care related to age in men with prostate cancer. Cancer 1991; 67:2633–2641.

49. West DW, Satariano WA, Ragland DR, Hiatt RA. Comorbidity and breast cancer survival: a comparison between black and white women. Ann Epidemiol 1996; 6:413–419.

50. Pearlman RA, Uhlman RF: Quality of life in chronic diseases: perceptions of elderly patients. J Gerontol 1988; 43:M25–30.

51. Slevin ML, Plant H, Lynch D, Drinkwater J, Gregory WM. Who should measure quality of life, the doctor or the patient? Br J Cancer 1988; 57:109–112.

52. Tsevat J, Cook EF, Green ML et al: Health values in the seriously ill. Ann Intern Med 1994; 122:514–520.

53. Bremnes RM, Andersen K, Wist EA. Cancer patients, doctors and nurses vary in their willingness to undertake cancer chemotherapy. Eur J Cancer 1995; 31A:1955–1959.
54. Coates A. Who shall decide? Eur J Cancer 1995; 31A:1917–1918.
55. Hürny C, Bernhard J, Bacchi M, van Wegberg B, Tomamichel M, Spek U, Coates A, Castiglione M, Goldhirsch A, Senn HJ, et al. The Perceived Adjustment to Chronic Illness Scale (PACIS): a global indicator of coping for operable breast cancer patients in clinical trials. Support Care Cancer 1993; 1:200–208.
56. Deyo RA. Pitfalls in measuring the health status of Mexican Americans: comparative validity of the English and Spanish Sickness Impact Profile. Am J Public Health 1984; 74:569–573.
57. Lawton MP, Brody EM. Assessment of older people: self-maintaining and instrumental activities of daily living. Gerontologist 1969; 9:179–186.
58. Reuben DB. What's wrong with ADLs? J Am Geriatr Soc 1995; 43:936–937.
59. Finkelstein DM, Ettinger DS, Ruckdeschel JC: Long-term survivors in metastatic non–small cell lung cancer: an Eastern Cooperative Oncology Group Study. J Clin Oncol 1986; 4:702–709.
60. Coates A, Gebski V, Signorini D, Murray P, McNeil D, Byrne M, Forbes JF. Prognostic value of quality-of-life scores during chemotherapy for advanced breast cancer. Australian New Zealand Breast Cancer Trials Group. J Clin Oncol 1992; 10:1833–1838.
61. Tamburini M, Brunelli C, Rosso S, Ventafridda V. Prognostic value of quality of life scores in terminal cancer patients. J Pain Symptom Manage 1996; 11:32–41.
62. Murphy E, Smith R, Lindesay J, Slattery J. Increased mortality rates in late-life depression. Br J Psychiatry 1988; 152:347–353.
63. Ganzini L, Smith DM, Fenn DS, Lee MA. Depression and mortality in medically ill older adults. J Am Geriatr Soc 1997; 45:307–312.
64. Lobato-Mendizabal E, Ruiz-Arguelles GJ, Marin-Lopez A. Leukemia and nutrition I: malnutrition is an adverse prognostic factor in the outcome of treatment of patients with standard-risk acute lymphoblastic leukemia. Leukemia Res 1989; 13:899–906.
65. Stuck AE, Siu AL, Wieland D, Adams J, Rubenstein LZ: Comprehensive geriatric assessment: a meta-analysis of controlled trials. Lancet 1993; 342:1032–1036.
66. Rich MW, Beckham V, Wittenberg C, Leven CL, Freedland KE, Carney RM. A multidisciplinary intervention to prevent the readmission of elderly patients with congestive heart failure. N Engl J Med 1995; 333:1190–1195.
67. Loprinzi CL, Ravdin PM, De Laurentiis M, Novotny P: Do American oncologists know how to use prognostic variables for patients with newly diagnosed primary breast cancer? J Clin Oncol 1994; 12:1422–1426.
68. Schipper H, Olweny CLM, Clinch JJ. A mini-handbook for conducting small-scale clinical trials in developing countries. In: Bert Spilker, ed. Quality of Life and Pharmacoeconomics in Clinical Trials. 2nd Ed. Philadelphia: Lippincott-Raven, 1996:669–680.
69. Ganz PA, Schag CA, Lee JJ, Sim MS. The CARES: a generic measure of health-related quality of life for patients with cancer. Qual Life Res 1992; 1:19–29.
70. Osoba D, Zee B, Pater J, Warr D, Kaizer L, Latreille J. Psychometric properties and responsiveness of the EORTC Quality of Life Questionnaire (QLQ-30) in patients with breast, ovarian, and lung cancer. Qual Life Res 1994; 3:353–364.

71. Cull AM. Cancer-specific quality of life questionnaires: the state of the art in Europe. Eur J Cancer 1997; 33(Suppl 6):S3–S7.

72. Cella DF, Tulsky DS, Gray G, Sarafian B, Linn E, Bonomi A, Silberman M, Yellen SB, Winicour P, Brannon J, Eckberg K, Lloyd S, Purl S, Blendowski C, Goodman M, Barnicle M, Stewart I, McHale M, Bonomi P, Kaplan E, Taylor IV S, Thomas Jr CR, Harris J. The Functional Assessment of Cancer Therapy Scale: development and validation of the general measure. J Clin Oncol 1993; 11:570–579.

73. Schipper H, Clinch J, McMurray A, Lewitt M. Measuring the quality of life of cancer patients: the Functional Living Index—Cancer: development and validation. J Clin Oncol 1984; 2:472–483.

74. Ware, J, and Sherbourne, CD. The MOS 36-Item Short-Form Health Survey (SF-36). I. Conceptual framework and item selection. Med Care 1992; 30:473–483.

20
Comorbidities and Cancer

William A. Satariano
University of California
Berkeley, California

I. INTRODUCTION

It has been said that just as children should not be viewed simply as young versions of adults, neither should the elderly be considered as simply old adults (1). This means that the study of aging, health, and disease requires an understanding of the special physiological, psychosocial, and pathological characteristics of aging, an understanding that is critical for the management of cancer in older populations.

It is well known that the risk of most forms of cancer increases markedly with chronological age (2, 3). Sixty percent of all cancer occurs among people aged 65 years and older (4). Although it is very important to understand the reasons for the association between aging and cancer incidence, the study of cancer in the elderly involves much more. One of the special characteristics of older people is that they are not only at elevated risk for single conditions but also for multiple concurrent health conditions as well. As people age, they are likely to develop more than one chronic health condition, also known as *comorbidity*. For example, results from the National Health Interview Survey indicate that the percentage of people aged 60 years and over who reported having two or more of the nine most common conditions increased steadily with age (5). Specifically, the percentage of women who reported two or more conditions increased from 45% among those aged from 60 to 69 years, to 61% for those aged from 70 to 79, to 70% for those aged 80 years and over. Among men, the percentages were 35, 47, and 53% respectively. These results provide compelling evidence that comorbidity is not unusual or atypical in older populations. Quite the contrary. For most older people, comorbidity may provide the best characterization of general health. It is not surprising, therefore, that older people with cancer are likely to have other concurrent health conditions. The results of one national study indicate that many older people with cancer are currently being treated for other conditions that include arthritis, heart conditions, and hypertension (6, 7).

The presence of multiple, concurrent health conditions has significant implications for the management of cancer in older populations. This is reflected in the growing number of studies in this area. MEDLINE, for example, lists over 200 scientific articles published on comorbidity and cancer since 1993 compared to only about 50 articles that appeared between 1980 and 1992. In addition to a growing number of publications, at least two scientific meetings have been devoted to the topic of comorbidity. In 1994, the scientific meetings of the American College of Epidemiology addressed the topic of "Rethinking Disease: Implications for Epidemiology" (8). The meetings included scientific presentations devoted to theoretical and methodological issues associated with the study of comorbidity in epidemiology, including three papers dealing with cancer treatment and survival. In 1996, the Netherlands Organization for Scientific Research initiated a national research program on the causes and consequences of comorbidity, which included the convening of an international conference on the state of research and research methods associated with the study of comorbidity in older populations (9).

With the growing interest in comorbidity, the purpose of this chapter is to review current research on the effects of comorbidity on cancer management in older populations. Special attention will be given to the major comorbidities and their impact on decisions regarding cancer diagnosis, screening, and treatment strategies for selected cancers. The following issues will be addressed: (a) definition and measurement of comorbidity, (b) sources of information and timing of assessment, (c) overview of research results, and (d) recommendations for future research.

II. DEFINITION AND MEASUREMENT OF COMORBIDITY

Comorbidity is typically defined as the presence of multiple, concurrent health conditions found in one individual (9–14). There are two general areas of research. The first area includes studies of the prevalence of multiple conditions among a sample of people from the general population (11, 15–17). Differences in the number of comorbid conditions and in the number of specific combinations of conditions have been presented by age group, gender, race, and, in some cases, socioeconomic status. Studies in this area also have examined the risk of disability and death by level of comorbidity. The second area of research includes studies of the incidence and/or prevalence of the number and types of comorbid conditions found among people diagnosed with a specific "index condition," such as breast or prostate cancer (10, 13, 18).

There is general agreement that the diagnosis, treatment, and prognosis of cancer patients are affected by the presence of concurrent conditions. Indeed, Feinstein and colleagues have proposed that measures of comorbidity, together with measures of performance status and reported symptoms, be used to expand the criteria for cancer staging to provide a better assessment of prognosis following diagnosis and treatment (19–23). Despite general agreement about the importance of comorbidity, there is no clear consensus about the number and types of conditions that should be included in measures of comorbidity; nor is there agreement about the criteria for the differential "weighing" of those conditions for the development of a comorbidity index. Four indexes of comorbidity that have been used in studies of cancer patients are presented to illustrate some of these differences (24–27).

1. Kaplan–Feinstein Index. This early comorbidity index was originally designed to summarize the effects of comorbid conditions on vascular complications among people diagnosed with adult-onset diabetes (24). Building on the earlier work of Feinstein, clinical judgment was used first to identify a list of comorbid conditions from a review of medical records that would be sufficiently severe to affect the prognosis adversely, either directly or indirectly, by elevating the susceptibility to other fatal ailments. The Kaplan-Feinstein Index has since been used in a variety of studies of cancer treatment and prognosis (28–30).

For this index, each condition is given a score of 1–3, based on the level or severity of the condition in the individual patient (grade 1 = slight; grade 2 = impaired; grade 3 = full or most severe). In general, the final comorbidity score is based on the patient's most severe condition (grade 0 = none; grade 1 or 2 = moderate; grade 3 = severe).

2. Charlson Index. This comorbidity index is clearly the most commonly used scale in studies of cancer patients (25). It provides an overall score based on a composite of values weighted by level of severity and assigned for any of 19 selected conditions reported in the medical records.

Each condition is assigned a severity score. The score for each condition is based on the results of an earlier study of the 1-year, age-adjusted risks of death for hospitalized patients with selected conditions. A score of 1 was assigned to those conditions with an adjusted relative risk of 1.2–1.5 (e.g., myocardial infarction); a score of 2 for those conditions with a relative risk of 1.5–2.5 (e.g., diabetes with end organ damage); and a score of 3 for conditions with risks from 2.5 to 6.0 (e.g., moderate or severe liver disease). A score of 6 was assigned to two conditions (acquired immunodeficiency syndrome [AIDS] and other metastatic cancer) with an adjusted risk of 6 or more. Conditions with a relative risk of less than 1.2 were excluded. Scores for most conditions ranged from 1 to 3. Using these severity weights, the overall comorbidity score is based on the sum of the scores for the individual conditions.

3. Greenfield Index. This comorbidity index, also known as Index of Coexistent Disease (ICED), was developed originally to assess the effects of coexisting conditions on the level and types of treatment for cancer patients (26, 31). Later, it was used to examine the process of recovery among patients treated for hip surgery (32).

For Greenfield and colleagues, comorbidity is defined as the overall severity of illness due to diseases other than the index condition and consists of two components: individual disease severity and functional status. Individual disease severity (IDS) represents the physiological severity of 12 categories of specific conditions. Each condition is assigned a stage based on symptoms, signs, and laboratory tests: IDS of 0 indicates absence of a coexistent disease; IDS of 1, an asymptomatic or mildly symptomatic condition (e.g., controlled hypertension with no medications, diabetes, sporadic urinary tract infections); IDS of 2, a mild to moderate condition that is generally symptomatic and requires medical intervention or a past condition, presently benign, that presents a moderate risk of morbidity (e.g., hypertension or asthma controlled with medications, history of myocardial infarction with no residual effects); IDS of 3, an uncontrolled condition which causes moderate to severe disease manifestations (e.g., chronic renal or hepatic failure, symptomatic coronary heart disease); and IDS of 4, an uncontrolled condition which causes severe manifestations requiring immediate intervention and carrying an extremely high risk of mortality (e.g., respiratory failure, coma, diabetic ketoacidosis). Functional status (FS) measures the global impact of all conditions, diagnosed or not, on the patient's functional ability. Ten functional areas are included, each area rank ordered in terms of three levels of severity. Patients are given the highest IDS and FS scores achieved in any of the categories, the final index being assigned according to the combination of both IDS and FS scores.

4. NIA/NCI Cancer and Comorbidity Index. The most recent comorbidity index was developed for a collaborative study organized and funded by the National Institute on Aging and the National Cancer Institute (6, 7). The study, known as the NIA/NCI SEER (Surveillance, Epidemiology, and End Results [Program]) Study, represented six geographical areas of the NCI SEER network of population-based cancer registries and included approximately 7600 patients newly diagnosed with any of seven primary cancer sites: breast, cervix, ovary, prostate, colon, stomach, and urinary bladder. Data on comorbidity were obtained from a review of medical records, primarily the physician's notes, anesthesia notes, nursing notes, discharge summaries, and reports from departments of radiology and other laboratories. The number and severity of comorbid conditions were found to predict early mortality among patients with colon cancer after adjusting for age, gender, and disease stage (27). To date, this index has been used only in the NIA/NCI SEER Study.

The index includes 27 major medical categories. Illness severity is based on whether the condition is current and whether the patient is receiving active treatment. Four categories are used to summarize the level of severity: code 1, current medical management or diagnostic problem; code 2, condition noted; no medical management, no diagnostic problem; code 3, history of condition only; or code 4, condition noted but unknown whether it is a current or past condition. The "comorbidity burden" is further weighted by its potential impact on short-term survival. The weights, referred to as potential "life threat," are based on clinical judgment and a review of data on disease-specific mortality.

A. Comorbidity Indexes: A Comparison

Each of the four comorbidity indexes provides a summary score that reflects the overall severity of conditions for subjects with an index condition. The more severe the level of comorbidity, the poorer the chances for survival. Although each index predicts cancer survival, there are differences. The overall scores for the Kaplan-Feinstein and Greenfield indexes are based on the individual's most severe condition or state. In contrast, the Charlson and NIA/NCI Indexes are derived from a total of the values for each individual health condition. The Greenfield Index includes functional status as a measure of severity; the others do not. The composite indexes assume an additive relationship between conditions; none of the indexes are designed to capture possible multiplicative or synergistic effects.

There have been several systematic comparisons of the Kaplan-Feinstein, Charlson, and Greenfield Indexes. In most cases, the Charlson Index is reported to have better interrater reliability and to be easier to use. For example, Newschaffer and colleagues report that the Charlson Index has better interrater agreement and cross-source agreement (Medicare claims vs medical record) than the Kaplan-Feinstein Index in a group of 404 elderly, incident breast cancer cases identified from the Virginia Cancer Registry (28). In a study of patients with head and neck cancer, Singh and colleagues indicate that although both the Kaplan and Feinstein and Charlson Indexes independently predicted tumor-specific survival, the Charlson Index could be more readily applied (29). Finally, Albertson and colleagues examined the effects of comorbidity on the long-term survival of men with localized prostate cancer (30). The prognostic significance of Kaplan-Feinstein, Charlson, and Greenfield Indexes were examined and reported to be comparable, although no data were provided (30).

III. SOURCES OF INFORMATION AND TIMING OF ASSESSMENT

A. Medical Records

Most assessments of comorbidity, including the four comorbidity indexes described previously, are based on data obtained from the patient's medical record. The medical record is generally regarded to be the most complete and authoritative source of information on the patient's past and current health status. Although it is possible that comorbid conditions may be antecedent, concurrent, or subsequent to the index cancer, data on comorbidity are typically drawn from the medical records of the hospitalization for the first cancer treatment.

Although the medical record represents the most common source of data for comorbidity, concerns have been expressed about its use. One concern is that specific information may not be consistently available. For example, the Greenfield Index requires an assessment of functional status that is usually measured in terms of the patient's level of activities of daily living (ADL). Results from the NIA/NCI study indicate, however, that data on functioning were not consistently available across hospitals and patients (6). Another concern is possible selection bias. Differences in the number and types of comorbidity may reflect the number of physician visits and hospitalizations rather than actual health differences between people. A subject who has more physician visits and hospitalizations has a greater chance of having a comorbid condition identified. This may be especially problematic in case-control studies (33). In a case-control study, it is necessary to record the number and type of concurrent health conditions in a similar fashion for both cases and controls. By definition, medical records for the cases are available at least for the hospitalization associated with the initial treatment. This may not always be the case for the controls, especially in a population-based study in which the controls are identified through telephone random-digit dialing or from a community census. Even if medical records are available for the controls, those records may not be associated with a recent hospitalization. A final concern is that a review of medical records may be too time consuming and costly. With regard to this point, alternative sources of data have been proposed to improve the efficiency of the medical review.

There has been extensive discussion, for example, about the use of administrative medical record databases as sources of data on comorbidity. The size and complexity of the databases range from computerized discharge summaries of individual hospitals to the computerized records of the Medicare and Medicaid populations. In 1993, Deyo and colleagues (34) adapted and evaluated the Charlson Index for an outcome study of Medicare beneficiaries who underwent lumbar spine surgery. Later, Romano and colleagues (35, 36), although acknowledging the prognostic significance of the Charlson Index, expressed reservations about the accuracy of the correspondence or translation as proposed by Deyo and colleagues (34) between the items in the Charlson Index and the ICD-9-CM administrative data. Romano and colleagues (35, 36) also argued that the Charlson Index, based on an examination of a hospitalized population in New York, may not be completely generalizable to other patients with other conditions, a concern also expressed by others (37). Finally, Romano and colleagues (35, 36) were concerned that a summary index, such as provided by the Charlson Index, may not reflect the interaction, that is, multiplication of effects, between individual conditions, a position echoed in a recent article by Elixhauser and colleagues (38). This concern, of course, could be legitimately expressed about any of the common comorbidity indexes that are based on additive scales. Despite these concerns, data from medical records, either obtained from special reviews or from computerized, administrative records, remain the leading source of information about multiple health conditions of cancer patients.

B. Personal Interviews

Personal interviews also have been used as sources of information on comorbidity, especially in studies that are designed to estimate the prevalence of comorbid conditions in the general population (11, 16). Katz and colleagues, for example, have developed an interview-based version of the Charlson Index (39). Although personal interviews have been used in general population surveys, they are less likely to be used in studies of comorbidity in cancer patients. There are exceptions. In one study of breast cancer patients, comorbidity was restricted to diagnosed conditions that were reported by the subject to limit daily activities (40, 41). Women with breast cancer who reported two or more limiting conditions were 2.5 times more likely than those without limiting conditions to die in a follow-up period, adjusting for age, stage of disease, and treatment (40). In a separate study, subjects were classified as having medical comorbidity if they indicated that they saw a physician in the year prior to their cancer diagnosis (cancers of the breast, colon, or prostate) for any of 11 common medical conditions perceived as having limited their activity during that year (42). In a multivariate analysis, this measure of comorbidity was marginally associated with subsequent survival.

The use of the interview as a source of data on comorbidity has several advantages. First, it is an efficient and less costly procedure than a review of medical records. Second, in a case-control study, it ensures that data on comorbidity are obtained in the same manner for both cancer patients and controls (33). Third, it provides an opportunity to obtain alternative data on severity. Unlike an index that uses the risk of death as the sole measure of severity, an interview-based system also may use the subject's reported functional limitations to establish severity (40, 41).

Despite these advantages, it has been argued that subjects may misreport either the nature or dates of diagnosis (27). Results from validity studies suggest, however, that there is reasonably good correspondence between health conditions reported by subjects and the conditions found on medical records (43). In general, the more serious the condition, the greater the correspondence (44). It has been argued that this may be due to the fact that the most serious chronic diseases are usually homogeneous with clear diagnostic criteria (45). It remains to be seen, however, how well subjects can recall accurately the dates of diagnosis.

C. Death Certificates

The presence of comorbidity also has been inferred from multiple cause of death data (46–48). If a condition, such as cancer, is listed as the underlying cause of death on the death certificate, that means the cancer was judged to be the condition that began the chain of events that ultimately lead to the patient's death. More specifically, the cause of death was determined to be from the cancer if the death occurred as a result of a complication directly related to the primary or metastatic cancer process. Examples include (a) wasting, weakness, or malnutrition due to metastatic cancer that lead to a reduced ability to fight infection and eventual death from pneumonia, sepsis, or other generalized infection; and (b) malnutrition from the cancer leading to electrolyte imbalance, arrhythmias, and cardiac death in the absence of acute ischemic disease. The death certificate also includes space for the listing of associated causes of death. The associated causes of death are comorbid conditions that may have theoretically contributed to the chain of events leading to death. The advantages of this source of comorbidity data are that it is widely available and it can be linked programmatically to demographical and clinical data from population-based cancer surveillance systems. It may be, however, that the listing of associated causes at the time of death may not always be reliable nor reflect the full range or timing of comorbid conditions that affected the decedent.

Although medical records, personal interviews, and death certificates all represent possible sources of data on comorbidity, each source has potential strengths and limitations.

IV. COMORBIDITY, MULTIPLE PRIMARIES, AND RISK OF CANCER

A number of studies have identified associations between selected health conditions and different forms of cancer. These associations, known as "cluster comorbidity," occur more frequently than would be expected by chance (9). Diabetes, for example, has been shown to be associated with primary endometrial, liver, and pancreatic cancers (49–51). Other combinations of comorbidity and cancer include hepatitis C viral infection and liver cancer, papilloma viral infection and cervical cancer, and a history of kidney stones and renal cell cancer (52–54). There are also reports that specific chemotherapeutic agents, such as doxorubicin, and radiotherapy for left-sided breast cancer, under certain circumstances, may have cardiac side effects (55–58). For the most part, however, it has not been established how the risk of cancer associated with these conditions and treatments is affected by age or gender.

There is also an extensive literature on multiple primary cancers (59). The term *multiple primary cancers* refers to the occurrence of more than one primary cancer in the same individual, not including the presence of cancers that have metastasized to another anatomical site (59). People who have developed their first primary cancer early in life are at greater risk for developing a subsequent primary cancer in later years (60). There are also specific associations between multiple primary sites. Women with breast cancer, for example, are at elevated risk for developing a subsequent breast cancer and endometrial, ovarian, or colon cancers (60). Breast cancer patients who received radiotherapy are at approximately a threefold risk of developing lung cancer over a 15-year period (61). In a separate study, close associations were reported between kidney and bladder cancers and between head and neck and esophageal cancers (62). Despite the growing number of studies in this area, it is unknown whether people at risk for multiple primary cancers are also at risk for developing other comorbid conditions.

V. COMORBIDITY, SCREENING, AND STAGE OF DISEASE

The relationship between comorbidity and screening practices is presently unclear. Although Crawford and Cohen (63) argue that cancer screening is not likely to be performed in elderly patients under medical attention for other health problems, Feinstein speculates that the presence of comorbid conditions may actually improve the chances of diagnosing a cancer at an earlier stage (10). There is evidence to suggest that women who report a history of any diagnosed medical condition, especially breast cancer, are more likely than women without previously diagnosed conditions to practice breast self-examination and obtain annual mammograms (64, 65). However, in a study of older black women, those least likely to accept a mammogram were those with multiple health problems (66). In the NIA/NCI SEER (National Institute on Aging/National Cancer Institute Surveillance, Evaluation, and End Results [Program]) study, no association was found between comorbidity and breast cancer stage (6). In contrast, there is evidence from another study of a trend, although not statistically significant, between increasing levels of comorbidity and an increase in the percentage of women diagnosed with localized breast cancer ($P = .15$) (67). Specifically, the percentage of women diagnosed with localized disease increased from 52.4% among those with no comorbid conditions to 53.8% for those with one condition, to 56.5% for those with two conditions, and 61.0% for those with three or more conditions. Interestingly, there was also evidence of an increase in the percentage of women with remote disease with increasing levels of comorbidity. For each level of comorbidity (0, 1, 2, 3+), the percentage of women diagnosed with remote disease was 5.0, 3.8, 8.9, and 9.8, respectively (67). The same general pattern was found in a study of breast cancer among female members of a health maintenance organization (HMO) in the San Francisco Bay Area (68). With increasing levels of comorbidity, as measured by the Charlson Index, the more likely women were to be diagnosed with either localized disease or remote disease (66).

There are several possible explanations for this association. First, the association may depend more on the specific combination of comorbid conditions than on the absolute number. It may be that some conditions, perhaps those that are either more disabling or whose signs and symptoms are more obscure or more likely to be confused with cancer signs, are more likely to be associated with later stage disease. In contrast, those conditions that require regular monitoring may be more likely to be associated with localized disease. It also may be that physicians, patients, or family members are less likely to endorse regular screening for people who have health problems that are associated with reduced life expectancy. Second, the association may depend on the relative access of the person to health screening. Those people with comorbid conditions who have regular access to health care may be more likely to be diagnosed with localized disease. On the other hand, those with comorbid conditions who do not have such access may be more likely to be diagnosed with later stage disease.

VI. COMORBIDITY AND CANCER TREATMENT

A. Patterns of Care

A variety of studies indicate that older people are less likely than younger people to receive definitive cancer therapy (69–75). For cancers of most sites, the proportion of patients who receive curative therapy for either local or regional stage disease declines with age (69–75). There is also evidence that cancers diagnosed in older people are less likely than cancers in younger people to be microscopically confirmed (76).

It has been hypothesized that comorbidity may account, at least in part, for this age pattern (26, 31). Specifically, the presence of comorbid conditions that are found in older patients, such as heart disease and diabetes, and their associated medications may elevate the risks associated with the most definitive or invasive procedures. As a result, physicians are less likely to recommend those procedures for their older patients. This hypothesis has been tested directly with mixed results.

In several studies, comorbidity was found to explain part, but not all, of the association between chronological age and the approach to cancer treatment. Chronological age remained an independent predictor of both the extent and type of treatment. In one study, a smaller proportion of women aged 50 years and over with moderate to severe concurrent conditions (58.9%) received appropriate therapy for breast cancer compared with women who had only slight or no comorbidity (81.3%) (26). Despite the significance of comorbidity, age was still predictive of the type of treatment after adjustment for comorbidity and the stage of disease. In a separate study, age was negatively associated with any surgical treatment, breast-conserving procedures when surgery was done, and radiotherapy following breast-conserving surgery (77). Although comorbidity, as measured with the Charlson Index, was associated with both older age and less invasive treatment, chronological age remained a correlate of the type of treatment. In another study, Medicare claims were linked to data from the SEER program to examine factors associated with surgical and radiation therapy for early-stage breast cancer in older women (78). Comorbidity was again measured by the Charlson Index; this time with a version for use with automated claims data. The results indicated that the frequency of breast-conserving surgery was highest among women aged 80 years or more who had two or more comorbid conditions and stage I disease. In general, however, the receipt of radiation therapy among patients undergoing breast-conserving surgery declined markedly with age irrespective of the comorbidity status and disease stage. Even after adjustment for comorbidity, age remained an important independent factor associated with the receipt of radiation therapy after breast-conserving surgery among women aged 65 years or more who were diagnosed with early-stage breast cancer. Similar findings were reported in a study of treatment for prostatic cancer (31). Prostatic cancer patients aged 75 years and older had significantly less intensive work-ups for clinical staging and the use of surgical and radiation therapies compared with younger patients. Although differences in levels of comorbidity were found to be associated with intensity of treatment, they did not account for the differences in treatment by age group.

In contrast to these studies where comorbidity was associated with less intensive treatment, other researchers report no association between comorbidity and the type of treatment. Goodwin and colleagues examined the determinants of cancer therapy in elderly New Mexico residents diagnosed with breast, prostatic, or colorectal cancers (79). Comorbidity was collected through personal interview and summarized as either the presence or absence of one or more selected conditions. In a multivariate analysis, only advanced age and decreased mental status remained significant predictors of nonreceipt of definitive therapy. Similar results have been reported from a Dutch study of age and treatment for breast cancer. The study consisted of a medical record review of breast cancer patients treated at the Netherlands Cancer Institute (80). Like the New Mexico study, comorbidity was defined as the presence or absence of selected chronic conditions.

Differences in the definition and measurement of comorbidity may explain the variations in research findings. In studies in which an association is reported between comorbidity and the extent of treatment, the measurement of comorbidity is more detailed and classified by level of severity (26, 31, 77, 78). In contrast, when comorbidity is measured as a dichotomous variable (present/absent), no association is found (79, 80). It is important to emphasize again, however, that even in those studies in which comorbidity was associated with less invasive therapy, differences in comorbidity could not completely account for age differences in the treatment approach. This finding may suggest that either there are other factors associated with age, such as functional status, that account for the differences in treatment or that current measures of comorbidity are not sufficiently detailed or sufficiently sensitive to explain the findings.

B. Prescriptions for Care

There is a growing interest in learning whether particular cancer therapies for patients with comorbid conditions improve either their duration or quality of life (81–88). Although clinical trials have not been conducted, observational studies have examined the prognostic significance of treatment among patients with different levels of comorbidity. Decision analyses also have been used to compare medical outcomes among patients undergoing different therapies for cancer by level of comorbidity (89–93). Decision analysis provides a means of incorporating data from a variety of clinical and epidemiological sources to model and compare the outcomes of different clinical options (94).

Most of the work has focused on older men with prostatic cancer and whether those with the disease should receive radical prostatectomy or be monitored so that the progression of the tumor can be assessed ("watchful waiting"). Comorbidity is important for several reasons. First, prostatic cancer is typically a cancer of older men (2). As such, prostatic cancer patients are likely to have concurrent health conditions. Second, the presence of the conditions may adversely affect the duration or quality of life of men undergoing radical prostatectomy. Third, older men diagnosed with prostatic cancer are more likely to die of a comorbid condition than the prostatic cancer (95).

For prostatic cancer, the research suggests that watchful waiting is more appropriate than other treatment strategies for older men with comorbid conditions. In one study in which patients undergoing transurethral resection of the prostate were older and sicker than patients undergoing open prostatectomy (96), some of the difference in the 5-year survival still seemed to be due in part to differences in comorbidity (96). In a different study, the level of comorbidity elevated the risk of death among men who received conservative treatment for localized disease (30).

In addition to the observational studies, two decision analyses have been conducted to examine treatment outcomes among men with clinically localized prostatic cancer (89, 93). It is reported that the chances of survival would be better among men under the age of 70 years with low to moderate comorbidity if they underwent a radical prostatectomy rather than watchful waiting. In contrast, men older than 70 years with a high level of comorbidity would fare better with watchful waiting (93). In a separate decision analysis, estimated survival was compared among men with clinically localized disease undergoing one of three treatments: radical prostatectomy, external-beam radiation therapy, and watchful waiting, with delayed hormonal therapy if metastatic disease developed (89). The investigators concluded that invasive treatment may be harmful to men over the age of 70 years.

VII. COMORBIDITY AND CANCER SCREENING

A. Prescriptions for Care

It is also important to determine whether diagnosing cancer at an earlier stage improves the chances for survival among people with background levels of comorbidity as it does among people in the general population. One study suggested that diagnosing breast cancer at an early stage may not confer the same advantage for women with severe comorbidity as it does for women with fewer or no concurrent medical conditions (67). As expected, breast cancer patients with distant disease had a lower probability of survival than did patients with local or regional disease. However, among patients with three or more comorbid conditions, the stage of disease seemed to have little additional effect on survival.

Two decision analyses of screening for cancer also have been conducted (97, 98). The utility of breast cancer screening was compared in a decision analysis study among four groups of women aged 65–85 years or more: average health (all races), mild hypertension, congestive heart failure, and average-health black women alone (97). The results indicated that screening improved the chances for survival at all ages among patients studied. Although the potential for improvement in survival was highest for black women, it decreased with increasing age and comorbidity. A decision analysis also was used to assess the clinical and economic effects of screening for prostatic cancer (98). Three screening methods were examined: prostate-specific antigen (PSA), transrectal ultrasound (TRUS), and digital rectal examination (DRE). In unselected men between the ages of 50 and 70 years, screening with PSA or TRUS prolonged unadjusted life expectancy but reduced quality of life. Screening with DRE alone did not improve life expectancy in any age group. It was concluded that screening in general improved life expectancy, decreased quality of life, and increased costs. It was also concluded that combinations of comorbidity, risk attitude, valuation of sexual function, probability of iatrogenic impotence, and time dependence of utilities may make screening more or less desirable for selected individuals.

VIII. COMORBIDITY AND SURVIVAL

As noted previously, comorbidity has been shown consistently to elevate the risk of death of cancer patients, adjusting for other prognostic indicators (23). In fact, the relative risk of death is the most common criterion for establishing the severity of individual comorbid conditions (25).

Measures of comorbidity also have been used to help explain racial and socioeconomic differences in survival. In a Dutch study, it has been reported that the prevalence of comorbidity was greatest among patients of lower socioeconomic status with selected cancers, including cancers of the breast and lung (18). Also, there is evidence, for example, that racial differences in disease burden among people in the general population is explained in part by differences in levels of comorbidity (99). Eley and colleagues report that black women with breast cancer had a greater number of comorbid conditions than white women with the disease (100). Comorbidity was defined in terms of the presence or absence of selected conditions found in the medical record that included diabetes mellitus, systemic arterial hypertension, heart disease, lung disease, and renal disease. In addition, any residual condition was included that potentially could affect treatment or survival. Overall comorbidity was measured in terms of the total number of conditions. Although the level of comorbidity was not associated with death from breast cancer, it was associated with the risk of death from all causes. In addition, comorbidity, in conjunction with other sociodemographic factors, helped to explain some of the racial differences in survival that could not be explained by the stage of disease and other clinical variables. In a separate study, comorbidity, as measured by the Charlson Index, had the same independent effect on the 10-year survival among both black and white women diagnosed with breast cancer after adjustment for age, stage, tumor size, and treatment (68).

IX. MECHANISMS OF SURVIVAL

It is important to consider the reasons why cancer patients with comorbidity are at elevated risk of death. One hypothesis is that comorbidity aggravates the course of the index cancer, in part, by a reduction of functional reserves and/or by a modification of standard therapies. An alternative hypothesis is that the index cancer actually aggravates the course of the comorbid conditions; again, either through the reduction of functional reserves or a modification of standard therapies for the comorbid condition. It is fair to say that the specific interaction between the index cancer and the set of comorbid conditions would depend on the relative severity and temporal sequence of each condition.

There is evidence that patients with comorbid conditions are more likely to die with an underlying cause of death other than the index cancer (47, 67, 95). In a national study, Manton and colleagues reported that cancer is often found on death certificates as contributing to the risk of noncancer causes of death. The occurrence of cancer as a nonunderlying cause of death increased with age and was highest for treatable and slowly growing tumor types (47). Breast cancer patients from the Detroit metropolitan area who had three or more of seven selected comorbid conditions had a 20-fold higher rate of mortality from causes other than breast cancer and a 4-fold higher rate of all-cause mortality when compared with patients who had no comorbid conditions (67).

In a recent study of the cause of death among men diagnosed with prostatic cancer in Kaiser hospitals in the San Francisco Bay Area, increasing age and comorbidity, in particular, cardiovascular comorbidity, were independently associated with death due to a cause other than prostatic cancer (95).

The results suggest that the index cancer may aggravate the course of the comorbid condition. It may be that the index cancer reduces the patient's functional reserves and elevates the risk of death. It also may be that the diagnosis and treatment of the index cancer leads to a modification of the treatment protocol for a preexisting comorbid condition, such as treatment for diabetes. This modification, in turn, may inadvertently have a negative effect on the patient's prognosis (95).

X. CONCLUSIONS AND RECOMMENDATIONS

Research on comorbidity and cancer is at a crossroads. It is clear that comorbidity is an important variable; it affects cancer diagnosis, treatment, and prognosis in older populations. It also contributes to our understanding of racial and socioeconomic differences in the stage of disease at diagnosis as well as differences in treatment and survival. Unfortunately, the research on comorbidity to date has not been sufficiently detailed to lead to recommendations about the management of cancer in older patients with specific concurrent conditions. The following recommendations are proposed to expand the research agenda in this area.

1. Future studies should be designed (a) to examine the independent effects of individual comorbid conditions in conjunction with specific forms of cancer on the duration and quality of life and (b) to determine to what extent the nature of those prognostic effects vary by the patient's age, gender, race, or socioeconomic status (14, 38, 95). Cardiovascular diseases and diabetes should be given special attention. In addition to being relatively common, standard criteria are available to measure the level of severity. Psychiatric conditions also should be investigated. With the possible exception of depression, these conditions typically are not included in measures of comorbidity among cancer patients even though there is a substantial literature on psychiatric comorbidity (101–103). Disease algorithms also should be developed for the clear and consistent identification of individual comorbid conditions (104).

This recommendation is not intended to underestimate the significance of summary measures of comorbidity. Quite the contrary. Summary measures, such as the Charlson Index (25), have played a key role in the assessment of comorbidity. It is necessary, however, to obtain more detailed information about the effects of specific sets of conditions so that more refined summary measures can be developed (10, 14, 38). As noted previously, most summary measures are additive. Little is known about whether specific combinations of comorbid conditions have multiplicative or synergistic effects on either the quality or duration of life. In one of the few studies of the multiplicative effects of comorbidity, Verbrugge and colleagues present results from a national study that indicate that cancer and ischemic heart disease have a synergistic effect on disability (11). More research in this area needs to be conducted.

2. Examinations of different methods of assessment of comorbidity should be conducted, including comparisons of the strengths and limitations of medical records, personal interviews, and death certificates as sources of data on comorbidity. Special attention should be given to assessments of automated databases, such as the hospital discharge summary, and strategies for regular linkage to clinical and demographical data from population-based cancer registries, such as the National Cancer Institute's SEER Program.

3. Studies of treatment should be expanded to include examinations of the effects of cancer diagnosis and treatment on the management of preexisting comorbid conditions; for example, whether the diagnosis and treatment of breast cancer leads to a modification in the management plan for preexisting diabetes and whether that modification affects subsequent survival. Most of the studies on patterns of care have neglected this issue, focusing instead on whether preexisting comorbidity affects cancer treatment. This research should contribute to a more comprehensive understanding of the prognostic significance of comorbidity.

4. The evaluation of analytical and statistical issues associated with comor-

bidity should be conducted (105, 106). This should include the development of parsimonious strategies to summarize additive and multiplicative effects of concurrent health conditions and to incorporate data on the temporal sequence of concurrent conditions.

5. The effects of comorbidity on medical practice and patient preferences need to be investigated in greater detail (107, 108). This could involve the use of factorial experiments in which physicians are presented with hypothetical cases that differ systematically by the index cancer, the number, and type of concurrent conditions, as well as by the patient's age, gender, and socioeconomic status. For each case, the physician is then asked to recommend treatment. These "simulations" could contribute useful information about the basis of physician decision making (107, 109, 110). In addition to the effects of comorbidity, the receipt of less aggressive treatment in older patients may be due to the belief (justified or not) that cancer at old ages is less aggressive than at younger ages.

6. The epidemiology of comorbidity needs to be developed. Just as the etiology of single, categorical conditions is presently investigated, it is necessary in the future to examine the etiology of multiple conditions. For example, why are some women at elevated risk for breast cancer, whereas other women are at elevated risk for breast cancer and diabetes? In one study, a history of cigarette smoking, recent alcohol consumption, and obesity were associated with comorbidity among women with breast cancer (40). Research in this area will contribute to programs of primary and secondary prevention.

7. New designs for clinical trials should be considered. Often subjects with comorbid conditions are not included in clinical trials (111, 112). This approach is used to minimize the risks to the patients and to preserve the "internal validity" of the study. Unfortunately, by excluding subjects with comorbidity, it is difficult to generalize the results of the trial to a population of older people who typically have comorbid conditions. The external validity of the study is compromised. As more refined measures of comorbidity are developed, it may be possible to conduct clinical trials in which subjects are stratified by level of comorbidity (67). Within each stratum, subjects could be randomly assigned to different protocols. It would be possible then to generalize the results of the trial to people with a given level of background comorbidity. It must be emphasized that a clinical trial of this kind would require a larger sample size than is typically used in more conventional trials. Finally, these recommendations are all contingent on first ensuring the subjects' safety.

In conclusion, research on comorbidities and cancer must be conducted on many fronts and involve the collaboration of researchers in a variety of fields that include, but are not limited to, gerontology and geriatrics, oncology, cancer biology, therapeutics, epidemiology, and public health. New strategies of linking automated comorbidity data with data from population-based cancer registries are very promising and should be expanded. The NIA/NCI SEER study, for example, has demonstrated the feasibility of obtaining data on comorbid conditions as part of regular cancer surveillance (7). Finally, research in this area should lead to the development of better strategies of management of cancer in older populations that are based on the special physiological, psychosocial, and pathological characteristics of the aging process.

ACKNOWLEDGMENTS

I wish to thank Francois Schellevis, Trudi van den Bos, and Rosemary Yancik for their review and critique of an earlier version of this chapter.

REFERENCES

1. Rowe J. Health care of the elderly. N Engl J Med 1985; 312:826–835.
2. Miller BA, Ries LAG, Hankey BF, Kosary CL, Harras A, Devesa SS, Edwards BK, eds. SEER cancer statistics review 1973–1990. NIH Publication Number 93-2789. Bethesda, Maryland: National Cancer Institute, 1993.
3. Coebergh JWWW. Significant trends in cancer in the elderly. Eur J Cancer 1996; 32A: 569–571.
4. Yancik R. Cancer burden in the aged: an epidemiologic and demographic overview. Cancer 1997; 80:1273–1283.
5. Guralnik JM, LaCroix AZ, Everett DF, Kovar MG. Aging in the eighties: the prevalence of comorbidity and its association with disability. Hyattsville, MD: National Center for Health Statistics, Advanced Data from Vital and Health Statistics, No. 170, 1989.
6. Havlik RJ, Yancik R, Long S, Ries L, Edwards B. The National Institute on Aging and the National Cancer Institute SEER collaborative study on comorbidity and early diagnosis of cancer in the elderly. Cancer 1994; 74(Suppl):2101–2106.
7. Yancik R, Havlik RJ, Wesley MN, Ries L, Long S, Rossi WK, Edwards BK. Cancer and comorbidity in older patients: a descriptive profile. Ann Epidemiol 1996; 6(Special):399–412.
8. Satariano WA. Foreward. Rethinking disease: implications for epidemiology. Ann Epidemiol 1996; 6(Special):377.
9. Schellevis FG, Bos GAM van den, Tijssen JGP, Grobbee DE, Heinsbroek RPW. Comorbidity and chronic diseases: a report of the workshop, Comorbidity and Chronic Diseases. The Hague, The Netherlands: Council for Medical Research, The Netherlands Organization for Scientific Research, November, 1997.
10. Feinstein AR. The pre-therapeutic classification of co-morbidity in chronic disease. Chron Dis 1970; 23:455–469.
11. Verbrugge LM, Lepkowski JM, Imanaka Y. Comorbidity and its impact on disability. Milbank Q 1989; 67:450–484.
12. Cornoni-Huntley JC, Foley DJ, Guralnik JM. Co-morbidity analysis: a strategy for understanding mortality, disability and use of health care facilities of older people. Int J Epidemiol 1991; 20:S8–S15.

13. Satariano WA. Comorbidity and functional status in older women with breast cancer: implications for screening, treatment, and prognosis. J Geront 1992; 47(Special):24–31.

14. Guralnik JM. Assessing the impact of comorbidity in older populations. Ann Epidemiol 1996; 6(Special):376–380.

15. Wilson LA, Lawson IR, Brass W. Multiple disorders in the elderly: a clinical and statistical study. Lancet 1962; 2:841–843.

16. Seeman TE, Guralnik JM, Kaplan GA, Knudsen L, Cohen R. The health consequences of multiple morbidity in the elderly: the Alameda County Study. J Aging Health 1989; 1:50–66.

17. Schellevis FG, Veldin J van der, Lisdonk E van der, Eijk J th M van, Weel C van. Comorbidity of chronic diseases in general practice. J Clin Epidemiol 1993; 46:469–473.

18. Schrijvers CTM, Coebergh JWWW, Mackenbach JP. Socioeconomic status and comorbidity among newly diagnosed cancer patients. Cancer 1997; 80:1482–1488.

19. Feinstein AR, Schimpff CR, Andrews JF, Wells CK. Cancer of the larynx: a new staging system and a re-appraisal of prognosis of treatment. J Chron Dis 1977; 30:277–305.

20. Feinstein AR, Schimpff CR, Hall EW. A reappraisal of staging and therapy for patients with cancer of the rectum: I: development of two new systems of staging. Arch Intern Med 1975; 135:1441–1453.

21. Peipert JF, Wells CK, Schwartz PE, Feinstein AR. The impact of symptoms and comorbidity on prognosis in stage IB cervical cancer. Am J Obst Gynecol 1993; 169:598–604.

22. Piccirillo JF, Wells CK, Sasaki CT, Feinstein AR. New clinical severity staging system for cancer of the larynx. Ann Otol Rhinol Laryngol 1994; 103:83–92.

23. Piccirillo JF, Feinstein AR. Clinical symptoms and comorbidity: significance for the prognostic classification of cancer. Cancer 1996; 77:834–842.

24. Kaplan MH, Feinstein AR. The importance of classifying initial comorbidity in evaluating the outcome of diabetes mellitus. J Chron Dis 1974; 27:387–404.

25. Charlson ME, Pompei P, Alex KL, MacKenzie CR. A new method of classifying prognostic comorbidity in longitudinal studies: development and validation. J Chron Dis 1987; 40:373–383.

26. Greenfield S, Blanco DM, Elashoff RM, Ganz PA. Patterns of care related to age of breast cancer patients. JAMA 1987; 257:2766–2770.

27. Yancik R, Wesley MN, Ries LAG, Havlik RJ, Long S, Edwards BK, Yates JW. Comorbidity and age as predictors of risk for early mortality in male and female colon carcinoma patients: a population-based study. Cancer 1998; 82:2123–2134.

28. Newschaffer CJ, Bush TL, Penberthy LT. Comorbidity measurement in elderly female breast cancer patients with administrative and medical records data. J Clin Epidemiol 1997; 50:725–733.

29. Singh B, Bhaya M, Stern J, Roland JT, Zimbler M, Rosenfeld RM, Har-El G, Lucente FE. Validation of the Charlson comorbidity index in patients with head and neck cancer: a multi-institutional study. Larynogoscope 1997; 107:1469–1475.

30. Albertson PC, Fryback DG, Storer BE, Kolon TF, Fine J. Long-term survival among men with conservatively treated localized prostate cancer. JAMA 1995; 274:626–631.

31. Bennett CL, Greenfield S, Aronow HU, Ganz P, Vogelzang NH, Elashoff RM. Patterns of care related to age of men with prostate cancer. Cancer 1991; 67:2633–2441.

32. Greenfield S, Apolone G, McNeil BJ, Cleary PD. The importance of co-existent disease in the occurrence of postoperative complications and one-year recovery in patients undergoing total hip replacement. Med Care 1993; 31:141–154.

33. Satariano WA, Ragland DR, DeLorenze GN. Limitations in upper-body strength associated with breast cancer: a comparison of black and white women. J Clin Epidemiol 1996; 49:535–544.

34. Deyo RA, Cherkin DC, Clol MA. Adapting a clinical comorbidity index for use with ICD-9-CM administrative databases. J Clin Epidemiol 1992; 45:613–619.

35. Romano PS, Roos LL, Jollis JG. Adapting a clinical comorbidity index for use with ICD-9-CM administrative data: differing perspectives. J Clin Epidemiol 1993a; 46:1075–1079.

36. Romano PS, Roos LL, Jollis JG. Further evidence concerning the use of a clinical comorbidity index with ICD-9-CM administrative data. J Clin Epidemiol 1993b; 46:1085–1090.

37. Ghali WA, Hall RE, Rosen AK, Ash AS, Moskowitz MA. Searching for an improved comorbidity index for use with ICD-9-CM administrative data. J Clin Epidemiol 1996; 49:273–278.

38. Elixhauser A, Steiner C, Harris DR, Coffey RM. Comorbidity measures for use with administrative data. Med Care 1998;36:8–27.

39. Katz JN, Chang LC, Sangha O, Fossel AH, Bates DW. Can comorbidity be measured by questionnaire rather than medical record review? Med Care 1996; 34:73–84.

40. Satariano WA, Ragheb NE, Dupuis ME. Comorbidity in older women with breast cancer: an epidemiologic approach. In: Yancik R, Yates JW, eds. Cancer in the Elderly: Approaches to Early Detection and Treatment. New York: Springer, 1989:71–107.

41. Satariano WA. Aging, comorbidity, and breast cancer survival: an epidemiologic view. Adv Exp Med Biol 1993; 330:1–11.

42. Goodwin JS, Samet JM, Hunt WC. Determinants of survival in older cancer patients. J Natl Cancer Inst 1996; 88:1031–1038.

43. Bush TL, Miller SR, Golden AL, Hale WE. Self-report and medical record report agreement of selected medical conditions in the elderly. Am J Public Health 1989; 79:1554–1556.

44. Meltzer JW, Hochstim JR. Reliability and validity of survey data on physical health. Public Health Rep 1970; 85:1075–1086.

45. Velden J van der, Abrahamse HphH, Donker G, Steen J van der, Sonsbeek JLA van, Bos GAM van den. What do health interview surveys tell us about the prevalences of somatic chronic diseases? A study into concurrent validity. Eur J Public Health 1998; 8:52–58.

46. Israel RA, Rosenberg HM, Curtin LR. Analytical potential for multiple cause-of-death data. Am J Epidemiol 1986; 124:161–179.

47. Manton KG, Wrigley JM, Cohen HJ, Woodbury MA. Cancer mortality, aging, and patterns of comorbidity in the United States: 1968 to 1986. J Gerontol Soc Sci 1991; 46:S225–S234.

48. Mackenbach JP, Kunst AE, Lawtenbach H, Bijlsma F, Gei YB. Competing causes of death: an analysis using multiple-cause-of-death data from the Netherlands. Am J Epidemiol 1995; 141:466–475.

49. Centers for Disease Control Cancer Steroid Hormone (CASH) Study. Oral contraceptive use and the risk of endometrial cancer. JAMA 1983; 249:1600–1604.
50. Adami HO, Chjow W-H, Nyren O, Berne C, Linet MS, Ekbow A, Wolk A, McLaughlin JK, Fraumeni JF. Excess risk of primary liver cancer in patients with diabetes mellitus. J Natl Cancer Inst 1996; 88:1472–1477.
51. Everhart J, Wright D. Diabetes mellitus as a risk factor for pancreatic cancer: a meta-analysis. JAMA 1995; 273:1605–1609.
52. Tanaka H, Hiyama T, Okubo Y, Kitada A, Fujimoto I. Primary liver cancer incidence-rates related to hepatitis-C virus infection: a correlational study in Osaka, Japan. Cancer Causes Control 1994; 5:61–65.
53. Tindle RW. Immunomanipulative strategies for the control of human papillomavirus associated with cervical cancer. Immun Res 1997; 16:387–400.
54. Schlehofer B, Pommer W, Mellemgaard A, Stewart JH, McCredie M, Niwa S, Lindblad P, Mandel JS, McLaughlin JK, Wahrendorf J. International renal-cell-cancer study. VI. The role of medical and family history. Int J Cancer 1996; 66:723–726.
55. Unverferth DV, Magoricn RD, Leier CV, Balcerzak SP. Doxorubicin cardiotoxicity. Cancer Treat Rev 1982; 9:149–164.
56. Von Hoff DD, Layard MW, Basa P, Davis HL, Von Hoff AL, Rozencweig M, Muggia FM. Risk factors for doxorubicin-induced congestive heart failure. Ann Intern Med 1979; 91:710–717.
57. Gyenes G, Fornander T, Carlens P, Rutqvist LE. Morbidity of ischemic heart disease in early breast cancer 15-2-years after adjuvant radiotherapy. Int J Radiat Oncol Biol Phys 1994; 28:1235–1241.
58. Wei JY. Cardiovascular comorbidity in the older cancer patient. Semin Oncol 1995; 22(Suppl)1:9–10.
59. Schottenfeld D. Multiple primary cancers. In Schottenfeld D, Fraumeni JF, eds. Cancer Epidemiology and Prevention. Philadelphia: Saunders, 1982:1025–1038.
60. Schwartz AG, Ragheb NE, Swanson GM, Satariano WA. Racial and age differences in multiple primary cancers after breast cancer: a population-based analysis. Breast Cancer Res Treat 1989; 14:245–254.
61. Inskip PD, Stovall M, Flannery JT. Lung cancer risk and radiation dose among women treated for breast cancer. J Natl Cancer Inst 1994; 86:983–988.
62. Begg CB, Zhang Z-F, Sun M, Herr HW, Schantz SP. Methodology for evaluating the incidence of second primary cancers with application to smoking-related cancers from the Surveillance, Epidemiology, and End Results (SEER) Program. Am J Epidemiol 1995; 142:653–665.
63. Crawford J, Cohen HJ. Aging and neoplasia. Ann Rev Geront Geriatr 1985; 4:3–32.
64. Chao A, Paganini-Hill A, Ross RK, Henderson BE. Use of preventive care by the elderly. Prev Med 1987; 16:710–722.
65. Burack RC, Liang J. The early detection of cancer in the primary care setting: factors associated with the acceptance and completion of recommended procedures. Prev Med 1987; 16:739–751.
66. Burack RC, Liang J. The acceptance and completion of mammography by older black women. Am J Public Health 1989; 79:721–726.
67. Satariano WA, Ragland DR. The effect of comorbidity on 3-year survival of women with primary breast cancer. Ann Intern Med 1994; 120:104–110.
68. West DW, Satariano WA, Ragland DR, Hiatt RA. Comorbidity and breast cancer

survival: a comparison between black and white women. Ann Epidemiol 1996; 6(Special):413–419.

69. Allen C, Cox EP, Manton KG, Cohen HJ. Breast cancer in the elderly: current patterns of care. J Am Geriatr Soc 1986; 34:637–642.

70. Samet J, Key C, Hunt W, Goodwin JS. Choice of cancer therapy varies with age of the patient. JAMA 1986; 255:3385–3390.

71. Chu J, Diehr P, Feigl P, Glaefke G, Begg C, Glicksman A, Ford L. The effect of age on the care of women with breast cancer in community hospitals. J Gerontol 1987; 42:185–190.

72. Guadagnoli E, Weitberg A, Mor V, Silliman RA, Glicksman AS, Cummings FJ. The influence of patient age on the diagnosis and treatment of lung and colorectal cancer. Arch Intern Med 1990; 150:1485–1490.

73. Satariano ER, Swanson GM, Moll PP. Non-clinical factors associated with surgery received for treatment of early-stage breast cancer. Am J Public Health 1992; 82:195–198.

74. Ganz PA. Age and gender as factors in cancer therapy. Clin Geriatr Med 1993; 9:145–155.

75. August DA, Rea T, Sondak VK. Age-related differences in breast cancer treatment. Ann Surg Oncol 1994; 1:45–52.

76. Saftlas A, Satariano WA, Swanson GM, Roi L, Albert S. Methods of cancer case selection: implications for research. Am J Epidemiol 1983; 118:852–855.

77. Newschaffer CJ, Penberthy L, Desch CD, Retchin SM, Whittemore M. The effect of age and comorbidity in the treatment of elderly women with nonmetastatic breast cancer. Arch Intern Med 1996; 156:85–90.

78. Ballard-Barbash R, Potosky AL, Harlan LC, Nayfield SG, Kessler LG. Factors associated with surgical and radiation therapy for early stage breast caner in older women. J Natl Cancer Inst 1996; 88:716–726.

79. Goodwin JS, Hunt WC, Samet J. Determinants of cancer therapy in elderly patients. Cancer 1993; 72:594–601.

80. Bergman L, Dekker G, van Kerhoff EHM, Peterese HL, van Dongen JA, van Leeuwen FE. Influence of age and comorbidity on treatment choice and survival in elderly patients with breast cancer. Breast Cancer Res Treat 1991; 18:189–198.

81. Silliman RA, Balducci L, Goodwin JS, Holmes FF, Lewenthal EA. Breast cancer in old age: what we know, don't know, and do. J Natl Cancer Inst 1993; 85:190–199.

82. Singletary SE, Shallenberger R, Guinee VF. Factors influencing management of breast cancer in elderly women. Clin Geriatr Med 1993; 9:107–113.

83. Ershler WB, Balducci L. Treatment considerations for older patients with cancer. In Vivo 1994; 8:737–744.

84. McKenna RJ. Clinical aspects of cancer in the elderly: treatment decisions, treatment choices, and follow-up. Cancer 1994; 74:2107–2017.

85. Taplin SH, Barlow W, Urban N, Mandelson MT, Timlin DJ, Ichikawa L, Nefey P. Stage, age, comorbidity, and direct costs of colon, prostate, and breast cancer care. J Natl Cancer Inst 1995; 87:417–426.

86. Graves TA, Bland KI. Comorbidity risk parameters associated with advanced breast cancer and systemic disease: management of nonbreast disease. Surg Oncol Clinic North America 1995; 4:633–656.

87. Bennahum DA, Forman WB, Vellas B, Albarede JL. Life expectancy, comorbidity,

and quality of life: a framework of reference for medical decisions. Clin Geriatr Med 1997; 13:33–53.

88. Kimmick GC, Gleming R, Muss HB, Balducci L. Cancer chemotherapy in older adults: a tolerability perspective. Drugs Aging 1997; 10:34–49.

89. Fleming C, Wasson JH, Albertson PC, Barry MJ, Wennberg JE. A decision analysis of alternative treatment strategies for clinically localized prostate cancer. JAMA 1993; 269:2650–2658.

90. Simpson KN. Problems and perspectives on the use of decision-analysis from prostate cancer. J Urol 1994; 152:1888–1893.

91. Robinson BE, Balducci L. Breast lump in an 85-year-old women with dementia: a decision analysis. J Am Geriatr Soc 1995; 43:282–285.

92. Ravdin PM. A computer program to assist in making breast cancer adjuvant therapy decisions. Semin Oncol 1996; 23:43–50.

93. Katton MW, Carven ME, Miles BJ. A decision analysis for treatment of clinically localized prostate cancer. J Gen Intern Med 1997; 12:299–305.

94. Pauker SG, Kassirer JP. Decision analysis. N Engl J Med 1987; 316:250–258.

95. Satariano WA, Ragland K, Van Den Eeden S. Cause of death in men diagnosed with prostate carcinoma. Cancer 1998; 83:1180–1188.

96. Concato J, Horwitz RI, Feinstein AR, Elmore JG, Schiff SF. Problems of comorbidity in mortality after prostatectomy. JAMA 1992; 267:1077–1082.

97. Mandelblatt JS, Wheat ME, Monane M. Breast cancer screening for elderly women with and without comorbid conditions: a decision model. Ann Intern Med 1992; 116: 722–730.

98. Krahn MD, Mahjoney JE, Eckman MH, Trachtenberg J, Pauker SG, Detsky AS. Screening for prostate cancer: a decision analytic view. JAMA 1994; 272:773–780.

99. McGee D, Cooper R, Liao Y, Durazo-Arvizu R. Patterns of comorbidity and mortality risk in blacks and whites. Ann Epidemiol 1996; 6(Special):381–385.

100. Eley JW, Hill HA, Chen VW, Austin DF, Wesley MN, Muss HB, Greenberg RS, Coates RJ, Correa P, Redmond CK, Hunter CP, Herman AA, Kurman R, Blacklow R, Shapiro S, Edwards BK. Racial differences in survival from breast cancer: results of the National Cancer Institute Black/White Cancer Survival Study. JAMA 1994; 272:947–954.

101. Ferentz K. The primary care setting: managing medical comorbidity in the elderly depressed patient. Geriatrics 1995; 50:S25–S31.

102. Harrison J, MacGuire P. Predictors of psychiatric morbidity in cancer patients. Br J Psychiatry 1994; 165:593–598.

103. McDaniel JS, Musselman DL, Porter MR, Reed DA, Nemeroff CB. Depression in patients with cancer: diagnosis, biology, and treatment. Arch Gen Psychiatry 1995; 52:89–99.

104. Fried LP, Kasper JD, Williamson JD, Skinner EA, Morris CD, Hochberg MC for the Disease Ascertainment Working Group. Disease ascertainment algorithms. In: Guralnik JM, Fried LP, Simonsick EM, Kasper JD, Lafferty ME, eds. The Women's Health and Aging Study: Health and Social Characteristics of Older Women with Disability. NIH Pub No. 95-4009. Bethesda, MD: National Institutes of Health, 1995.

105. Kraemer HC. Statistical issues in assessing comorbidity. Stat Med 1995; 14:721–733.

106. Gill TM, Horwitz RI. Evaluating the efficacy of cancer screening: clinical distinctions and case-control studies. J Clin Epidemiol 1995; 48:281–292.

107. McKinlay JB, Burns RB, Feldman HA, Freund EM, Irish JT, Easten LE, Moskowitz MA, Potter DA, Woodman K. Physician variability and uncertainty in the management of breast cancer: results from a factorial experiment. Med Care 1998; 36:385–396.

108. Yellen SB, Cella DF, Leslie WT. Age and clinical decision making in oncology patients. J Natl Cancer Inst 1994; 86:1766–1770.

109. Rossi PH, Anderson AB. The factorial survey approach: an introduction. In: Rossi PH, Nock SL, Eds. Measuring Social Judgments: the Factorial Survey Approach. Beverly Hills, CA: Sage, 1982; 15–67.

110. Hennessy CH. Modelling care management decision-making in a prepaid long-term care program for the elderly. DrPH dissertation, University of California at Berkeley, Berkeley, CA, 1990.

111. Trimble EL, Carter CL, Cain D, Freidlin B, Ungerleider RS, Friedman MA. Representation of older patients in cancer treatment trials. Cancer 1994; 74:2208.

112. Muss HB. Breast cancer in older women. Semin Oncol 1996; 23(Suppl):82–88.

21
Health Service Issues and the Elderly Cancer Patient

Shulamit L. Bernard
Research Triangle Institute
Research Triangle Park, North Carolina

Stephen A. Bernard and Arnold D. Kaluzny
University of North Carolina at Chapel Hill
Chapel Hill, North Carolina

I. INTRODUCTION

Elderly cancer patients often require a range of health care services for the management and treatment of their disease. Malignancy in the older person is often accompanied by a number of other chronic conditions and comorbidities that may cause cognitive impairment, frailty, and diminished capacity for independent function. Ideally, health care services for older adults would provide a coordinated continuum of care ranging from acute care to supportive or long-term-care services. Although the elderly cancer patient would greatly benefit from such an approach with a multidisciplinary care team for disease treatment and management, too often the reality consists of a health care delivery and financing system that is fragmented and confusing. The system often discourages coordination of services and offers little incentive to integrate acute, subacute, and long-term care services (1).

Three financing sources, Medicare, Medicaid, and private payment out-of-pocket or through insurance represent the basic structure of payment of health care–related services for the elderly. These have been termed ''public-private partnership'' (2), because the amount of coverage by Medicare impacts on how much financial and care-giving resources must be expended by the consumers of health care on uncovered services, with the most costly being long-term care (2).

Cancer has often been called the disease of old age because of its increased age-specific incidence and mortality among the elderly. Demographical forecasts project growth in the older population well into the 21st century and suggest that cancer care and treatment will present financial and organizational challenges to the health care system; particularly, for an entitlement program such as Medicare which must provide the needed medical and palliative care services. Strain will also be felt by providers, who are often constrained by ongoing changes in the financing and delivery of health care; by elderly patients, who must often pay high out-of-pocket costs; and by families, who must fill gaps in services (1).

Policymakers have been focusing attention on maintaining the viability of the Medicare system by emphasizing cost containment. Traditionally, cost containment efforts attempted to manipulate services covered by type of payer. More recent efforts, such as the emphasis on Medicare managed care, attempt to alter the type, amount, and setting of care. Current funding for health care emphasizes acute and institutional care. However, because of advances in the diagnosis and treatment of cancer, elderly patients are living longer with their disease and require long-term care and other community-based supportive services. In this chapter, we will explore the organization and financing of health care services, how these factors influence treatment and delivery of care to the elderly cancer patient, and the range of formal and informal services available to the elderly cancer patient.

II. ORGANIZATIONAL FINANCING AND ARRANGEMENTS OF HEALTH CARE SERVICES

A variety of political, social, and economic factors are driving important changes in the way in which health care services are provided to elderly Americans (3). Technical and demographical changes, expanding information processing capability, growing demand for value, and a fundamental redefinition of health care as an economic good or commodity are restructuring the health care–delivery system (4). Historically composed of autonomous providers and financial components, increasingly, hospitals, physicians, and health-financing mechanisms are being organized in ways that were unimaginable just a few years ago. The growth of managed care continues across the country, and it is becoming increasingly prevalent among elderly Medicare beneficiaries. Accompanying the anticipated funding reductions in Medicare and Medicaid, and consistent with the ongoing pressure to reduce prices, there will undoubtedly be a continuation of recent efforts to encourage enrollment in Medicare managed care plans (1) in which care is provided through an integrated network of primary and specialist physicians who have ready access to a population and an existing information system to monitor and coordinate care delivery (3).

The dynamic character of the health care–delivery system seems likely to continue for some years to come (5). Capitation, expected targets, and global budgets are the watchwords of the changing health care system. Although quality continues to be the rhetoric, increasing emphasis is given to the reality of cost, not quality (6). Although the changes occurring within health services provide some unique opportunities, these changes produce significant challenges for cancer prevention, care, and treatment for elderly patients.

III. FINANCING OF HEALTH CARE

The funding for health care in the United States has changed dramatically over the past decade. The traditional fee-for-service (FFS) system, where the patient or payer pays the health care provider for each item, encounter, or service provided, that existed through the mid-1980s is no longer predominant. Today, financial arrangements in health care include a variety of plans, managed care organizational arrangements, and alternative payment systems. Some of the fundamental issues in managed care financing include prospective pricing, capitated financing, and bundling of services.

Prospective pricing is the process of establishing a negotiated price before delivery of the services. This method of payment requires that the provider of services control cost and utilization so that, on average, the total cost will be less than the prospective price. The best example of prospective pricing is the Health Care Financing Administration (HCFA) Medicare Prospective Payment System that outlines a payment scheme for specific groups of services known as Diagnosis-Related Groups (DRGs). In Medicare DRGs, not only are the reimbursement rates prospectively determined at a fixed rate, but services provided are bundled (i.e., the payment rate includes a group of services such as the hospital stay, laboratory and diagnostic testing, medications, and other services).

The financing structure of health care is rapidly changing. Despite failed efforts to institute formal national health care reform in the early years of the Clinton administration, reform is underway. Most states have made fundamental changes in the funding arrangements for state Medicaid programs; many going to capitated payment systems. In response to these continued and inevitable changes, providers are rapidly forming alliances, affiliations, and mergers to increase their market share and competitiveness. These changes will undoubtedly affect the ability for older cancer patients to access new, innovative treatments and procedures.

Reimbursement issues are of significance in the management of cancer. For example, although the elderly enjoy nearly universal health insurance because of the Medicare system, cost remains a factor in the choice and availability of medications to treat cancer and the side effects of treatment. Most cancer patients should be able to have pain management medication available on an outpatient basis. However, Medicare does not routinely reimburse the patient for the cost of outpatient oral analgesics, although it does cover the cost of inpatient medications. The cost for drugs prescribed in the outpatient setting must be borne by the elderly patient. This approach results in situations where patients may not fill prescriptions for optimal treatment or limit the amount of pain medication because of their inability to afford the cost of the drugs (7). Elderly cancer patients who are enrolled in a managed care program that provides outpatient drugs as a benefit may still have limited access to certain newer, higher cost medications. The managed care insurance may provide drugs for standard pain management but may exclude from coverage newly developed more costly drugs.

A. Medicare

For elderly Americans, health care financing is almost synonymous with the Medicare program. Medicare has contributed substantially to the well-being of America's oldest and most disabled citizens (8), and it is critical for cancer-related care. In 1994, elderly Medicare beneficiaries with the principal diagnostic classification of malignant neoplasm accounted for about 6% of all Medicare-covered hospital discharges. The average length of stay for these patients was 8.9 days, which was 19% above the Medicare average. Their Medicare program payment per discharge was 35% above the mean averaging $8627 (9). Overall cancer accounts for nearly 18% of total deaths of Medicare beneficiaries and approximately 28% of total Medicare health care expenditures (10).

Medicare and Medicaid were established by Congress in 1965 by the addition of Titles 18 and 19 to the Social Security Act. Medicare is the largest public health care program in the United States, providing the major source of insurance for acute care for the elderly and disabled. The Medicare program is divided into two parts. Part A, hospital insurance, covers hospital, skilled nursing facility (SNF), and home health care services. Hospital and SNF care are limited within a given spell of illness and after 60 days of hospital and 20 days of SNF care are subject to substantial coinsurance. Home health care, intended to be for skilled needs only, requires no beneficiary contributions. In addition, a limited hospice benefit is also available under Part A. Part B, Supplementary Medical Insurance, covers physician services, outpatient hospital services, and other ambulatory care for those who wish to enroll. Physician services and most of the other Part B services require a 20% coinsurance payment and a deductible.

Part A is mainly funded by payroll tax contributions of workers and by a part of the revenues collected from the taxation of the Social Security benefits. Beneficiaries aged 65 years and older are automatically eligible if they are eligible for Social Security benefits. Part B is funded by a combination of general revenues and premium contributions from beneficiaries. Those eligible for Part A can choose to enroll in Part B and about 98% opt to do so.

Some of the recent changes in Medicare, Medicaid, private insurance, and the managed care climate directly affect cancer patients and cancer-detection efforts. For example, the change from the previous cost-based reimbursement mechanism to the current Prospective Payment System (PPS), along with the passage of the

Medicare hospice benefit in 1983, resulted in shifting many hospital-based services for the care of terminally ill patients to the community and nursing homes (11). Since 1983, hospice and home health care benefits and services have expanded dramatically and now offer a wide range of services for the terminally ill.

Medicare physician reimbursements have also undergone significant change in recent years. HCFA has instituted caps for physicians who do not accept Medicare assignment such that they cannot charge a patient more than 115% of the Medicare-approved charge. This policy has resulted in a number of physicians dropping Medicare patients from their practice or not accepting any new Medicare patients (10).

A 1992 report to the Senate Committee on Finance by the General Accounting Office summarized factors that influence where oncologists treat Medicare patients and the variation in the cost of chemotherapy treatment by setting (12). The following three findings were highlighted: (a) some oncologists treat cancer patients in hospital settings both as inpatients and outpatients when these patients could have received treatment in the physician's office; (b) financial factors influence the oncologist's choice of treatment settings; and (c) treatment in the hospital inpatient setting was the most expensive. The Government Accounting Office (GAO) concluded that the HCFA's chemotherapy reimbursement policies have unintended consequences and affect where a cancer patient receives treatment and as a result the cost of that treatment (10).

B. Medigap Policies

Because Medicare leaves a number of gaps in coverage, a market for private supplemental insurance, often referred to as Medigap, has grown up around Medicare (8). In addition to Medicare Part B, elderly Medicare beneficiaries can purchase Medigap insurance to cover out-of-pocket costs that result from deductibles, coinsurance, and uncovered benefits such as private nursing and medications. Approximately three fourths of older adults have some form of a Medigap policy (13). Older adults who are eligible for income support under the Supplemental Security Income program and those who have very high medical expenses that leave them with very low incomes after accounting for medical costs may have gaps in Medicare covered by the Medicaid program. Even with Medicare, Medicaid, and private insurance, elderly patients face substantial out-of-pocket expenses for medical care. On average, these costs consume 21% of the income of a typical person over the age of 65 years (8), and can be particularly burdensome for the elderly cancer patient undergoing treatment.

C. Managed Care

Managed care is one of the most common and rapidly expanding forms of health insurance in the United States. More than 100 million Americans are now enrolled in some form of managed care. Medicare is also experiencing rapid growth in managed care enrollment. More than 4 million beneficiaries, about 11% of all Medicare enrollees, are now enrolled in managed care plans. Enrollment of older people in health maintenance organizations and other managed care arrangements has increased rapidly in recent years (14), and this is likely to continue. Acceptance of the program is high, particularly among Medicare beneficiaries with modest incomes, because of additional benefits that typically include prescription drugs. Enrollment in a Medicare managed care plan is voluntary for beneficiaries. In order to attract Medicare beneficiaries, many plans offer, in addition to prescription drugs, medical services such as preventive care, eye examinations and lenses, and hearing tests and aids. Managed care options have been incorporated as a limited feature of Medicare since the inception of the program in 1965 (15); however, it is only in recent years that enrollment has increased from 3.5% of all enrollees in 1985 to 7.1% in 1993 and continues to increase annually. As of June 1996, there were almost 4.3 million Medicare beneficiaries enrolled in managed care plans accounting for 11.2% of the total Medicare population (Health Care Financing Review, Statistical Supplement, 1996; p.127) Medicare beneficiaries who enroll in managed care plans must select their health care provider from a panel approved by the plan. However, unlike most of the non–Medicare population who are "locked in" for a year, Medicare beneficiaries may disenroll at any time with 1 month's notice.

Managed care refers to prepaid coverage of health care services that are provided through specific benefits designs. In exchange for a predetermined monthly fee, managed care members are guaranteed access to a range of health services with only limited additional out-of-pocket expense (1) provided the member receives care from an approved panel of providers. Managed care includes methods for achieving increased efficiency, such as increasing beneficiary cost sharing, controlling inpatient admissions and lengths of stay, establishing cost-sharing incentives for physicians, selectively contracting with physicians, and directly managing high-cost cases. Managed care capitalizes on the ability of managed "competition" to reduce costs. Cost-reducing efforts in managed care may also take the shape of attempts to alter provider or patient behaviors. In terms of providers, efforts to alter practice to reduce costs and ensure an appropriate quality of care include peer review, utilization review, and, in some cases, practice guidelines. In each case, the extent of utilization of services and types of services provided to patients covered by the managed care plans are reviewed prospectively or retrospectively to assess the appropriateness of care and to assess the efficiency and cost effectiveness of care delivery (14).

In a managed care plan, the providers of care are held responsible for some share of the financial risk involved with service delivery. The purest form of managed care is capitation, a practice in which a provider, or managed care company, agrees to furnish a given set of services (or benefits) for a fixed price per person, thereby assuming the entire financial risk (1). As it has evolved, managed care has come to mean health insurance with some form of active oversight through case management or special contracts with providers. Managed care has largely focused on acute care; however, as boundaries between acute and chronic care become less clear, long-term care will be affected. Already nursing homes are being used by some managed care companies to provide subacute services previously provided more expensively in hospitals (1).

Managed care organizations, in theory, are more interested in and place more emphasis on the prevention of disease and the prevention of the need for health care services. In fact, Medicare managed care does emphasize cancer screening procedures such as mammography. By encouraging healthy lifestyles and providing preventative services, managed care organizations can potentially reduce future need for cancer care among the younger cohort and increase early diagnosis of cancer among the older cohort.

This move from fee-for-service to capitated reimbursement changes the fundamental rules of reimbursement incentives (16). What was once considered a revenue-generating activity under cost-based reimbursement in a managed care environment becomes a cost center with incentives directed to increasing efficiency and decreasing cost. Many managed care systems position the primary care physician as a gatekeeper. Individuals with malignant diseases seek and receive care from a range of health care providers, including medical oncologists, surgeons, and radiation oncologists. The primary care physician must be able to make timely referrals, as outcomes are often influenced by timing of diagnosis and treatment.

The reality of finances and incentives under a capitation system means that some procedures and treatments that are regarded as being dubious or involving high cost and providing marginal effectiveness will be discouraged or not covered. Consequently, the elderly cancer patient who is enrolled in a managed care plan may be at risk for limited access to cutting edge treatments (e.g., some clinical trials) that the plan either does not cover or deems unnecessary. In addition, most managed care companies will have a formulary for approved drugs. The formulary may provide generic drugs or exclude newer, expensive drugs. Specific disagreements between the managed care plan and patient treatment preferences must be resolved quickly to avoid an unnecessary treatment delay or harm to the patient. Under managed care, the primary care physician cannot always be assumed to be the patient's advocate in these situations, so that there is a compelling need to establish mechanisms of appeal for resolving denial of treatment problems quickly and fairly (5). Most managed care plans have mechanisms that provide for a second medical opinion at the request of a member. Because consumers have also been advocates for external reviews by doctors not affiliated with the plan to ensure objectivity, Medicare managed care plans established an external appeals process. Elderly cancer patients in managed care may need to test the boundaries of coverage when they desire treatments that tend to be denied.

Managed care systems mainly save on the costs of care by reducing use. This strategy may reduce unnecessary care, but it can also cut into important services as well. Consequently, such organizations make it necessary that patients and families be diligent and aggressive advocates for justifiable care. The barriers to care that HMOs and others establish to discourage overuse may be intimidating, particularly for the very old or frail (8).

D. Long-Term Care

Elderly cancer patients are often in need of long-term care (17). Although long-term care is often equated with nursing homes, the nursing home is not, however, the major site of long-term care delivery, particularly for the cancer patient. Relatively few elderly persons with cancer are admitted to nursing homes and the stays of those admitted are brief (17).

In assessing the need for formal long-term care services in institutions or in the community, the physician or health provider must consider both the functional abilities of the elderly patient and the coping capability of the social support system (17). In addition, community resources must be considered as well. Urban settings generally provide more choices for patients with cancer, including hospice and home health care, whereas rural settings often present additional challenges (18). Rural families caring for older cancer patients frequently face barriers to the availability and accessibility of health care services, including long distances to treatment facilities and the lack of community-based supportive services.

Delivery of care in the home or the community is commonly preferred to institutional care, and there is a strongly held belief that home- and community-based services can limit the rapid rise in nursing home costs without an equally large increase in alternative care costs (2). Numerous demonstration projects, however, found that these services tend to be an add-on cost to the system because of the difficulty in targeting services to those who will use them effectively to delay or avoid institutionalization.

At present, long-term care is funded mainly by the federal/state Medicaid program and by individuals and their families. Medicare plays only a limited role in nursing home care. Over the last decade, private insurance has emerged as another means for spreading the risk of long-term care. As of 1993, nearly 3.4 million Americans purchased private long-term care insurance policies (19). Since costs for nursing home care, in 1996 dollars, often exceed $35,000 per year, and can be well over $15,000 for extensive home care services (8), these expenses can be devastating to the majority of families who do not have private long-term care insurance. For that reason, many older adults ''spend down'' and ultimately turn for help to the Medicaid program.

The Medicaid program, which was originally established to help low-income families meet acute care needs, has become the most important public program funding long-term care for the elderly and disabled. Medicaid provides mostly nursing home coverage; however, eligibility is limited to individuals who have spent down their income and assets to very low levels. Medicaid then offers protection once catastrophe has already occurred (8). Nonetheless, it is the only public program to offer substantial coverage to older adults needing nursing home care (2).

A substantial number of demonstration projects are underway to test various approaches to integrating acute care and long-term care services (20). An integrated delivery system would be ideal for the typical elderly cancer patient who could benefit from additional support services both in the home and in long-term care facilities. For reasons of both cost and quality, there is increasing interest in approaches that integrate acute care and long-term care services for frail older adults (20). The rapid growth in the costs of long-term care have also led states to focus on holding down the number of nursing home beds, to limit reimbursement for nursing homes, and to restrict their programs to institutional settings as additional ways to limit spending.

E. Home Health Care Services

Changes in health care financing have led to reductions in the length of hospital stays for patients with cancer. As a direct result, elderly cancer patients are now discharged in a more unstable condition and require that services once given in the hospital, postacute care and rehabilitation, be given in alternative settings (21). These patients are discharged from hospitals with increasingly complex and sophisticated technological equipment and require interventions that necessitate ongoing monitoring and medical treatments. Cancer patients and their families often find themselves being responsible for these complex cancer care–related tasks for which they often receive little or no advanced preparation or training during the brief hospital stay (22). Home health services have been found to be a vital resource in assisting families to assume caregiving roles by teaching them the skills required to manage the patient effectively (22).

Home health services, the provision of medical and rehabilitation services to patients in their own homes, as an alternative to or following a hospital stay, is one of the fastest growing sectors of the health care market (23, 24). In 1994, Medicare program payments for home health benefits totaled $12.7 billion; an increase of more than 550% since 1988 (9) and 8.6% of all Medicare payments. In 1995, elderly cancer patients constituted 7.2% of all persons served by a home health agency; averaging 40 visits and $2595 per elderly cancer patient served (9).

Users of home care services generally fall into several categories (24): (a) persons who require assistance with activities of daily living (ADL), including elderly cancer patients with other chronic disorders; (b) persons requiring rehabilitation, monitoring, and nursing care posthospitalization (25); and (c) persons requiring the administration of complicated treatments, medications, and procedures (26). Patients with both early and progressive cancer report high levels of symptom distress, limited self-care and functional abilities, and poor health perceptions following a hospitalization (22). Referral to home care services following a hospitalization has been shown to be an effective means to address the care needs of elderly cancer patients and their families (22, 26). Home care interventions have demonstrated an improvement in patients' mental health status and preservation of functional abilities. Results of clinical trials also suggest that patients receiving home care experience a reduction of symptoms associated with cancer treatments and the progression of disease (22).

Despite demonstrated benefits of home care services, a number of studies have identified barriers to the receipt of home care services by patients with cancer (26). Lack of effective discharge planning by the hospital accompanied by a lack of the patient's and family's knowledge regarding services results in patients being discharged without an adequate referral (27). Alternatively, patients and families may decline home care referral because of doubts about the benefits of services, prejudice against receiving formalized help, or a reluctance to accept assistance from anyone other than family members (26, 28).

Cost concerns may also present a barrier to home care. Although Medicare currently reimburses for skilled services in the home, these are often restricted in duration or the number of visits permitted. Home care is often cited as a less expensive alternative to hospital or nursing home care; however, the costs of home care to the families are typically underestimated. When family labor is included in the cost calculations, average cancer home care costs for a 3-month period are not much lower than the costs of nursing home care (29). The strength of the elderly patient's support system, the home environment to which a patient is being discharged, and the appropriate community resources must be assessed prior to discharge (26). This process is particularly important for patients who live in rural areas where such services may not be available (30).

As illness and disability increase, the need for both formal (e.g., home health) and informal care (from family and friends) increases. ''Moreover, the amount of informal care received increases with disability at a much greater rate than does formal care under the same circumstances. This suggests that as care needs increase, family and friends step in to provide the bulk of care'' (31).

IV. SOCIAL SUPPORT AND INFORMAL CARE

Individuals are protected or positively prepared to cope with a health event by their support relationships prior to its occurrence. Studies of the buffering effect of social support suggest that social relations help the older individual cope with pre- and postcrises events; people in crises are better able to cope with and recover from these events when they have good supportive relationships (32).

In general, older patients resist the use of formal support preferring instead immediate family (33). Research findings demonstrate that caregiving by the informal network, family and friends, is the primary source of assistance given to frail and ill older adults (34). When health deteriorates, the informal network tends to provide the needed care; the preponderance of home health care for older people is provided by families rather than through service agencies (35, 36, 54).

Informal assistance, care, and support refer to a variety of activities. Frequently, the family is called on to assist with activities of daily living ranging from instrumental activities (e.g., meal preparation, shopping, and transportation) to more personal activities (e.g., bathing, toileting, and transferring). As discussed in Section III.E under home care services, the policy of hospital reimbursement based on DRGs has lead to earlier hospital discharge. This resulted in the need for greater involvement by the family in treatments and tasks that had previously been done in the hospital. In the case of the elderly cancer patient, in addition to dealing with the debilitation due to cancer or other chronic diseases, the family may also be called on to assist with monitoring devices for infusions for chemotherapy or other technological and intensive interventions.

By and large, older adults are not left alone and isolated by their families. However, social support and informal long-term care provision is often a matter of one older person providing care for another (17). In general, there is a hierarchical selection of caregivers determined by the primacy of the relationship between the caregiver and the elderly patient. There is generally one main helper—one person who provides most of the caregiving (34). When available, the spouse is typically the caregiving individual most preferred, followed by daughters, sons, siblings, and other relatives, friends, and neighbors. Thus, the spouse usually plays a pivotal role in providing support for the ill partner. Because women tend to marry men older than themselves and because women have a greater life expectancy, they are more likely than their husbands to assume the caregiving role. Children rank second to the spouse as caregivers for elderly parents, especially when the spouse is too frail to assume caregiving responsibilities. Despite our mobile society, the majority of the current cohort of older adults live close to at least one child. The caregiving roles played by sons and daughters differ and are often gender based. In general, daughters are more likely to provide the day-to-day hands-on care, whereas sons are more likely to provide supervision and financial assistance (34).

In the future, given today's demographical trends for smaller families, and the rise in divorce rates, the support systems of the elderly cancer patient may be increasingly limited to only one individual. Patients with such a vulnerable support system would benefit from extended community-based services to assist and support the lone caregiver, thereby extending the role of the lone caregiver and increasing the likelihood that the patient will be able to remain at home.

In conjunction with physical support, the need for emotional support is well recognized (36). The informal support often provides the elderly cancer patient with companionship and intimacy. However, a cancer diagnosis may evoke fear and feelings of inadequacy on the part of informal caregivers. Some cancer treatment may be particularly debilitating and require additional assistance with personal care and household tasks. Care must be taken by the health care providers to evaluate the stability and capacity of the informal system to provide the patient with the needed services; particularly if the caregiver is an elderly, frail, spouse (33, 36).

V. HOSPICE

Hospice is a treatment philosophy oriented toward the care of the dying. The hospice movement in the United States developed as an alternative to traditional medicine's emphasis on intensive technology and a hospital-oriented approach to care at the end of life (7). Under the Medicare Hospice Act, hospice became a Medicare-covered service effective November 1983. This funding mechanism provides for hospice care to elderly terminally ill patients and includes both home care and inpatient care. The Medicare program pays a per diem during the benefit program, and allows a hospice to provide services not typically covered by Medicare, including homemaker services and counseling. There are no additional costs for the patient under this program, with the exception of small coinsurance amounts for outpatient drugs and inpatient respite care.

During the past decade, hospice benefits under the Medicare program experienced a rapid growth. Although the program Medicare benefit payments in 1986 for hospice care totaled $77 million, by 1994 hospice payments had increased to $1.6 billion; more than a 20-fold difference. This growth is accounted for mostly by increases in the number of beneficiaries using this program (9). Hospice care is provided by facilities certified as hospices by Medicare and meeting certain standards and conditions of participation. A hospice may be freestanding, home health agency based, hospital based or skilled nursing facility based. Licensed hospice providers are paid a per diem payment to provide care to patients with less than 6 months to live. It is anticipated that patients will be managed at home, thus avoiding more costly inpatient care (7).

Hospice, as currently designed, is not for everyone. Not only must patients be ready to acknowledge that they are dying, they must also meet certain criteria specified by HCFA. Hospice is a Medicare benefit, for which Medicare patients are eligible if they are terminally ill with a life expectancy of 6 months or less, are unable to benefit from further curative therapy, are able to receive 80% of their care at home, and have a caregiver who will assume the responsibility for custodial care. Patients can have their hospice benefits terminated if the benefit period exceeds the 6-month limit. These restrictions preclude the use of hospice for many patients. In addition, some physicians are reluctant to discuss dying far enough in advance for plans to be made to institute hospice, believing that it "robs patients of hope" (37).

There are several additional barriers to the use of hospice by the elderly patient (38). The program requires the availability of a primary care giver in the patient's home. However, approximately 30% of the U.S. elderly live alone, the majority of whom are women. Many of the patients who do not live alone live with an elderly spouse who may have frailties and functional limitations due to chronic illness in addition to which caregiving becomes another burden. Additional barriers to hospice care are suggested by the low utilization of hospice services by minority elderly perhaps resulting from cultural issues; for example, inadequate availability of services in areas with either a high concentration of minority older adults or the lack of primary caregivers (7, 38). The Medicare Hospice Act requires that a hospice provider be licensed, a relative barrier to hospice services in rural areas, where services are often fragmented and less available (39).

In order for a patient to be eligible for hospice care, the physician must agree that the patient has an estimated life expectancy of less than 6 months. This estimation is often difficult to make with any reliability and may present an additional barrier to these services for elderly cancer patients, or it may result in the late referral of patients when they could have benefited by hospice care. The late referral is suggested by the relatively short mean survival of patients admitted to hospice (7).

It is estimated that only 10% of deaths in the United States occur under the care of hospice (7). Approximately 80% of hospice patients (around 220,000) are Medicare beneficiaries (40). Christakis and Escarce reviewed 1990 Medicare claims data from five states, Texas, Florida, California, Illinois, and New York, and found that the mean age of the patients was 76.4 years and that 80% of those receiving hospice benefits were cancer patients (40). The median survival of the patients admitted to hospice was 36 days, and 15.6% of the patients died within 7 days of admission. These figures have not changed since the late 1970s and 1980s, when the National Hospice Study found that the median length of survival was 35 days, and 20 percent of patients died within 7 days of admission to hospice (41). Current estimates indicate that nearly a third of cancer deaths in the United States will occur in patients under the care of a hospice (42), although many of these patients continue to have short lengths of stay (50% for less than 1 month) (7). However, despite these statistics, the majority of cancer patients over the age of 65 years have not received hospice care at the end of life (17), indicating that a greater emphasis should be placed on palliative care and hospice care.

In October 1996, the HCFA announced the approval of a new diagnosis code for palliative care, which was included in the International Classification of Disease, 9th Revision, Clinical Modification (ICD-9-CM) (37). The new code will allow hospitals to indicate that palliative care was delivered during a hospital stay enabling the HCFA to study the feasibility of creating a DRG that allows payment for end-of-life care for people who die in hospitals or require hospitalization for palliative care close to the end of life. The intent of this code is to legitimize and encourage the use of palliative care.

VI. THE CARE PROCESS: SELECTED ISSUES

Financing and various service delivery arrangements provide the organizational context through which care is provided. Care is a process and the process is characterized by a number of issues that are central to the provision of care to elderly cancer patients.

A. Patient Delay in Seeking Medical Care

Many older adults delay seeking care for medical problems (43), often resulting in a cancer diagnosis made at an advanced stage (44). Some of the reasons for delay are attributable to a general lack of awareness of the signs and symptoms of cancer— symptoms such as pain, a breast lump, blood in the sputum or stool may be ignored by the patient—whereas more nonspecific symptoms such as weakness or fatigue or loss of appetite may be attributed to old age. Some of the causes for the delay may be attitudinal (43). These include concern about the cost of a doctor visit and subsequent treatment, educational barriers to relevant information, social isolation, and pessimism about cancer and its treatment (44, 43). The current cohort of older adults lived the majority of their lives during the years in which cancer cures were infrequent, and they may consequently perceive treatment to be debilitating and ineffective.

B. Treatment Decisions

Older adults have the right to take part in the decision-making process about treatment for cancer. Elderly patients need to be informed of treatment options and the advantages and disadvantages of each choice in terms of both the expected length and quality of life. Clinical judgment must be used in elderly patients who are frail, cognitively impaired, or have a known limited life expectancy. The goal of treatment should be to provide the best quality of life for the longest duration of life, taking into account acceptable risks to the patient (45). Age alone should not be the basis for treatment plans (46), and each treatment plan must be individualized. The presence of frailty, a reduced functional reserve, may compromise the tolerance of treatment and may indicate the need for alternative forms of cancer management (47). Even among otherwise robust individuals, the functional reserve of many organ systems, and consequently the ability to cope with the stress of cancer and treatment, is decreased (47). The most important determinant of life expectancy among elderly cancer patients is not age; it is the presence and severity of comorbidity and functional status (48, 49).

The patient and the physician must weigh the risks and benefits of treatment with the complications of cancer. Physiological age is more important than chronological age in guiding decisions for cancer prevention and treatment (44, 50). Treatment decisions must acknowledge the tremendous variability in health and in age-related declines in functioning (47). Many older cancer patients have concurrent chronic conditions that contribute to decreased physical, cognitive, and physiological functioning (50, 51). It is not fully known to what extent concurrent health problems complicate cancer management in the older person (50).

The availability of social support is an important factor in predicting whether or not an individual will decide to see a physician in response to cancer-suspicious symptoms (52). Discussion of a cancer symptom with a supportive other increases the likelihood that medical attention will be sought for that symptom. The availability of family and other social support is critical to the treatment of the elderly cancer patient. In the case of the patient who is cared for by an elderly spouse, treatment options must be weighed with consideration to whether the spouse or others in the support network are able to transport the patient to and from treatment and whether someone will be available to assist with medications at home. Lacking this type of support, patients may miss therapy, forget to take medications, or take them improperly (46).

Efforts to diagnose, treat, and rehabilitate elderly cancer patients must consider the presence of other chronic diseases (e.g., arthritis, cardiovascular disorders, diabetes, neurological disorders) along with physical and cognitive dysfunction (53). The complexities of treatment decisions for cancer in the elderly patient are intensified by the presence of chronic illness that is often present in the older individual.

There is no debate about the importance of providing comfort and palliative care (e.g., relief of pain, family and patient support services). However, as the expected benefits from disease-oriented treatment lessen, no clear guidelines exist to help physicians, patients, and families decide when further treatment should be limited to relief of symptoms (53). A thoughtful geriatrician, Dr. Mary Gillik, recommends a paradigm that considers the patient's functional and cognitive status and weighs the potential benefits and hazards resulting from treatment. She recommends that as long as the elderly patient is vigorous, the goals of medical care should be the same as they have always been: to cure disease and to ameliorate suffering. Once the patient begins a downward slide, the goals of medical treatment begin to change; they focus on maintaining dignity and independence, helping the patient remain at home, optimizing the ability to care for self, and continuing to socialize with family and friends. At this stage of treatment, the effect of medical interventions on the quality of life becomes an ever more important factor in the decision to treat aggressively or not (51). Patients often need guidance in deciding how much and what kind of medical intervention to accept. They frequently cannot anticipate the effect of treatment until they are in the midst of a crisis (51, 53). "Elderly persons are concerned about body image, disfigurement, and pain. They grapple with issues about quality versus quantity of life. They have fears and misinformation about cancer; the particular content of these fears is shaped by culture and age cohort. Like other persons with cancer, the elderly fare best when they retain control over their lives'' (17). These patients need to be given information that will enable them to make decisions about desirable forms of treatment. They should be helped to decide what forms of long-term care are preferable to themselves and their family.

Treatment of cancer for patients with advanced senile dementia presents a formidable challenge for informed consent, health care ethics, and design of supportive care. Frequently, the decision maker is the one with power of attorney. This individual may opt for aggressive therapy to avoid feelings of guilt and helplessness.

VII. CONCLUSIONS

It is difficult, if not impossible, to predict the exact form that health services will take in the years ahead. The amount of fundamental change just within the past few years has been unprecedented and is likely to continue into the foreseeable future. The movement toward managed care, the ascendance of for profit health care organizations, and the emergence of specialty product service lines and/or clinical product companies (56) are vivid reminders that change is reality. What was at one point thought impossible within health services is often occurring.

Yet, the challenges are clear. Regardless of the structure and programmatic nature of health services, the future will witness an aging population and an increasing burden of cancer arising in this population group. Although technological advances in both the basic and clinical sciences will occur, the fundamental challenge that will accompany the millennium will be how well we are able to translate that technology into actual service delivery and the extent to which it will reduce morbidity and mortality and improve the quality of life.

REFERENCES

1. Polich C, Parker M, Chase D, Hottinger M. Managing Health Care for the Elderly. New York: Wiley, 1993.
2. Meiners M. The Financing and Organization of Long-Term Care. In: Binstock RH, Cluff LE, von Mering O, eds. The Future of Long-Term Care: Social and Policy Issues. Baltimore, MD: Johns Hopkins University Press, 1996.
3. Kaluzny AD. Prevention and Control Research within a Changing Health Care System. Prevent Med 1997; 26:S31–S35.
4. Shortell S, Gillies R, Anderson D, Morgan-Erickson K, Mitchell J. The Transformation of American Health Care: Building Organized Delivery Systems. San Francisco: Jossey-Bass, 1996.
5. Rother J. Consumer protection in managed care: a third-generation approach. Generations 1996; 20:42–46.
6. Kaluzny AD, Zuckerman HS, Rabiner DJ. Interorganizational factors affecting the de-

livery of primary care to older Americans. Health Serv Res 1998; 33, (2 pt 2):381–400.

7. Cleary JF, Carbone PP. Palliative medicine in the elderly. Cancer 1997; 80:1335–1347.
8. Moon M, Mulvey J. Entitlements and the Elderly: Protecting Promises, Recognizing Realities. Washington, DC: Urban Institute; 1996.
9. Medicare and Medicaid Statistical Supplement, 1996. Health Care Finan Rev 1996, Supplement.
10. Jackson R. The Role of Third-Party Support in the Detection and Treatment of Cancer in the Elderly. Cancer 1994; 74(Suppl):2200–2203.
11. McMillan A, Mentnech RM, Lubitz J, McBean AM, Russell D. Trends and patterns in place of death for medicare enrollees. Health Care Finan Rev 1990; 12:1–7.
12. Office UGA. Medicare: Reimbursement Policies Can Influence the Setting and Cost of Chemotherapy. Report to the Chairman, Committee on Finance, US Senate; 1992.
13. Chullis GS, Eppig FJ, Hogan MO, Waldo DR, Arnet RH. Health insurance and the elderly: data from MCBC. Health Care Finan Rev 1993; 14:163–81.
14. Fox PD, Fama T. Managed care and the elderly: performance and potential. Generations 1996; 20:31–36.
15. Leading Short-Stay Hospital Principal Diagnoses. Health Care Finan Rev 1996; Medicare and Medicaid Statistical Summary, 52–53.
16. Kane RL. The Evolution of the American Nursing Home. In: Binstock RH, Cluff LE, von Mering O, eds. The Future of Long-Term Care: Social and Policy Issues. Baltimore, MD: Johns Hopkins University Press, 1996.
17. Kane RA. Coordination of Cancer Treatment and Social Support for the Elderly. In: Yancik R, Carbone PP, Patterson WB, Steel K, Terry WD, eds. Perspectives on Prevention and Treatment of Cancer in the Elderly. New York: Raven Press, 1983.
18. Krout JA. Providing Community-Based Services to the Rural Elderly. Thousand Oaks, CA: Sage, 1994.
19. Coronel S, Fulton D. Long-Term Care Insurance in 1993. Washington, DC: Health Insurance Association of America; 1995.
20. Wiener JM. Managed care and long-term care: the integration of financing and services. Generations 1996; 20:47–52.
21. Shaughnessy PW, Kramer AM. The increased needs of patients in nursing homes and patients receiving home health care. N Engl J Med 1990; 322:21–23.
22. McCorkle R, Jepson C, Malone D, et al. The impact of posthospital home care on patients with cancer. Res Nursing Health 1994; 17:243–251.
23. Bishop C, Skwara KC. Recent growth of medicare home health. Health Affairs 1993; fall:95–110.
24. Repetto L, Granetto C, Venturino A. Home care in the older person. Clin Geriatr Med 1997; 13:403–413.
25. Koren MJ. Home care—who cares? N Engl J Med 1986; 314:917–919.
26. Yost LS. Cancer patients and home care: extent to which services are not received. Cancer Pract 1995; 3:83–87.
27. Wolock I, Schlesinger E, Dinerman M, Seaton R. The posthospital needs and care of patients: implications for discharge planning. Soc Work Health Care 1987; 12:61–76.
28. Simmons WJ. Planning for discharge for the elderly. Q Rev Bull 1986; 12:68–71.
29. Stommel M, Given CW, Given BA. The cost of cancer home care to families. Cancer 1992; 71:1867–1874.

30. Buehler JA, Lee HL. Exploration of home care resources for rural families with cancer. Cancer Nurs 1992; 15:299–308.
31. Kemper P. The use of formal and informal home care by the disabled. Health Serv Res 1992; 27:421–51.
32. Antonucci T. Social supports and social relationships. In: Binstock RH, George LK, eds. Handbook of Aging and the Social Sciences. New York: Academic Press, 1990.
33. Litwak E. Helping the elderly: the complemetary role of informal networks and formal systems. New York: Guilford, 1985.
34. Chappell NL. Aging and social care. In: Binstock R, George L, eds. Handbook of Aging and the Social Sciences. 3rd ed. New York: Academic Press, 1990.
35. Wettle T. The social and service context of geriatric care. In: Rowe J, Besdine R, eds. Geriatric Medicine. 2nd ed. Boston: Little Brown, 1988.
36. Kane RA, Penrod JD. Family Caregiving in an Aging Society. Thousand Oaks, CA: Sage, 1995.
37. Cassel CK, Vladeck BC. ICD-9 Code for Palliative or Terminal Care. N Engl J Med 1996; 335:1232–1234.
38. Miller PJ, Mike PB. The Medicare Hospice Benefit. Death Studies 1995; 19:531–42.
39. Coward RT, Netzer JK, Peek CW. Obstacles to creating high-quality long-term care services for rural elders. In: Rowles GD, Beaulieu JE, Myers WW, eds. Long-Term Care for the Rural Elderly. New York: Springer, 1996.
40. Christakis N, Escare JJ. Survival of Medicare patients after enrollment in hospice programs. N Engl J Med. 1996; 335:172–8.
41. Greer D, Mor V, Sherwood S, Kidder D, Birnbaum H. An alternative in terminal care: results of the National Hospice Study. J Chronic Dis 1986; 39:9–26.
42. Hunt R, McCaul K. A population-based study of the coverage of cancer patients by hospice services. Palliat Med 1996; 10:5–12.
43. Bernard SL. Racial Differences in Perceptions of Access to Health Care Among the Elderly. New York: Garland, 1997.
44. McKenna RJ. Clinical aspects of cancer in the elderly: treatment decisions, treatment choices, and follow-up. Cancer 1994; 74(Suppl):2107–2117.
45. Singletary SE, Shallenberger R, Guinee VF. Factors influencing management of breast cancer in the elderly woman. Clin Geriatr Med 1993; 9:107–113.
46. Lichtman SM, Bayer RL. Gastrointestinal cancer in the elderly. Clin Geriatr Med 1997; 13:307–326.
47. Balducci L, Lyman GH. Cancer in the elderly: epidemiologic and clinical implications. Clin Geriatr Med 1997; 13:1–14.
48. Siu AL, Hays RD, Ouslander JG. Measuring functioning and health in the very old. J Gerontol Med Sci 1993; 48:M10–14.
49. Siu AL, Kravitz RL, Keeler E, Postdischarge geriatric assessment of hospitalized frail elderly. Arch Intern Med 1996; 156:76–81.
50. Yancik R, Ries LA. Cancer in older persons: magnitude of the problem—how do we apply what we know. Cancer 1994; 74(Suppl):1995–2003.
51. Gillick M. Choosing Medical Care in Old Age. Cambridge, MA: Harvard University Press, 1994.
52. Antonucci TC, Kahn RL, Akiyama H. Psychosocial factors and the response to cancer symptoms. In: Yancik R, Yates JW, eds. Cancer in the Elderly. New York: Springer, 1989:40–52.

53. Patterson WB, Williams TF. Epilogue: future directions for cancer control in older persons. In: Yancik R, Yates JW, eds. Cancer in the Elderly. New York: Springer, 1989: 224–231.

54. Binstock RH, Cluff LE, Von Mering O, eds. The Future of Long-Term Care: Social and Policy Issues. Baltimore: Johns Hopkins University Press, 1996.

55. The Advisory Board Company. The Great Product Enterprise: Future State for the American Health System, Washington, DC, 1997.

22

Assessment of Health Status and Outcomes: Quality of Life and Geriatric Assessment

Patricia A. Ganz and David B. Reuben
University of California
Los Angeles, California

I. INTRODUCTION

Quality of life considerations have been brought to the forefront of health care research in the late 20th century as a result of the convergence of several important factors. These include (a) prolonged life expectancy, from the eradication of many infectious diseases and the successful treatment of other conditions (e.g., diabetes, kidney failure); (b) the appearance of many new chronic diseases (e.g., arthritis, heart disease, cancer, and human immunodeficiency virus (HIV) infection); (c) the increasing cost and toxicities of some treatments; and (d) the concern about health outcomes other than mortality. Coincident with these circumstances has been an emerging science of outcomes assessment (1), which borrows extensively from concurrent methodological advances in the social sciences enabling the quantification and evaluation of the quality of life outcomes of diseases and their treatments. In this chapter, we will examine the intersection of these events from the perspective of cancer in the elderly.

There are numerous textbooks and reviews that devote considerable time to the examination of quality of life assessment (2–6). This chapter cannot cover all of the important topics that a reader may be interested in, and, therefore, reference will be made to more detailed texts, but we will provide sufficient information to allow discussion of critical issues relevant to older persons with cancer. We will review the following aspects of quality of life assessment: the definition and conceptualization of quality of life; methods of measuring quality of life; the role of quality of life assessment in the elderly cancer patient; special aspects of quality of life in the elderly; and future directions for research and application.

In parallel with the developments in quality of life assessment, the field of geriatrics has been rapidly expanding and systematizing the approach to the evaluation of the older person. There are many parallels between geriatric assessment and quality of life assessment in that they are multidimensional and broad. Both utilize standardized instruments that frequently rely on patient perceptions and other ''biologically soft'' measures. Moreover, they share many dimensions (Fig. 1) and focus on issues that are among the most important to older persons, particularly the ability to function fully in social roles and participate in activities consistent with their desires. On the other hand, some differences between the two constructs illustrate that the two are not synonymous. For example, quality of life is best assessed by the patient, whereas functional status and other dimensions of geriatric assessment may be better assessed by clinicians or proxies such as family members.

We believe that there are considerable opportunities to integrate many of the components of quality of life assessment with geriatric assessment. Knowledge about both of these disciplines will facilitate better care of the older cancer patient, and has great promise for improving the quality of cancer research conducted with older patients. In this chapter, we provide an introduction to both of these approaches

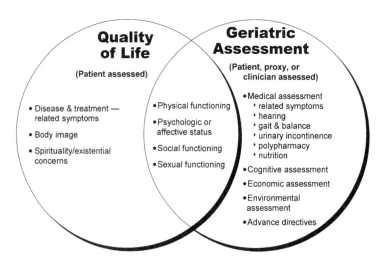

Figure 1   Intersection of quality of life assessment and geriatric assessment.

to evaluation of health status and outcomes, as well as propose strategies for integrating the two methods of assessment in practice with the older cancer patient.

II. QUALITY OF LIFE ASSESSMENT IN THE CANCER PATIENT

A. Definition and Conceptualization of Quality of Life

1. Definition and History

Although most of us intuitively understand what the term *quality of life* connotes, it has been exceedingly difficult for social scientists, health services researchers, and clinicians to define precisely. Often "quality of life" is used by the authors of scientific papers without explicit definition, and a wide range of variables are used as measures of quality of life (QOL) (from physiological indicators such as weight loss to standardized psychological measures of emotional distress) (7). "Quality of life" has been a frequently abused catch phrase; however, there is growing consensus about its definition. Two research groups have proposed definitions: (a) "Quality of life is the subjective evaluation of life as a whole" (8); and (b) Quality of life "refers to patients' appraisal of and satisfaction with their current level of functioning compared to what they perceive to be possible or ideal" (9). The first definition emphasizes the subjectivity of the measurement, as well as the importance of a global assessment or summary score. The second definition also highlights the subjectivity of QOL assessment, as well as the preference or value given to the person's current health state. For example, two people with the same disability may place a different value on their current health state. Conceptually, both of these definitions contribute to our understanding of the phrase "quality of life"; however they do not necessarily indicate how one should measure it.

Many recent reviews and papers have focused on the evolving conceptualization of QOL (10–13). The concept of QOL has broad, general meaning based on roots in ancient philosophical works (14). Contemporary definitions of QOL and measurement strategies derive from historical efforts designed to measure the well-being of the population using social indicators such as general satisfaction and happiness, as well as satisfaction with, for example, housing, employment, or income (15–17). The World Health Organization (WHO) definition of health as a "state of complete physical, mental, and social well-being and not merely the absence of disease" (18) is central to current work designed to measure health-related quality of life. Although the WHO definition was considered impossible to operationalize and measure at the time of its publication, contemporary QOL assessment tools focus on these three critical dimensions of health and QOL. Current conceptualization of QOL as measured in relationship to disease and treatment is called health-related quality of life (HRQOL), as it tends to limit the focus to dimensions of QOL that are directly affected by health and/or disease states (11, 19).

In oncology practice, the Karnofsky Performance Status scale (20) was one of the earliest tools used to measure the functional performance of cancer patients. Although this tool does not meet our current idea of a QOL instrument, it was an early attempt to obtain data on a nonmortality endpoint. The scale was developed by clinicians primarily to collect and record information that was thought to be important for diagnosis, treatment, and clinical response. Although widely accepted clinically, the reliability of clinically rated scales like the Karnofsky scale tends to be poor (21), which limits their use for monitoring health care outcomes and QOL. Although the Karnofsky Performance Status scale correlates highly with the physical functioning dimension of QOL questionnaires in some studies, it does not seem to correlate well with overall measures of QOL in cancer patients (22). The measure is limited further by being clinician rather than patient rated. However, it has the advantage of being brief, acceptable in the clinical setting, and has a clear relationship to other important clinical variables such as mortality (20, 21).

Early in the 1980s, Spitzer and colleagues developed a tool specifically to evaluate the QOL of cancer patients (23). This instrument contains a uniscale for the global evaluation of QOL along with separate components that evaluate the physical and emotional aspects of QOL. This latter 10-point scale is appealing because of its simplicity, as well as the ease with which it can be rated by an observer. For this reason, it was extensively used in cancer research during the 1980s (e.g., the National Hospice Study) (23a). However, during the past decade, there was growing consensus that QOL should be rated by the patient rather than by a clinician or proxy (24). Thus, many new tools have been developed to capture the patient's own assessment of QOL. The National Cancer Institute has had two workshops (1990 and 1995) on the topic of QOL assessment in clinical trials (25), and now each of the clinical trial's cooperative groups has clinical investigators and staff devoted to consideration of inclusion of QOL endpoints in clinical treatment trials. In addition, many pharmaceutical companies are routinely including QOL measures as part of the evaluation of new drugs. Recently, improvements in QOL (including pain and symptom relief) have been acknowledged as being relevant endpoints in the new drug-approval process.

2. Multidimensionality of Quality of Life

Most experts in this field perceive QOL as a multidimensional construct that includes several key dimensions (12, 13, 19, 26, 27). These include *physical functioning* (performance of self-care activities, functional status, mobility, physical activities, and role activities such as work or household responsibilities); *disease- and treatment-related symptoms* (specific symptoms from the disease such as pain or shortness of breath or side effects of drug therapy such as nausea, hair loss, impotence, or sedation); *psychological functioning* (anxiety or depression that may be secondary to the disease or its treatment); *social functioning* (disruptions in normal social activities). Additional considerations in the evaluation of QOL may include spiritual or existential concerns, sexual functioning and body image, and satisfaction with health care.

Whenever possible, QOL should be assessed by the patient (7, 28) and should reflect the evaluation of a number of dimensions affecting his or her life at that moment. Although the specific dimensions that are the most satisfactory or unsatisfactory at any point in time may vary, the individual's QOL may in fact remain stable or change depending on how these dimensions fluctuate and interact. For this reason, some have argued that both the component dimensions of QOL as well as a global assessment should be considered (29). Therefore, in the research or clinical setting, one should always ask what specific dimensions of QOL are likely to be affected and choose a QOL tool based on its content relevance to the questions of interest.

B. Measurement of Quality of Life

1. Data Collection Methods

Although there is consensus that the patient should assess QOL, there are a variety of ways in which this information can be obtained. The clinical interview (using structured questions from a validated instrument) is the most comprehensive approach in that it allows participation of the greatest number of individuals (e.g., those who cannot read or write or those with visual impairment or frailty). However, the clinical interview is more costly in personnel and time, and there may be some bias introduced through in person interaction. Interviews can be conducted in person or by telephone, and they can assure less missing data. For geriatric research, the clinical interview is a standard approach for a variety of reasons, but most often it is used because of the frailty of the target population. However, geriatric assessment also relies heavily on self-administered questionnaires (especially in healthier older persons) and performance-based measures in which patients are directly observed completing tasks. Geriatric assessment also frequently uses data sources other than the patient, particularly caregivers, family members, and nursing staff.

In contrast, most of the research on QOL with cancer patients has focused on self-administered questionnaires. This has occurred primarily because of an interest in the inclusion of QOL assessments in clinical trials. In this setting, there are few personnel available for conduct of clinical interviews. The advantages of the self-administered format include limited need for personnel to collect data, more accurate responses for sensitive information, and administration at a time and place that are convenient for the patient. However, there are important limitations to self-administered instruments that include a requirement for literacy and sometimes language translation, familiarity with completion of pencil and paper tests, and the increased likelihood of missing data when compared to interview-obtained information. In addition, very ill patients (e.g., Karnofsky score less than 60) may have difficulty completing more than the briefest scales (30).

Ideally, a combination of these two approaches should be used in the assessment of QOL in cancer patients. One can start with the self-administered format, and reserve the structured research interview for those patients who are unable to complete the written form without assistance. Even when a self-administered format is used, however, it is important to review all questionnaires for missing data. Thus, the combination of the two approaches can lead to the greatest efficiency in terms of data completeness and personnel time. In the Medical Outcomes Study, which included a sizeable portion of outpatients over 65 years of age, their fairly lengthy survey was self-administered by the majority of subjects, with telephone interviews being required in the remainder (31). Although, in general, results from self-report and telephone interviews are similar, there can be some variation, especially on sensitive topics, and researchers should track the mode of administration. In research studies with older cancer patients, an attempt should be made to collect the data in a single systematic format, but assistance of an interviewer after an attempt at completion may be most realistic in older cancer patients. If resources permit, the interview may be the best approach to ensure inclusion of all eligible older patients.

2. Choice of Instruments

In the field of QOL assessment, there is controversy about the use of instruments that are highly specific to the research or clinical question at hand (e.g., a unique toxicity for a treatment) versus the use of a tool that has been widely used with other samples of cancer patients or patients with other chronic conditions (e.g., diabetes, arthritis, heart disease). The debate revolves around the use of generic measures or cancer-specific/cancer site and phase-specific tools (Table 1). In considering the geriatric cancer patient, one must also consider a whole body of geriatric assessment tools (e.g., Mini-Mental Status Examination Geriatric Depression Scale), and these will be discussed later in this chapter. However, for the purpose of this discussion, we will focus on QOL instruments that have been used in a broad range of populations.

Generic instruments such as the RAND measures (31–33), the Dartmouth COOP charts (34), and the Duke scales (35) all have considerable value if one wishes to compare the general impact of differing diseases/conditions on QOL. From a policy standpoint, this may be important in terms of preventing discrimination against cancer patients, as their functional status and QOL may exceed patients with other chronic conditions (36). On the other hand, the information obtained from these scales often lacks the sensitivity to detect impairments from cancer treatments (37, 38)

In contrast, the cancer-specific QOL instruments [e.g., Functional Living Index—Cancer (FLIC), European Organization for Research and Treatment of Cancer (EORTC), Cancer Rehabilitation Evaluation System (CARES), Functional Assessment of Cancer Therapy (FACT)] that have been developed during the past decade have high reliability and validity and are responsive to changes from treat-

Table 1 Examples of Health-Related Quality of Life
Instruments Used with Cancer Patients

Generic health status measures
  Sickness Impact Profile (SIP)
  RAND Health Insurance Experiment Measures
  Medical Outcomes Study (MOS) Instruments
  Nottingham Health Profile
  Psychosocial Adjustment to Illness Scale (PAIS)
  Dartmouth COOP Charts
Generic Cancer-Specific Instruments
  Quality of Life Index (Spitzer)
  Quality of Life Index (Padilla and Grant)
  Functional Living Index—Cancer (FLIC)
  European Organization for Research and Treatment of
    Cancer Quality of Life Questionnaire (EORTC-QLQ)
  Cancer Rehabilitation Evaluation System (CARES)
  Functional Assessment of Cancer Therapy (FACT)
Cancer Site-Specific Instruments
  Breast Cancer Chemotherapy Questionnaire
  Linear Analogue Self-Assessment (LASA) for Breast Cancer
  Performance Parameter (Head & Neck)
  Site-specific modules for the FACT and the EORTC-QLQ
Symptom-Oriented Scales
  Rotterdam Symptom Checklist
  Symptom Distress Scale (McCorkle)
  Memorial Pain Assessment Card
  Morrow Assessment of Nausea and Emesis (MANE) Scale

---

ments (39). In addition, they are more likely to capture the known toxicities and concerns related to cancer treatment. Therefore, they should be a preferred choice in the comparative evaluation of cancer treatments. However, one must recognize that each of these generic cancer-specific instruments may need to be supplemented with disease-specific modules (e.g., for breast cancer, prostatic cancer, or leukemia) or condition-specific questions that target specific QOL issues (e.g., pain, nausea, or sexual functioning). Thus, in designing a QOL assessment, one must carefully define the expected impacts of the disease and its treatment on QOL and use a battery of assessment tools that are likely to reflect these effects.

In considering how to assess QOL in the geriatric cancer patient, one must follow the same general principles as for other populations; however, special issues may arise in very frail elderly samples, especially those who are not routinely included in clinical trials because of other exclusion criteria. Relatively little research has been conducted with this group of cancer patients, and it is unclear whether other chronic conditions (e.g., dementia, arthritis, heart, pulmonary, or neurological disease) will overwhelm any specific contribution made by the cancer. This is clearly an area ripe for further research, and it is beginning to receive attention from several investigators (40, 41).

C. Role of Quality of Life Assessment in Cancer Treatment

Assessment of QOL can be used for a variety of purposes: to describe the impact of cancer and its treatment on patients; to compare the outcome of different treatments in clinical trials; to identify unanticipated benefits or toxicities of treatment; and to inform future treatment planning through modification of aspects which detract from QOL. Information gained from prior QOL research can help inform treatment decisions. For example, multiple studies have shown that overall QOL, and most of its dimensions, differ little among women who choose mastectomy over lumpectomy in the primary treatment of breast cancer (42). Therefore, a woman who is considering alternative surgical treatments for breast cancer can be reassured that her subsequent adjustment will not be dependent on the type of surgery she receives. However, since research has shown that there is much more body image disruption from mastectomy compared to lumpectomy (43), a woman who expresses concerns about her body image should be encouraged to consider a lumpectomy.

Several studies have also demonstrated that QOL is an important prognostic factor for survival (30, 44). Although this should not be the only variable used in considering whether a patient should receive aggressive cancer therapy, assessing patient-rated QOL could help physicians determine more systematically when only palliative care should be offered.

For example, patients with poor physical functioning are not likely to have substantial improvement from treatment of tumors for which treatment response rates are marginal (e.g., metastatic cancers of the lung or pancreas or melanoma). Therefore, serious consideration should be given to avoiding the additional toxicity of chemotherapy. In this regard, there is mounting evidence that physicians regularly ignore the advance directives or expressed wishes of patients regarding end of life support (45). Regular evaluation of a patient's QOL over time can capture functional deterioration, which physician's poorly assess (28). Physician reluctance to engage in discussions with seriously ill patients is likely to be enhanced by more objective and quantified measures of outcome. Although these issues are relevant to all cancer patients, they are particularly salient for the elderly, who experience the majority of cancer deaths.

D. Special Relevance of Quality of Life in the Geriatric Cancer Patient

Often there have been assumptions made about the QOL impact of cancer and its treatment on older patients. These include the belief that older patients suffer more side effects from treatment or have more difficulty adjusting to a cancer diagnosis. As indicated earlier, the elderly are quite heterogeneous, and one cannot assume that chronological age is the primary factor affecting functioning or well-being. In a study by Kahn and colleagues (46), 300 matched pairs of adult patients with cancer and their physicians were interviewed concerning the effects of disease and treatment on the patients' QOL. The physicians overestimated the problems of the elderly cancer patients, whereas in actuality younger patients reported more difficulties. These investigators suggest that physicians need to become more sensitized to the individualized, personal nature of their patients' QOL and the factors that may shape or modify it (46). Thus, it is critical that health care providers assess the individual patient's QOL; there is no room for paternalistic decision making for older adults simply because of their age.

Where side effects of cancer treatment have been examined (e.g., nausea and vomiting), older patients often fare better than younger patients, requiring less antiemetic therapy (47). Some side effects, such as diarrhea (and resultant dehydration), may be more of a problem in the older cancer patient receiving chemotherapy. Pain is an important symptom that may detract from the QOL (48, 49), and care should be given to provide adequate education and treatment for this problem. Although pain research specific to the elderly is sparse (50, 51), older persons with cancer are the majority of those cared for in hospice programs where excellent palliative care is a primary goal.

Several studies have documented better mental health in the elderly in general, with consistent findings among older cancer patients (36). Life experiences, as well as familiarity with the health care setting, may allow older cancer patients to cope with a cancer diagnosis with more resiliency. With fewer responsibilities to juggle (e.g., child care or work), as well as awareness that this is a disease experience their peers have had, older cancer patients often are not as distressed as younger cancer patients. A specific issue for the elderly, however, may be their need for assistance of various types. In a detailed study of determinants of need and unmet need among cancer patients residing at home, Mor and colleagues (52) found that physiological factors (metastases, disease stage, and functional status) were associated with the need for assistance in the areas of personal care, instrumental tasks, and transportation. Also, older age (over 65 years old) and low-income predicted the need for help with personal care, and women were more likely than men to report an illness-related need for assistance with instrumental tasks and transportation. Unmet needs were primarily associated with the patients' social support system (52). Again, there may be considerable variation in the degree of social support among elderly cancer patients, and this may influence the patient's functioning and well-being. Health care providers should include evaluation of social support when considering treatment decisions as well as the patient's subjective assessment of well-being. Geriatric assessment, described in the following section, is critical to the translation of information from QOL assessment into active interventions for the older cancer patient.

III. FEATURES OF GERIATRIC ASSESSMENT

A. Definition of Geriatric Assessment

Geriatric assessment extends beyond the traditional medical evaluation of older persons' health to include assessment of cognitive, affective, functional, social, economic, and environmental status, as well as a discussion of patient preferences regarding advance directives (Table 2). For younger and healthier seniors, simple probes for the presence of common geriatric problems may suffice. Those who are frail or at high risk for functional decline or nursing home placement should receive more extensive evaluation conducted by individual practitioners or by a multidisciplinary team of health care professionals (comprehensive geriatric assessment). For the oncologist, referral for comprehensive geriatric assessment might be considered when an elderly patient's cancer is well controlled but the patient is failing to thrive.

Validated assessment instruments that focus on specific components of the health of older persons can be included as part of a questionnaire (which can be administered before the visit) by office staff or by the clinician. These instruments can be used to guide these brief evaluations but must be interpreted in the context of their limitations. They are rarely, if ever, diagnostic tests. Rather they indicate the need for further evaluation. Nor do they substitute for good clinical skills and judgment, including the skill of eliciting important items from the patient's history

Table 2 Assessment of the Elderly Oncology Patient

Dimension	Brief screening test	Potential referral resource
Medical		
Nutrition	BMI serum albumin and cholesterol	Dietitian
Mobility/balance	Time up & Go (5), office-based maneuvers	Physical therapist
Visual impairment	Snellen eye chart	Optician, ophthalmologist
Hearing impairment	Audioscope	Audiologist
Urinary incontinence	Two-questions (8)	Geriatrician, urologist, gynecologist
Cognitive	Three item recall, Mini-Mental State Examination (9)	Geriatrician, psychiatrist, neurologist
Affective	Geriatric Depression Scale (12)	Geriatrician, psychiatrist
Functional status	BADL, IADL, AADL questions	Geriatrician, social worker, physical therapist, occupational therapist
Social support	Specific questions	Social worker
Economic	Specific questions	Social worker
Environment	Home Safety Checklist	Physical therapist, home health nurse, social worker
Advance directive	Specific questions	Social worker

BMI, body mass index; BADL, basic activities of daily living; IADL, instrumental or intermediate activities of daily living; AADL, advanced activities of daily living.

and physical examination. However, information obtained from assessment instruments can be used quickly to direct the clinician's attention to issues that are particularly relevant to an individual patient. The clinician must also be able to act on the information obtained by seeking additional diagnostic tests, by implementing therapy for problems detected, or by referring patients to appropriate professionals for additional evaluation and management. Although detailed discussion of the management of problems identified through assessment instruments is beyond the scope of this chapter, possible referral resources are indicated in Table 2. The remainder of this chapter will focus on the initial multidimensional assessment and assumes that the oncologist is the primary care physician.

B. Assessment for Geriatric Conditions

1. Medical Assessment

a. Malnutrition/Weight Loss.

Among oncology patients, the most common nutritional disorder is energy undernutrition (including protein-energy undernutrition). New patients can be asked on a previsit questionnaire about weight loss within the previous 6 months, and all patients should be weighed at every office visit. Height should also be measured on the initial visit to allow calculation of body mass index (weight in kilograms/height in meters^2) and probably yearly because of changes in height due to thinning of vertebral disks with age and possible changes due to vertebral compression fractures. Healthy older adults should have a body mass index (BMI) between 22 and 27.

Energy undernutrition states include adult marasmus (energy undernutrition) and adult kwashiorkar (protein-energy undernutrition). Protein-energy undernutrition is defined by the presence of clinical (physical signs such as wasting or low BMI) *and* biochemical (albumin or other protein) evidence of insufficient intake. Recently, the importance of low serum albumin (56) and low cholesterol (57) as prognostic factors for mortality in community-dwelling older persons has been demonstrated. It is probably appropriate to order these tests as baseline and screening tests for oncological patients (58), particularly those for whom chemotherapy, radiation therapy, or surgery is being considered. For patients who are undergoing intensive treatment, nutritional status can be monitored using prealbumin, which has a half-life of 2 days, or transtergin, which has a half-life of 7 days. Both may be more sensitive to change compared to albumin, which has a half-life of 21 days.

b. Mobility and Balance Disorders/Fall Risk.

As a result of other age-related diseases and the burden of their malignancy and associated treatments, older persons cared for by oncologists may be at high risk for falling and subsequent consequences (e.g., hematomas and hip fractures). Accordingly, the assessment of fall risk by assessing balance, gait, lower extremity strength, and a history about previous falls is quite valuable.

A question about falls may be included on a previsit questionnaire. A positive response to the question "During the past 12 months have you fallen all the way to the ground or fallen and hit something like a chair or stair?" should prompt subsequent questions by the clinician, such as those that assess the likelihood of injurious falls (e.g., loss of consciousness, long lie of 5 min or more before arising, or frequent falls). Balance and gait disorders are best assessed by observing a patient perform tasks. The "Up & Go" test is a timed measure of the patient's ability to rise from an arm chair, walk 3 m (10 ft), turn, walk back, and sit down again; those who take longer than 20 s to complete the test merit further evaluation (53). It can be administered by office staff prior to the clinician's visit. The Performance-Oriented Assessment of Mobility instrument is a standardized instrument that measures gait and balance (59) that has been used in research and some clinical settings.

All clinicians should learn to conduct a basic evaluation of gait and balance, which requires little time and provides an excellent assessment of the patient's mobility and risk of falling. Once trained, the alert clinician can perform a gait evaluation while the patient is entering or leaving the examining room. Several tests of balance and mobility can also be performed quickly in the office and provide substantial clinical information. These include the ability to maintain a tandem or semitandem stand for 10 s, resistance to a sternal nudge, and observation of a 360-degree turn. Quadriceps strength can be briefly assessed by observing an older person arising from a hard armless chair without the use of his or her hands.

c. Polypharmacy.

Because older persons often receive care from multiple providers who may not communicate with each other and because they may fill prescriptions at several pharmacies, each patient should be told to bring in all their current medications to each visit. This is particularly important when the oncologist co-manages a patient with another primary care physician. Office personnel can check these against the medication list in the medical record and discrepancies can be brought to the clinician's attention at the time of the patient encounter. Several drug-interaction programs are commercially available to check for potential drug–drug interactions.

d. Visual and Hearing Impairment.

When the oncologist is the primary care physician, several other dimensions of the medical assessment need to be included. Too often these problems go unnoticed and missed, because older patients fail to report them spontaneously. For example, they may not recognize that hearing loss can be treated, with subsequent improvement in health-related QOL. In addition, they may attribute some symptoms (e.g., loss of hearing) to normal aging and believe that there is no effective treatment.

Therefore, systematic assessment of remediable problems with vision and hearing should be undertaken.

Office staff should be trained to test visual acuity using a Snellen Eye Chart, which requires the patient to stand 20 ft from the chart and read letters, using their best corrected vision. Patients who are unable to read all the letters on the 20/40 line should be referred to an opthalmologist or optometrist for further evaluation.

Several methods to screen for hearing loss are available that can be administered by office staff or can be included on a questionnaire. The most accurate of these is the Welch Allyn Audioscope (Welch Allyn, Inc., Skaneateles Falls, NY), a hand-held otoscope with a built-in audiometer. The audioscope can be set at several different levels of intensity, but it should be set at 40 dB to evaluate hearing in older persons. A pretone at 60 dB is delivered and then four tones (500, 1000, 2000, and 4000 Hz) at 40 dB are delivered. Patients fail the screen if they are unable to hear either the 1000- or 2000-Hz frequency in both ears or both the 1000- and 2000-Hz frequencies in one ear (60).

Office staff can also administer the whispered voice test by whispering three to six random words (numbers, words, or letters) at a set distance (6, 8, 12, or 24 in) from the person's ear and then asking the patient to repeat the words. The examiner should be behind the person to prevent speech reading and the opposite ear should be occluded during the examination. Further evaluation is indicated for those who cannot repeat 50% of the whispered words correctly (60).

A self-administered test of emotional and social problems associated with impaired hearing, the Hearing Handicap Inventory for the Elderly-Screening Version (HHIE-S), can be included as part of a questionnaire. However, it is less accurate than the audioscope (60).

e. Urinary Incontinence.

Although patients are frequently embarrassed to verbalize spontaneously that they have incontinence, this problem can be uncovered by inclusion of two questions on a previsit questionnaire: (a) "In the last year, have you ever lost your urine and gotten wet?" and (b) "Have you lost urine at least 6 separate days?" Answering "yes" to both questions indicates a potential problem with urinary incontinence that needs further investigation by the clinician (54).

2. Cognitive Assessment

Because the prevalence of Alzheimer's disease and other types of dementia rises considerably with advancing age, the yield of screening for cognitive impairment will be highest in the 85 years and older age group. The most commonly used screen is the Mini-Mental State Examination, a 30-item interviewer-administered assessment of several dimensions of cognitive function (61). Several shorter screens have also been validated, including recall of three items at 1 min, the clock drawing test, and the serial sevens test (patients are asked to subtract 7 from 100 five times) (62).

Although normal results on these tests vastly reduce the probability of dementia and abnormal results increase the odds of dementia, these tests are neither diagnostic for dementia nor do normal results exclude the possibility of this disorder. Shortcomings include their lack of relevance to functional activities of daily life and their failure to account for educational level, languages other than English, and cultural differences.

3. Affective Assessment

Affective assessment is particularly important in oncology patients, because the complications of malignant diseases, particularly those that are incurable, may lead to depressive symptoms. For example, increased dependency or the anticipation of reduced life expectancy may precipitate adjustment disorders or major depression. Older patients can be asked about depression on a previsit questionnaire using the question "Do you often feel sad or depressed?" (63). This single question, however, tends to be overly sensitive and may be better used in tandem with a second screen such as the Geriatric Depression Scale, which has 15- and 30-item versions (55).

4. Assessment of Function

Measurement of functional status is a cardinal component of assessment of older persons. Fortunately, the importance of functional status has been recognized by oncologists for decades and has been used to provide prognostic information (see earlier discussion on Karnofsky Performance Status in Sec. II.A.1). For elderly populations, functional status is regarded as an important outcome measure, particularly because survival may not be prolonged in this age group. In many respects, the patient's ability to function is among the most important measures of the overall impact of his or her diseases and disorders. From a clinical perspective, the major shift for the oncologist is to measure not only functional status for prognostic or outcome purposes, but to attempt also to remediate functional impairment as part of the management plan. As such, changes in functional status may prompt further diagnostic evaluation and intervention, monitor response to treatment, and provide a prognosis and plan for long-term care.

Functional status can be assessed at three levels: basic activities of daily living (BADL), instrumental or intermediate activities of daily living (IADL), and advanced activities of daily living (AADL) (64). BADL assess the ability of the patient to complete basic self-care tasks (e.g., bathing, dressing, toileting, continence, feeding, and transferring). IADL measure the patient's ability to maintain an independent household (e.g., shopping for groceries, driving or using public transportation, using the telephone, meal preparation, housework, handyman work, laundry, taking medications, and handling finances). AADL measure the patient's ability to fulfill societal, community, and family roles as well as participate in recreational or occupational tasks. These advanced activities vary considerably from individual to individual, but they may be exceptionally valuable in monitoring functional status prior to the development of disability.

Questions that ask about specific BADL and IADL function can be incorporated into a previsit questionnaire. some AADL (e.g., exercise and leisure time physical activity) can also be ascertained in this manner, but open-ended questions about how older persons spend their days may provide a better assessment of function in healthier older persons.

5. Assessment of Social Support

The older patient's family structure can be assessed by a few questions on a previsit questionnaire; however, the quality of these relationships must be assessed by the clinician during the patient encounter. Many larger oncological clinics have nurse clinicians or social workers who routinely assess for potential problems in this domain. In smaller practices, it becomes incumbent on the physician or office staff to probe systematically into the adequacy of social support. For very frail older persons, the availability of assistance from family and friends is frequently the determining factor of whether a functionally dependent older person remains at home or is institutionalized. If dependency is noted during functional assessment, the clinician should inquire as to who provides help for specific BADL and IADL functions and whether these persons are paid or voluntary help. Even in healthier older persons, it is often valuable to raise the question of who would be available to help if the patient becomes ill; early identification of problems with social support may prompt planning to develop resources should the necessity arise.

6. Environmental Assessment

Environmental assessment encompasses two dimensions: the safety of the home environment and the adequacy of the patient's access to needed personal and medical services. Particularly among the frail and those with mobility and balance problems, the home environment should be assessed for safety. Although most physicians do not personally conduct environmental assessments, the National Safety Council has developed a Home Safety Checklist that patients and their families can complete. For those at high risk of recurrent falls, home health agencies can send health professionals to inspect homes for safety and can recommend installation of adaptive devices (e.g., shower bars or raised toilet seats).

Older persons who begin to develop IADL dependencies should be evaluated for the geographical proximity of necessary services (e.g., grocery shopping or banking), their need for the use of such services, and their ability to utilize these services in their current living situations. Transportation needs may be exceptionally important among oncological patients who may need frequent medical visits for radiation therapy.

7. Advance Directives

Although important in all practices of medicine, discussions of advance directives are particularly important for oncological patients who have life-threatening tumors.

When treating cancer patients in ambulatory settings, the oncologist needs to begin early on to discuss the patient's goals and preferences for care should she or he become unable to speak for themselves because of progressive cognitive impairment or acute illness. The durable power of attorney for health care, which asks the patient to designate a surrogate to make medical decisions if the patient loses decision-making capacity, is often less emotionally laden than specifying treatments that the patient may or may not want. Although it is often difficult to find time to discuss advance directives in detail during the initial office visit, a revisit questionnaire can determine whether the patient already has such a directive and patients can be given information to read at home in preparation for subsequent discussions.

Oncologists must also be careful not to equate these preferences for advance directives with preferences for aggressiveness of treatment for the tumor. These are separate issues, and it should be made clear that discussions of advance directives should not be interpreted by patients or oncologists as "giving up on a patient." For example, a patient may want all available treatment for a cancer yet may not want to be resuscitated should a cardiac arrest occur. As such, discussions about advance directives should not be reserved for the days when death is imminent but rather be addressed early on. These should be reassessed as more medical information becomes available and as patients may revise their thoughts about the benefits of treatment.

C. Special Relevance of Geriatric Assessment to the Cancer Patient

Older persons account for approximately 40% of visits to internists' offices. Although specific estimates for oncologists are not available, there is ample support for the importance of older persons in the oncologist's practice. For example, the probability that a man 60–79 years of age will develop an invasive cancer is one in three; for women, it is one in four (65). For both genders, cancer is among the top two causes of deaths (heart disease is the other) among persons 55 years of age or older, and the three leading causes of cancer death in this age group are lung, colorectal, and breast (in women) carcinomas. Moreover, the proportion of oncological practice that will focus on older persons will increase, as demographical trends indicate substantial growth in the elderly population, particularly after the year 2010.

Clinicians caring for older persons must recognize the heterogeneity of the elderly population and focus the assessment and care plan accordingly. For the youngest group of geriatric patients who are in good health or have few chronic conditions, the focus is geared toward preventive geriatrics (i.e., lifestyle modifications, chemoprophylaxis, immunizations, and screening for diseases) and brief screening for potential geriatric problems. In contrast, for those above the age of 85 years and those with multiple complex health and social problems, a more extensive assessment is indicated.

For the patient with advanced cancer or whom cancer is the major health problem, the oncologist frequently becomes the primary care physician. It should be noted that the medical and functional impairments caused by many systemic cancers and their treatments precipitate typical geriatric problems. Thus, the oncologist needs to be more familiar than most specialists with the multidimensional components of the assessment of the older patient. In other cases, the care of the patient is shared with a primary care physician, who may occasionally be a geriatrician. This primary care physician will likely attend to the geriatric aspects of the patient. Regardless of which role the oncologist plays for a particular patient, his or her responsibilities should be delineated clearly early in the relationship.

IV. STRATEGIES FOR COMBINING THESE APPROACHES IN THE FUTURE

In summary, cancers are particularly common among older persons. As the population ages and the relative percentage of the elderly increases, the oncologist's role in caring for older persons will assume increasing importance. Unfortunately, many of the health problems associated with aging are precipitated earlier and are amplified by malignancies and their treatment. By broadening the oncologist's assessment skill to include domains that are beyond traditional internal medicine and oncology training, the profession can better serve their older cancer patients.

Although the majority of cancer patients are over 60 years of age, the elderly are not always adequately represented in clinical trials or QOL research. In particular, patients with comorbid conditions or physiological abnormalities of aging (e.g., decreased renal function) usually are excluded from clinical treatment trials. Therefore, it may be difficult to extrapolate information obtained in clinical trials to the general elderly population. There is increasing awareness of the need for effectiveness studies (examination of what clinical practices work in the real world) to determine which treatments are best for the general community of older cancer patients. Similarly, QOL studies in older cancer patients should be conducted to understand better their values and estimation of QOL. These studies are particularly necessary because of the exclusion of these patients from usual clinical cancer research. Observation and community-based studies of elderly cancer patients will be critical for increasing our understanding of the specific needs of this population.

From our vantage point, there seems to be considerable promise in beginning to integrate some of the formal aspects of geriatric assessment into the management of the older cancer patient. In particular, oncologists could adapt some components of geriatric assessment in their evaluation of newly diagnosed older patients. This can provide more accurate information on the hardiness of patients who are planning to undergo treatment, as well as to identify concomitant geriatric problems that should be attended to (e.g., cognitive problems, functional limitations, and social support) that would enhance the likelihood of successful cancer treatment. This approach could also be used to screen patients for eligibility for cancer treatment trials to ensure that representative numbers of older cancer patients are treated to inform clinical practice in the future. It would seem that the time is ripe for more active collaboration among oncologists and geriatricians to merge their skills and common interests in the older patient with cancer.

ACKNOWLEDGMENT

Supported in part by a grant from the National Institute on Aging, AG13095.

REFERENCES

1. Ellwood PM. Shattuck Lecture. Outcomes management: A technology of patient experience. N Engl J Med 1988; 318:1549–1556.
2. Aaronson NK, Beckmann J, eds. The Quality of Life of Cancer Patients. New York: Raven Press, 1987.
3. McDowell I, Newell C. Measuring Health: A Guide to Rating Scales and Questionnaires, Second Edition. New York: Oxford University Press, 1996.
4. Tchekmedyian NS, Cella DF, eds. Quality of life in current oncology practice and research. Oncology 1990; 4(Suppl 5):11–232.
5. Tchekmedyian NS, Cella DF, Winn RT, eds. Economic and quality of life outcomes in oncology. Oncology 1995; 9(Suppl 11):3–215.
6. Osoba D, ed. Effect of Cancer on Quality of Life. Boca Raton, FL: CRC Press, 1991.
7. Hollandsworth JG Jr. Evaluating the impact of medical treatment on the quality of life: a five year update. Soc Sci Med 1988; 26:425–434.
8. De Haes JCJM. Quality of life: conceptual and theoretical considerations. In: Watson M, Greer S, Thomas C, eds, Psychosocial Oncology. Oxford, UK: Pergamon Press, 1988:61–70.
9. Cella DF, Cherin EA. Quality of life during and after cancer treatment. Compr Ther 1988; 14:69–75.
10. Cella DF, Tulsky DS. Quality of life in cancer: definition, purpose, and method of measurement. Cancer Invest 1993; 11:327–336.
11. Guyatt GH, Feeny DH, Patrick DL. Measuring health-related quality of life. Ann Intern Med 1993; 118:622–629.
12. Aaronson NK. Quality of life: What is it? How should it be measured. Oncology 1988; 2:69–74.
13. De Haes JCJM, Van Knippenberg FCE. The quality of life of cancer patients: a review of the literature. Soc Sci Med 1985; 20:809–817.
14. Aristotle. Ethics. Harmondsworth, UK: Penguin Books, 1976.
15. Andrews FM, Withey SB. Social Indicators of Well Being: Americans' Perception of Life Quality. New York: Plenum Press, 1976.
16. Campbell A. Subjective measures of well-being. Am Psychol 1974; 31:117–124.
17. Campbell A. The Sense of Well-being in America: Recent Patterns and Trends. New York: McGraw-Hill, 1981.

18. World Health Organization. Constitution in Basic Documents. Geneva: World Health Organization, 1948.

19. Ware JE Jr. Conceptualizing disease impact and treatment outcomes. Cancer 1984; 53(Suppl):2316–2323.

20. Karnofsky DA, Burchenal JH. The clinical evaluation of chemotherapeutic agents in cancer. In: Macleod, CM, ed. Evaluation of Chemotherapeutic Agents. New York: Columbia University Press, 1949:199–205.

21. Patrick DL, Deyo RA. Generic and disease-specific measures in assessing health status and quality of life. Med Care 1989; 27:S217–S232.

22. Adams SG Jr, Britt DM, Godding PR, Khansur TI, Bulcourf BB. Relative contribution of the Karnofsky Performance Status scale in a multi-measure assessment of quality of life in cancer patients. Psycho-oncology 1995; 4:239–246.

23. Spitzer WO, Dobson AJ, Hall J, Chesterman E, Levi J, Shepherd R, Battista RN, Catchlove BR. Measuring the quality of life of cancer patients. J Chronic Dis 1981; 34:585–597.

23a. Greer DS, MORV, Sherwood S, Morris JN, Birnbaum H. National Hospice Study Analysis Plan. J Chronic Dis 1983; 36(1):737–780.

24. Moinpour CM. Quality of life assessment in Southwest Oncology Group Trials. Oncology 1990; 4:79–89.

25. Nayfield SG, Hailey BJ. Quality of Life Assessment in Cancer Clinical Trials. Report of the Workshop on Quality of Life Research in Clinical Trials held July 16–17, 1990. Bethesda, MD: U.S. Dept. of Health & Human Services, Public Health Service, National Institutes of Health.

26. Patrick DL, Erickson P. Assessing health-related quality of life for clinical decision making. In: Walker, SM, and Rosser, RM, eds. Quality of Life: Assessment and Application. Lancaster, UK: MTP Press, 1988:9–49.

27. Schipper H, Clinch J, McMurray A, Levitt M. Measuring the quality of life of cancer patients: The Functional Living Index—Cancer: Development and Validation. J Clin Oncol 1984; 2:472–483.

28. Slevin ML, Plant H, Lynch D, Drinkwater J, Gregory WM. Who should measure quality of life, the doctor or the patient? Br J Cancer 1988; 57:109–112.

29. DeHaes JCJM, van Knippenberg FCE. Quality of life instruments for cancer patients: Babel's tower revisited. J Clin Epidemiol 1989; 42:1239–1241.

30. Ganz PA, Haskell CM, Figlin RA, LaSoto N, Siau J. Estimating the quality of life in a clinical trial of patients with metastatic lung cancer using the Karnofsky Performance Status and the Functional Living Index—Cancer (FLIC). Cancer 1988; 61:849–856.

31. Stewart AL, Ware JE, eds. Measuring Function and Well-Being. The Medical Outcomes Study Approach. Durham, NC: Duke University Press, 1992.

32. Ware JE, Sherbourne CD. The MOS 36-Item Short-Form Health Survey (SF-36): I. Conceptual framework and item selection. Med Care 1992; 30:473–483.

33. Hays RD, Sherbourne CD, Mazel RM. The RAND 36-Item Health Survey 1.0. Health Economics 1993; 2:217–227.

34. Nelson E, Wasson J, Kirk J, Keller A, Clerk D, Dietrich A, Stewart A, Zobkoff M. Assessment of function in routine clinical practice: description of the COOP chart method and preliminary findings. J Chronic Dis 1987; 40(Suppl):55S–69S.

35. Parkerson GR, Broadhead WE, Tse CJ. The Duke Health Profile: a 17-item measure of health and dysfunction. Med Care 1990; 28:1056–1072.

36. Cassileth BR, Lusk EJ, Strouse TB, Miller DS, Brown LL, Cross PA, Tenaglin AN. Psychosocial status in chronic illness. N Engl J Med 1984; 311:506–511.

37. Litwin MS, Hays RD, Fink A, Ganz PA, Leake B, Leach GE, Brook RH. Quality-of-life outcomes in men treated for localized prostate cancer. JAMA 1995; 273:129–135.

38. Ganz PA, Coscarelli A, Fred C, Kahn B, Polinsky ML, Petersen L. Breast cancer survivors: psychosocial concerns and quality of life. Breast Can Res Treat 1996; 38:183–1991.

39. Cella DF, Bonomi AE. Measuring quality of life: 1995 update. Oncology 1995; 9(Suppl 11):47–60.

40. Silliman RA, Balducci L, Goodwin JS, Holmes FF, Leventhal EA. Breast cancer care in old age: what we know, don't know, and do. J Natl Cancer Inst 1993; 85:190–199.

41. Goodwin JS, Hunt WC, Samet JM. Determinants of cancer therapy in elderly patients. Cancer 1993; 72:594–601.

42. Kiebert GM, de Haes JCJM, van de Velde CJH. The impact of breast-conserving treatment and mastectomy on the quality of life of early-stage breast cancer patients: a review. J Clin Oncol 1991; 9:1059–1070.

43. Ganz PA, Schag CAC, Lee JJ, Polinsky ML, Tan S-J. Breast conservation versus mastectomy: is there a difference in psychological adjustment or quality of life in the year after surgery? Cancer 1992; 69:1729–1738.

44. Coates A, Gebski V, Bishop JF, Jeal PN, Woods RL, Snyder R, Tattersall MH, Byrne M, Harvey V, Gill G. Improving the quality of life during chemotherapy for advanced breast cancer. A comparison of intermittent and continuous treatment strategies. N Engl J Med 1987; 317:1490–1495.

45. The SUPPORT Principal Investigators. A Controlled trials to improve care for seriously ill hospitalized patients. The Study to Understand Prognoses and Preferences for Outcomes and Risks of Treatments (SUPPORT). JAMA 1995; 274:1591–1598.

46. Kahn SB, Houts PS, Harding SP. Quality of life and patients with cancer: A comparative study of patient versus physician perceptions and its implications for cancer education. J Cancer Ed 1992; 7:241–249.

47. Nerenz DR, Love RR, Leventhal H, Easterling DV. Psychosocial consequences of cancer chemotherapy for elderly patients. Health Serv Res 1986; 20(6 Pt 2):961–976.

48. Hillier R. Control of pain in terminal cancer. Br Med Bull 1990; 46:279–91.

49. Stein WM, Miech RP. Cancer pain in the elderly hospice patient. J Pain Symptom Manage 1993; 8:474–82.

50. Portenoy RK. Pain management in the older cancer patient. Oncology 1992; 6(Suppl 2):86–98.

51. Ferrell BR, Ferrell BA, Ahn C, Tran K. Pain management for elderly patients with cancer at home. Cancer 1994; 74(Suppl 7):2139–2146.

52. Mor V, Allen SM, Siegel K, Houts P. Determinants of need and unmet need among cancer patients residing at home. Health Serv Res 1992; 27:337–360.

53. Podsiadlo D, Richardson S. The timed "UP & Go": a test of basic functional mobility for frail elderly persons. J Am Geriatr Soc 1991; 39:142–148.

54. Diokno AC, Brown MR, Brock BM, Herzog AR, Normolle DP. Clinical and cystometric characteristics of continent and incontinent noninstitutionalized elderly. J Urol 1988; 140:567–571.

55. Yesavage JA, Brink TL, Rose TL, Lum O, Huang V, Adey M, Leirer VO. Development and validation of a geriatric depression screening scale: a preliminary report. J Psychiatr Res 1983; 17:37–49.

56. Corti M, Guralnik JM, Salive ME, Sorkin JD. Serum albumin level and physical disability as predictors of mortality in older persons. J Am Med Assoc 1994; 272:1036–1042.

57. Noel MA, Smith TK, Ettinger WH. Characteristics and outcomes of hospitalized older patients who develop hypocholesterolemia. J Am Geriatr Soc 1991; 6:249–258.

58. Reuben DB, Greendale GA, Harrison GG. Nutrition screening in older persons. J Am Geriatr Soc 1995; 43:415–425.

59. Tinetti ME. Performance-oriented assessment of mobility problems in elderly patients. J Am Geriatr Soc 1986; 34:119–126.

60. Mulrow CD, Lichtenstein MJ. Screening for hearing impairment in the elderly. J Gen Int Med 1991; 6:249–258.

61. Tombaugh TN, McIntyre NJ. The Mini-Mental State Examination: a comprehensive review. J Am Geriatr Soc 1992; 40:922–935.

62. Siu AL. Screening for dementia and investigating its causes. Ann Intern Med 1991; 115:122–132.

63. Lachs MS, Feinstein AR, Cooney LM Jr, Drickamer MA, Marottoli RA, Pannill FC, Tinetti ME. A simple procedure for general screening for functional disability in elderly patients. Ann Intern Med 1990; 112:699–706.

64. Reuben DB, Wieland DL, Rubenstein LZ. Functional status assessment of older persons: concepts and implications. In: Abarede JL, Garry PJ, and Vellas B, eds. Facts and Research in Gerontology. New York: Springer, 1993; 7:231–240.

65. Landis SH, Murray T, Bolden S, Wingo PA. Cancer statistics, 1999. Ca Cancer J Clin 1999; 49:8–31.

23

Management of the Terminally Ill Patient

Linda M. Sutton
Duke University Medical Center
Durham, North Carolina

Elizabeth C. Clipp
Veterans Administration Medical Center and
Duke University Medical Center
Durham, North Carolina

Eric Paul Winer
Dana–Farber Cancer Institute and
Harvard Medical School
Boston, Massachusetts

I. INTRODUCTION

Advances in the treatment of cancer have occurred at a dramatic pace over the past 50 years. Although many patients, particularly those with early-stage disease, will be cured, over 500,000 persons die of cancer-related deaths each year in the United States. Those over the age of 55 years accounted for over 87% of cancer deaths in 1993, with 39% aged 75 years or greater (1). The majority (62%) of deaths in the United States occur in hospital, with 16% in nursing homes and only 17% at home. The underlying illness as well as age and marital status influence where an individual dies. The proportion of individuals dying at home is slightly higher among those with cancer (26%) (2). It is estimated that 33% of cancer deaths in the United States will occur in patients under hospice care where palliative care is the focus.

The World Health Organization (WHO) has defined *palliative care* as the active total care of patients whose disease is not responsive to curative treatment. The goal of palliative care is to allow the terminally ill patient to live until death by achieving the best possible quality of life for the patient and family through control of physical symptoms with attention to psychological, social, and spiritual issues. Hospice care seeks to affirm life and regards dying as a normal part of living; neither hastening nor postponing death. Proponents of hospice care regard the family—at whose center the patient exists—as the unit of treatment (3).

Although the principles of palliative care are applicable early on in the disease process, it is usually not until quite late in the disease process that a referral to hospice care is made. A study conducted in the late 1970s and early 1980s by the National Hospice Organization pointed out that 20% of patients admitted to hospice services died within 7 days, with a median length of survival of 35 days (4). One of the purported reasons for this is the difficulty in predicting when a patient is "terminal." The Tax Equity and Fiscal Responsibility Act of 1982 firmly established the role of palliative care when it created the Medicare Hospice Benefit for eligible patients who are terminally ill with a "prognosis of 6 months or less." Nevertheless, a useful definition of terminally ill has been elusive. McCusker has suggested that the terminal period begins with the physician's recognition that progressive, uncontrollable disease is present (5). However, it is well documented that physicians and care providers have difficulty accurately predicting when patients are likely to die. The length of survival for patients defined as terminal in one study ranged from 1 to 1320 days, with a median of 45 days and a mean of 94 days.

Attempts to better define prognosis employed the Karnofsky Performance Status (KPS) scale. This 11-point scale scored patients on the basis of functionality. Patients with low KPS scores were less functional and had shorter life expectancy than those with higher scores and better function in daily living. Very low scores (10–20) were associated with death within 3 months. Early studies suggested that the KPS more accurately predicted the length of survival than did physicians. More careful scrutiny of the question suggested that the accuracy of the clinician prediction had a direct relationship with the degree of clinical experience with the population (6). Nonetheless, as death approaches, the predictive value of the KPS wanes. Other factors that might be informative regarding prognosis include mental status deterioration and consequences of impaired nutrition such as xerostomia, dysphagia, anorexia, cachexia, and weight loss. Den Daas suggests that problematic nutrition and functional status fit into a condition of general debilitation and wasting termed the terminal cancer syndrome. An Italian study of 530 terminally ill patients with solid tumors attempted to correlate easily obtainable biological parameters with survival. With multiple regression analysis, only the white blood cell, lymphocyte percentage, and pseudocholinesterase levels were independent predictors of survival (7).

II. TERMINALLY ILL ELDERLY PATIENT

During the last half of the 20th century, improvements in health care and sanitation have led to large gains in life expectancy in industrialized countries. The boom in

U.S. births following World War II combined with improved life expectancy has significantly increased the proportion of elderly persons in the population. Over the next several decades, this proportion will expand further. In the United States, the percentage of elderly people (aged 65+ years) is expected to jump from 12.6% in 1990 to nearly 20% in the year 2020 (8).

A significant majority of elderly patients are likely to suffer from one or more chronic medical conditions. By the age of 80+ years, only 10% of women and 19% of men are free of chronic illnesses (9). The presence of chronic comorbid illness complicates palliative care in several ways. Elderly cancer patients often will have symptoms associated with other illnesses that need to be considered in the overall palliative plan. Elderly patients are more likely to be taking one or more medications to manage these preexisting conditions. While managing symptoms in terminal care, the clinician must be vigilant for the possibility of adverse drug reactions and interactions. Aging has important effects on drug handling. Alterations in body composition, metabolic rate, hepatic mass, and blood flow as well as the glomerular filtration rate effect how the body absorbs, distributes, and eliminates exogenous chemicals. Consequently, the effects of drugs may be exaggerated or more dramatic in the elderly. In addition, the elderly may occasionally experience side effects not routinely associated with use of a particular drug in a younger population. For example, the incidence of peptic ulcer disease following use of nonsteroidal anti-inflammatory drugs (NSAIDs) increases significantly in those over the age of 60 years but is relatively uncommon in younger patients (10).

Although it is important to monitor for adverse effects of medications, this should not translate into an avoidance of therapeutic interventions. Clinicians are frequently reluctant to provide medications with potential adverse effects to elderly patients. For example, commonly held misconceptions regarding opioids by elderly patients also hinder effective palliation, particularly of pain. As a result, the elderly are at particular risk for inadequate symptom management, the price of which may be considerable. The elderly who suffer from cancer pain are at an increased risk of suicide. Great care must be exercised to achieve symptom control, whereas avoiding unwanted consequences of medical therapy.

An additional area of concern for the terminally ill elderly patient is the relative paucity of caregivers. Changes in societal norms and shifts in demographics have led to an increasing proportion of elderly without siblings or children available to provide emotional or financial support. The relative poverty and isolation of many elderly patients also challenges optimal medical management.

III. SYMPTOM MANAGEMENT IN THE TERMINALLY ILL

The variability in the range of symptoms experienced by terminally ill patients is tremendous. Seale and Cartwright surveyed a large number of patients in Britain for the presence of symptoms during the year before death (11). These investigators studied both the incidence of symptoms in patients near death and the effect of age on these symptoms. Two separate cohorts were studied in 1969 and 1987, with 785 and 639 patients, respectively. The 10 most commonly reported symptoms are listed in Table 1. Approximately 85% of cancer patients in both cohorts experienced pain, whereas 60–65% of noncancer patients experienced pain. It is of interest that there was no difference in the incidence of pain with age. Nonetheless, elderly patients were more likely to experience mental confusion, loss of bladder control, auditory and visual deficits, and dizziness. In addition, the number of symptoms reported increased with age from 5.7 in those under 65 years old to 7.4 in those over 85 years old. Despite having more symptoms, elderly patients were less likely to report their symptoms as ''very distressing.'' Symptoms tended to be present for longer in older patients; perhaps facilitating coping mechanisms and thereby decreasing the inherent distress of individual symptoms.

Successful management of symptoms requires thorough and repeated assessment. Cancer-related symptoms are dynamic. As the disease progressess, symptoms may change dramatically. A patient with tumor encasement of a nerve may experience significant pain that escalates as the tumor causes increasing nerve impingement. However, that same pain may decline dramatically if the function of the nerve becomes sufficiently compromised; blocking transmission of both sensory and motor stimuli. New sites of disease may appear over time as cancer growth continues.

Clinicians who care for the terminally ill must make a point of regularly inquiring about the status of existing symptoms. There are reliable assessment tools that allow repeated evaluations of the presence and intensity of symptoms such as pain. However, experience with these tools, particularly with the debilitated, is limited. These tools include the pain-grading scale of 0–10 and visual analogue scales, as well as tools for patients who are verbally challenged. One scale that was originally

Table 1   Ten Most Common Symptoms in Terminally Ill Patients

---

Pain
Loss of appetite
Sleeplessness
Vomiting/feeling sick
Trouble breathing
Constipation
Depression
Loss of bladder control
Mental confusion
Loss of bowel control

Source: Seal C, Cartwright A. The Year Before Death. Brookfield, VT: Ashgale, 1994.

devised for children uses a series of faces with expressions of increasing distress to correlate to pain intensity. This tool is also quite useful for elderly patients with mild dementia or previous cerebrovascular accidents. There are also scales based on facial expression and body language of the patient that may be most useful in severely cognitively impaired patients. However, for the majority of symptomatology in the terminally ill, no such tools exist. The clinician is dependent on his or her own assessment skills.

Once the presence and severity of a particular symptom is identified, there should be an assessment of the cause. Treatment directed at the cause of a symptom is more likely to alleviate the suffering it engenders. In the terminally ill, the cause of most symptoms is multifactorial. Reversal of one or more of the underlying factors may provide considerable symptomatic benefit.

The mainstay of terminal symptom management is drug therapy. Regularly scheduled administration of medications is more likely to maintain control of many symptoms. The dosing interval will depend on the plasma half-life of the drug used. The oral route is preferred. Useful therapeutic adjuncts include nondrug methods such as diversional therapy, breathing exercises, and relaxation techniques. Therapeutic options must be individualized.

A. Pain Management

Seale and Cartwright, as well as others, have documented a very high prevalence of pain in terminally ill patients. There are well-described pain syndromes that commonly occur in cancer patients throughout the course of their disease. The pain that accompanies spinal cord compression is just one example. Prompt recognition of these syndromes will often alleviate real and potential suffering. Table 2 outlines the common pain syndromes present in cancer patients. However, the majority of patients with advanced cancer have pain at multiple sites with multiple potential mechanisms. Cancer patients often have both nociceptive and neuropathic pain simultaneously. Direct tumor involvement is the most common cause of pain; present in approximately 67% of patients with pain from metastatic cancer. Tumor invasion of bone accounts for pain in approximately 50% of patients with breast and prostatic carcinoma, as well as those with multiple myeloma. The remaining 50% experience tumor-related pain that is due to nerve compression or infiltration or involvement of the gastrointestinal tract or soft tissue. Up to 25% of patients may have pain related to their therapy (12).

Persistent posttherapy pain accounts for up to 20% of those patients who report pain with metastatic cancer. Begg and Carbone assessed the effect of aging on the toxicities of chemotherapy in 25,000 patients who participated in clinical trials conducted by the Eastern Cooperative Oncology Group (ECOG). They concluded that elderly patients appeared more susceptible to certain types of toxicities, such as the frequently painful neuropathy associated with cisplatin and the vinca alkaloids (13).

Progression of neoplastic growth correlates with the increasing incidence of

Table 2 Common Cancer Pain Syndromes

Bone metastases
Epidural metastases/spinal cord compression
Plexopathies
  Cervical
  Brachial
  Lumbosacral
Peripheral neuropathies
  Nerve infiltration by tumor
    Craniai
  Postsurgical
    Radical neck dissection
    Mastectomy
    Thoracotomy
    Nephrectomy
    Limb amputation
  Treatment related
    Chemotherapy; e.g., with taxol, cisplatin
    Radiation
  Acute and postherpetic
Abdominal pain
Mucositis

Source: Adapted from Clinical Practice Guideline No. 9: Management of Cancer Pain, Agency for Health Care Policy and Research, US Department of Health and Human Services, 1994.

pain. Only 15% of patients with localized disease had pain associated with their tumor at the time of diagnosis (12), whereas the incidence increases to 74% with metastatic disease and up to 87% prior to death (14). In addition, the prevalence of painful comorbidities, such as osteoarthritis, is much greater for an older population. The predominant cause of pain in the elderly is musculoskeletal, with 80% of the people older than 65 years old suffering with arthritis. The prevalence of pain in those older than 60 years is 250/1000; double that of those less than 60 years old (15). Although elderly patients may not identify their pain as ''very distressing,'' data suggests that biological aging has no impact on the perceived unpleasantness of pain (16).

Thus, it is not surprising that pain in elderly patients with cancer is inadequately treated. In a study of pain management in outpatients with metastatic cancer who participated in ECOG clinical trials at multiple centers, at least 42% of those with pain did not receive the type of analgesics recommended by standard cancer pain management guidelines. Patients age older than 70 years were among specific populations at greater risk of inadequate analgesia. The persons at greatest risk of inadequate analgesia were elderly, female patients from a minority racial group (17).

The assessment of pain and suffering should be global, including the emotional, psychosocial, and spiritual aspects of the pain. In the terminally ill, the impact of emotional or spiritual distress may increase as death approaches. Therapeutic intervention with medications may be fruitless if these aspects are ignored. Few physicians are equipped to manage all of the aspects of pain and suffering in the terminally ill. Multidisciplinary teams, as provided by hospice care, are better prepared to address the global aspects of pain.

1. Management Suggestions

In 1990, the WHO introduced a simple but reliable method of pain management based on the WHO analgesic ladder (Fig. 1). This method has effectively alleviated pain for approximately 90% of patients with cancer and 75% of terminally ill cancer patients (18, 19). The Agency for Health Care Policy and Research in the United

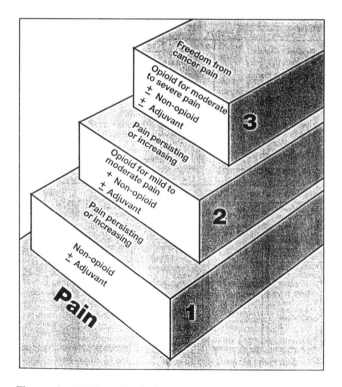

Figure 1 WHO analgesic ladder (Source: World Health Organization, 1990. Used with permission.)

States (AHCPR) has incorporated the WHO analgesic ladder into the Clinical Practice Guideline for the Management of Cancer Pain, which was published in March 1994 (20). Hwang and his colleagues have demonstrated an average of 50% pain reduction in cancer patients within 1 day of implementation of AHCPR guidelines. By the end of 1 week, pain was reduced by an average of 80% in these patients with moderate to severe pain (21).

The most fundamental principle of pain management is that it must be individualized. This is particularly important in the elderly for whom there are age-associated changes in drug metabolism. The potential impact of age on drug metabolism was initially demonstrated for morphine. Systemic clearance of opioids is diminished in patients older than 50 years; largely due to diminished first-pass metabolism resulting from alterations in liver mass and blood flow that occur with age (22). In addition, decreased glomerular filtration rates and an increased fat to lean body mass in the elderly may allow accumulation of biologically active opioid metabolites such as morphine-6-glucuronide or normeperidine. The increased bioavailability of morphine allows a greater analgesic effect for elderly subjects in response to a standard dose of morphine compared to younger individuals. Studies have also demonstrated that a prolonged duration of pain relief is experienced by the elderly following administration of graded doses of morphine. A corollary of this is that the elderly are also more prone to the adverse effects of narcotic analgesics, particularly opioid-naïve patients. Consequently, the use of short half-life opioids such as hydromorphone, morphine, or oxycodone, may be more prudent in the elderly rather than long half-life opioids such as methadone or levorphanol, particularly when initiating therapy.

As the experience of pain is inherently subjective, treatment should be initiated based on the patient's report of both the intensity and frequency of pain. Using the guidelines of the WHO and AHCPR, mild pain may be treated with acetaminophen or NSAID's. These agents have a ceiling dose beyond which no further analgesic effect is achieved. For pain that is incompletely responsive to these agents or moderate to severe in nature, narcotics are the agents of choice. Combinations of opioids with nonopioid analgesics in fixed doses are available for moderate pain. Opioids such as codeine, dihydrocodiene, hydrocodone, oxycodone, and propoxyphene are combined with nonopioids such as acetominophen, ibuprofen, and aspirin. These agents are useful in that analgesia is effected by two separate mechanisms. However, the efficacy of the fixed-combination agents is limited by the maximal dose and frequency of administration associated with the nonopioid. These agents may also be more difficult to administer to the elderly given the increased susceptibility to peptic ulcer disease following NSAIDs in this population (23). Severe pain should be treated with opioid analgesics that are not limited by fixed combinations.

Analgesics should be administered at regularly scheduled intervals (25). The interval between doses of analgesics should depend on the half-life of the individual drug rather than on preconceived notions of how often patients should take pain medicine. There are several long-acting narcotic preparations available to decrease

Table 3 Long-Acting Narcotic
Preparations

Agent	T (peak plasma concentration) (h)
MS Contin	~4.0 h
Oramorph	3.8 h
Oxycontin	~3.0 h
Duragesic	~12–78 h
Kadian[a]	8.6 h
Methadone[b]	
Levorphanol[b]	

[a] Kadian is a controlled-release morphine preparation that comes in a once per day capsule, the contents of which may be sprinkled on food for consumption.

[b] Although both methadone and levorphanol have long serum half-lives, the duration of analgesic effect is considerably shorter, predisposing patients to the adverse effects of drug accumulation.

the frequency at which analgesics are scheduled (Table 3). The dose of analgesics administered at regularly scheduled intervals in a 24-h period is the baseline dose, often referred to as the around the clock (ATC) dosage. Additional doses of analgesics should be allowed for pain that ''breaks through'' the threshold systemic level of analgesic. Analgesics chosen for rescue or breakthrough should have a relatively rapid onset of action and systemic half-life that allows dosing every 1–2 h as needed. The recommended dose of analgesic that should be given as a rescue or breakthrough dose is somewhat controversial. Cherny and Portenoy recommend that 5–15% of the baseline 24-h dose be given for breakthrough every 1–2 h (25). Levy recommends that the dose be one third of the 12-h dose (26). Others have suggested a dose equivalent to 1 h's worth of the baseline dose. However, these recommendations are largely based on experience rather than scientific study. Once a clinician gains experience with an individual patient, a more rational recommendation is that the rescue dose be sufficient to provide maximal analgesia with minimal side effects (27).

Opioids are available as a variety of agents that can be delivered by almost any route imaginable. Morphine, the main naturally occurring alkaloid of opium, is the prototypical agent. Table 4 lists the opioids commonly used in the treatment of cancer pain and the routes by which they may be administered. Agonist–antagonist opioids should generally be avoided in this population. The oral route is considered the optimal route of delivery when it is effective given the convenience, cost effi-

Table 4 Opioids in Cancer Pain

Agent/Combination Agent	Route
Morphine	Oral
	Subcutaneous
	Intravenous
	Rectal
Hydromorphone	Oral
	Subcutaneous
	Intravenous
	Rectal
Oxymorphone	Rectal
	Parenteral
Oxycodone	Oral
OxyIR	
Roxicodone	
Percocet/Percodan	
Tylox	
Others	
Hydrocodone	Oral
Lorcet/Lortab	
Vicodin	
Vicoprofen	
Others	
Not recommended[a]	
Propoxyphene	
Wygesic	
Darvocet/Darvon	
Mepergan (meperidine + promethizine)	
Meperidine	

[a] These agents are of low potency and provide poor analgesia. Chronic meperidine use predisposes to accumulation of toxic metabolites.

cacy, and minimal invasion required. When the oral route is unavailable, other less invasive routes of administration, such as rectal or transdermal, should be considered. Subcutaneous and intravenous administration opioids provide rapid relief of pain but are invasive, relatively expensive, and frequently inconvenient to both the patient and health care system. Patient-controlled anesthesia (PCA) has been shown to be safe and effective for postoperative pain relief in the elderly (28), but it has not been studied extensively for long-term use with chronic pain in elderly patients with cancer pain. Intramuscular (im) injection of opioids is not recommended, as the absorption is erratic and produces unreliable analgesia. Absorption that does occur produces an analgesic effect that parallels the oral administration of an equivalent dose of the same drug. Patients with unmanageable opioid side effects may benefit from epidural or intrathecal administration of opioids, as centrally administered opioids produce minimal serum concentrations. The dose of an opioid administered epidurally is usually considerably smaller than that required intravenously to achieve analgesia.

Successful management of cancer pain requires aggressive upward titration with ongoing assessment of the efficacy of therapy. Titration of a short-acting opioid may occur relatively quickly. Levy suggests that the dose of morphine be increased every 24 hs by 50–100% in patients with severe unrelieved chronic pain and by 25–50% in those with moderate unrelieved pain (26). Titration with long-acting opioids is a more prolonged process and is not practical in managing an acute pain crisis or rapidly changing pain. There is no ceiling or maximal dose of narcotics; the appropriate dose is that dose which produces acceptable analgesia with manageable side effects for each individual patient. Failure with one opioid does not preclude success with another. When switching from one opioid to another, it is important to bear in mind that there is incomplete cross tolerance among opioids. That is to say, tolerance to a given dose of one opioid does not guarantee tolerance to an equianalgesic dose of another.

Opioids should be dose escalated in the elderly with caution owing to the alterations in morphine bioavailability previously discussed. The caution against overtreatment of pain should be as vigilant as the caution against undertreatment. Uncontrolled pain may manifest as psychiatric symptoms in elderly patients. At least one study suggests that diminished cognitive function in older adult (aged 50–80 years) patients following total hip replacement surgery was related to the experience of pain rather than to the analgesic intake (29). As previously discussed, the dose of opioids should initially be smaller in the elderly or dosing intervals increased to achieve the same analgesic effect as in younger patients (30–32).

Opioid dose titration should take into account not only analgesic effects but also side effects. Such side effects may include urinary retention (particularly a problem for elderly males with prostatic hyperplasia), constipation and intestinal obstruction, or respiratory depression and cognitive impairment. Anticipatory management of side effects such as constipation should be inherent in every opioid-based analgesic regimen. The elderly are particularly prone to the constipating side effects of the narcotics because of the alterations in gut motility and splanchnic blood flow. Concern over respiratory depression as a potential side effect is often given as a reason to withhold narcotic medications in the elderly. Respiratory capacity is usually preserved with increased tidal volumes despite a decreased respiratory rate in patients using opioids. It is important to note that respiratory patterns may be altered in the elderly. The Cheyne–Stokes respiratory pattern is not unusual in the elderly during sleep, and its presence does not mandate automatic discontinuation of an opioid (33).

Despite aggressive titration, opioids may not eliminate painful suffering. Adjuvant analgesics may enhance the analgesic efficacy of opioids, particularly for certain types of cancer pain. NSAIDs and corticosteroids are particularly helpful for bone pain or pain associated with inflammation of tumor-infiltrated tissues. Neuropathic pain may be effectively treated by tricyclic antidepressant agents, anticonvulsants, local anesthetic agents, or antiarrhythmic agents. The anticonvulsants are best suited for treatment of lancinating neuropathic pain, whereas the antidepressant medications are better employed for continuous neuropathic pain (34). Pain associated with edema may improve with corticosteroids. Meticulous attention to side effects must be practiced when these agents are administered to the elderly given the potential for adverse effects and drug interactions. The increased risk of gastric toxicity from NSAIDs has been discussed previously. NSAIDs with lower gastric toxicity (e.g., choline magnesium trisalicylate) should be employed when possible, and the administration of misoprostol as gastric mucosal protectant should be considered. The incidence of other unusual side effects such as cognitive impairment, constipation, and headache is also increased among elderly patients (35). Adjuvant medications may result in a decrease in opioid dose with an associated decrease in side effects.

B. Anorexia/Cachexia Syndrome

The anorexia/cachexia syndrome is a collection of symptoms at the core of which is anorexia. The prevalence of anorexia in cancer patients ranges from 15 to 40% at cancer diagnosis and goes up to 80% in the advanced stage (36). The presence of anorexia with concomitant weight loss portends a poor prognosis (37). Chronic nausea and vomiting, early satiety, constipation, malnutrition, and asthenia contribute to the profound debilitation seen in those patients who experience this syndrome. Other clinical features of the syndrome include abnormalities in carbohydrate, fat, protein, and energy metabolism that result in loss of adipose tissue and skeletal muscle. The link between the clinical manifestations and the aberrant metabolism is unclear. Some of the symptoms such as nausea, vomiting, early satiety, and constipation with resulting malnutrition suggest an abnormality in gastrointestinal motility that may be associated with autonomic failure related to the presence of the cancer. Similar symptoms are frequently observed in patients receiving opioids (38, 39). Associated with the aberrant changes in metabolism are anemia, hypertriglyceridemia, hypoalbuminemia, hypoproteinemia, hyperlacticacidemia, and intolerance of glucose.

How the presence of cancer induces these changes is under investigation. Studies in animals demonstrate that a tumor will grow at the expense of the host, increasing in size while the host consumes less and less (40). Endogenously produced cytokines such as tumor necrosis factor, interleukin-1, and interleukin-6 as well as others may contribute to cancer-related cachexia but are not universally present. In addition, this syndrome is not unique to cancer patients. Persistent anorexia and inanition appears to be a marker for the terminal stage of progressive dementia (41) and may reflect a final common pathway to death.

1. Management Suggestions

The anorexia/cachexia syndrome is difficult to palliate. Effective palliation generally requires successful treatment of the underlying cancer, and this is not an option for the terminally ill. Although anorexia and the resulting malnutrition seem to be at the core of the syndrome, the pathophysiology is extraordinarily complex. The inability to take in adequate food to satisfy perceived nutritional requirements is often given as a justification for parenteral as well as enteral tube feedings. It is far from clear that nutritional supplementation reverses the process or improves the quality of life, comfort, or overall outcome. In a review of randomized clinical trials of parenteral nutrition in patients with advanced cancer, Koretz found no improvement in survival for those receiving the supplemental nutrition (42). Other studies suggest an increase in infections and decreased survival (43). More to the point for terminal patients, there is a paucity of data examining the impact of supplemental nutrition of any type on the quality of life. It is possible that enteral or parenteral feeding may have a negative impact on the quality of life through the discomfort and side effects inherent to its administration. Elderly patients with delirium or advanced dementia might be unable to report hunger or thirst. This same population of patients would also be unable to report satiety or adverse symptoms from supplemental feeding. Occasionally, the risk of aspiration pneumonia is sometimes given as justification for enteral tube feeding in the terminally ill. However, there is no evidence that tube feeding reduces the risk of aspiration pneumonia. Indeed among 42 patients whose cause of death was given as pneumonia, 55% died with feeding tubes in place compared with 22% of patients listed as dying of other causes (44). A more rational approach to palliation for patients experiencing this syndrome is to address the symptoms most bothersome to the patient and caregivers. The following sections will outline measures that may improve individual symptoms.

a. Anorexia

Many patients want to eat, often for social or cultural reasons. Pharmacological measures may improve appetite as well as the quality of life. However, the efficacy is often transient, with less benefit being seen as death approaches.

Corticosteroids were the first agents identified as appetite stimulants that also improved the overall sense of well-being in patients with advanced cancer. Long-term use of corticosteroids is compromised by waning efficacy as well as increased side effects such as weakness, gastric irritation, delirium, osteoporosis, and immunosuppression. Despite a long history of availability, the optimal agent, dose, and duration of corticosteroids as appetite stimulants require further study. Nonetheless, corticosteroids may be useful for selected patients who may benefit from short periods of their use.

Progestational agents such as megestrol acetate and medroxyprogesterone were pressed into service for the treatment of anorexia following recognition that they produced significant weight gain as an unpleasant side effect when used for the treatment of hormone-responsive cancers. Several studies have demonstrated increased appetite, improved quality of life, and non–fluid weight gain in patients with advanced cancer (45, 46). There appears to be a dose response to megestrol acetate up to 800 mg/day. Beyond this dose the incidence of side effects appears to increase with no further benefit. Although generally well tolerated, there are reports that the use of megestrol acetate as an appetite stimulant may be associated with decreased survival (47).

The cannabinoids, marijuana and dronabinol, also have weight gain as a side effect of use. Clinical trials in cancer patients have documented improvement in appetite and mood with dronabinol at doses of 5 mg/24 h. Although the rate of weight loss appeared to decline, many patients in one trial continued to lose weight. Nearly 20% of patients discontinued use because of unpleasant side effects (48).

Additional agents tested in clinical trials include pentoxifylline, hydrazine sulfate, and cyproheptadine. Pentoxifylline failed to improve appetite and weight despite its ability to decrease tumor necrosis factor mRNA levels in cancer patients (49). There is convincing data from randomized placebo control trials that hydrazine sulfate and cyproheptadine provide no benefit whatsoever in patients with advanced cancer (50, 51).

b. Nausea and Vomiting

Nausea with or without vomiting is a frequent problem in cancer patients, occurring in one half to three quarters of patients with advanced cancer. Chronic nausea plays an important role in the anorexia/cachexia syndrome. In terminal cancer patients, nausea is likely the result of one or more of the factors listed in Table 5. A careful

Table 5   Common Causes of
Nausea/Vomiting in the Terminally Ill

Gastrointestinal
Constipation
Bowel Obstruction
Peptic Ulcer Disease
Hepatic dysfunction/enlargement
Metabolic
Hypercalcemia
Uremia
Medication effects
Narcotics
Chemotherapy
Others
Increased intracranial pressure
Radiation effects
Autonomic failure

Table 6 Pathophysiological Mechanisms of Nausea/Vomiting

Category	Stimuli	Anatomic location	Neurotransmitter receptor[a]
Visceral	Gastric irritation, abdominal cancer, obstruction, constipation, liver disease, GB/GU distention, gastric distention	Vagal and sympathetic afferents	D2, 5HT4
Chemical	Drugs, biochemical disorders, toxins	Chemoreceptor trigger zone	D2, 5HT3
Vestibular	Motion and positional sickness	Vestibular nuclei	M, H1
CNS	Pain, emotional factors, CNS cancer, raised intracranial pressure	CNS	H1
Vomiting Center	Visceral, chemical, vestibular CNS processes	CNS	H1, M, 5HT3

GB/GU, gallbladder/genitourinary; CNS, central nervous system.
[a] D2, dopamine D2; H, histamine H1; M, muscarinic cholinergic; 5HT3, serotonin group 3; 5HT4, serotonin group 4.
Source: Adapted from Lichter I. Which antiemetic? J Palliat Care, 1993; 9(1):42–50.

history and physical examination are mandatory to identify the physical, psychological, and emotional contributants to nausea. Once the components are identified, knowledge of the responsible pathophysiological mechanisms allows tailored symptom management as outlined in Table 6. Aggressive titration of the medication dose with ongoing evaluation of efficacy is required for optimal palliation. As nausea is often the result of multiple causes, multiple targeted interventions are frequently necessary. Cessation of offending medications should be considered. Drug-induced nausea is often promptly reversible with the withdrawal of the offending agent. Narcotic-induced nausea may be eliminated with the use of an alternative narcotic. The nausea associated with constipation and bowel obstruction are better managed with decompression. Adjunctive therapies such as relaxation techniques and imagery may be appropriate for individual patients. Dietary and psychological modifiers of nausea should also be addressed if success is to be achieved.

c. Constipation

Constipation is relatively common in the elderly. Although not part of the normal aging process, constipation appears to be more common in the elderly; perhaps due to the prevalence of chronic illnesses that affect gut homeostasis. The prevalence of constipation is high among terminally ill patients, approaching 50% in those with cancer. Gut dysfunction, as a result of autonomic failure, medications (such as narcotics), comorbid illnesses, or the cancer itself, underlies the development of constipation in many terminally ill patients. This may be exacerbated by the general debility of the terminally ill with poor oral intake and limited mobility. Untreated constipation in an elderly patient may be life threatening or cause severe disability.

Constipation is best managed through prevention. Terminally ill patients should be assessed regularly for bowel function. Assessment of bowel function in the elderly may be challenging, particularly in patients with cognitive or neurological impairment. The presentation of constipation in the elderly may be more subtle, manifesting as anorexia, depression, or a decline in functional status. Ambulatory patients should be encouraged to be as active as possible and maintain adequate fluid and fiber intake. Patients who are less functional may benefit from a regular program of being out of bed to sit in a chair or limited ambulation with assistance. Even completely bed-bound patients can benefit from regular turning and positioning to stimulate gut motility. Laxative therapy should be initiated in high-risk patients, such as those with predisposing medical conditions or medication regimens, before the onset of symptoms.

Identification of constipation should prompt consideration of the underlying etiology. Frequently, over-the-counter medications as well as prescription medications may be the culprit. Alternative agents may need to be considered. Progressive tumor growth, particularly in the setting of gastrointestinal or gynecological cancers, also may be responsible. There are a host of agents broadly classified as hydrophilic agents, osmotic agents, contact stimulant agents, stool softeners, lubricants, and physical agents. The hydrophilic agents, such as bran, psyllium, or methylcellulose promote bulk formation within the stool by retaining water within the colon. These agents are taken with large volumes of liquid and begin to stimulate bowel movement approximately 12–72 h postingestion. They are best suited to highly ambulatory patients with adequate oral intake. Osmotic agents include magnesium hydroxide, magnesium citrate, or magnesium sulfate. These agents promptly increase the intracolonic water content through an osmotic gradient, again increasing bulk formation within the stool. The onset of action is approximately 0.5–3.0 h. The increased bulk created with hydrophilic and osmotic agents creates distention of the intestinal wall, encouraging peristalsis. However, when transit through the colon is obstructed by a stricture or impaction, for example, bulk-forming agents should be avoided. Caution also should be exercised with use of osmotic agents in patients with renal compromise.

Stool softeners such as docusate sodium, lactulose, or polyethylene glycol electrolyte solutions soften the stool by promoting the mixture of fat and water into the stool. Polyethylene glycol electrolyte solutions (GoLytely, Colyte) are frequently used for bowel preparation and may be useful in fecal impaction. Although large volumes of fluid are ingested, there are no major shifts of intrinsic electrolytes or fluid. Consequently, these agents are useful in elderly patients who have little tolerance for excess fluid volume because of underlying congestive heart failure or renal insufficiency. Lubricating agents include mineral oil or glycerin which facilitate physical elimination. Coating fecal material with these agents also prevents absorption of water from the stool by the colonic wall and promote elimination within 6–8 h of administration. Contact stimulant agents also affect electrolyte and water secretion. These agents, such as bisadocyl, as found in Dulcolax and Carter's Little Pills, or phenolphthalein, as contained in Ex-Lax, Correctal, and others, stimulate bowel movement within 6–12 h. Prunes contain a derivative of phenolphthalein.

These agents are useful in patients with compromised neurological gut function. Patients with diminished rectal reflex or perineal and abdominal wall muscle strength may benefit from the stimulant effect of these agents. Overuse is a potential problem; these agents are most frequently implicated in the cathartic bowel syndrome. Of note, Dulcolax and Ex-Lax require adequate biliary function for activity. Finally, enemas and suppositories stimulate reflex elimination following colorectal distention. These techniques have a prompt onset of action within 2–60 min and are best suited to the management of acute constipation or impaction. Both enemas and suppositories may cause local burning and irritation. Soap enemas in particular are best avoided, particularly in the elderly because of the potential for severe irritation.

Fecal impaction is a dreaded complication of constipation. Unrecognized, fecal impaction may have catastrophic consequences such as bowel perforation, peritonitis, and sepsis. The impacted bowel may present as a complete lack of bowel elimination associated with nausea, crampy abdominal pain with distention, and occasionally fever. Diarrhea may accompany impaction as liquefaction of the impacted stool produces a flow of watery fecal material. Every assessment of constipation, particularly severe symptoms, should include an evaluation for fecal impaction. Digital rectal examination will reveal the presence of a low-lying impaction. Radiographs may be helpful when a more proximal impaction is suspected.

C. Dyspnea

Dyspnea, or the subjective sensation of difficulty in breathing, is one of the most common symptoms among the terminally ill. In the National Hospice Study, dyspnea was reported in 70% of patients receiving hospice care in the final 6 weeks of life (52). The prevalence is affected by disease site, with the highest prevalence being in lung cancer. In one study of patients in a home hospice care setting, dyspnea was the main symptom for 78% of lung cancer patients but only for 6% of those with genitourinary cancers and none of those with gastrointestinal cancers (53).

The causes of dyspnea in the terminally ill are legion. Therapeutic interventions are frequently best selected on the basis of etiology and underlying performance status. Dyspnea may be caused by intrathoracic as well as extrathoracic disease. Within the thorax, causes of respiratory distress may be related to pulmonary, cardiac, pleural, or chest wall processes. Pulmonary processes are widely varied, including chronic obstructive pulmonary disease (COPD)/asthma, pneumonia, tracheobroncheal tumors, lymphangitic carcinomatosis, radiation, or chemical toxicities, as well as pulmonary emboli. Ischemic heart disease, superior vena cava obstruction, congestive heart failure, or pericardial disease may underlie dyspneic symptoms. Extrathoracic disease processes such as anemia, progressive neuromuscular compromise, or paraneoplastic syndromes may also contribute to dyspnea in the terminally ill cancer patient.

The mechanics of pulmonary ventilation are altered with the aging process. The function of the skeleton, respiratory muscles, and lung elasticity is compromised by the aging process. Consequently, the elderly have smaller lung volumes, falling to a quarter of the values for healthy young adults. This may be exacerbated by the long-term effects of chronic illness and smoking (54). Diffusion capacity and gas exchange are also reduced with age (55). In addition, the impact of malnutrition on respiratory muscle strength may be considerable, with more than a 40% reduction (56).

1. Management Suggestions

Initial assessment of dyspnea in the terminal patient should seek reversible causes. What is reversible will vary with the performance status and immediate prognosis of the patient. Investigations that may be useful include a thorough history and physical examination. Plain radiographs of the chest in conjunction with ultrasound or ventilation-perfusion scanning play a role in evaluating intrathoracic disease. Ultrasound may help locate either a pleural or pericardial effusion. An arterial blood gas and blood count (CBC) are simple laboratory studies that may point to an etiology. Pulmonary function studies may provide a useful diagnostic adjunct. The most common causes of dyspnea in the terminally ill include COPD, pneumonia, lung cancer, cardiac failure, anemia, and anxiety. Frequently these causes coexist. Reversible causes of dyspnea should be treated as long as the potential for worthwhile benefit exists.

When alleviation of the symptom is desired, but treatment of the underlying cause of dyspnea is no longer possible or feasible, medical management is directed toward the relief of the subjective sensation of uncomfortable breathing. Bronchodilators (β-agonists, anticholinergics, and methylxanthines), diuretics, corticosteroids, and oxygen therapy are familiar agents in the treatment of respiratory embarrassment. These etiology-directed agents clearly have an important role in the management of dyspnea. Other agents such as the opioids, benzodiazepines, phenothiazines, and cannabinoids have the ability to suppress the uncomfortable respiratory sensation whatever the source of respiratory compromise. Most clinical experience is with the opioids.

The opioids effectively reduce dyspnea through several mechanisms. Opioids are anxiolytic, provide cerebral sedation, and decreased sensitivity to hypercapnia while providing analgesia and decreased cardiac preload through vasodilatation. In addition, the opioids may reduce metabolic requirements such that respiratory suppression may be an appropriate physiologic response. Patients with chronic obstructive pulmonary disease have improved exercise tolerance following administration of an oral morphine solution despite rising P_{CO_2} and falling P_{O_2} (57). Patients with intermittent dyspnea are best served with intermittent, "as needed" dosing of oral morphine. As dyspnea becomes more pervasive for individual patients, continuous delivery of morphine will provide better relief. This can be achieved with long-acting oral agents or infusion pumps. The baseline dose should be supplemented with intermittent doses as needed.

Opioids may be delivered via nebulization as well as the more conventional oral and parenteral routes. The systemic absorption of nebulized morphine is low but not insignificant, with pharmacokinetic studies demonstrating a 1:6 difference in peak plasma levels compared with intramuscular morphine (58). Theoretically, the relatively low systemic availability should favorably effect side effects. Unfortunately, the superiority of nebulized morphine over conventional routes has not, as yet, been convincingly demonstrated. In addition, nebulized morphine may induce bronchospasm in some individuals, requiring prompt bronchodilatory treatment.

Studies in patients with COPD demonstrate the efficacy of the benzodiazepines and phenothiazines in alleviating breathlessness (59, 60). Lorazepam is a short-acting benzodiazepine with a rapid onset to a peak within 2 h of oral administration. Lorazepam may be administered orally, sublingually, and intravenously. In healthy volunteers, lorazepam has a tranquilizing effect on the central nervous system with no appreciable effect on the respiratory or cardiovascular systems. The usefulness of the phenothiazines in the terminally ill, on the other hand, is limited by extrapyramidal and autonomic nervous system side effects.

The cannabinoids have important respiratory effects as well as the potent antiemetic and appetite stimulatory properties for which they are better known. The cannabinoids produce bronchodilatation and may enhance ventilatory response to rising P_{CO_2}. Nabilone, a synthetic cannabinoid available outside of the United States, has been used sporadically for relief of dyspnea in anxious, continuously dyspneic patients at the end stage of the terminal process. The doses required are considerably less than those required for an antiemetic effect (61). However, nabilone and other cannabinoids such as dronabinal, which is available in the United States should be used with caution in the elderly. The elderly are more sensitive to the psychotropic effects of these agents. In addition, the reflex tachycardia and hypotension which accompanies the use of these agents are often poorly tolerated in elderly patients, particularly those with underlying cardiovascular disease.

As death becomes imminent, many patients will experience difficulty clearing upper respiratory secretions. The accumulated secretions create turbulence as air passes over and through, producing noisy respirations that are often referred to as the "death rattle." Anticholinergic agents such as hyoscine (scopolamine) will decrease the volume of upper respiratory secretions, decreasing the noise of respiration, without compromising respiratory function. Of note, hyoscine and similar agents are less effective in decreasing the production of bronchial secretions. Hyoscine may be administered subcutaneously at 0.8–2.4 mg/24 h as a continuous infusion, as intermittent injections of 0.4–0.6 mg, or transdermally (62).

IV. PSYCHOSOCIAL ISSUES SURROUNDING TERMINAL CANCER IN LATER LIFE

The literature on the terminally ill cancer patient is noteworthy in its focus on the care of the patient in the context of the patient's family. The Institute of Medicine's Committee on Care at the End of Life recently adopted, as one of its guiding principles, that "care for those approaching death should involve and respect both patients and those close to them" (63). This moves beyond the widely acknowledged notion that caring for the dying patient means caring for the family to a heightened sensitivity that clinicians need to view their terminally ill patients in the context of their close relationships, their culture, values, and resources. "Family" from this perspective includes not only the traditional family in the sense of spouses, children, parents, and siblings but also friends, confidants, and partners who share significant and meaningful ties with patients. From this broadened perspective, families are increasingly regarded by clinicians and researchers as not only the primary source of support to terminally ill patients, but *as* the patient (64).

Families caring for older terminally ill members experience unique challenges and problems related to the developmental stage of the patient family member. For older individuals, the developmental tasks of later life include preparation for death, coping with multiple losses, and recognizing the possibility that formal care will be needed. These are common concerns of many older people despite a marked heterogeneity in their physical limitations, psychological stresses, and social resources. Among the current cohort of elderly cancer patients, normal developmental tasks are intensified, because many older persons equate cancer with death, intractable pain and suffering, loss of control, family burden, and feelings of abandonment. These associations stem from experiences that occurred decades earlier when a cancer diagnosis was a veritable death sentence. The elderly person today remembers clearly that prior to the early 1950s, few people survived a cancer diagnosis (65). The existential question of "how will I die" in the current cohort of elderly cancer patients takes on different meaning because of this collective memory.

In addition, the elderly cancer patient's adjustment is complicated by a host of age-related factors such as comorbid illnesses, diminished financial resources, and multiple psychosocial losses that increase the potential for isolation at a time when social support is especially needed (66–68). Berkman notes that increased age among cancer patients correlates with a decreasing support system either due to death, mobility, or an inability to render care (66). Because older cancer patients also face age-related issues, additional research is needed to explore the relationships between the usual developmental milestones in later life and the terminal cancer experience. A significant number of elderly cancer patients experience, in addition to their cancer and treatment, multiple comorbid conditions with associated functional decline, impairments, and age-related disabilities. To date, however, most studies of elderly cancer patients focus on single problems (69).

Interestingly, and despite the many challenges facing cancer patients and families in the terminal phase, studies suggest that older patients have healthier psychological profiles and better mental well-being than younger cancer patients. Cassileth et al. studied approximately 1200 cancer patients in three age groups (70). Those in the oldest group (60 years and older) had significantly better mental health scores. Similarly, Ganz and colleagues (71) found that older patients experienced less severe psychosocial problems than younger patients. A third study, by Maisiak and colleagues (72), found that elderly patients had better psychosocial status and were less likely to be depressed than younger cancer patients despite having lower incomes and education.

What accounts for this apparent psychological advantage among our older patients? Cassileth and Chou raise the interesting possibility that older people may have genetic dispositions to cope well with life's problems (65). More apparent, however, is the fact that elderly cancer patients are veterans in coping with adversity and health limitations. More so than younger adults, they have already experienced the cessation of relationships and bereavement through deaths of age peers, friends, and family. Many have survived multiple acute illnesses and surgeries and functional declines associated with chronic conditions. They also are less likely than younger patients to experience additional stress related to work and family demands. Moreover, in facing developmental tasks of later life, many older patients have thought seriously about death and regard it as a natural, or expected, occurrence or "on-time" event (73).

Despite what may be superior coping abilities among older cancer patients, their families generally struggle with a number of challenging end of life issues. Central among these are the patient's complete dependency and impending death (74). From this reality springs feelings of uncertainty and fear and issues of separation, grief, resolution of mourning, and concerns about the resumption of normal family life after the older person's death. Consequently, anxiety and depression are often more severe among family members than among patients (75). Spouses, often elderly themselves, are particularly concerned with their loved ones' emotional responses to the disease and their own physical illnesses (76–79). However, most families' single greatest concern in the terminal stage is the comfort of their dying loved ones. This was reported in studies of families using hospice care (64) and families not using hospice services (80).

In describing families whose loved ones are dying, Rolland (81) stresses the importance of families successfully shifting their anticipation from the possibility, to the probability, to the inevitability of death. Clinicians should look for this pattern and expect intense grieving related to decisions to stop aggressive care. As families enter the terminal phase, they need to understand that they will be in more frequent contact with health care providers but the care orientation in this phase will be different. In making this transition, some families that previously handled skillfully the day-to-day practical tasks of cancer illness management may find the emotional coping necessary for terminal care more difficult. Therefore, families who tend to avoid communication about emotional issues may be unable to adapt to the terminal phase without therapeutic intervention (81).

Family members should not feel compelled to initiate discussions with the older patient about dying. According to Holland (82), not all patients want to engage in such discussions. If they do, patients tend to identify select family members, who know them well, to share these feelings. In many cases, however, communication in the terminal stage between older patients and their families may be complicated by patients' cognitive dysfunction. This is important for families to know, because cancer-related cognitive deficits in older patients may be overlooked or attributed to aging (83).

Among patients with minimal or no cognitive dysfunction, communication among family members may be enhanced through the process of advanced care planning. Such planning involves ongoing discussions with the patient and family about what the future holds and what the patient and family want to achieve as life ends. General elements of advance care planning include the options available to the family and the costs and benefits of those options; family preferences that should guide decisions; practical issues that should be anticipated; and what immediate steps should be taken by families should certain events occur. According to the Institute of Medicine's Committee on the Care at the End of Life, advance care planning provides a cooperative effort to understand individuals' physical, emotional, practical, and spiritual concerns, serves to prevent distressing and unwanted interventions, and makes clear what the patient, family, and provider team consider a good death (63).

V. INFORMAL CAREGIVING CHALLENGES IN THE DYING TRAJECTORY

Older people with cancer and other disabling chronic conditions receive most of their care during the period just prior to death from family members (63). The most important ingredients for providing terminal care in the home is a genuine desire on the part of patients and families to carry out this work, recognition that death is the outcome, and a commitment to face and solve any problems that arise (84). In reality, families taking on this challenge are often unprepared and unskilled in handling the complex problems and demanding tasks they face (63). Families that want more guidance about the experience they are embarking on can be referred to Dying at Home: A Family Guide to Caregiving by Andrea Sankar (85).

As direct care tasks increase, elderly patients become highly dependent on their focal or primary caregivers, usually spouses or daughters. Recent work by Stetz and Brown emphasize, in addition to the burden of direct care tasks, the emotional work required of caregivers in managing the psychosocial demands or suffering associated with end-stage disease (86). In response to these demands, most studies examining caregiver needs in the terminal phase have found that caregivers believed that they lacked the skills and emotional resources required during this difficult time (87). It is not surprising that many studies have found that the intensity of dying patients' care needs has been linked empirically to caregiver distress (88–92). As illness proceeds, caregivers tend to call on formal support for medical or palliative interventions.

Families need to anticipate that normative family roles that have shifted gradually over the cancer experience will become permanently disrupted in the terminal phase. The healthy reciprocity that sustained and nourished family relationships or friendships prior to the illness become strained in the transformation to caregiver–patient relationships. Caregivers assume responsibilities that were formerly held by their patients or delegate these responsibilities to other family members. According to Rolland, a new version of balance needs to be negotiated such that old relationship rules do not continue to operate, creating role strain (81). Even the strongest relationships are strained by such shifts. Caregivers also assume new roles, including that of emotional counselor, patient protector, and family spokesperson. Tasks related to these new roles include monitoring visitations and calls to the patient, promoting the completion of any unfinished family business, emotionally supporting the terminally ill member, and helping the family to live together as fully as possible in the time remaining. Caregivers also serve as key facilitators in the process of family reorganization (81). However, clinicians should note that as patients withdraw and begin to take leave, caregivers' feelings of isolation and loneliness peak. Some caregivers also may become the focus of concern in the dying phase.

VI. FAMILY RESPONSES TO PROVIDING TERMINAL CARE

Families provide the context for elderly cancer patients' progression along the dying trajectory. Much of what we know about the impact on informal caregivers of cancer care comes from the more general literature on family caregiving in the context of chronic illness. After nearly two decades of empirical research on the challenges inherent in dementia caregiving, there is little question that caregiving constitutes a chronic stress. This process has been conceptualized as caregiver strain (81, 93–95), caregiver stress (96, 97), and caregiver burden (98, 99) with identified adverse outcomes in caregivers' physical health (100–102), emotional health (103, 104), family relations (105, 106), and social and recreational activities (101). Given the fact that cancer is a disease of later life (107), the caregiver spouses of patients are usually elderly themselves with significant physical and psychosocial problems related to their own developmental stage (64).

Caregivers report that caring for the dying person is the single most exhausting experience of their entire lives (85). Sleep deprivation over a long period is one of the most difficult aspects of caring for the terminally ill patient. Other studies have shown that the negative consequences for caregivers of family members dying of cancer include anxiety (108), stress (92), demands and difficulties (109), perceived declines in health (109), uncertainty (84, 110), role conflicts (110), feelings of harm or loss (92), and strain (111).

Some families find it necessary to turn to institutionalization in the terminal phase of care. Recent statistics show that most deaths in this country occur in hospitals followed by nursing homes (63). The number of people dying at home in the care of their families is increasing; only a minority of deaths involve hospice programs (63). Berkman and associates (66) identified risk factors for institutionalization when the cancer patient was elderly. An accumulation of stresses rather than specific problems move families to seek formal care, including increases in caregiving requirements at home, cognitive impairment, and escalating psychosocial problems.

Clearly, ongoing psychosocial support and education about terminal care should be provided to families that are caring for an aged loved one in advanced-stage disease. This is the responsibility of health care providers, hospitals, hospices, support programs, and the public media. Given the projected expansion of the older population with cancer by the turn of the century (69), numerous clinical and research agendas such as those developed by Yancik (69), Given and Keilman (107), and Boyle (112) that bridge geriatrics, gerontology, and oncology are needed immediately to increase the understanding of older cancer patients' and their families lived experiences. More than a decade ago, Oberst and James (113, p. 56) noted that "learning to live with cancer is clearly no easy task. Learning to live with someone else's cancer may be even more difficult precisely because no one recognizes just how hard it really is." Unfortunately, this statement remains true today. We will never fully understand the impact of cancer on families without the knowledge of the informal caregiving context. What families know and have experienced, how they cope, and what they expect will inform providers and ultimately improve care at the end of life.

REFERENCES

1. Parker SL, Tong T, Bolden S, Wingo PA. Cancer Statistics, 1997. Ca Can J Clin 1997; 47:5–27.
2. Lubitz JD, Riley GF. Trends in Medicare payments in the last year of life. N Engl J Med 1993; 328:1092–1096.
3. World Health Organization Expert Committee. Cancer Pain Relief and Palliative Care. Technical Report series 804. Geneva: World Health Organization, 1990.
4. Greer DS, Mor V, Morris JN, Sherwood S, Kidder D, Birnbaum H. An alternative in terminal care; results of the National Hospice Study. J Chron Dis 1986; 39:9–26.
5. McCusker J. The terminal period of cancer: definition and descriptive epidemiology. J Chron Dis 1984; 37:377–385.
6. Den Daas, N. Estimating length of survival in end stage cancer: a review of the literature. J Pain Symptom Manage 1995; 10(7):548–555.

7. Maltoni M, Pirovano M, Nanni O, Marinari M, Indelli m, Gramazio A, Terzoli E, Luzzani M, De Marinis F, Caraceni A, Labianca R. Italian multicenter study group on palliative care. Biological indices predictive of survival in 519 Italian terminally ill cancer patients. J Pain Symptom Manage 1997; 13(1):1–9.

8. U.S. Bureau of the Census, International Data Base on Aging; and United Nations Department of International Economic and Social Affairs (1989). Global estimates and projections of population by sex and age, the 1988 revision, ST/ESA/SER. R/93, New York.

9. Brody JA, Freels S, Miles TP. Epidemiological issues in the developed world. In: Evans JG, Williams TF, eds. Oxford Textbook of Geriatric Medicine. Oxford, UK: Oxford University Press, 1992:14–20.

10. Meyer BR, Reidenberg MM. Clinical pharmacology and ageing. In: Evans JG, Williams TF, eds. Oxford Textbook of Geriatric Medicine. Oxford, UK: Oxford University Press, 1992:107–116.

11. Seal C, Cartwright A. The Year before Death. Brookfield, VT: Ashgale, 1994.

12. Foley KM, The treatment of cancer pain. NEJM 1985; 313:84–95.

13. Begg CB, Carbone PP. Clinical trials and drug toxicity in the elderly. The experience of the Eastern Cooperative Oncology Group. Cancer 1983; 52(11):1986–1992.

14. Seale C, Cartwright A. The year before death. Brookfield, VT: Ashgate, 1994.

15. Crook J, Rideout E, Browne G. The prevalence of pain complaints in a general population. Pain 1984; 18(3):299–314.

16. Harkins SW, Kwentus J, Price DD. Pain and suffering in the elderly. In: Bonica J, Febiger L, eds. The Management of Pain. Philadelphia: Lea and Febiger, 1990:552–559.

17. Cleeland CS, Gonin R, Hatfield AK, Edmonson JH, Blum RH, Stewart JA, Pandya KJ. Pain and its treatment in outpatients with metastatic disease N Engl J Med 1994; 330:592–596.

18. Ventafridda GV, Caraceni AT, Gamba A. Field testing of the WHO Guidelines for Cancer Pain Relief: summary report of demonstration projects. In: Foley KM, Bonica JJ, Ventafridda V, eds. Proceedings of the Second International Congress on Pain. Vol. 16. Advances in Pain Research and Therapy. New York: Raven, 1990:451–464.

19. Grond S, Zech D, Schug SA, Lynch J, Lehmann KA. Validation of World Health Organization Guidelines for Cancer Pain Relief during the last days and hours of life. J Pain Symptom Manage 1991; 6(7):411–422.

20. Agency for Health Care Policy and Research. Clinical Practice Guideline for the Management of Cancer Pain. U.S. Department of Health and Human Services, AHCPR publication No. 94-0592, March 1994.

21. Hwang SS, Chang VT, Corpion C, Kasimis B. Outcomes of cancer pain management based upon AHCPR guidelines: pain relief and quality of life (QOL). Proc Am Soc Clin Oncol 1998; 17:61a.

22. Meyer BR, Reidenberg MM. Clinical pharmacology and ageing. In: Evans JG, Williams TF, eds. Oxford Textbook of Geriatric Medicine. Oxford, UK: Oxford University Press, 1992:107–116.

23. Roth SH. From peptic ulcer to NSAID gastropathy. An evolving nosology. Drugs Aging 1995; 6(5):358–367.

24. Portenoy RK, Hagen NA. Breakthrough pain: definition, prevalence and characteristics. Pain 1990; 41:273–281.

25. Cherny NI, Portenoy RK: Cancer pain management. Cancer 72:3393–3415, 1993.

26. Levy MH. Pharmacologic treatment of cancer pain. N Engl J Med 1996; 335:1124–1132.

27. Cleary JF. Pharmacokinetic and pharmacodynamic issues in the treatment of breakthrough pain. Semin Oncol 1997; 24(5 Suppl 16):S16-13–S16-19.

28. Egbert AM, Parks LH, Short LM, Burnett ML. Randomized trial of postoperative patient-controlled analgesia vs intramuscular narcotics in frail elderly men. Arch Intern Med 1990; 150:1897–1903.

29. Duggleby W, Lander J. Cognitive status and postoperative pain: older adults. J Pain Symptom Manage 1994; 9:19–27.

30. Owen JA, Sitar DS, Gerger L, Brownell L, Duke PC, Mitenko PA. Age related morphine kinetics. Clin Pharmacol Ther 1993; 34:364–368.

31. Kaiko RF, Wallenstein SL, Rogers AG, Houde RW. Sources of variation in analgesic responses in cancer patients with chronic pain receiving morphine. Pain 1983; 15:191–200.

32. Berkowitz BA, Ngai SH, Yang JC, Hempstead BS, Spector S. The disposition of morphine in surgical patients. Clin Pharmacol Ther 1975; 17:629–635.

33. Kaiko RF. Age and morphine analgesia in cancer patients with post-operative pain. Clin Pharmacol Ther 1980; 28(6):823–826.

34. Cherny NI, Foley KM. Current approaches to the management of cancer pain: a review. Ann Acad Med Singapore 1994; 23:139–159.

35. Roth SH. Merits and liabilities of NSAID therapy. Rheum Dis Clin North Am 1989; 15(3):479–498.

36. Nelson K, Walsh D, Sheehan F. Assessment of upper gastrointestinal motility in the cancer associated dyspepsia syndrome. J Palliat Care 1993; 9:1:27–30.

37. DeWys WD, Begg D, Lavin PT, Band PR, Bennett JM, Bertino JR, Cohen MH, Douglass HO Jr, Engstrom PF, Ezdinli EZ, Horton J, Johnson GH, Moertel CG, Oken MM, Perlia C, Rosenbaum C, Silverstein MN, Skeel RT, Sponzo RW, Tormey DC. Prognostic effects of weight loss prior to chemotherapy in cancer patients. Am J Med 1980; 69:491–497.

38. Bruera E, Fainsinger RL. Clinical management of cachexia and anorexia. In: Doyle D, Hanks G, MacDonald N, eds. Oxford Textbook of Palliative Medicine. Oxford, UK: Oxford Medical Publications, 1993:330–337.

39. Alexander HR, Norton J. Pathophysiology of cancer cachexia. In: Doyle D, Hanks G, MacDonald N, eds. Oxford Textbook of Palliative Medicine. Oxford, UK: Oxford Medical Publications 1993:316–329.

40. Moley JF, Morrison SE, Norton JA. Preoperative insulin reverses cachexia and decreases mortality in tumor-bearing rats. J Surg Res 1987; 43:21–28.

41. Blandford G, Watkins L, Mulvihill M, Taylor B. Correlations of aversive feeding behavior in dementia patients (abstr). J Am Geriatr Soc 1995; 43:SA10.

42. Koretz R. Parenteral nutrition: is it oncologically logical? J Clin Oncol 1984; 2:534–538.

43. American College of Physicians: Parenteral nutrition in patients receiving cancer chemotherapy—position paper. Ann Intern Med 1989; 110:734–736.

44. Ahronheim JC. Nutrition and hydration in the terminal patient. Clin Geriatr Med. 1996; 12(2):379–391.

45. Bruera E, Macmillan K, Hanson J, Kuehn N, MacDonald RN. A controlled trial of

megestrol acetate on appetite, caloric intake, nutritional status, and other symptoms in patients with advanced cancer. Cancer 1990; 66:1279–1282.

46. Loprinzi C, Ellison, NM, Goldberg RN. Alleviation of cancer anorexia and cachexia. Studies of the Mayo Clinic and the North Central Cancer Treatment Group. J Natl Cancer Inst 1990; 82:1127–1132.

47. Reynolds R, Khojasteh A, Ben-Jacob A. Contribution of progestational agents (PA) to cancer fatigue syndrome (CFS)—a double-edged sword phenomenon. Proc Am Soc Clin Oncol 1998; 17:67a.

48. Wadleigh R, Spaulding GM, Lumbersky B, Zimmer M, Shepard K, Plass T. Dronabinol enhancement of appetite and cancer patients (abstr). Proc Am Soc Clin Oncol 1990; 9:1280–1331.

49. Goldberg RM, Loprinzi CL, Mailliard JA, O'Fallon FR, Krook JE, Ghosh C, Hestorff RD, Chong SF, Reuter NF, Shanahan TG. Pentoxifylline for treatment of cancer anorexia and chachexia? A randomized, double-blind placebo-controlled trial. J Clin Oncol 1995; 13:2856–2859.

50. Kardinal CG, Loprinzi C, Shaid DF, Hass AC, Dose AM, Athmann LM, Mailliard JA, McCormack GW, Gerstner JB, Schray MF. A controlled trial of cyproheptadine in cancer patients with anorexia. Cancer 1990; 65:2657–2662.

51. Loprinzi CL, Kuross SA, O'Fallon JR, Gesme DH Jr, Gerstner JB, Rospond RM, Cobau CD, Goldberg RM. Randomized placebo-controlled evaluation of hydrazine sulfate in patients with advanced colorectal cancer. J Clin Oncol 1994; 12:1121–1125.

52. Ventafridda V, de Conno F, Ripamonti C, Gamba A, Tamburine M. Quality of life assessment during a palliative care programme. Ann Oncol 1990; 1:415–420.

53. Higginson I, McCarthy M. Measuring symptoms in terminal cancer; are pain and dyspnoea controlled? J R Soc Med 1989; 82:264–267.

54. Sykes DA, Mohanaruban K, Finucane P, Sastry BSD. Assessment of the elderly with respiratory disease. Geriatr Med 1989; 19:49–54.

55. Mahler DA, Cunningham LN, Curfman GD. Aging and exercise performance. Respir Dis 1986; 2:433–452.

56. Mier A. Respiratory muscle weakness. Resp Med 1990; 84:351–359.

57. Light RW, Muro JR, Sato RI, Stansbury DW, Fischer CE, Brown SE. Effects of oral morphine on breathlessness and exercise tolerance in patients with chronic obstructive pulmonary disease. Am Rev Respir Dis 1989; 139:126–133.

58. Young IH, Daviskas E, Keena VA. Effect of low dose nebulised morphine on exercise endurance in patients with chronic lung disease. Thorax 1989; 44:387–390.

59. Woodcock A, Gross E, Geddes D. Drug treatment of breathlessness: contrasting effects of diazepam and promethazine in pink puffers. Br Med J 1981; 283:343–346.

60. Wedzicha JA, Wallis PJW, Ingram DA, Empey DW. Effect of diazepam on sleep in patients with chronic airflow obstruction. Thorax 1988; 43:729–730.

61. Ahmedzai S. Palliation of respiratory symptoms. In: Doyle D, Hanks GWC, MacDonald N, eds. Oxford Textbook of Palliative Medicine. 2nd ed., Oxford, UK: Oxford University Press, 1998: 583–616.

62. Bennett MI, Death rattle: An audit of hyoscine (scopolamine) use and review of management. J Pain Symptom Manage 1996; 12(4):229–233.

63. Field M, Cassel C, eds. Approaching Death; Improving Care at the End of Life. Washington, DC: National Academy Press, 1997.

64. Kristjanson L, Ashcroft T. The family's cancer journey: a literature review. Cancer Nurs 1994; 17:1–17.
65. Cassileth B, Chou J. Psychosocial Issues in the Older Patient with Cancer. In: Balducci L, Lyman G, Ershler W, eds. Geriatric Oncology. Philadelphia: Lippincott, 1992:311–313.
66. Berkman B, Stolberg C, Calhoun J. Elderly cancer patients: factors predictive of risk for institutionalization. J Psychosoc Oncol 1983; 1:85–100.
67. Ganz P, Schag C, Heinrich R. The psychological impact of cancer on the elderly. J Am Geriatr Soc 1985; 33:429–435.
68. Gwyther L, Matteson M. Care for the caregivers. J Gerontol Nurs 1983; 9:72–95.
69. Yancik R. Integration of Aging and Cancer Research in Geriatric Medicine. J Gerontol Medi Sci 1997; 52A:M329–M332.
70. Cassileth B, Lusk E, Brown L, Cross P, Walsh W. Factors associated with psychological distress in chronically ill patients. Med Pediatr Oncol 1986; 14:251–254.
71. Ganz P, Coscarelli C, Heinrich R. The psychosocial impact of cancer on the elderly: a comparison with younger patients. J Am Geriatr Soc 1985; 33:420–435.
72. Maisiak R, Gams R, Lee E. The psychosocial support status of elderly cancer outpatients. In: Engstrom P, Anderson P, Mortenson L, eds. Advances in Cancer Control: Research and Development. New York: Liss, 1985:395–399.
73. Neugarten B. Dynamics of transition of middle age to old. J Geriatr Psychiatry 1970; 4:71–87.
74. Schulz K, Schulz H, Schulz O, Kerekjarto MV. Family structure and psychosocial stress in families of cancer patients. In: Baider L, Cooper C, De-Nour AK, eds. Cancer and the Family. New York: Wiley, 1996:226–255.
75. Vaile I. Hospice or rehabilitation hospital? Alternatives for the terminally ill. Can Med Assoc J 1979; 120:1291–1292.
76. Krant M, Johnson L. Family member's perception of communication in late stage cancer. Int J Psychiatry Med 1977; 8:203–216.
77. Woods NF, Lewis FM, Ellison ES. Living with cancer. Family experiences. Cancer Nurs 1989; 12:28–33.
78. Kristjanson L. Quality of terminal care: salient indicators identified by families. J Palliat Care 1989; 5:21–30.
79. Kristjanson L. Indicators of quality care from a family perspective. J Palliat Care 1986; 1:8–17.
80. Ferrell B, Taylor E, Grant M, Fowler M, Corbisiero R. Pain management at home: struggle, comfort, and mission. Cancer Nurs 1993; 16:169–178.
81. Rolland J. Families, Illness, & Disability. New York: Basic Books, 1994.
82. Holland J. Clinical course of cancer. In: Holland J, ed. Handbook of Psychooncology. New York: Oxford University Press, 1989:75–100.
83. Silverfard P, Oxman T. The effects of cancer therapies on the central nervous system. Adv Psychosom Med 1988; 18:13–25.
84. Coyle N, Loscalzo M, Bailey L. Supportive home care for the advanced cancer patient and family. In: Holland J, Rowland J, eds. Handbook of Psychooncology: Psychological Care of the Patient with Cancer. New York: Oxford University Press, 1989:598–606.
85. Sankar A. Dying at Home: A Family Guide for Caregiving. Baltimore. Johns Hopkins University Press, 1991:257.

86. Stetz K, Brown M. Taking care: caregiving to persons with cancer and AIDS. Cancer Nurs 1997; 20:12–22.

87. Biegel D, Sales E, Schulz R. Caregiving in Cancer. Family Caregiving in Chronic Illness. Newbury Park, CA: Sage, 1991:62–104.

88. Baider L, DeNour K. Couples' reactions and adjustments to mastectomy. Int J Psychiatry Med 1984; 14:265–276.

89. Cassileth B, Lusk E, Brown L, Cross P. Psychosocial status of cancer patients and next of kin. J Psychosoc Oncol 1985; 3:99–105.

90. Mor V, Guadagnoli E, Wool M. An examination of the concrete service needs of advanced cancer patients. J Psychosoc Oncol 1987; 5:1–17.

91. Cassileth B, Lusk E, Struse T, Miller D, Brown L, Cross P. A psychological analysis of cancer patients and their next-of-kin. Cancer 1985; 55:72–76.

92. Oberst M, Thomas S, Gass K, Ward S. Caregiving demands and appraisal of stress among family caregivers. Cancer Nurs 1989; 12:209–215.

93. Select Committee on Aging. Exploding the Myths: Caregiving in America. Washington DC: US Government Printing Office No. 99–611, 1987.

94. Cantor H. Strain among caregivers: study of experience in the United States. Gerontologist 1983; 1983.

95. Morycz R. Caregiving strain and the desire to institutionalize family members with Alzheimer's disease. Res Aging 1985; 7:329–361.

96. Stephens M, Kinney J, Ogrocki P. Stressors and well-being among caregivers to older adults with dementia: the in-home vs. nursing home experience. Gerontologist 1991; 31:217–223.

97. Pearlin L, Mullan J, Semple S, Skaff M. Caregiving and the stress process: an overview of concepts and their measures. Gerontologist 1990; 30:583–591.

98. Morycz R, Malloy J, Bozich M, Martz P. Racial differences in family burden: clinical implications for social work. Gerontol Soc Work 1987; 10:133–154.

99. Zarit S, Reever K, Bach-Peterson J. Relatives of the impaired elderly: Correlates of feelings of burden. Gerontologist 1980; 20:649–655.

100. George L, Gwyther L. Caregiver well-being: A multidimensional examination of family caregivers of demented adults. Gerontologist 1986; 26:253–259.

101. Deimling G, Bass D. Symptoms of mental impairment among elderly adults and their effects on family caregivers. J Gerontol 1986; 41:778–784.

102. Kiecolt-Glaser J, Dura J, Speicher C, Trask J, Glaser R. Spousal caregivers of dementia victims: longitudinal changes in immunity and health. Psychosom Med 1991; 53:345–362.

103. Kiecolt-Glaser J, Dyer C, Shuttleworth E. Upsetting social interactions and distress among Alzheimer's disease family caregivers: a replication and extension. Am J Comm Psych 16(6):825–837, 1988.

104. Haley W, Levine E, Brown S, Bartolucci A. Stress, appraisal, coping, and social support as predictors of adaptation outcome among dementia caregivers. Psychol Aging 1987; 2:323–330.

105. Archold P. The impact of parent caring on women. Fam Rel 1983; 32:39–45.

106. Stephens S, Christianson J. Care of the Elderly. Lexington, MA: Lexington Books, 1986.

107. Given B, Keilman L. Cancer in the elderly population: research issues. Oncol Nurs Forum 1990; 17:121–123.

108. Hays J. Patients' symptoms and family coping: predictors of hospice utilization patterns. Cancer Nurs 1986; 9(6):317–325.

109. Stetz K. The relationship among background characteristics, purpose in life, and caregiving demands on perceived health of spouse caregivers. Scholar Inq Nurs Pract 1989; 3:133–153.

110. Blank J, Clark L, Longman A, Atwood J. Perceived home care needs of cancer patients and their caregivers. Cancer Nurs 1989; 12:78–84.

111. Bass D, Bowman K. The transition from caregiving to bereavement: the relationship of care-related strain and adjustment. Gerontologist 1990; 30:35–42.

112. Boyle D. Realities to guide novel and necessary nursing care in geriatric oncology. Cancer Nurs 1994; 17:125–136.

113. Oberst M, James R. Going home: patient and spouse adjustment following cancer surgery. Top Clin Nurs 1985; 7:46–57.

24
Health Policy Issues and Cancer in the Elderly in the 21ˢᵗ Century

Mary S. Harper
University of Alabama
Tuscaloosa, Alabama

I. INTRODUCTION

Cancer, the second leading cause of death in the United States, will be diagnosed in an estimated 1.2 million men and women in the year 1999, with 563,000 deaths due to this disease (1). Nearly 60% of all cancers occur in elderly Americans over the age of 65 years, a group that accounted for 12.5% of the U.S. population in 1990 (2, 3). By the year 2030, men and women over the age of 65 years are projected to account for 20% of the U.S. population. The cancer burden among the elderly is projected to increase during this period due, in part, to a greater number of people and longer life expectancy.

The prevention and control of cancer and other chronic diseases are of paramount importance to the public health and to the economic well-being of our nation. Overall, data about trends in morbidity, mortality, and disability present a disturbing picture of health and aging. They show an overall increase in life expectancy for the elderly, with only a modest addition to the years of active life expectancy, but a substantial increase in the number of years lived with disabilities. It has been estimated by Brody et al. that for each good, active functional year of life gained, about 3.5 compromised years are added to the life span [4]. The paradox of longer life with poorer health and quality of life will greatly impact future policies for the elderly in the 21ˢᵗ century, because this expanding population could be living longer with increased limitations in activities of daily living, have less support due to shrinking family size, and have a higher probability of living alone.

Economically the total health expenditure in the United States in 1993, estimated by the Health Care Finance Administration (HFCA), was \$884.2 billion, and this represented 13.9% of the gross domestic product. Thom's review of health expenditures [5] showed that substantial economic resources are necessary for the treatment of cancers, arteriosclerotic diseases, and diabetes (direct costs)—illnesses which account for two-thirds of all deaths in the United States each year. Substantial productivity is also lost owing to morbidity and mortality from these three diseases (indirect costs). Estimates of costs for these chronic diseases from the 1993 national health expenditures from the HCFA and survey data from the National Center for Health Statistics show that direct costs are \$37 billion for neoplasms, \$126 billion for arteriosclerosis, and \$15 billion for diabetes. Indirect costs are \$70, \$83, and \$5 billion, respectively [5]. Consequently, it is apparent that a significant proportion of health care costs is expended to prevent and treat cancer and other chronic diseases in the elderly.

As the 21st century unfolds, the problem of cancer in men and women over 65 years old is juxtaposed against major advancements in the prevention and treatment of cardiovascular disease over the past 50 years that have led to reductions in deaths due to heart disease and stroke. Overall, both men and women are benefitting from several decades of scientific achievements in cancer diagnostic capabilities, better health promotion campaigns and prevention interventions, more effective treatments, and improved quality of cancer care. Significantly, cancer incidence and mortality data from 1990 to 1995 show that although overall cancer rates are decreasing in most age groups, the rates in men and women aged 65–74 years are declining at a slower rate than for persons aged 35–44 years or 75 years and older [6]. However, within our multicultural society, cancer also causes a disproportionate excess in morbidity and mortality among some racial and ethnic cultural groups such as African-Americans and Native Hawaiians and among socioeconomically disadvantaged populations. The prevention, treatment, and control of cancer and its associated disabilities profoundly impact the individual and family unit, as well as the accessibility and availability of health care resources in the community. Greater demands will be placed on policy makers to make decisions and allocate resources that address the expanding needs and cancer services for a diverse, elderly population.

II. GENERAL HEALTH CARE POLICY ISSUES

Health policy issues establish the framework of health for all people and acknowledge the principles of equity, accessibility, and quality of care [7]. Health policy is one component of a broader social policy, which is concerned with the ideology and principles of redistribution of separate social welfare measures, such as income, housing, transportation, employment, entitlement, and about methods and procedures involved in determining access and the allocation and utilization of benefits [8]. Most health policies are oriented toward acute illness and institutionalization despite the facts that approximately 75% of the nation's elderly have a chronic illness [9] and only 5% are in institutions. Consequently, health care policies and budgetary expenditures are frequently focused on the 5% of the elderly population confined to institutions but not on the 95% who are living in the community, usually with one to three limitations in activities of daily living. With the advent of managed care, the average length of stay in hospitals is 3.7 days. Most policies pertaining to care and reimbursement relate to hospital care and not to home care or to community-based or other enabling community services. Therefore, policies and budgets should be refocused to include the community where most of the elderly live.

Government policies and those of other institutions are generally based upon some normative assumptions that have been shaped by perceptions of how, why, and where people and their needs are distributed around those norms. In a heterogeneous society, many of these assumptions are strained. Policies based upon them are sometimes imperfect and occasionally "sidetracked" by "special interest groups." Aside from the usual normative assumptions, health policies typically consider access, cost, and acute managed care, but they seldom deal with quality of care, chronic conditions, or the social forces which can also determine health status for the elderly. Studies of cancer and other chronic diseases indicate that survival outcome may be related, in part, to various factors such as one's position in society stratified along the lines of age, race, sex, ethnicity, gender, cultural orientation, socioeconomic status, occupation, living arrangements, and political structure. For example, a study of breast cancer management by physicians confirmed earlier suspicions that older, poorer, and minority women are likely to be offered less aggressive care, given identical symptoms, family history, and test results. Age and race biases were found to be minimal when the patient was assertive in requests for treatment [10].

Most health policies focus on cost, utilization reviews, formularies, outcomes, and guidelines but not on quality. There is no question that there are high users of health care who remain morbid or comorbid. Only recently have researchers and policy makers focused on quality. Between 1996 and 1998 a special task force called The Roundtable on Health Care Quality was convened by the Institute of Medicine of the National Academy of Sciences. It was composed of 20 representatives from the health care industry, media, business, consumers, academia, advocacy, and federal programs for the purpose of identifying issues related to the quality of health care in the United States, including its measurement, assessment, and improvement requiring actions by health care professionals and other constituencies in the public and private sectors [11]. This task force concluded that serious and widespread quality problems—classified as misuse, overuse, and underuse—exist throughout American medicine. These problems occur in both large and small communities throughout the country, and with approximately equal frequency in managed care and fee-for-service systems of care. They further concluded that quality of care, not managed care, is a problem in the United States. The task force recommended a major overhaul of how we deliver health care services, educate and train clinicians, and assess and improve quality for our citizens [11]. Assessing quality requires attention to both outcomes, process, and structure—key elements that policies should focus on.

There is a need to examine the relationship between policy and the distribution of health access in all settings (i.e., managed care, fee-for-services, institution- and community-based programs administered by health professionals, as well as home health care services delivered by families). Changes in demographics, socioeconomic, and health care trends frequently give rise to new health policy issues, such as the reimbursement or provision of other support to family caregivers, who provide nearly 80% of long-term care for the chronically ill [9, 12–14]. Policies, therefore, should reflect an understanding not only of individual lifestyle and risk-related behaviors but also of the relationships among social characteristics, the structure of the medical system, and health. This approach involves the examination of the broad economic, political, and social processes that not only shape the life events of individuals but also the nation's approach and definition of public health problems.

III. SELECTED HEALTH CARE POLICY ISSUES IN ELDERLY CANCER PATIENTS

Future advancements in technology and health care delivery services will result in improved health outcomes. Economic constraints in health expenditures will require policy makers to rethink the appropriate allocation of limited resources. The report of the panel on Statistics for the Aging Population [14] strongly recommended that efforts be expended to improve data bases necessary for formulating health policies for an aging population. Some of the key health policy questions to be addressed for the elderly include the following:

- Who will pay for cancer health care for the elderly and how will it be financed (those without entitlement of Medicare, Medicaid, social security, pensions, financial savings and assets, the uninsured, the new immigrant, the recently unemployed without benefits, and those below the poverty level)?
- What alternative health care system should be developed in the next millennium to meet the cancer care needs for the elderly as it becomes inflated by the "baby boomers"?
- How can health promotion, disease prevention, disease management, and self-care/patient/family education be advanced for the elderly in the 21st century?
- What data are necessary to plan for the 59 million elderly by the year 2040?
- What will be the differences in health status among women, cultural, racial, and ethnic subgroups and other vulnerable populations?

- What policies are needed to ensure that the elderly with cancer receive appropriate quality of care?
- What provisions are needed for subgroups to assure access to evidence-based technology in appropriate diagnosis, treatment, and rehabilitation?
- Are there unintended effects of public policy that foster fraud, abuse, and a sick role?
- Will the 21st century focus policies on the care of chronically ill and social support that is essential to comprehensive treatment outcomes?
- Will policies of the 21st century recognize and reward nonmedical health care providers as well as family caregivers?

Selected health care issues that need to be examined for elderly cancer patients and individuals at risk for cancer include the need to monitor trends in cancer and health care outcomes, clinical trials participation, screening, coverage, unpaid medical care (self-care), education and training, and the dissemination of genetic information to the elderly.

A. Monitoring Trends in Cancer and Health Care Outcomes

To formulate appropriate health policies, health analysts need to be able to detect trends in cancer and to forecast changes in the health status of individuals affected by and at risk for cancer and to monitor changes in the utilization of health care services and expenditures. For example, as successful risk reduction occurs secondary to smoking cessation and prevention, chemoprevention, and early detection, the prevalence and stage of cancers in the elderly population will change, reflecting the impact of these interventions on disease outcome. Such effects must be tracked. Also, the elderly population is heterogeneous. Geriatricians and gerontologists often subdivide the population to discern better functional changes and responses. There are clear age-related differences in different age subsets: young-old (age 65–74), old (age 75–84), and oldest-old (age 85 and older) [14, 15]. The marked effect of age itself on disability, morbidity, and mortality points to the need to divide the over age 65 population into two, if not three, groups in order to better understand the complex interaction and dynamic processes of aging and cancer. Within each age subgroup, individual biological responses to aging are affected by a range of physiological, genetic, socioeconomic, and environmental factors (such as nutrition, smoking, obesity) as well as access to medical care.

B. Clinical Trial Participation

It has become well recognized that among individuals over age 65 years, physiological age is not invariably linked to chronological age. The design and eligibility criteria of early clinical research protocols disallowed many elderly men and women age 70 years and older from participation owing, in large part, to concerns about associated comorbid conditions and the risk of excess morbidity due to toxicity from chemotherapy. Early clinical cooperative group studies suggested that, for some cancers, the incidences of severe toxic reactions as well as response rates were comparable in elderly patients compared to nonelderly controls [16, 17]. By 1989, the National Cancer Institute guidelines had changed so that age was no longer recognized as a factor in selecting patients for clinical research studies. This policy change preceded the more recent legislative requirements to include women and minorities in clinical studies [18]. Although cancer policy does not exclude the elderly, proportionally fewer individuals participate in clinical research. Increased educational awareness and efforts are needed to design studies to address issues in this group.

C. Screening

Although the elderly are at greatest risk of developing and dying of cancer, screening occurs less often in older persons. There is no clear consensus on the appropriate use of screening services in the elderly. The lack of consensus is important, because identification of a demographic group with low utilization may have limited policy or clinical implications if there is no agreement that the use of the procedure for screening has a positive impact on health. Among women above age 75 years and older in the 1987–1988 National Health Interview Survey (NHIS), 83.5% of black women and 93.2% of Hispanic women had never had a mammogram as compared to 75% of the white women. The most common reason given for not having a mammogram among black women 65 years and older was that a physician did not recommend it. For Hispanic and white women, the most common reason was that they thought a mammogram was not needed or was unnecessary [19]. Elderly Hispanic women are also less likely than whites or blacks to have received a Pap smear within the preceding 3-year period [20]. Vulnerable elderly populations other than black, Hispanic, or white should be assessed. For example, nursing home residents, some of whom might benefit from cancer screening provided they have cognitive ability to understand the screening methods and implications, no comorbid illnesses that would preclude treatment, and at least 5 years of life expectancy [21].

Utilization of cancer screening tests (mammography, clinical breast exam, Pap smear, fecal occult blood test, and digital rectal examination) according to health care coverage was evaluated by Potosky and colleagues using data from a 1992 nationally representative survey [22]. Among persons aged 65 years and older, those who had supplemental private fee-for-service insurance in addition to Medicare were more likely to receive five of the six tests than those with Medicare and Medicaid or Medicare alone. Managed care enrollees were 10% more likely to receive screening tests than persons enrolled in fee-for-service plans. There was no overall difference in the use of cancer screening tests between managed care and fee-for-service in 1992 when compared to earlier usage of preventive services in health maintenance organizations with fee-for-service care.

Evidence-based screening policies should be developed for cancers of the breast, cervix, prostrate, colon, skin, and mouth, sites for which screening has benefit. Consumers (male and female elderly) should be involved in the development of these policies. Robinson and Beghe [23] have suggested that policies pertaining to screening in later life should focus on screening test performances (sensitivity, specificity, cost), the burden of investigation, the effectiveness of early detection (improved survival and reduced morbidity), the duration of detectable preclinical phase, an estimation of survival independence for the target conditions, and the philosophy of individual regarding life prolongation. Policies must ensure access for vulnerable groups in rural as well as urban areas. There must be mechanisms for follow-up, a report of findings to the client, and counseling if necessary. Physicians must be provided with clear guidelines for specific age groups and organ sites. Evidence-based screening is derived from the results of appropriately conducted studies in the target population. However, few studies directed toward screening in the elderly have been done. Until such studies are conducted, there will be a lack of evidence-based cancer screening policies for the elderly.

D. Coverage and "Carve-Out"

Health care policies are needed to cover "carve-outs." Carve-outs are defined by a written contract which specifies the type of services to be provided, guidelines for services, financial and service risks, projected outcomes, and cost per patient. It is one strategy used by managed care health plans, employers, and payers to contract with specialty providers to care for particular groups of patients; for example, cancer care, surgical procedures, and mental health and cardiovascular disease care [24, 25]. In assessing carve-outs, a distinction must be made between a carve out created by an employer which separates behavioral health and medical care versus a contract that creates a partnership between behavioral and medical specialties.

In the 1998 workshop on carve-outs convened by the Agency for Health Care Policy and Research, Kurowski reviewed the evolution, effectiveness, and prognosis of cancer carve-outs [26]. As noted in this report, the success of cancer carve-outs has been modest even though cancer might appear to be an ideal condition for a carve-out. Cancer represents a complex array of over 100 different types of diseases. Owing to this complexity, a patient's preferences and clinician decisions that incorporate them are likely to vary significantly. Given the seriousness of the disease, these preferences are hard to ignore or structure. Thus, treatment guidelines are difficult to establish and follow. There are also financial incentives and disincentives of cancer carve-outs. For example, treatment of a single patient can involve a number of specialties that are difficult to include in a single price package.

E. Unpaid Medical Care (Self-care)

The World Health Organization has defined unpaid medical care as activities of individuals, families, and communities undertaken with the intention to enhance health, prevent disease, limit illness, and restore health so that patients are able to live more independently. These activities can be refined by knowledge and skills obtained from an interaction between health care professional and lay people. They are undertaken by lay people on their own behalf either separately or in collaboration with professionals. Policies seldom are made pertaining to unpaid medical care. Such policies are appropriate when one considers the number of elderly persons who are disabled and limited in the performance of three of the seven activities of daily living. In addition, the number of elderly cancer patients cared for by family caregivers contributes to the need for policies which support the training of elderly and family caregivers in self-care procedures. Such a policy would enhance the independence, autonomy, and self-esteem of the elderly cancer patients [7, 27].

F. Training and Education

Formal training that educates health care professionals about the process of policy making should be included in the curricula for training all health care providers. Health care policies are major determinants of access to care as well as the quality of care experienced by the American elderly. Policies frequently determine the length of hospital stay in a community-based health care program, the type of provider who will perform the health care services, or whether the care will be given or denied in an institutional or community-based health care setting. Health care policies play a major role in health care access, delivery, and financing, yet few publications exist pertaining to health policy for chronic diseases such as cancer. Likewise, health policies, social policies, and the financing of health care are seldom included in the curricula which prepare health care providers in medicine, nursing, social work, psychology, physical therapy, and other disciplines. An unprepared health provider team is ill equipped to deal promptly and judiciously with the demands of a dynamic and changing society that impacts health overall. This is an oversight that could benefit from correction in the new millennium.

G. Dissemination of Genetic Information

The frontiers on health policy are being greatly expanded by scientific advancements in cancer genetics research. Just as public health policies are expected to protect society at large, these same policies should also protect elderly consumers in their use of services such as those made available through technological advancements in genetics research, especially genetic testing for the diagnosis and management of cancer and carcinogenesis. Since the early 1990s, consumers, including the elderly, have been bombarded with reports about the discovery of new genes and disease markers and other research test capabilities to determine genetic susceptibility for breast and colon cancer, Alzheimer's disease, and other conditions. A 15-year international effort to map and sequence the entire human genome is sponsored by the Human Genome Project. Tremendous scientific advances are being made in understanding gene structure and function and molecular alterations related to diseases such as cancer. The rapidity with which new genetic discoveries are being made and disseminated is changing the landscape of health policy and the role and composition of policy makers who make decisions. Elderly persons frequently are not aware of the significance of the genetic information [28]. For the elderly, the legal, ethical, and social issues for relatives may take on greater significance. In this rapidly changing arena, policies must be developed and implemented to educate the elderly consumer as to the risks and benefits from genome research that may impact their lives and that of family members.

IV. CANCER HEALTH POLICY IN THE NEW MILLENNIUM

In 1979, then Congressman Claude Pepper held a hearing before the Select Committee on Aging, of the U.S. House of Representatives to discuss "Frontiers in Cancer Research for the Elderly." This landmark hearing marked the first time such a session on cancer in the elderly had been held. During the past quarter century, federal agencies such as the National Cancer Institute and the National Institute on Aging, nonprofit organizations such as the American Society of Clinical Oncology, and the President's Cancer Panel have initiated efforts to expand knowledge, stimulate research, and address specific health issues in elderly cancer patients.

In 1997, the President's Cancer Panel sponsored a national meeting on "Cancer and the Aging Population" [29]. Key issues raised at that session included the need to develop a coordinated research agenda in the oncology and geriatric disciplines to address the impact that cancer in the aging population will have in the coming millennium. Emphasis was placed on the need to examine the pharmacological properties and toxicity of cancer drugs administered to older patients, as well as the need to individualize drug therapy to address the diversity and changes in physiological function that occur in older age. Greater attention to the benefits of cancer prevention, including screening and early detection, clinical trials involvement, and quality of care issues, were also stressed. Other initiatives, such as the development of recommended cancer surveillance guidelines for colorectal cancer by the American Society of Clinical Oncology in 1999, although not specifically directed to the elderly, provide important information that should be utilized by health care practitioners in the care and treatment of elderly patients at risk for cancer. Future attention to cancer issues that will advance the nation's effort for the elderly by the newly established National Cancer Policy Board is encouraged.

According to the Public Policy and Aging Report (February 1999) [30], the elderly of the 21st century will be better educated, have higher income, be healthier, and will be productively employed longer than the present cohorts of elderly. To obtain these goals in the new millennium, health policies will need to target issues such as equity in health, quality of life, promotion of lifestyles conducive to health, and healthy environments. The need for appropriate care must be acknowledged and delivered in a way that is sensitive to cultural, racial, ethnic, and religious beliefs and ideologies, as well as to gender, socioeconomic status, and geographic setting (rural, overcrowded urban, suburban). The problems of cancer survivors and those with disabilities will need to be met. To meet these goals, frequent analyses, monitoring, and revision of health policies will be necessary, as well as the involvement of health care stakeholders, consumers, and families in the development and assessment of health policies. Effective policy making will require access to accurate data, systems for collecting data, staff to monitor and assess the development and implementation of policies, methods to measure implementation and outcomes, and adequate levels of statistical and analytic support for publications and forecasting of cancer trends in the elderly population.

In the next millennium, cancer will provide many challenges and enormous opportunities. Future progress in addressing cancer in the elderly must (a) build on scientific advancements in basic, behavioral, and clinical research, (b) disseminate information on effective prevention interventions and treatments to health care professionals and the lay community, (c) ensure the quality of cancer care and the quality of life, and (d) protect the public health of all citizens.

REFERENCES

1. Landis SH, Murray T, Bolden S, Wingo PA. Cancer statistics, 1999. CA Cancer J Clin 1999; 49:8–31.
2. U.S. Bureau of the Census. Current Population Reports, Special Studies, P23-190, 65+ in the United States. U.S. Government Printing Office, Washington, DC, 1996.
3. Devesa S, Hunter CP. The Burden of Cancer in the Elderly. In: Hunter CP et al., eds. Cancer in the Elderly. New York: Marcel Dekker, 1999:1–24.
4. Brody JA, Brock DB, Williams TF. Trends in the health of the elderly populations. In Breslow L., ed. Annual Review of Public Health. Vol 8. Palo Alto, CA, 1987:211–234.
5. Thom TJ. Economic costs of neoplasms, arteriosclerosis, and diabetes in the United States. In Vivo 1996;10:255–260.
6. Wingo PA, Reis LAG, Rosenberg HM, Miller DS, Edwards BK. Cancer incidence and mortality, 1973–1995. A report card for the U.S. Cancer 1998; 82:1197–1207.
7. World Health Organization. Health for All Targets: Health Policy for Europe, European Health for All, Series, No. 4, WHO Regional Office, Copenhagen, Denmark, Scherfigsv 8, D K-2100 Copenhagen, Denmark, 1993:122.
8. Harper MS. Mental health and social policy. In: Ruiz DS, ed. Handbook of Mental Health and Mental Disorders Among Black Americans. Westport, CN: Greenwood, 1990:229–251.
9. AAHP Fact Sheet, Chronic Care, American Association of Health Plans, Washington, DC, July 29, 1997.
10. McKinlay JB, Burns RB, Feldman HA, Freund KM, Kasten LE, Meskowitz M, Potter DA, Woodman K. Physician variability and uncertainty in the management of breast cancer—results from a factorial experiment. Med Care 1998; 36:385–396.

11. Chassin MR, Galvin RW. The urgent need to improve health care quality. Institute of Medicine National Roundtable on Health Care Quality. JAMA 1998; 280:1000–1005.

12. McGlynn EA. Quality of care for women: where are we now and where are we headed? J Women's Health Iss 1999; 9(2):65–80.

13. Estes CL, Rundall TG. Social characteristics, social structure, and health in the aging population. In: Ory MG, et al. eds. Aging Health and Behavior. Newbery Park, CA: Sage, 1992:299–326.

14. Gilford DM. The Aging Population in the Twenty-First Century—Statistics for Health Policy, National Academy Press, Institute of Medicine, Washington, DC, 1998:1–15.

15. Gioranazzi-Gannon S, Rademaker A, Lai G, et al. Treatment tolerance of elderly cancer patients entered into phase II clinical trials: an Illinois Cancer Center study. J Clin Oncol 1994; 12:2447–2452.

16. Begg CB, Cohen JL, Ellerton J. Are the elderly predisposed to toxicity from cancer chemotherapy? Cancer Clin Trials 1980; 3:269–377.

17. Begg CB, Carbone PP. Clinical trials and drug toxicity in the elderly: the experience of the Eastern Cooperative Oncology Group. Cancer 1983; 52:1986–1992.

18. NIH Guidelines on the Inclusion of Women and Minorities as Subjects in Clinical Research. Fed Reg 1994; 59:March 28.

19. Caplan LS, Wells BL, Haynes S. Breast cancer screening among older racial/ethnic minorities and whites: barriers to early detection. Jl Gerontol 1992; 47(Spec Iss):101–110.

20. Harlan LC, Bernstein AB, Kessler LG. "Cervical cancer screening. Who is not screened and why?" Am J Public Health 1991; 81:885–890.

21. Caranasas GJ. Prevalence of cancer in older persons living at home and in institutions. In: Balducci L ed. Cancer in the Elderly. Part I. Clin Geriatr Med 1997; 13:15–31.

22. Potosky AL, Breen N, Graubard BI, Parsons PE. The association between health care coverage and the use of cancer screening tests. Results from the 1992 National Health Interview Survey. Med Care 1998; 36:257–270.

23. Robinson B, Beghe C. Cancer screening in the older patient. In: Balducci L ed. Cancer in the Elderly. Part I. Clin Geriatr Med 1997; 13:97–118.

24. Fine A. Strategic viability of oncology carve-outs. Adm Radiol J 1996; 15:12–17.

25. AAHCPR Research Activities. Workshop Highlight Pros and Cons of Carve Outs Contract for Specialty Care, AHCPF Publication #98-0050, Vol. 218, Rockville, MD, August 1998;12–13.

26. Kurowski B. Cancer carve-outs, specialty networks, and disease management: a review of their evolution, effectiveness, and prognosis. Am J Manag Care 1998; 4:SP71-89.

27. Ory MG, DeFriese GH, Duncker AP. Introduction: the nature, extent, and modifiability of selfcare in later life. In: Ory MG et al, eds. Selfcare in Later life: Research, Program and Policy Issues. New York: Springer, 1998, pp. 1–8.

28. Mogilner A, Otten M, Cunningham JD, Brower ST. Awareness and attitudes concerning BRCA gene testing. Ann Surg Oncol 1998; 5:607–612.

29. President's Cancer Panel. Concerns of Special Populations in the National Cancer Program. Cancer and the Aging Population. Ann Arbor, MI, July 31, 1997.

30. Public Policy and Aging Report. Is Demography Destiny. National Academy on an Aging Society, Policy Institute, Vol. 9, No. 4, p. 8. Washington, DC, February, 1999.

Index

About the Editors

CARRIE P. HUNTER is Special Assistant to the Director, Office of Research on Women's Health, National Institutes of Health, Bethesda, Maryland. The author or coauthor of over 20 peer-reviewed articles, papers, and abstracts, Dr. Hunter is a member of the American Society of Clinical Oncology, the American Society of Preventive Oncology, the American Public Health Association, and the International Society of Preventive Oncology. She received the B.S. degree (1967) from Tougaloo College, Tougaloo, Mississippi, the M.D. degree (1971) from New York University School of Medicine, New York, and the M.P.H. degree (1995) from the Johns Hopkins University School of Hygiene and Public Health, Baltimore, Maryland.

KAREN A. JOHNSON is Acting Chief, Breast and Gynecologic Cancer Research Group, Division of Cancer Prevention, National Cancer Institute, Bethesda, Maryland. The author or coauthor of over 35 peer-reviewed articles, papers, book chapters, reviews, and abstracts, Dr. Johnson is a member of the American Society of Clinical Oncology and the American Society of Preventive Oncology. She received the B.S. degree (1968) in chemistry from Washington College, Chestertown, Maryland, the Ph.D. degree (1972) in inorganic chemistry from the University of Delaware, Newark, the M.D. degree (1981) from Jefferson Medical College, Thomas Jefferson University, Philadelphia, Pennsylvania, and the M.P.H. degree (1995) from the Johns Hopkins University School of Hygiene and Public Health, Baltimore, Maryland.

HYMAN B. MUSS is Professor of Medicine, University of Vermont College of Medicine; Associate Director, Vermont Cancer Center; and Unit Director, Hematology/Oncology, Fletcher Allen Health Care, Burlington, Vermont. The author or co-author of more than 450 peer-reviewed articles, book chapters, and abstracts, Dr. Muss is a member of the American Society of Clinical Oncology, the American College of Physicians, the American Federation for Clinical Research, the International Association for Breast Cancer Research, the American Association for Cancer Research, and many other societies and associations. He received the B.A. degree (1964) in chemistry from Lafayette College, Easton, Pennsylvania, and the M.D. degree (1968) from the Downstate Medical Center, State University of New York, Brooklyn.